SALEM HEALTH

COMPLEMENTARY
& ALTERNATIVE
MEDICINE

SALEM HEALTH

COMPLEMENTARY
& Alternative Medicine

Volume 4

Editors

Richard P. Capriccioso, M.D.
University of Phoenix

Paul Moglia, Ph.D.
South Nassau Communities Hospital

SALEM PRESS
A Division of EBSCO Publishing
Ipswich, Massachusetts   Hackensack, New Jersey

Note to Readers

The material presented in *Salem Health: Complementary and Alternative Medicine* is intended for broad informational and educational purposes. Readers who suspect that they or someone they know has any disorder, disease, or condition described in this set should contact a physician without delay. This set should not be used as a substitute for professional medical diagnosis. Readers who are undergoing or about to undergo any treatment or procedure described in this set should refer to their physicians and other health care providers for guidance concerning preparation and possible effects. This set is not to be considered definitive on the covered topics, and readers should remember that the field of health care is characterized by a diversity of medical opinions and constant expansion in knowledge and understanding.

Library of Congress Cataloging-in-Publication Data

Complementary & alternative medicine / editors, Richard P. Capriccioso, Paul Moglia.
    p. ; cm. — (Salem health)
Complementary and alternative medicine
Includes bibliographical references and indexes.
    ISBN 978-1-58765-870-9 (set : alk. paper) — ISBN 978-1-58765-871-6 (vol. 1) — ISBN 978-1-58765-872-3 (vol. 2) — ISBN 978-1-58765-873-0 (vol. 3) — ISBN 978-1-58765-874-7 (vol. 4)
    I. Capriccioso, Richard P. II. Moglia, Paul. III. Title: Complementary and alternative medicine. IV. Series: Salem health (Ipswich, Mass.)
    [DNLM: 1. Complementary Therapies–Encyclopedias–English. WB 13]
    LCclassification not assigned
    615.503–dc23
                                                                                               2011051023

Contents

Appendixes

Indexes

Complete List of Contents

Volume 1

Volume 2

Volume 3

Volume 4

Complete List of Contents

SALEM HEALTH

COMPLEMENTARY
& Alternative Medicine

S

Saffron

CATEGORY: Herbs and supplements

RELATED TERM: *Crocus sativus*

DEFINITION: Herbal product promoted as a dietary supplement for specific health benefits.

PRINCIPAL PROPOSED USE: Depression

OTHER PROPOSED USES: Cancer prevention, high cholesterol, mental function enhancement

OVERVIEW

The Mediterranean herb saffron, long used in cooking, is made from the dried stigma (top of the female portion) of the *Crocus sativa* flower. Each flower has only three small stigmas, and about seventy-five thousand flowers are needed to produce 1 pound of saffron. As a cooking herb, saffron is valued for its intense orange-yellow color and its subtle flavor.

Medicinally, saffron has been used since ancient times for strengthening digestion, relieving coughs, smoothing menstruation, relaxing muscle spasms, improving mood, and calming anxiety. Saffron contains vitamin B_2 along with a yellow flavonoid called crocin, a bitter glycoside called picrocrocin, and the volatile, aromatic substance called safranal.

USES AND APPLICATIONS

The best evidence for medicinal effects of saffron involve the treatment of depression. According to five preliminary double-blind studies, the use of saffron at 30 milligrams (mg) daily is more effective than placebo and just as effective as standard treatment for major depression. However, all these studies were small and preliminary and were performed by a single research group in Iran. Larger studies and independent confirmation is necessary to determine whether this expensive herb is truly effective for depression.

Other proposed uses of saffron have even weaker supporting evidence. Test-tube and animal studies hint that saffron and its constituents may help prevent or treat cancer, reduce cholesterol levels, protect against side effects of the drug cisplatin, and enhance mental function.

DOSAGE

In the foregoing studies of depression, saffron was used at a dose of 30 mg daily as an alcohol-based extract.

SAFETY ISSUES

Saffron appears to be safe. One study found no serious adverse effects among healthy volunteers given up to 200 mg per day of saffron for one week. It is often said that very high doses of saffron can cause abortion and possible toxic symptoms, but there is no scientific documentation of these supposed effects. However, the so-called meadow saffron, *Colchicum autumnale*, is highly toxic, and sometimes people mistake one for the other. Also, the safety of saffron use in young children, pregnant or nursing women, and people with severe liver or kidney disease has not been established.

EBSCO CAM Review Board

FURTHER READING

Abdullaev, F. I., and J. J. Espinosa-Aguirre. "Biomedical Properties of Saffron and Its Potential Use in Cancer Therapy and Chemoprevention Trials." *Cancer Detection and Prevention* 28 (2004): 426-432.

Gout, B., C. Bourges, and S. Paineau-Dubreuil. "Satiereal, a *Crocus sativus* L. Extract, Reduces Snacking and Increases Satiety in a Randomized Placebo-Controlled Study of Mildly Overweight, Healthy Women." *Nutrition Research* 30 (2010): 305-313.

Modaghegh, M. H., et al. "Safety Evaluation of Saffron (*Crocus sativus*) Tablets in Healthy Volunteers." *Phytomedicine* 15 (2008): 1032-1037.

Noorbala, A. A., et al. "Hydro-alcoholic Extract of *Crocus sativus* L. Versus Fluoxetine in the Treatment of Mild to Moderate Depression." *Journal of Ethnopharmacology* 97 (2005): 281-284.

See also: Cancer risk reduction; Cholesterol, high; Depression, mild to moderate; Herbal medicine; Memory and mental function impairment.

Sage

CATEGORY: Herbs and supplements
RELATED TERMS: *Salvia lavandulaefolia, S. officinalis*
DEFINITION: Natural plant product used to treat specific health conditions.
PRINCIPAL PROPOSED USES: Dyspepsia, excessive perspiration (hyperhidrosis), sore throat
OTHER PROPOSED USES: Alzheimer's disease, anxiety, breast-feeding support (reducing breast engorgement during weaning), enhancement of mental function, herpes

OVERVIEW

The herb sage has a long history of use in food and medicine. In Mediterranean cultures it has traditionally been used internally to treat excessive menstrual bleeding, increase fertility, aid memory, reduce symptoms of arthritis, and reduce breast engorgement during weaning. It has been used topically for treatment of wounds, sprains, and muscle injuries, and as a gargle for sore throat, hoarseness, and cough.

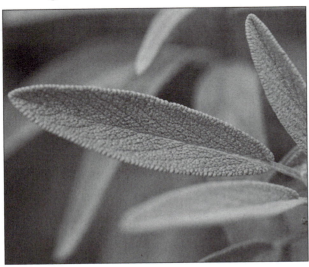

In Mediterranean cultures, sage has long been used for various ailments. (Voisin/Phanie/Photo Researchers, Inc.)

THERAPEUTIC DOSAGES

For use as tea or gargle, one can steep 1 to 3 grams of dried sage in a cup of water three times daily. The equivalent dose of tincture or extract may also be used.

THERAPEUTIC USES

Sage has been approved by Germany's Commission E for internal use in the treatment of dyspepsia (non-specific digestive distress) and excessive sweating, and for topical use in the treatment of inflammation of the mucous membranes of the throat and nose. However, only double-blind, placebo-controlled studies can prove that a treatment really works, and no studies of this type have been performed using sage for any of these purposes other than sore throat.

SCIENTIFIC EVIDENCE

A double-blind study of 286 people found that a throat spray made using sage at a 15 percent concentration significantly reduced sore-throat pain compared with placebo. Additionally, in double-blind trials performed in Iran, 42 people with Alzheimer's disease were given either a sage extract or placebo for four months. The results appeared to suggest a modest improvement in mental function in the sage group compared with the placebo group.

In another double-blind, placebo-controlled study, either placebo or sage essential oil was given to twenty-four healthy people using a crossover design. The results showed possible improvement in some, but not all, aspects of mental function, but the design of the study was such that the results are difficult to trust. The same is true for another small study involving twenty older healthy subjects who took various doses of sage extract. Short-term benefit was seen at a dose of 333 milligrams (mg) per day. A similar-sized study (with similar flaws) found weak hints that sage leaf might improve mood and reduce anxiety level.

Much weaker evidence, too weak to rely upon at all, hints that sage might have liver-protective, anti-cancer, immunomodulatory (alters immune function), antimicrobial, antianxiety, and anti-inflammatory activity. One study failed to find that sage cream provided more than very modest benefits for treatment of herpes.

SAFETY ISSUES

As an herb widely used in foods, sage is thought to have a relatively high level of safety. However, comprehensive safety studies have not been performed. Sage essential oil contains the neurotoxic substance thujone. Maximum safe doses in young children, pregnant or nursing women, and people with severe liver or kidney disease have not been established.

EBSCO CAM Review Board

Further Reading

Akhondzadeh, S., et al. "*Salvia officinalis* Extract in the Treatment of Patients with Mild to Moderate Alzheimer's Disease." *Journal of Clinical Pharmacy and Therapeutics* 28 (2003): 53-59.

Capek, P., and V. Hribalova. "Water-Soluble Polysaccharides from *Salvia officinalis* L. Possessing Immunomodulatory Activity." *Phytochemistry* 65 (2004): 1983-1992.

Kavvadias, D., et al. "Constituents of Sage (*Salvia officinalis*) with In Vitro Affinity to Human Brain Benzodiazepine Receptor." *Planta Medica* 69 (2003): 113-117.

Kennedy, D. O., et al. "Effects of Cholinesterase Inhibiting Sage (*Salvia officinalis*) on Mood, Anxiety, and Performance on a Psychological Stressor Battery." *Neuropsychopharmacology* 31 (2006): 845-852.

Rota, C., et al. "In Vitro Antimicrobial Activity of Essential Oils from Aromatic Plants Against Selected Foodborne Pathogens." *Journal of Food Protection* 67 (2004): 1252-1256.

Tildesley, N. T., et al. "Positive Modulation of Mood and Cognitive Performance Following Administration of Acute Doses of *Salvia lavandulaefolia* Essential Oil to Healthy Young Volunteers." *Physiology and Behavior* 83 (2005): 699-709.

Vujosevic, M., and J. Blagojevic. "Antimutagenic Effects of Extracts from Sage (*Salvia officinalis*) in Mammalian System In Vivo." *Acta Veterinaria Hungarica* 52 (2004): 439-443.

See also: Colds and flu; Dyspepsia; Strep throat.

Salacia oblonga

Category: Herbs and supplements
Related term: Ekanayaka
Definition: Natural plant product used to treat specific health conditions.

Principal proposed use: Diabetes
Other proposed uses: Complications of diabetes, weight loss

Overview

Salacia oblonga has a long history of use in the traditional Ayurvedic medicine system of India. Its bark has been used for treating diabetes, diarrhea, fever, arthritis, gonorrhea, and skin diseases.

Therapeutic Dosages

A typical dose of *S. oblonga* is 2.5 to 5.0 grams (g) daily of the whole herb, or a comparable amount as extract. The root bark is the part of the plant used.

Therapeutic Uses

Since the late 1990s, *S. oblonga* has undergone modern research that has, to a certain highly preliminary extent, substantiated its traditional reputation as a treatment for diabetes and obesity. *S. oblonga* may work similarly to the standard diabetes drug acarbose, used in type 2 diabetes. Acarbose inhibits the intestinal enzyme alpha-glucosidase, an enzyme responsible for helping the body digest carbohydrates. When alpha-glucosidase is inhibited, carbohydrate absorption is slowed, thereby reducing the rise in blood sugar that follows a meal.

Scientific Evidence

A double-blind, placebo-controlled study published in 2005 evaluated the effects of *S. oblonga* extract taken at a dose of 1,000 milligrams (mg) daily. In this study, forty-three healthy people were given a high-carbohydrate beverage with or without addition of the herb. The results showed that when the herbal extract was included, the normal rise in blood sugar and insulin following consumption of the beverage was significantly decreased. Additional evidence collected in this study (breath hydrogen levels) supported the hypothesis that *S. oblonga* works by inhibiting alpha-glucosidase.

Another double-blind study compared the effectiveness of various doses of *S oblonga* extract: 0, 500, 700, or 1,000 mg daily. Again, participants were given a high-carbohydrate beverage. The results in these thirty-nine people showed that the highest dose, but not the lower doses, significantly improved postmeal blood sugar and insulin levels. This type of "dose-related" effect, where higher doses have a greater effect, tends to bolster the confidence researchers can place in the results of a study.

However, neither of the studies described above involved people with diabetes. Further research will be necessary to determine whether *S. oblonga* is actually a useful treatment for people with this condition.

Aside from effects on carbohydrate absorption, some evidence weakly hints that *S. oblonga* might inhibit the enzyme aldose reductase. In theory, this effect could mean that use of the herb might help prevent certain complications of diabetes, such as cataracts, peripheral neuropathy, and retinopathy. However, the evidence to support this possibility remains far too preliminary to rely upon at all.

S. oblonga has been marketed for preventing type 2 diabetes as well as for aiding in weight loss. However, there is no evidence whatsoever that it offers either of these benefits.

SAFETY ISSUES

S. oblonga is believed to be relatively safe. Some evidence suggests that *S. oblonga* does not damage DNA. Studies in rats have shown a good safety profile. In human studies, the primary side effects seen are identical to the side effects of standard alpha-glucosidase inhibitors: gas and cramping. Maximum safe dosages are not known for pregnant or nursing women or for people with severe liver or kidney disease.

EBSCO CAM Review Board

FURTHER READING

Collene, A. L., et al. "Effects of a Nutritional Supplement Containing *Salacia oblonga* Extract and Insulinogenic Amino Acids on Postprandial Glycemia, Insulinemia, and Breath Hydrogen Responses in Healthy Adults." *Nutrition* 21 (2005): 848-854.

Flammang, A. M., et al. "Genotoxicity Testing of a *Salacia oblonga* Extract." *Food and Chemical Toxicology* 44 (2006): 1868-1874.

Heacock, P. M., et al. "Effects of a Medical Food Containing an Herbal Alpha-Glucosidase Inhibitor on Postprandial Glycemia and Insulinemia in Healthy Adults." *Journal of the American Dietetic Association* 105 (2005): 65-71.

Li, Y., T. H. Huang, and J. Yamahara. "Salacia Root, a Unique Ayurvedic Medicine, Meets Multiple Targets in Diabetes and Obesity." *Life Sciences* 82 (2008): 1045-1049.

Matsuda, H., et al. "Antidiabetic Principles of Natural Medicines. IV. Aldose Reductase and Alpha-Glucosidase Inhibitors from the Roots of *Salacia oblonga* Wall. (Celastraceae): Structure of a New Friedelane-Type Triterpene, Kotalagenin 16-Acetate." *Chemical and Pharmaceutical Bulletin* (Tokyo) 47 (2000): 1725-1729.

Wolf, B. W., and S. E. Weisbrode. "Safety Evaluation of an Extract from *Salacia oblonga*." *Food and Chemical Toxicology* 41 (2003): 867-874.

See also: Diabetes; Diabetes, complications of; Obesity and excess weight.

Salt bush

CATEGORY: Herbs and supplements
RELATED TERM: *Atriplex halimus*
DEFINITION: Natural plant product used to treat specific health conditions.
PRINCIPAL PROPOSED USE: Diabetes

OVERVIEW

Salt bush is a shrub that grows throughout the Mediterranean region, in the Middle East, northern Africa, and southern Europe. As its name suggests, it is especially common in areas where the soil is saline. Salt bush is a nutritious plant, high in protein; vitamins C, A, and D; and minerals such as chromium. It is also fairly tasty–shepherds as well as their flocks enjoy eating salt bush.

THERAPEUTIC DOSAGES

No standard dosage of salt bush has been established. Diabetes is a serious disease that should be treated only under medical supervision. Salt bush cannot be used as a substitute for insulin. Blood sugar levels should also be closely monitored.

THERAPEUTIC USES

Salt bush may prove useful in the treatment of type 2 (non-insulin-dependent, or adult-onset) diabetes. This idea came to the attention of medical researchers in 1964, when they discovered that a rodent called the sand rat (*Psammomys obesus*) is highly susceptible to developing diabetes. However, wild sand rats, which regularly consume salt bush, never show any signs of diabetes; instead, they tend to develop it in response to being fed regular laboratory food. As a result, scientists have explored the possibility that salt bush has an antidiabetic effect.

The results of animal studies and preliminary human trials suggest that salt bush does indeed have antidiabetic effects. However, while these studies are certainly intriguing, only double-blind, placebo-controlled studies can prove a treatment effective, and none have been reported. For this reason, the use of salt bush for diabetes remains highly speculative.

Some animal researchers speculate that the effect of salt bush (if, indeed, it has one) may be partly due to the chromium it contains. Considerable evidence indicates that chromium supplementation can improve blood sugar control, especially in type 2 diabetes. However, there could be other active ingredients in salt bush as well.

SAFETY ISSUES

As a plant food commonly consumed by animals and humans, salt bush appears to be relatively safe. However, no comprehensive safety testing of salt bush has been performed. For this reason, it should not be used by young children, pregnant or nursing women, or people with severe liver or kidney disease.

It should be noted that if salt bush is effective in lowering blood sugar, the result might be excessive lowering of blood sugar levels. For this reason, people with diabetes who take salt bush should do so only under a physician's supervision.

EBSCO CAM Review Board

FURTHER READING

Stern, E. "Successful Use of *Atriplex halimus* in the Treatment of Type 2 Diabetic Patients." Zamenhoff Medical Center, Tel Aviv, 1989.

See also: Diabetes; Diabetes, complications of.

SAMe

CATEGORY: Herbs and supplements
RELATED TERMS: Ademetionine, S-adenosylmethionine
DEFINITION: Natural substance used as a dietary supplement for specific health benefits.
PRINCIPAL PROPOSED USES: Depression, osteoarthritis

OTHER PROPOSED USES: Chronic viral hepatitis, cirrhosis and other forms of liver disease, fibromyalgia, Parkinson's disease

OVERVIEW

The chemical structure and name of S-adenosylmethionine, usually called SAMe, are derived from two materials: methionine, a sulfur-containing amino acid, and adenosine triphosphate (ATP), the body's main energy molecule. SAMe was discovered in Italy in 1952. It was first investigated as a treatment for depression, but along the way it was accidentally noted to improve arthritis symptoms–a kind of positive side effect.

SOURCES

The body makes all the SAMe it needs, so there is no dietary requirement. However, deficiencies in methionine, folate, or vitamin B_{12} can reduce SAMe levels. SAMe is not found in appreciable quantities in foods, so it must be taken as a supplement. It has been suggested that the supplement trimethylglycine might indirectly increase SAMe levels and provide similar benefits, but this effect has not been proven.

THERAPEUTIC DOSAGES

A typical full dosage of SAMe is 400 milligrams (mg) taken three to four times per day. As little as 200 mg twice daily may suffice to keep a person feeling better once the full dosage has "broken through" the symptoms.

However, some people develop mild stomach distress if they start full dosages of SAMe at once. To avoid this side effect, one may need to start low and work up to the full dosage gradually.

SAMe is on the market in the United States at a recommended dosage of 200 mg twice daily. This dosage labeling makes SAMe appear more affordable, but it is unlikely that SAMe will actually work when taken at such a low dosage.

THERAPEUTIC USES

A substantial amount of evidence suggests that SAMe can be an effective treatment for osteoarthritis, the "wear and tear" type of arthritis that many people develop as they get older. Also, a moderate amount of evidence suggests that SAMe might be helpful for depression.

Weak and inconsistent evidence hints that SAMe might be helpful for a variety of liver conditions such as cirrhosis, chronic viral hepatitis, pregnancy-related jaundice, and Gilbert's syndrome. SAMe also may help the chronic, painful muscle condition known as fibromyalgia.

SAMe has undergone some investigation as a possible supportive treatment for Parkinson's disease. One study suggests that it may reduce the depression

so commonly associated with the disease. In addition, the drug levodopa, used for Parkinson's disease, depletes the body of SAMe. This suggests that taking extra SAMe might be helpful. However, it is also possible that SAMe could interfere with the effect of levodopa, requiring an increase in dosage. Finally, preliminary evidence suggests that SAMe can protect the stomach against damage caused by alcohol.

SCIENTIFIC EVIDENCE

Osteoarthritis. A substantial body of scientific evidence supports the use of SAMe to treat osteoarthritis. Double-blind studies involving a total of more than one thousand participants suggest that SAMe is about as effective as standard anti-inflammatory drugs. In addition, evidence from studies of animals suggests that SAMe may help protect cartilage from damage.

For example, a double-blind, placebo-controlled Italian study tracked 732 people taking SAMe, naproxen (a standard anti-inflammatory drug), or placebo. After four weeks, participants taking SAMe or naproxen showed about the same level of benefit compared with each other and a superior level of benefit compared with those in the placebo group.

A later double-blind study compared SAMe with celecoxib (Celebrex), a member of the newest class of nonsteroidal anti-inflammatory drugs. Celecoxib produced more rapid effects than SAMe, but over time, SAMe appeared to catch up. However, the lack of a placebo group makes these results less than fully reliable.

Another double-blind study compared SAMe with the anti-inflammatory drug piroxicam. Forty-five people were followed for eighty-four days. The two treatments proved equally effective. However, the SAMe-treated persons maintained their improvement long after the treatment was stopped, whereas those on piroxicam quickly started to hurt again.

Similarly long-lasting results have been seen with glucosamine and chondroitin. This pattern of response suggests that these treatments are somehow making a deeper impact on osteoarthritis than simply relieving symptoms. However, while there is some direct evidence that glucosamine and chondroitin can slow the progression of osteoarthritis, the evidence regarding SAMe is more hypothetical. In other double-blind studies, oral SAMe has shown benefits equivalent to those of various doses of indomethacin, ibuprofen, and naproxen.

SAMe Study Results

The supplement S-adenosylmethionine (SAMe) was compared with celecoxib (Celebrex), a nonsteroidal anti-inflammatory drug, in a study published in 2004. The supplement and the drug, and their effect on osteoarthritis, are discussed in brief here.

Given the limitations of the established osteoarthritis medications/treatments, and the recent explosion of information and interest in complementary and alternative medicine (CAM), the public has turned their attention to CAM and is exploring safer alternatives to manage their symptoms. . . . S-adenosylmethionine (SAMe) is one of the dietary supplements that gained popularity, and was recently reported to be effective in the management of depression, liver disease, and arthritis. . . .

SAMe is helpful for the management of pain in osteoarthritis, and demonstrates similar effectiveness as a currently accepted COX-2 inhibitor, celecoxib. Results from this study add and confirm results from prior studies indicating a possible role for SAMe in the management of osteoarthritis. It is clear however, that many questions remain unanswered. Prime among these questions is: What is the optimal (effective and safe) dose of SAMe in the management of osteoarthritis? Other questions that should be explored are: What is the long-term effectiveness and safety of SAMe? What is the mechanism of action of SAMe? Does SAMe affect the disease progression or could it reverse the disease process? and finally Is the combination of SAMe and a COX-2 inhibitor more effective than either alone in the management of osteoarthritis?

Source: Wadie I. Najm et al., "S-Adenosyl Methionine (SAMe) Versus Celecoxib for the Treatment of Osteoarthritis Symptoms," *BMC Musculoskeletal Disorders* 5 (2004). This open-source article is available at http://www.biomedcentral.com/1471-2474/5/6.

Depression. The evidence for SAMe for the treatment of depression is provocative but far from definitive. Several double-blind, placebo-controlled studies have found SAMe effective in relieving depression, but most were small and poorly reported, and many used an injected form of the supplement. Furthermore, a late trial, a double-blind, placebo-controlled study of 133 people with depression, failed to find intravenous SAMe more effective than placebo. (Researchers resorted to questionable statistical manipulation of the data to show benefit.)

Other trials compared SAMe to standard antidepressants rather than to placebo. The best of these trials was a six-week, double-blind trial of 281 people with mild depression that compared oral SAMe to imipramine. The results indicated that the two treatments were about equally effective. However, the absence of a placebo group makes this study less than fully definitive.

Other studies have also compared the benefits of oral or intravenous SAMe to those of tricyclic antidepressants and have also found generally equivalent results; however, again, poor reporting and inadequacies of study design (such as too limited a treatment interval) mar the meaningfulness of the reported outcomes.

Fibromyalgia. Four double-blind trials have studied the use of SAMe for fibromyalgia, three of them finding it to be helpful. Most of these studies, however, used SAMe given either intravenously or as an injection into the muscles, sometimes in combination with oral doses. Injected medication has effects that can be quite different from those of the same medications taken orally. For this reason, these studies are of questionable relevance.

Nonetheless, the one double-blind study that used only oral SAMe did find positive results. In this trial, forty-four people with fibromyalgia took 800 mg of SAMe or placebo for six weeks. Compared with the group taking placebo, those taking SAMe had improvements in disease activity, pain at rest, fatigue, and morning stiffness, and in one measurement of mood. In other respects, such as the amount of tenderness in their tender points, the group taking SAMe did no better than those taking the placebo. It is not clear whether SAMe is helping fibromyalgia through its antidepressant effects or by some other mechanism.

Parkinson's disease. Evidence suggests that levodopa (the drug used to treat Parkinson's disease) can reduce brain levels of SAMe. This depletion may contribute to the side effects of levodopa treatment and to the depression sometimes seen with Parkinson's disease. One study found that SAMe taken orally improved depression without changing the effectiveness of levodopa. However, it is also possible that over time, taking extra SAMe could interfere with levodopa's effectiveness.

SAFETY ISSUES

SAMe appears to be quite safe, according to both human and animal studies. The most common side effect is mild digestive distress. However, SAMe does not actually damage the stomach.

Like other substances with antidepressant activity, SAMe might trigger a manic episode in those with bipolar disease. Also, safety in young children, pregnant or nursing women, or those with severe liver or kidney disease has not been established.

SAMe might interfere with the action of the Parkinson's drug levodopa. In addition, there may be risks involved in combining SAMe with standard antidepressants. For this reason, one should not try either combination without physician supervision.

IMPORTANT INTERACTIONS

One should not take SAMe except on a physician's advice if already taking standard antidepressants, including monoamine oxidase inhibitors, selective serotonin reuptake inhibitors, and tricyclics. Also, SAMe might help relieve the side effects of levodopa for Parkinson's disease. However, it might also reduce levodopa's effectiveness over time.

EBSCO CAM Review Board

FURTHER READING

Fava, M. "Using Complementary and Alternative Medicines for Depression." *Journal of Clinical Psychiatry* 71 (2010): e24.

Hosea Blewett, H. J. "Exploring the Mechanisms Behind S-adenosylmethionine (SAMe) in the Treatment of Osteoarthritis." *Clinical Reviews in Food Science and Nutrition* 48 (2008): 458-463.

Najm, W. I., et al. "S-adenosyl Methionine (SAMe) Versus Celecoxib for the Treatment of Osteoarthritis Symptoms." *BMC Musculoskeletal Disorders* 5 (2004): 6.

Porter, N. S., et al. "Alternative Medical Interventions Used in the Treatment and Management of Myalgic

Encephalomyelitis/Chronic Fatigue Syndrome and Fibromyalgia." *Journal of Alternative and Complementary Medicine* 16 (2010): 235-249.

See also: Cirrhosis; Depression, mild to moderate; Fibromyalgia: Homeopathic remedies; Hepatitis, viral; Liver disease; Osteoarthritis; Parkinson's disease.

Sampson, Wallace

CATEGORY: Biography
IDENTIFICATION: American medical doctor and critic of alternative medicine
BORN: March 29, 1930; Los Angeles, California

OVERVIEW

Wallace Sampson, a retired American professor, hematologist-oncologist, and editor in chief of the *Scientific Review of Alternative Medicine*, is best known for investigating and teaching about medical systems or practices that could be classified as unscientific. These practices include complementary and alternative medicine (CAM). His work also focuses on the exploration of aberrant medical claims.

Sampson has been affiliated with the National Council Against Health Fraud and many other organizations working to protect the public from bogus medical practices and products. In line with the sentiments of many other critics of CAM, Sampson is reported as saying of alternative medicine that "It doesn't exist." He added that "We've looked into most of the practices and, biochemically or physically, their supposed effects lie somewhere between highly improbable and impossible."

In 1952, Sampson obtained an undergraduate degree from the University of California, Berkeley, and in 1955, he received his medical degree from the University of California, San Francisco School of Medicine. He was the chief of medical oncology at the Santa Clara Valley Medical Center and a clinical professor emeritus of medicine at the Stanford University School of Medicine. He has been a contributor to the Web site Science-Based Medicine, which evaluates, from a scientific perspective, medical treatments and products of interest to the public.

Sampson has been especially critical of acupuncture, arguing that acupuncture triggers a response similar (in terms of endorphin release) to "a walk in the woods, a 5-mile run, or a pinch on the butt." He claims that acupuncture has no effect on disease processes but adds that it could serve as a type of distraction from a person's primary health complaint.

In a 2005 online article, Sampson wrote that the U.S. Congress should cease funding the National Center for Complementary and Alternative Medicine (NCCAM) because, he suggests, the center has failed to prove the effectiveness of any alternative method. The money required for the operation of this center, he further argues, could be applied more effectively to proven research endeavors. He further states that NCCAM is ridden with potential and actual conflicts of interest and that most recipients of money from this branch have consistently failed to deliver positive results.

Brandy Weidow, M.S.

FURTHER READING

Harmanci, Reyhan. "Healthy Doubts: Wallace Sampson—Alternative Medicine Doesn't Exist and Acupuncture Is Useless, He Says." *San Francisco Gate*, August 31, 2006. http://articles.sfgate.com/2006-08-31/entertainment/17309357_1_acupuncture-alternative-medicine-western-medicine.

Sampson, Wallace. "Whatever Happened to Plausibility as the Basis for Clinical Research and Practice After EBM and CAM Rushed In?" Medscape, January 26, 2007. http://www.medscape.com/viewarticle/548128.

See also: Acupuncture; Barrett, Stephen; Clinical trials; Dawkins, Richard; National Center for Complementary and Alternative Medicine; Popular practitioners; Pseudoscience; Scientific method.

Sandalwood

CATEGORY: Herbs and supplements
RELATED TERM: *Santalum album*
DEFINITION: Natural plant product used to treat specific health conditions.
PRINCIPAL PROPOSED USE: Supportive treatment of urinary tract infections
OTHER PROPOSED USES: Peptic ulcers, skin conditions

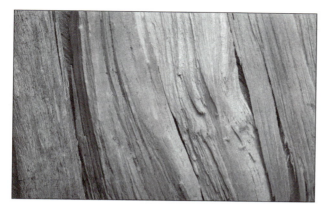

Wood from the white sandalwood tree is used to make sandalwood oil. (Pascal Goetgheluck/Photo Researchers, Inc.)

OVERVIEW

The oil of the sweet-smelling sandalwood tree has a long history of use as a perfume and incense fragrance. Sandalwood oil also has a medicinal tradition in various countries, having been used for digestive distress, liver problems, acne and other skin problems, gonorrhea, anxiety, and insomnia. Additionally, it has played a role in some Hindu religious ceremonies and has been used as a meditation aid.

THERAPEUTIC DOSAGES

According to Germany's Commission E, sandalwood oil should be taken at a dose of 1 to 1.5 grams daily in enteric-coated form for supportive treatment of urinary tract infections. (Enteric-coated products are designed so they do not open up and release their contents until they reach the small intestine.) However, this is a relatively high dose for an essential oil and should be used only under the supervision of a physician. Non-enteric-coated products may cause stomach distress. For external use in skin conditions, a few drops of the oil are added to a cup of water.

THERAPEUTIC USES

Sandalwood oil has been approved by Germany's Commission E for treatment of bladder infections. It is not recommended as a sole treatment, but rather as an accompaniment to conventional care. However, there is no meaningful evidence that it is effective for this purpose. Only double-blind, placebo-controlled studies can prove that a treatment really works, and no studies of this type have been performed with sandalwood.

Weak evidence, far too preliminary to rely upon, hints that sandalwood may have antiviral, anti-*Helicobacter pylori* (*H. pylori* is the underlying cause of most stomach ulcers), sedative, and cancer-preventive properties.

SAFETY ISSUES

Sandalwood oil appears to be relatively safe, but it has not undergone comprehensive safety testing; in general, essential oil can have toxic and even fatal effects when taken in sufficient doses, especially by children. Allergic reactions caused by direct contact with sandalwood oil occur relatively frequently. Sandalwood oil should not be used by young children, pregnant or nursing women, or people with severe liver or kidney disease.

EBSCO CAM Review Board

FURTHER READING

Frosch, P. J., et al. "Further Important Sensitizers in Patients Sensitive to Fragrances." *Contact Dermatitis* 47 (2003): 279-287.

Hongratanaworakit, T., et al. "Evaluation of the Effects of East Indian Sandalwood Oil and Alpha-Santalol on Humans After Transdermal Absorption." *Planta Medica* 70 (2004): 3-7.

Ochi, T., et al. "Anti-*Helicobacter pylori* Compounds from *Santalum album.*" *Journal of Natural Products* 68 (2005): 819-824.

See also: Bladder infection; Bladder infection: Homeopathic remedies; Peptic ulcer disease: Homeopathic remedies; Ulcers.

Sarsaparilla

CATEGORY: Herbs and supplements
RELATED TERMS: *Smilax officinalis*, other *Smilax* species
DEFINITION: Natural plant product used to treat specific health conditions.
PRINCIPAL PROPOSED USES: Antifungal, anti-inflammatory, cancer (anticancer), menstrual disorders, sexual dysfunction, sports and fitness support and performance enhancement

OVERVIEW

Vinelike plants in the sarsaparilla family are found in many parts of the world. The most common form, *Smilax officinalis*, is grown primarily in Jamaica. Other common forms include *S. glyciphylla* (Australia), *S. japicanga* (Brazil), *S. glabra* (Sri Lanka), *S. china* (China), and *S. luzonensis* (Malaysia). The root is the part of the plant that is used medicinally.

Traditionally, various forms of sarsaparilla have been use to treat cancer, psoriasis, eczema, and other skin diseases. These uses are all tied together by an outdated treatment concept known as blood purification. It was thought that numerous ailments, including skin diseases, cancer, and other conditions, were caused by impurities in the blood. Herbs said to have blood-purifying properties, such as sarsaparilla, were used to correct this traditionally acknowledged problem. Additionally, sarsaparilla was recommended for joint pain, "female problems," and syphilis.

An entirely different plant, *Aralia nudicaulis*, is sometimes called wild sarsaparilla. However, it is more closely related to ginseng than to the forms of sarsaparilla discussed here. Sarsaparilla should also not be confused with sassafras, a flavoring traditionally used in root beer.

THERAPEUTIC DOSAGES

A typical dose of sarsaparilla is 2 to 4 grams (g) three times per day. Various tinctures are also available; these should be taken according to label instructions.

THERAPEUTIC USES

There are no medicinal uses of sarsaparilla with meaningful scientific support. Extremely weak evidence, far too weak to be relied upon at all, hints at possible antifungal, anti-inflammatory, and anticancer effects.

Like numerous other herbs, sarsaparilla contains substances in the saponin family. One of these, sarsasapogenin, is often said to reproduce the effect of various hormones. However, there is no evidence whatsoever to support this claim.

Based on traditional usage, as well as unwarranted extrapolation from test-tube findings, sarsaparilla is sold today as a treatment for psoriasis and other skin problems, as well as cancer, menstrual disorders, and asthma. Other unsubstantiated uses include enhancement of sexual function, improvement of mental function in Alzheimer's disease, protection of the liver, and improvement of sports performance.

SAFETY ISSUES

Although the use of sarsaparilla has not been associated with any serious adverse consequences, comprehensive safety studies have not been performed. Sarsaparilla is traditionally not recommended for use during pregnancy or breast-feeding. Safety in young children and people with liver or kidney disease is also questionable.

As with most substances taken orally, sarsaparilla may cause gastrointestinal distress. Germany's Commission E also reports short-term "kidney irritation" as a side effect; precisely what this means, however, remains unclear.

Note that although various species of sarsaparilla are often used somewhat interchangeably, it is quite possible that some varieties of this plant are safer than others. Finally, some sarsaparilla products have been found to contain unsafe levels of lead.

EBSCO CAM Review Board

FURTHER READING

Cox, S. D., K. C. Jayasinghe, and J. L. Markham. "Antioxidant Activity in Australian Native Sarsaparilla (*Smilax glyciphylla*)." *Journal of Ethnopharmacology* 101 (2005): 162-168.

Kuo, Y. H., et al. "Cytotoxic Phenylpropanoid Glycosides from the Stems of *Smilax china*." *Journal of Natural Products* 68 (2005): 1475-1478.

Sautour, M., T. Miyamoto, and M. A. Lacaille-Dubois. "Steroidal Saponins from *Smilax medica* and Their Antifungal Activity." *Journal of Natural Products* 68 (2005): 1489-1493.

Shao, B., et al. "Steroidal Saponins from *Smilax china* and Their Anti-inflammatory Activities." *Phytochemistry* 68 (2007): 623-630.

Shu, X. S., Z. H. Gao, and X. L. Yang. "Anti-inflammatory and Anti-nociceptive Activities of *Smilax china* L. Aqueous Extract." *Journal of Ethnopharmacology* 103 (2006): 327-332.

Thabrew, M. I., et al. "Cytotoxic Effects of a Decoction of *Nigella sativa*, *Hemidesmus indicus*, and *Smilax glabra* on Human Hepatoma HepG2 Cells." *Life Sciences* 77 (2005): 1319-1330.

Xu, J., et al. "Anti-inflammatory Constituents from the Roots of *Smilax bockii* Warb." *Archives of Pharmacal Research* 28 (2005): 395-399.

See also: Cancer risk reduction; Sexual dysfunction in men; Sexual dysfunction in women; Sports and fitness support: Enhancing performance; Women's health.

Sassafras

CATEGORY: Herbs and supplements
RELATED TERM: *Santalum album*
DEFINITION: Natural plant product used to treat specific health conditions.
PRINCIPAL PROPOSED USES: The use of sassafras in any form is not recommended.

OVERVIEW

The sassafras tree, a native of North America, has a long history of use as both flavoring and medicine. The oil extracted from its root was one of the original constituents of herbal root beer. As medicine, it was used to treat influenza and other fever-producing infections, as well as arthritis, urinary tract infections, and digestive disorders. It was also commonly used as a "spring tonic" or "blood purifier."

However, in the 1960s, it was discovered that sassafras oil contains high levels of a liver toxin called safrole. When given to animals, safrole causes liver cancer, and even a single cup of sassafras tea contains dangerous levels of the substance. Because of this, sassafras has been banned for human consumption. Only safrole-free products containing sassafras can be sold; however, there may be other carcinogens in sassafras aside from safrole. Sassafras oil is also immediately toxic; a few drops can kill an infant, and a teaspoon can cause death in an adult.

EBSCO CAM Review Board

FURTHER READING

Foster, S., and V. E. Tyler. "Sassafras." In *Tyler's Honest Herbal: A Sensible Guide to the Use of Herbs and Related Remedies.* 4th ed. New York: Haworth Herbal Press, 1999.

Newall, C. A., et al. *Herbal Medicines: A Guide for Health-Care Professionals.* London: Pharmaceutical Press, 1996.

Tan, D., et al. "Both Physiological and Pharmacological Levels of Melatonin Reduce DNA Adduct Formation Induced by the Carcinogen Safrole." *Carcinogenesis* 15 (1994): 215-218.

See also: Liver disease.

Saw palmetto

CATEGORY: Herbs and supplements
RELATED TERMS: *Sabal serrulata, Serenoa repens*
DEFINITION: Natural plant product used to treat specific health conditions.
PRINCIPAL PROPOSED USE: Benign prostatic hyperplasia
OTHER PROPOSED USES: Hair loss, prostatitis

OVERVIEW

Saw palmetto is a native plant of North America, and it is still primarily grown in the United States. The saw palmetto tree grows to a height of 2 to 4 feet; it has fan-shaped serrated leaves and abundant berries. Native Americans used these berries for the treatment of various urinary problems in men, as well as for women with breast disorders. European and American physicians took up saw palmetto as a treatment for benign prostatic hyperplasia (BPH). In the 1960s, French researchers discovered that by concentrating the oils of saw palmetto berry, they could maximize the herb's effectiveness.

Saw palmetto contains many biologically active chemicals. It is unknown which among these chemicals are the most important. It is also not known precisely how saw palmetto works; the herb appears to interact with various sex hormones, but it also has many other complex actions that could affect the prostate.

THERAPEUTIC DOSAGES

The standard dosage of saw palmetto for the treatment of BPH is 160 milligrams (mg) twice a day of an extract standardized to contain 85 to 95 percent fatty acids and sterols. A single daily dose of 320 mg may be just as effective for this condition. However, taking more than this amount does not, on average, seem to produce better results. As with many other herbs, the quality of commercial saw palmetto products may vary widely. For this reason, it is recommended that individuals purchase only saw palmetto products that have been evaluated by an independent laboratory.

THERAPEUTIC USES

Saw palmetto oil is an accepted medical treatment for BPH in New Zealand and in France, Germany, Austria, Italy, Spain, and other European countries. Typical symptoms of BPH include difficulty starting urination, weak urinary stream, frequent urination,

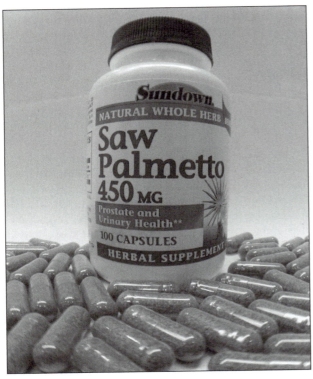

A bottle and pills of saw palemetto extract. (AP Photo)

dribbling after urination, and waking up several times at night to urinate. Most, though not all, research suggests that saw palmetto can markedly improve all these symptoms. Benefits require approximately four to six weeks of treatment to develop. It appears that about two-thirds of men respond reasonably well.

Furthermore, while the prostate tends to continue to grow when left untreated, saw palmetto causes a small but definite shrinkage. In other words, it appears that it does not just relieve symptoms but actually delays prostate enlargement. The drug Proscar does this too (and to a greater extent than saw palmetto), but other standard medications for BPH have no effect on prostate size.

Some studies suggest that saw palmetto is just as effective for reducing BPH symptoms as Proscar, and it has one meaningful advantage: It leaves prostate-specific antigen (PSA) levels unchanged. Cancer raises PSA levels, and lab tests that measure PSA are used to screen for prostate cancer. Proscar lowers PSA measurements, and therefore its use may have the unintended effect of masking prostate cancer. Saw pal-

metto does not do this. On the other hand, Proscar has been shown to reduce the need for surgery, unlike saw palmetto or any of the other drugs used for BPH. Saw palmetto may also be just as effective as another class of standard drugs known as alpha-blockers and may cause fewer side effects. Individuals should not self-treat with saw palmetto without first undergoing a proper medical evaluation to rule out prostate cancer.

Saw palmetto is also widely used to treat chronic prostatitis. An open trial that compared saw palmetto to the drug Proscar for the treatment of chronic nonbacterial prostatitis found that while the drug was effective, the herb was not. However, these results do not mean that saw palmetto is ineffective for prostatitis. Because this was an open study, researchers and participants knew who was getting saw palmetto and who was getting the drug. If there was any expectation that the drug would be more powerful than the herb, this in itself would have been sufficient to skew the results toward that outcome. Also, saw palmetto is sometimes recommended as a treatment for hair loss, but there is no evidence that it is effective for this purpose.

SCIENTIFIC EVIDENCE

The scientific evidence for the effectiveness of saw palmetto in treating prostate enlargement is inconsistent. A minimum of twelve double-blind studies involving a total of about nine hundred people have compared the benefits of saw palmetto against placebo over periods of one to twelve months. In all but three of these studies, the herb improved urinary flow rate and most other measures of prostate disease to a greater extent than did placebo. However, in the most recent and perhaps best designed of these studies, a one-year trial of 225 men, a saw palmetto product failed to prove more effective than placebo. Furthermore, a large review of fourteen trials with 5,222 men found that saw palmetto did not improve urinary symptom scores or peak urine flow compared with placebo. Subjects taking saw palmetto reported more overall symptom improvement than those taking placebo, but this result is questionable owing to inconsistencies among studies.

A double-blind study followed 1,098 men who received either saw palmetto or the drug Proscar for six months. (The study had no placebo group.) The treatments were equally effective, but while Proscar lowered PSA levels and caused a slight worsening of sexual function on average, saw palmetto caused no significant side effects. Both treatments caused the prostate to shrink, but Proscar had a greater effect.

A fifty-two-week double-blind study of 811 men compared saw palmetto to a standard drug in another class: the alpha-blocker tamsulosin. Once again, both treatments proved equally effective. However, saw palmetto caused fewer side effects than the drug. In addition, the herb caused some prostate shrinkage, while the drug caused a slight prostate enlargement.

A study involving 435 men found that the benefits of saw palmetto endure for at least three years. However, there was no control group in this study, making the results unreliable.

A forty-eight-week double-blind trial of 543 men with early BPH compared combined saw palmetto and nettle root against Proscar and found equal benefits. Benefits were also seen with a combination of saw palmetto and nettle root in a twenty-four-week placebo-controlled study of 257 men.

Finally, a six-month double-blind, placebo-controlled trial of 44 men given a saw palmetto herbal blend (containing, in addition, nettle root and pumpkin seed oil) found shrinkage in prostate tissue. No significant improvement in symptoms was seen, but the researchers pointed out that the study size was too small to statistically detect such improvements if they did occur.

SAFETY ISSUES

Saw palmetto is thought to be essentially nontoxic. In addition, in clinical trials, it has shown little to no adverse effect. For example, in a one-year randomized trial of 225 men, there was no significant difference in adverse events between the group receiving saw palmetto and the group receiving placebo. Also, in a three-year study, only 34 of the 435 participants had side effects, and these were primarily only of the usual nonspecific variety seen with all medications, such as mild gastrointestinal distress.

There are at least two case reports in which use of saw palmetto was linked to liver inflammation; however, a subsequent study in rats failed to find that even very high doses of saw palmetto are injurious to the liver. This case report might have been an instance of an allergic or other idiosyncratic reaction; alternatively, something other than saw palmetto may have gotten into the product. One of the above-mentioned cases also involved pancreatitis.

Finally, there is one report of saw palmetto apparently causing excessive bleeding during surgery. The significance of this isolated event is unclear, but it is probably prudent for individuals to avoid saw palmetto prior to and just after surgery, and during the period surrounding labor and delivery. Individuals with bleeding problems (such as hemophilia) should perhaps also avoid saw palmetto, as should those taking any drug that thins the blood, such as warfarin (Coumadin), heparin, aspirin, clopidogrel (Plavix), ticlopidine (Ticlid), or pentoxifylline (Trental).

Saw palmetto has no known drug interactions. Safety for pregnant or nursing women and those with severe kidney or liver disease has not been established.

EBSCO CAM Review Board

FURTHER READING

Avins, A. L., et al. "A Detailed Safety Assessment of a Saw Palmetto Extract." *Complementary Therapies in Medicine* 16 (2008): 147-154.

Bent, S., et al. "Saw Palmetto for Benign Prostatic Hyperplasia." *New England Journal of Medicine* 354 (2006): 557-566.

Jibrin, I., et al. "Saw Palmetto-Induced Pancreatitis." *Southern Medical Journal* 99 (2006): 611-612.

Kaplan, S. A., M. A. Volpe, and A. E. Te. "A Prospective, 1-Year Trial Using Saw Palmetto Versus Finasteride in the Treatment of Category III Prostatitis/Chronic Pelvic Pain Syndrome." *Journal of Urology* 171 (2004): 284-288.

Lopatkin, N., et al. "Long-Term Efficacy and Safety of a Combination of Sabal and Urtica Extract for Lower Urinary Tract Symptoms." *World Journal of Urology* 23 (2005): 139-146.

Tacklind, J., et al. "Serenoa Repens for Benign Prostatic Hyperplasia." *Cochrane Database of Systematic Reviews* (April 15, 2009), CD001423.

See also: Benign prostatic hyperplasia; Prostatitis.

Scar tissue

CATEGORY: Condition
RELATED TERM: Keloid scars
DEFINITION: Treatment of the fibrous tissue that naturally forms after surgery, disease, or a wound to the skin.

PRINCIPAL PROPOSED NATURAL TREATMENTS: None

OTHER PROPOSED NATURAL TREATMENTS: Acupuncture, allantoin, aloe vera, coconut oil, collagen, elastin, gotu kola, jojoba oil, lavender oil, magnet therapy, massage, selenium, snail extract, tamanu oil, vitamin A, vitamin C, vitamin E, zinc

INTRODUCTION

When the body repairs a wound, it often does so by creating fibrous scar tissue. Internal scars that may develop following surgery can cause significant pain. Surface scars are generally painless, but they may be cosmetically unpleasant. In some cases, scars on the skin can develop into a special form of oversized scar called a keloid. Keloids are generally red or pink and often form a ridge several millimeters above the skin. These scars occur when the body continues to fill the scar with collagen after it has healed. Darker-skinned people are more likely than others to develop keloids.

Conventional treatment of any type of scar is less than entirely satisfactory. Keloids and other scars on the skin may be reduced in size by freezing (cryotherapy), steroid injections, radiation therapy, or surgical removal. However, an even more visible scar may develop in place of the one that was removed. Similarly, the removal of painful internal scars may lead to the formation of new, painful scar tissue.

PROPOSED NATURAL TREATMENTS

The herb gotu kola is said to help remove keloid scars. When used for this purpose, it is taken orally, applied to the skin, or injected into the scar. However, there is no reliable evidence that it is effective.

According to some schools of acupuncture, surface scars impede the flow of energy and thereby cause various illnesses. Acupuncture treatment of both surface and internal scars is said to either shrink them or reduce their effects. However, there is no meaningful scientific evidence to indicate that acupuncture offers any benefits for scars.

Other natural treatments proposed for scars, but again without reliable supporting evidence, include aloe vera, allantoin, coconut oil, collagen, elastin, jojoba oil, lavender oil, massage, magnet therapy, selenium, snail extract, tamanu oil, vitamin A, vitamin C, vitamin E, and zinc.

EBSCO CAM Review Board

FURTHER READING

Aust, M. C., et al. "Percutaneous Collagen Induction Therapy: An Alternative Treatment for Burn Scars." *Burns* 36 (2010): 836-843.

Kartnig, T. "Clinical Applications of *Centella asiatica* (L.)." *Journal of Herbs, Spices, and Medicinal Plants* 3 (1988): 146-173.

Roseborough, I. E., M. A. Grevious, and R. C. Lee. "Prevention and Treatment of Excessive Dermal Scarring." *Journal of the National Medical Association* 96 (2004): 108-116.

See also: Aloe; Burns, minor; Injuries, minor; Peyronie's disease; Warts; Wounds, minor.

Schisandra

CATEGORY: Herbs and supplements

RELATED TERMS: *Fructus schizandrae*, gomishi, magnolia vine, *Schisandra chinensis*, wu-wei-zi

DEFINITION: Natural plant product used to treat specific health conditions.

PRINCIPAL PROPOSED USES: None

OTHER PROPOSED USES: Cancer prevention, enhancement of mental function, hepatitis, liver protection, enhancement of sports performance

OVERVIEW

Schisandra is a woody vine native to eastern Asia. It winds around the trunks of trees, covering the branches. The white flowers produce small red berries that may grow in clusters. Traditionally, the berries are harvested in the fall, dried, and then ground to make the powdered medicinal herb. The seeds of the fruit contain lignans, which are believed to be active constituents.

Schisandra has long been used in the traditional medicines of Russia and China for a wide variety of conditions, including asthma, coughs, and other respiratory ailments; diarrhea; insomnia; impotence; and kidney problems. Hunters and athletes have used schisandra in the belief that it will increase endurance and combat fatigue under physical stress. More recently, schisandra has been studied for potential liver-protective effects.

THERAPEUTIC DOSAGES

Schisandra comes in capsules, tinctures, powder, tablets, and extracts. Common dosages are 1.5 to 6 grams (g) daily.

THERAPEUTIC USES

Schisandra has not been proven effective for any condition. Research on the herb is limited to studies in animals, as well as human trials that are not up to modern scientific standards.

Animal studies suggest schisandra may protect the liver from toxic damage, improve liver function, and stimulate liver cell regrowth. These findings led to its use in human trials for treating hepatitis. In a poorly designed and reported Chinese study of 189 people with hepatitis B, those given schisandra reportedly improved more rapidly than those given vitamins and liver extracts.

Other animal studies of schisandra have found possible anticancer properties. Weak evidence hints that schisandra or its extracts might enhance sports performance and improve mental function.

SAFETY ISSUES

Studies in mice, rats, and pigs have found schisandra to be relatively nontoxic. Noticeable side effects are apparently rare, although upset stomach and allergic reactions have been reported. The safety of schisandra for pregnant or nursing women, children, or people with severe liver or kidney disease has not been established.

EBSCO CAM Review Board

FURTHER READING

Hancke, J. L., R. A. Burgos, and F. Ahumada. "*Schisandra chinensis* (Turcz.) Baill." *Fitoterapia* 70 (1999): 451-471.

See also: Cancer risk reduction; Sports and fitness support: Enhancing performance.

Schizophrenia

CATEGORY: Condition
DEFINITION: Treatment of a severe disease of the brain.
PRINCIPAL PROPOSED NATURAL TREATMENT: Glycine
OTHER PROPOSED NATURAL TREATMENTS: Coenzyme Q$_{10}$, creatine, D-serine, dehydroepiandros-

terone, eicosapentaenoic acid, folate, fish oil (and its constituents), ginkgo melatonin, milk thistle, repetitive transcranial magnetic stimulation, vitamin B$_3$ (niacin), vitamin B$_6$, vitamin C, yoga
HERBS AND SUPPLEMENTS TO AVOID: Chromium picolinate, dong quai, kava, phenylalanine, St. John's wort, yohimbe

INTRODUCTION

Schizophrenia is a chronic, severe, disabling brain disease. People with schizophrenia often have terrifying symptoms, such as hearing internal voices not heard by others or believing that other people are reading their minds, controlling their thoughts, or plotting to harm them. These symptoms may leave them fearful and withdrawn. Their speech and behavior can be so disorganized that they may be incomprehensible or frightening to others. Schizophrenia increases a person's risk of suicide, self-mutilation, substance abuse, and such social problems as unemployment, homelessness, and incarceration.

Schizophrenia is found in persons all over the world. The severity of the symptoms and the long-lasting, chronic pattern of schizophrenia often cause a high degree of disability. Approximately 1 percent of the population develops this condition during their lifetime; more than 2 million people in the United States have this illness in a given year. Although schizophrenia affects men and women with equal frequency, the disorder often appears earlier in men. Men are usually affected in their late teenage years or early twenties, while women are generally affected in their twenties to early thirties.

Researchers are not sure what causes schizophrenia. Problems with brain structure and chemistry are thought to play a role. There appears to be a strong genetic component, but some researchers believe that environmental factors may contribute. It is theorized also that a viral infection in infancy or extreme stress, or both, may trigger schizophrenia in people who are predisposed to the disease.

Conventional drug treatment for schizophrenia is moderately effective. Although it seldom produces a true cure, it can enable a person with schizophrenia to function in society.

Tardive dyskinesia (TD) is a potentially permanent side effect of drugs used to control schizophrenia and other psychoses. This late-developing (tardy, or tardive) complication consists of annoying, mostly uncontrollable movements (dyskinesias). Typical symptoms include repetitive sucking or blinking, slow twisting of the hands, and other movements of the face and limbs. TD can cause tremendous social embarrassment. Several natural treatments have shown promise for preventing or treating TD.

PRINCIPAL PROPOSED NATURAL TREATMENTS

Untreated schizophrenia is a very dangerous disease for which there is effective treatment, and for this reason it is not ethical to perform studies that compare a hypothetical new treatment with placebo. Therefore, studies of natural treatments for schizophrenia have looked at their potential benefit for enhancing the effects of standard treatment (or minimizing its side effects). No natural treatments have been studied as sole therapy for schizophrenia.

Glycine. Until recently, all common medications used for schizophrenia fell into a class called phenothiazines. These drugs are most effective for the positive symptoms of schizophrenia, such as hallucinations and delusions. (Such symptoms are called positive because they indicate the presence of abnormal mental functions, rather than the absence of normal mental functions.) In general, however, these medications are less helpful for the "negative" symptoms of schizophrenia, such as apathy, depression, and social withdrawal.

The supplement glycine might be of benefit here. A clinical trial enrolled twenty-two persons who continued to experience negative symptoms of schizophrenia despite standard therapy. In this double-blind, placebo-controlled crossover study, volunteers were randomly assigned to receive either 0.8 gram (g) of glycine per kilogram of body weight (about 60 g per day) or placebo for six weeks, along with their regular medications. The groups were then switched after a two-week "wash-out" period during which they all received placebo.

Significant improvements (about 30 percent) in symptoms such as depression and apathy were seen with glycine when compared with placebo. Additionally, glycine appeared to reduce some of the side effects caused by the prescription drugs. Furthermore, the benefits apparently continued for another eight weeks after glycine was discontinued.

No changes were seen in positive symptoms (for instance, hallucinations), but it is not possible to tell

---

Side Effects of Schizophrenia Drugs

Health professionals, including those practicing complementary and alternative medicine (CAM), are seeking ways to treat schizophrenia that avoid the severe side effects of antipsychotic drugs. One side effect is tardive dyskinesia, briefly discussed here. CAM treatments, such as dietary supplements, might offer some symptom relief without the major side effects of prescription drugs.

Tardive dyskinesia (TD) is a neurological syndrome caused by the long-term use of neuroleptic drugs. Neuroleptic drugs are generally prescribed for psychiatric disorders, including schizophrenia, as well as for some gastrointestinal and neurological disorders.

TD is characterized by repetitive, involuntary, purposeless movements. The movements commonly happen around the mouth. Features of the disorder may include grimacing, tongue protrusion, lip smacking, puckering and pursing, and rapid eye blinking. Rapid movements of the arms, legs, and trunk may also occur. Involuntary movements of the fingers may be present.

TD can range from mild to severe, and in some people the problem cannot be cured. Sometimes people with TD recover partially or fully after they stop taking the medication.

---

whether this was the case because these symptoms were already being controlled by prescription medications or because glycine simply has no effect on that aspect of schizophrenia.

Four other small, double-blind, placebo-controlled clinical trials of glycine together with standard drugs for schizophrenia (including the newer drugs olanzapine and risperidone) also found it to be helpful for negative symptoms. However, one small, double-blind, placebo-controlled trial (nineteen participants) suggests that adding glycine to the drug clozapine may not be a good idea. In this study, glycine was found to reduce the benefits of clozapine without helping to relieve the participants' negative symptoms. Lack of benefit, although no actual harm, was seen in two other double-blind, placebo-controlled trials of glycine and clozapine. Another, later study not specifically limited to clozapine also failed to find benefit with glycine. A natural substance (sarcosine) that blocks the action of glycine has also shown promise for the treatment of schizophrenia.

Other Proposed Natural Treatments

Numerous other natural therapies have shown promise for aiding various aspects of treatment for schizophrenia, but in most cases, the supporting evidence is weak at best.

Enhancing drug action. For a number of theoretical reasons, it has been suggested that fish oil and its constituents (especially a slightly modified constituent called ethyl-EPA) might enhance the effectiveness of standard drugs used for schizophrenia; however, evidence for benefit remains incomplete and inconsistent.

A small, six-week, double-blind, placebo-controlled study evaluated the potential effectiveness of the supplement dehydroepiandrosterone (DHEA) taken at a dose of 100 mg daily for enhancing the effectiveness of drug treatment for schizophrenia. The results indicated that the use of DHEA led to improvement in various symptoms, especially negative symptoms. However, in another double-blind, placebo-controlled study, the use of DHEA provided minimal benefits, if any. Preliminary evidence suggests that ginkgo, the amino acid D-serine, and N-acetylcysteine may also enhance the effectiveness of various antipsychotic drugs.

Drug side effects. Vitamin B_6 might also reduce symptoms of akathesia, a type of restlessness associated with phenothiazine antipsychotics. One small double-blind study found that the use of DHEA reduced the Parkinson-like movement disorders that may occur in people taking phenothiazine drugs. According to studies performed in China, the herb ginkgo may reduce various side effects caused by drugs used to treat schizophrenia.

Preliminary studies suggest that phenothiazine drugs might deplete the body of coenzyme Q_{10} (CoQ_{10}). While there is no evidence that taking this supplement provides any specific benefit for people using phenothiazines, supplementing with CoQ_{10} might be a good idea on general principles. The herb milk thistle might protect against the liver toxicity sometimes caused by phenothiazine drugs.

Other options. Preliminary evidence suggests that a special form of magnet therapy called repetitive transcranial magnetic stimulation (rTMS) may be useful for schizophrenia. However, not all studies have found benefits above the placebo effect; rTMS is not yet available outside a research setting.

A study of nineteen people with schizophrenia who had disturbed sleep patterns found that 2 mg of con-trolled-release melatonin improved sleep. Another small study failed to find the supplement creatine helpful for schizophrenia.

High doses of various vitamins, including folate, A, B_1, B_3 (niacin), B_6, B_{12}, C, and E, have been suggested for the treatment of schizophrenia, but the evidence that these vitamins offer any real benefit remains incomplete and contradictory at best. One trial of eighty-one adolescents and young adults (considered at very high risk for psychotic disorder) found that daily omega-3 fatty acid (fish oil) supplements for twelve weeks delayed the onset of a full schizophrenic episode. Larger trials are necessary before fish oil supplementation can be recommended for persons at risk for schizophrenia.

Yoga too has been studied for schizophrenia. In one small trial, persons who supplemented their regular treatment with a yoga program lasting four months had improved symptoms, were able to function better, and reported a better quality of life compared to those who did physical therapy alone.

Herbs and Supplements to Avoid

There are some indications that using the supplement phenylalanine while taking antipsychotic drugs might increase the risk of developing tardive dyskinesia. Antipsychotic drugs can cause dystonic reactions (sudden intense movements and prolonged muscle contraction of the neck and eyes.) There is some evidence that the herb kava can increase the risk or severity of this side effect.

Phenothiazine drugs can cause increased sensitivity to the sun. Various herbs, including St. John's wort and dong quai, can also cause this problem. Combined treatment with herb and drug might increase the risk further.

St. John's wort might also interact adversely with the newer antipsychotic drugs in the clozapine family. Persons who take any of these drugs and then start taking St. John's wort may see blood levels of the drug fall. However, if a person is already taking both the herb and the drug, but then stops St. John's wort, the level of drug in the body could reach the toxic point.

The supplement chromium is often sold as chromium picolinate. Because picolinate can alter levels of various neurotransmitters (substances that the brain uses to function), there are theoretical concerns that it could cause problems for people with schizophrenia.

The herb yohimbe is relatively toxic and can cause problems if used incorrectly. Also, phenothiazine medications may increase the risk of this toxicity.

EBSCO CAM Review Board

FURTHER READING

Amminger, G. P., et al. "Long-Chain Omega-3 Fatty Acids for Indicated Prevention of Psychotic Disorders." *Archives of General Psychiatry* 67 (2010): 146-154.

Buchanan, R. W., et al. "The Cognitive and Negative Symptoms in Schizophrenia Trial (CONSIST): The Efficacy of Glutamatergic Agents for Negative Symptoms and Cognitive Impairments." *American Journal of Psychiatry* 164 (2007): 1593-1602.

Duraiswamy, G., et al. "Yoga Therapy as an Add-On Treatment in the Management of Patients with Schizophrenia." *Acta Psychiatrica Scandinavica* 116 (2007): 226-232.

Holi, M. M., et al. "Left Prefrontal Repetitive Transcranial Magnetic Stimulation in Schizophrenia." *Schizophrenia Bulletin* 30 (2004): 429-434.

Kaptsan, A., et al. "Lack of Efficacy of 5 Grams Daily of Creatine in Schizophrenia." *Journal of Clinical Psychiatry* 68 (2007): 881-884.

Ritsner, M. S., et al. "Improvement of Sustained Attention and Visual and Movement Skills, but Not Clinical Symptoms, After Dehydroepiandrosterone Augmentation in Schizophrenia." *Journal of Clinical Psychopharmacology* 26 (2006): 495-499.

Tranulis, C., et al. "Should We Treat Auditory Hallucinations with Repetitive Transcranial Magnetic Stimulation?" *Canadian Journal of Psychiatry* 53 (2008): 577-586.

See also: Adolescent and teenage health; Anxiety and panic attacks; Bipolar disorder; Depression, mild to moderate; Glycine; Magnet therapy; Mental health; Tardive dyskinesia.

Sciatica

CATEGORY: Condition

RELATED TERM: Sciatic pain

DEFINITION: Treatment of irritation of the major nerve that extends from the lower spine to the lower buttocks, legs, and feet.

PRINCIPAL PROPOSED NATURAL TREATMENTS: None

OTHER PROPOSED NATURAL TREATMENTS: Acupuncture, Alexander technique, biofeedback, chiropractic, Feldenkrais method, massage, pilates, prolotherapy, Tai Chi, yoga

INTRODUCTION

Sciatica is the irritation of the sciatic nerve, a major nerve that passes down the back of each thigh. The sciatic nerve originates in the lower spine and travels deep in the pelvis to the lower buttocks. From there it passes along the back of each upper leg and divides at the knee into branches that go to the feet. Sciatica typically causes pain that shoots down the back of one thigh or buttock.

Anything that causes irritation or puts pressure on the sciatic nerve can cause sciatica. The most common cause is probably a sprain or strain of muscles or ligaments in the area, and for this reason sciatica is often associated with low back pain. The cushions between the bones of the spine (the disks) can also cause sciatica when they bulge out of place or degenerate. Other causes of sciatica include spinal stenosis (narrowing of the spinal canal in the lumbar area), spondylolisthesis (slippage of a bone in the low back) and, rarely, benign or malignant tumors.

Diagnosis of sciatica is made by symptoms, neurologic evaluation, and tests, such as a nerve conduction study, X rays, and a magnetic resonance imaging (MRI) scan. Common symptoms include burning, tingling, or a shooting pain down the back of one leg; pain in one leg or buttock that is worse with sitting, standing up, coughing, sneezing, or straining; and weakness or numbness in one leg or foot. More serious symptoms that sometimes occur in sciatica include difficulty walking, standing, or moving; increasing weakness or numbness in the leg or foot; and loss of bowel or bladder control.

In most cases, sciatic pain resolves on its own without specific treatment. Bed rest, although still sometimes recommended, is probably not helpful. However, physical therapy techniques and steroid injections have shown promise. If permanent nerve damage is threatened, surgery may be necessary.

Attacks of sciatica tend to recur. Certain commonsense steps that may help prevent recurrences include the following: When lifting, on should hold the object close to the chest, maintain a straight back, and use the leg muscles to slowly rise; practice good posture to reduce pressure on the spine; if possible, avoid sitting or standing in one position for prolonged periods; use low-back support during prolonged sitting; rest one foot on a low stool if standing for long periods; sleep on a firm mattress; exercise regularly a minimum of thirty minutes most days of the week (good exercise choices include walking, swimming, or exercises recommended by a doctor or physical therapist); and consider job retraining if working requires a lot of heavy lifting or sitting.

OTHER PROPOSED NATURAL TREATMENTS

Acupuncture has shown promise for sciatica, but the research evidence supporting its use remains preliminary. Similarly, biofeedback, chiropractic, massage, and prolotherapy, while sometimes advocated for sciatic pain, have not been proven effective.

The Alexander technique, Feldenkrais, pilates, Tai Chi, and yoga are thought to improve posture and movement habits. On this basis, these methods are advocated for preventing or treating sciatica, but again, proof of effectiveness is lacking.

EBSCO CAM Review Board

FURTHER READING

Allen, C., P. Glasziou, and C. Del Mar. "Bed Rest: A Potentially Harmful Treatment Needing More Careful Evaluation." *The Lancet* 354 (1999): 1229-1233.

Cherkin, D. C., Sherman, K. J., et al. "A Randomized Trial Comparing Acupuncture, Simulated Acupuncture, and Usual Care for Chronic Low Back Pain." *Archives of Internal Medicine* 169 (2009): 858-866.

Dagenais, S., et al. "Evidence-Informed Management of Chronic Low Back Pain with Prolotherapy." *Spine Journal* 8 (2008): 203-212.

Furlan, A. D., et al. "Massage for Low-Back Pain." *Cochrane Database of Systematic Reviews* (2008): CD001929. Available through *EBSCO DynaMed Systematic Literature Surveillance* at http://www.ebscohost.com/dynamed.

Longworth, W., and P. W. McCarthy. "A Review of Research on Acupuncture for the Treatment of Lumbar Disc Protrusions and Associated Neurological Symptomatology." *Journal of Alternative and Complementary Medicine* 3 (1997): 55-76.

Waddell, G., G. Feder, and M. Lewis. "Systematic Reviews of Bed Rest and Advice to Stay Active for Acute Low Back Pain." *British Journal of General Practice* 47 (1997): 647-652.

See also: Acupressure; Acupuncture; Back pain; Chiropractic; Exercise; Feldenkrais method; Massage therapy; Pain management; Prolotherapy; Soft tissue pain; Yoga.

Scientific method

CATEGORY: Issues and overviews

DEFINITION: A formal method for determining truth that involves the elements of laws, hypotheses, experiments, and theories.

OVERVIEW

The phrase "scientific method" is used in two contexts; the first is a formal method for determining truth. It involves the elements of laws, hypotheses, experiments, and theories. The second context of scientific method is how scientists actually work, and it seldom involves the first context.

Formal scientific method is no longer taught to aspiring scientists. Indeed, one survey of first-year college chemistry and physics textbooks showed no mention of the term. For many therapies and techniques in complementary and alternative medicine, the formal science is absent or less than adequate.

FORMAL SCIENTIFIC METHOD

A law, in formal scientific method, is something all persons believe to be true but which cannot be proven. The law of conservation of mass (that mass is neither created nor destroyed, but only transformed) was believed for more than a century, until nuclear reactions converted mass into energy. This law was then modified into the law of conservation of mass and energy (that the sum of mass and energy in the universe is a constant). One of the hallmarks of science is a willingness to change any aspect of a belief when enough evidence is available to a reasonable person that such change is appropriate; there are no absolutes in science.

A hypothesis is a verifiable statement about truth. An experiment is a test of whether a hypothesis is true, and a theory is a condensation of all the experiments that support the truthfulness of a hypothesis. A theory always has some reproducible, well-designed experiment in support of it, and some theories have hundreds of thousands of observations supporting them. This all sounds grand and ideal, but neither the formal scientific method nor any of the several other scientific methods proposed by philosophers of science are how science is actually done.

Modern science has amassed a virtually infinite body of knowledge. The chance that any scientist is really working on something new is small. In reality, for example, a young scientist joins a laboratory (such as a group studying the genetics of cholesterol metabolism) and is assigned a small bit of the laboratory's efforts (such as finding and isolating the gene that has changed in one patient's deviated cholesterol metabolism). There is no need for hypotheses, and the theory of genetics is already abundantly supported. What this young scientist is taught in exquisite detail, especially at higher levels of education, is appropriate experimental design.

A particular mistake often made in medicine and biology can be illustrated as follows: An experimenter mashes up the leaves of the herb in ethyl alcohol and filters the extract. He or she then applies the extract to a patient's rash; within two days the rash has been cured. This outcome sounds plausible: Something in the herb cured the rash.

Consider, however, this statement: A person's alarm clock goes off, and then the sun comes up. Even if the person observes this several days in a row, no cause-and-effect relationship exists between the alarm clock making a noise and the occurrence of dawn. One event followed by another event does not mean that the second event was caused by the first event. In the earlier example, it is not known if the ethyl alcohol cured the rash or if the rash would have cured itself in two days without intervention.

These types of errors can be subtle. For example, a study to find out if a certain drug had a curative effect on bedsores in hospitalized persons can be clouded by the fact that one-third of the persons with bedsores will be cured simply by signing up for the research and receiving no treatment whatsoever. Bedsores are caused by a lower standard of care and when persons cannot move around in bed.

DOUBLE-BLIND CLINICAL STUDY

The only acceptable experiment is the double-blind clinical study. In this type of study, the participant population must be large, and treatment and controls must be masked (blinded) so that neither the physician nor the participant knows who is receiving treatment versus control. These studies are the standard for acceptability to physicians and scientists, the final frail line that stands between science and pseudoscience.

Jack B. Robinson, Jr., Ph.D.

FURTHER READING

Iyioha, Ireh. "Law's Dilemma: Validating Complementary and Alternative Medicine and the Clash of Evidential Paradigms." *Evidence-Based Complementary and Alternative Medicine*, September 21, 2011. Available at http://www.ncbi.nlm.nih.gov/pmc/articles/pmc2952302.

Kantor, M. "The Role of Rigorous Scientific Evaluation in the Use and Practice of Complementary and Alternative Medicine." *Journal of the American College of Radiology* 6, no. 4 (2009): 254-262.

Neutens, James J., and Laurna Rubinson. *Research Techniques for the Health Sciences.* 4th ed. San Francisco: Benjamin Cummings, 2010.

Wilson, E. Bright. *An Introduction to Scientific Research.* 1952. New ed. New York: Dover, 1990.

See also: Alternative versus traditional medicine; CAM on PubMed; Clinical trials; Double-blind, placebo-controlled studies; National Center for Complementary and Alternative Medicine; Placebo effect; Pseudoscience; Regulation of CAM.

Scleroderma

CATEGORY: Condition

RELATED TERM: Systemic sclerosis

DEFINITION: Treatment of a disease that affects the connective tissues of the skin and various organs.

PRINCIPAL PROPOSED NATURAL TREATMENTS: None

OTHER PROPOSED NATURAL TREATMENTS: Acupuncture, beta-carotene, boswellia, danshen root, gotu kola, methyl sulfonyl methane, para-aminobenzoic acid, selenium, thymus extract, vitamin C, vitamin E, treatments for Raynaud's phenomenon, rheumatoid arthritis, esophageal reflux

HERBS AND SUPPLEMENTS TO AVOID: Combination therapy with 5-hydroxytryptophan and the drug carbidopa, L-tryptophan

INTRODUCTION

Scleroderma, technically called systemic sclerosis, is a disease of unknown cause that affects the connective tissues of the skin and various organs. Common symptoms include thickening and tightening of the skin (beginning with the extremities), Raynaud's phenomenon (a condition characterized by an exaggerated reaction in the fingertips to cold exposure), joint pain (especially in the fingers and knees), esophageal reflux (heartburn), calcium deposits under the skin, and telangiectasias (mats of enlarged small blood vessels). Scleroderma can lead to serious complications, such as fibrosis of the lungs, heart, and kidneys; for this reason, medical supervision is essential. There is no cure for scleroderma, although drugs may be used to alleviate the various individual symptoms of the disease.

PROPOSED NATURAL TREATMENTS

The supplement para-aminobenzoic acid has been suggested as a treatment for scleroderma. A four-month double-blind study of 146 people with long-standing, stable scleroderma failed to find any evidence of benefit. However, one-half of the participants in this trial dropped out before the end, making the results unreliable.

The herb gotu kola has a long history of use for various skin conditions; for this reason, it has been tried as a treatment for scleroderma. However, there is no meaningful evidence that it is effective. Other herbs and supplements that have been proposed for treatment of scleroderma (but do not have any significant supporting evidence) include boswellia, thymus extract, methyl sulfonyl methane, danshen root, and antioxidants (for example, the antioxidant vitamins C, E, and beta-carotene and the mineral selenium, which supports the body's own antioxidant defense system). One study, however, failed to find vitamin C helpful for the treatment of Raynaud's phenomenon associated with scleroderma.

One preliminary study suggests that acupuncture might have value for this condition. Finally, several herbs and supplements have shown promise for treating the individual symptoms of scleroderma.

HERBS AND SUPPLEMENTS TO AVOID

Combination therapy with the supplement 5-hydroxytryptophan (5-HTP) and the drug carbidopa has reportedly caused skin changes similar to those that occur in scleroderma. Furthermore, L-tryptophan, a supplement closely related to 5-HTP, has been taken off the market because it caused numerous

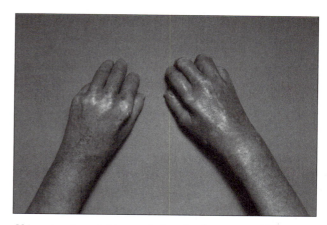

Shiny, toughened skin on the hands of someone afflicted with scleroderma. (SPL/Photo Researchers, Inc.)

cases of eosinophilia-myalgia syndrome, which is sometimes regarded as a close relative of scleroderma. It is thought that this outbreak was caused by a contaminant in a certain batch of the supplement, but some controversy about this explanation remains. Finally, various herbs and supplements may interact adversely with drugs used to prevent or treat scleroderma.

EBSCO CAM Review Board

FURTHER READING

Auffranc, J. C., et al. "Sclerodermiform and Poikilodermal Syndrome Observed During Treatment with Carbidopa and 5-Hydroxytryptophan." *Annals of Dermatology and Venereology* 112 (1985): 691-692.

Maeda, M., et al. "The Effect of Electrical Acupuncture-Stimulation Therapy Using Thermography and Plasma Endothelin (ET-1) Levels in Patients with Progressive System Sclerosis (PSS)." *Journal of Dermatologic Science* 17 (1998): 151-155.

Mavrikakis, M. E., et al. "Ascorbic Acid Does Not Improve Endothelium-Dependent Flow-Mediated Dilatation of the Brachial Artery in Patients with Raynaud's Phenomenon Secondary to Systemic Sclerosis." *International Journal for Vitamin and Nutrition Research* 73 (2003): 3-7.

See also: Bone and joint health; Dupuytren's contracture; Fibromyalgia: Homeopathic remedies; Gastroesophageal reflux; Lupus; Osteoarthritis; Pain management; Raynaud's phenomenon; Rheumatoid arthritis; Rolfing.

Sea buckthorn

CATEGORY: Herbs and supplements

RELATED TERM: *Hippophae rhamnoides*

DEFINITION: Natural plant product used to treat specific health conditions.

PRINCIPAL PROPOSED USES: None

OTHER PROPOSED USES: Prevention of colds, prevention of heart disease, treatment of stomach ulcers, reduction of side effects of cancer treatment

OVERVIEW

Sea buckthorn (not to be confused with common buckthorn) is a plant native to high-altitude regions of China and Russia, but today it is cultivated in many other areas, including the Saskatchewan province of Canada. The fruits of the plant have a long history of use as food. It was also used in ancient Chinese medicine for treating skin problems and digestive disorders. The whole berry and its oil extract are the parts used medicinally.

THERAPEUTIC DOSAGES

In the study of sea buckthorn for preventing colds noted below, the dose used was 28 grams (g) of frozen berry puree daily. Sea buckthorn oil is commonly recommended to be taken internally at a dose of 5 milliliters (ml) two to three times per day; it is also applied externally to lesions of the skin or mucous membranes. Other sea buckthorn products should be used according to label instructions.

THERAPEUTIC USES

Like many other berries, sea buckthorn berries are rich in vitamin C, vitamin A, and a variety of bioflavonoids and carotenoids. However, there are no well-established therapeutic uses of sea buckthorn. The only substantial, well-designed study of this herb examined its possible efficacy for reducing the frequency and duration of the common cold. This double-blind, placebo-controlled study of 254 people failed to find any evidence of benefit.

The study also found, rather incidentally, that use of sea buckthorn was associated with a reduction in C-reactive protein, an emerging marker for heart disease. However, contrary to widespread advertising, this incidental observation has no immediate practical meaning. High levels of C-reactive protein are, at present, only known to be associated with higher heart disease risk; it is not at all clear that deliberately reducing C-reactive protein will reduce heart disease risk. In fact, one of the leading theories is that high levels of C-reactive protein indicate the presence of a bacterium that is currently unidentified but that accelerates atherosclerosis. If this proves to be the case, it is no doubt possible to reduce the C-reactive protein levels that indicate the bacterium's presence without reducing the levels of the bacterium itself.

In other words, reducing C-reactive protein would only hide the signs of the problem rather than affect the problem. Furthermore, this study was designed to look at effects on the common cold, not effects on C-reactive protein. If one conducts a study and afterward goes on a hunt for something that is different between the treatment and placebo groups, the laws of chance alone guarantee that one will find some difference.

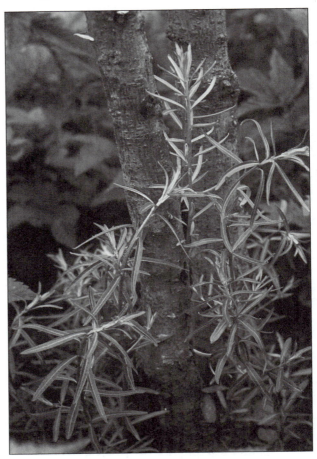

The stem and leaves of the sea buckthorn. (Adrian Thomas/ Photo Researchers, Inc.)

This is called data dredging, and it is a common cause of false conclusions.

To determine whether sea buckthorn actually affects C-reactive protein levels (something that itself may be altogether unimportant), a researcher would need to conduct a study designed at the outset to examine this question. Other evidence that is often cited to indicate that sea buckthorn can prevent or treat cardiovascular disease is similarly too preliminary to justify usage of the herb for this purpose.

The traditional use of sea buckthorn oil for stomach ulcers has been tested in a few studies, but all of them are far too preliminary to be relied upon at all. Other proposed uses of sea buckthorn that lack reliable supporting evidence include reducing the side effects of cancer treatment, treating liver cirrhosis, and aiding wound healing.

An often-cited study supposedly found that a sea buckthorn extract taken orally was helpful for eczema, but in fact placebo treatment proved equally or more effective.

SAFETY ISSUES

As a widely consumed food, whole sea buckthorn berries are presumed to be safe. Oil extracts of plants, however, are often much less safe than the whole plants, and the safety of sea buckthorn oil has not been established. The safety of use by pregnant or nursing women, young children, and people with liver or kidney disease has not been investigated.

EBSCO CAM Review Board

FURTHER READING

Eccleston, C., et al. "Effects of an Antioxidant-Rich Juice (Sea Buckthorn) on Risk Factors for Coronary Heart Disease in Humans." *Journal of Nutritional Biochemistry* 13 (2002): 346-354.

Goel, H. C., C. A. Salin, and H. Prakash. "Protection of Jejunal Crypts by RH-3 (a Preparation of *Hippophae rhamnoides*) Against Lethal Whole Body Gamma Irradiation." *Phytotherapy Research* 17 (2003): 222-226.

Goel, H. C., P. Indraghanti, et al. "Induction of Apoptosis in Thymocytes by *Hippophae rhamnoides*: Implications in Radioprotection." *Journal of Environmental Pathology, Toxicology, and Oncology* 23 (2004): 123-137.

Larmo, P., et al. "Effects of Sea Buckthorn Berries on Infections and Inflammation." *European Journal of Clinical Nutrition* 61 (2008): 1123-1130.

Li, Y., et al. "In Vitro Anti-*Helicobacter pylori* Action of Thirty Chinese Herbal Medicines Used to Treat Ulcer Diseases." *Journal of Ethnopharmacology* 98 (2005): 329-333.

Suomela, J. P., et al. "Absorption of Flavonols Derived from Sea Buckthorn (*Hippophae rhamnoides* L.) and Their Effect on Emerging Risk Factors for Cardiovascular Disease in Humans." *Journal of Agricultural and Food Chemistry* 54 (2006): 7364-7369.

Wang, Z. R., et al. "Effect of Total Flavonoids of *Hippophae rhamnoides* on Contractile Mechanics and Calcium Transfer in Stretched Myocyte." *Space Medicine and Medical Engineering* (Beijing) 13 (2000): 6-9.

See also: Citrus bioflavonoids.

Seasonal affective disorder

CATEGORY: Condition
RELATED TERMS: Seasonal depression, winter depression
DEFINITION: Treatment of a form of clinical depression most prominent in the late fall and winter months.
PRINCIPAL PROPOSED NATURAL TREATMENTS: None
OTHER PROPOSED NATURAL TREATMENTS: Melatonin, negative ions, St. John's wort, vitamin B_{12}, vitamin D

INTRODUCTION

In late fall, when the days get shorter, some people develop a special form of depression called seasonal affective disorder, or SAD. This condition should not be confused with mild winter blues. It is a real illness, as severely debilitating as any other form of clinical depression.

Symptoms are generally worse in January and February and begin to disappear as the days lengthen in the spring. SAD occurs most often in adolescents and women, but it is not limited to those groups. Up to 25 percent of the population may have a mild version of SAD, and perhaps 5 percent experience the full disorder.

The cause of SAD is not known, but it is believed to relate to the body's biological clock and the way it responds to sunlight. The hormones melatonin and serotonin are thought to be involved, although exactly in what manner remains unclear.

Conventional treatment for SAD focuses on increasing one's exposure to light. Ensuring that one gets outside during the brightest part of the day may help significantly. Bright artificial light sources (phototherapy) are also helpful. Antidepressant drugs may be used if these treatments prove ineffective.

PROPOSED NATURAL TREATMENTS

Vitamin D. The body creates vitamin D when it is exposed to the sun, and during the winter, vitamin D levels drop. For this reason, it seems logical that vitamin D supplements might help people with SAD. One double-blind, placebo-controlled trial conducted during winter with forty-four people without SAD found that vitamin D supplements produced improvements in various measures of mood. However, a double-blind, placebo-controlled study of women older than age seventy years failed to find benefit. It has been suggested that phototherapy for SAD works by raising vitamin D levels, but evidence indicates that this hypothesis is incorrect.

Melatonin. The hormone melatonin plays a major role in the daily biological clock. Human bodies are designed to manufacture melatonin at night and to stop making it when the sun rises. One study found that people with SAD had higher levels of melatonin than those without the condition. On this basis, it would seem that supplemental melatonin should worsen SAD symptoms. However, the evidence for such an effect is inconsistent. Some researchers have proposed that interaction between SAD and melatonin might be more complex than merely high or low levels, and that, when taken at certain times of the day, melatonin might help the condition. A small study found that when melatonin was given in the afternoon, it produced some benefit for people with SAD. However, a study of melatonin used in the early morning or the late evening failed to find any benefit.

OTHER PROPOSED NATURAL TREATMENTS

A small study failed to find vitamin B_{12} helpful for SAD. The herb St. John's wort has shown considerable promise for treating depression in general. However, the evidence that the herb is helpful for SAD consists only of studies too preliminary to prove much. It should be noted that combining St. John's wort with bright light therapy might not be safe. A substance called hypericin, which is found in most St. John's wort products, may cause the body to become

hypersensitive to light, increasing the risk of damage to the skin and eyes. Finally, for reasons that are not clear, the use of a device that produces negative ions may help SAD symptoms, according to two preliminary controlled studies.

EBSCO CAM Review Board

FURTHER READING

Dumville, J. C., et al. "Can Vitamin D Supplementation Prevent Winter-Time Blues? A Randomised Trial Among Older Women." *Journal of Nutrition, Health, and Aging* 10 (2006): 151-153.

Karadottir, R., and J. Axelsson. "Melatonin Secretion in SAD Patients and Healthy Subjects Matched with Respect to Age and Sex." *International Journal of Circumpolar Health* 60 (2001): 548-551.

Terman, M., J. S. Terman, and D. C. Ross. "A Controlled Trial of Timed Bright Light and Negative Air Ionization for Treatment of Winter Depression." *Archives of General Psychiatry* 55 (1998): 875-882.

Wheatley, D. "Hypericum in Seasonal Affective Disorder (SAD)." *Current Medical Research and Opinion* 15 (1999): 33-37.

See also: Bipolar disorder; Depression, mild to moderate; Melatonin; Mental health; St. John's wort; Vitamin B_{12}; Vitamin D.

Seborrheic dermatitis

CATEGORY: Condition
RELATED TERMS: Cradle cap, dandruff, seborrhea
DEFINITION: Treatment of inflammation of the upper layers of the skin.
PRINCIPAL PROPOSED NATURAL TREATMENT: Aloe
OTHER PROPOSED NATURAL TREATMENTS: Folate, tea tree oil, vitamin B_6

INTRODUCTION

Seborrheic dermatitis is an inflammation of the upper layers of the skin that causes scales on the scalp, face, and other parts of the body. When it affects newborns, it is called cradle cap.

Seborrheic dermatitis starts gradually. In adults, it often first appears as a condition similar to dandruff but involves more inflammation of the scalp; itching, burning, or hair loss may occur. Seborrhea may also affect the skin behind the ears, on the eyebrows, on the bridge of the nose, around the nose, or on the trunk.

Besides inflammation of the scalp, newborns with cradle cap might get red bumps on their faces, scaling behind the ears, or a persistent diaper rash. Older children with seborrheic dermatitis may develop a thick, flaky rash.

Seborrhea tends to run in families and often worsens during cold weather. Researchers do not know what causes the condition, and they have not found a cure. There are, however, ways to control the condition. Special shampoos containing selenium sulfide, pyrithione zinc, salicylic acid, sulfur, or tar may be helpful for adult dandruff associated with seborrhea.

Corticosteroids may be used for intensely inflammatory lesions. Milder treatments, such as salicylic acid in mineral oil or medicated baby shampoo, are used to treat young children and infants who have scalp rashes.

PRINCIPAL PROPOSED NATURAL TREATMENTS

There is some evidence that the herb aloe might offer some relief to people with seborrheic dermatitis.

Aloe. The gel inside the cactus-like leaves of the aloe plant (aloe vera) has traditionally been used to treat burns and cuts. While it may not be effective for this purpose, one late study indicates that aloe may help relieve the symptoms of seborrheic dermatitis. In this double-blind, placebo-controlled study, forty-four adults with seborrheic dermatitis applied either an aloe ointment or a placebo cream to affected areas two times daily for four to six weeks. Compared to the placebo group, those who used aloe reported that their symptoms improved significantly (62 versus 25 percent). Doctors who examined the participants also concluded that those using aloe had a significant decrease in scaliness, itching, and number of affected areas.

OTHER PROPOSED NATURAL TREATMENTS

In a four-week, placebo-controlled study of 126 people with mild to moderate dandruff, the use of 5 percent tea tree oil shampoo significantly reduced dandruff symptoms. This study, however, was not double-blind: The researchers knew which participants were receiving tea tree oil and which were receiving placebo. For this reason, the test's results cannot be taken as completely reliable.

One small double-blind study found benefit for dandruff with an extract made from the traditional Mexican herb *Solanum chrysotrichum.* Essential fatty acids, zinc, iron, and vitamins A, C, D, E, B_1, and B_2 have also been suggested as treatments for seborrheic dermatitis, but there is no real evidence that these treatments work.

HOMEOPATHIC REMEDIES

In a small, double-blind, placebo-controlled study, the oral use of a low-dilution homeopathic remedy containing potassium bromide, sodium bromide, nickel sulfate, and sodium chloride significantly improved symptoms of seborrheic dermatitis, including dandruff.

EBSCO CAM Review Board

FURTHER READING

Brenner, S., and C. Horwitz. "Possible Nutrient Mediators in Psoriasis and Seborrheic Dermatitis II: Nutrient Mediators–Essential Fatty Acids; Vitamins A, E and D; Vitamins B_1, B_2, vitamin B_6, Niacin, and Biotin; Vitamin C Selenium; Zinc; Iron." *World Review of Nutrition and Dietetics* 55 (1988): 165-182.

Herrera-Arellano, A., et al. "Clinical and Mycological Evaluation of Therapeutic Effectiveness of *Solanum chrysotrichum* Standardized Extract on Patients with Pityriasis Capitis (Dandruff): A Double Blind and Randomized Clinical Trial Controlled with Ketoconazole." *Planta Medica* 70 (2004): 483-488.

Satchell, A. C., et al. "Treatment of Dandruff with 5 Percent Tea Tree Oil Shampoo." *Journal of the American Academy of Dermatology* 47 (2002): 852-855.

Smith, S. A., et al. "Effective Treatment of Seborrheic Dermatitis Using a Low Dose, Oral Homeopathic Medication Consisting of Potassium Bromide, Sodium Bromide, Nickel Sulfate, and Sodium Chloride in a Double-Blind, Placebo-Controlled Study." *Alternative Medicine Review* 7 (2002): 59-67.

Vardy, D. A., et al. "A Double-Blind, Placebo-Controlled Trial of an Aloe Vera (*A. barbadensis*) Emulsion in the Treatment of Seborrheic Dermatitis." *Journal of Dermatological Treatment* 10 (1999): 7-11.

See also: Aloe; Children's health; Corticosteroids; Eczema; Folate; Hives; Psoriasis; Tea tree; Vitamin B_6.

Selenium

CATEGORY: Functional foods

RELATED TERMS: Selenite, selenium dioxide, selenized yeast, selenomethionine

DEFINITION: Natural substance essential for health and promoted as a dietary supplement for specific health benefits.

PRINCIPAL PROPOSED USE: Cancer prevention

OTHER PROPOSED USES: Acne, anxiety, asthma, cataracts, cervical dysplasia, depression, diabetic neuropathy, fibromyalgia, general well-being, gout, heart disease prevention, human immunodeficiency virus support, male infertility, multiple sclerosis, osteoarthritis, psoriasis, rheumatoid arthritis, ulcers

OVERVIEW

Selenium is a trace mineral that the body uses to produce glutathione peroxidase. Glutathione peroxidase is part of the body's antioxidant defense system; it works with vitamin E to protect cell membranes from damage caused by dangerous, naturally occurring substances known as free radicals.

China has very low rates of colon cancer, presumably because of the nation's low-fat diet. However, in some parts of China, where the soil is depleted of selenium, the incidence of various types of cancer is much higher than in the rest of the country. This fact has given rise to a theory that selenium deficiency is a common cause of cancer and that selenium supplements can reduce this risk. There is some preliminary evidence that selenium supplements might provide some protection against some types of cancer among people living in the United States, but this evidence is far from definitive.

REQUIREMENTS AND SOURCES

The official U.S. and Canadian recommendations for daily intake (in micrograms) of selenium are as follows: infants to six months of age (15) and seven to twelve months of age (20), children one to three years of age (20) and four to eight years of age (30), children nine to thirteen years of age (40), children and adults aged fourteen years and older (55), pregnant females (60), and nursing females (70).

The selenium content of food varies depending on the selenium content of the soil in which it was grown. Studies suggest that many people in certain developed countries, including New Zealand, Belgium, and Scandinavia, do not get enough selenium in their diets. However, most people in the United States and Canada are believed to consume more than enough selenium.

Foods containing significant and reliable amounts of selenium include animal products, such as meat, seafood, and dairy foods, and whole grains and vegetables grown in selenium-rich soils. These include wheat germ, nuts (particularly Brazil nuts), oats, whole-wheat bread, bran, red Swiss chard, brown rice, turnips, garlic, barley, and orange juice.

Certain digestive conditions, such as Crohn's disease, short-bowel syndrome, and ulcerative colitis may impair selenium absorption. In addition, medications that reduce stomach acid, such as proton pump inhibitors or H_2 blockers, may reduce the body's absorption of selenium.

THERAPEUTIC DOSAGES

In controlled trials of selenium, typical dosages were 100 micrograms (mcg) to 200 mcg daily. The two general types of selenium supplements available to consumers are organic and inorganic forms. These two terms have a very specific chemical meaning and have nothing to do with "organic" foods. In chemistry, "organic" means that a substance's chemical structure includes carbon. "Inorganic" chemicals have no carbon atoms.

The inorganic form of selenium, selenite, is essentially selenium atoms bound to oxygen. Some research suggests that selenite is harder for the body to absorb than are organic forms of selenium, such as selenomethionine (selenium bound to methionine, an essential amino acid) or high-selenium yeast (which contains selenomethionine). However, other research on both animals and humans suggests that selenite supplements are about as good as organic forms of selenium. These contradictory results suggest that any differences in absorption, if they exist, are relatively minor.

THERAPEUTIC USES

Preliminary studies hint that supplemental selenium may help prevent some forms of cancer. However, this evidence cannot be taken as reliable.

Selenium is required for a well-functioning immune system. Based on this, selenium has been suggested as a treatment for human immunodeficiency virus (HIV) infection. Early studies showed little to no

Selenium, Antioxidants, and the Fight Against Cancer

Although selenium is a mineral and not an antioxidant nutrient, it is nonetheless a component of antioxidant enzymes—proteins that speed up chemical reactions in the body. Antioxidants are substances that may protect cells from the damage caused by unstable molecules known as free radicals. Free radical damage may lead to cancer. Antioxidants interact with and stabilize free radicals and may prevent some of the damage free radicals might otherwise cause.

benefit. In a large trial reported in 2007, the use of selenium supplements reduced viral load. However, this study had numerous flaws in its statistical methods. For reasons that are not clear, another study found that selenium supplements decreased symptoms of psychological anxiety in HIV-positive persons undergoing highly active retroviral therapy.

One study of healthy people in the United Kingdom (where marginally low selenium intake is common) found that the use of selenium supplements improved general immune function, as measured by response to poliovirus immunization. A preliminary double-blind trial suggests that selenium supplements may improve fertility in males who are selenium deficient. Weak evidence suggests that selenium might be helpful for diabetic neuropathy.

Selenium has also been recommended for many other conditions, including acne, anxiety, cataracts, cervical dysplasia, fibromyalgia, gout, multiple sclerosis, osteoarthritis, psoriasis, and ulcers, but there is no real evidence that it is helpful for these conditions.

A small study among nursing home residents found that low levels of the mineral selenium were associated with depression. Moreover, eight weeks of supplementation tended to improve the mood of the most seriously depressed persons with low selenium levels. The same was not true of the two other nutrients investigated, folate and vitamin C.

Evidence regarding the use of selenium for preventing heart disease is more negative than positive. Also, a large (about five hundred participants), double-blind, placebo-controlled study failed to find that the use of selenium supplements at 100, 200, or 300 mcg daily improved mood or general well-being.

A study of 197 people with moderately severe asthma failed to find benefit with selenium (100 mcg daily). Low selenium levels have been associated with increased likelihood of developing certain kinds of rheumatoid arthritis. However, selenium supplements do not appear to help rheumatoid arthritis once it has developed. Despite hopes to the contrary, it does not appear that selenium supplements can help prevent type 2 diabetes; rather they might increase the risk of developing the disease.

SCIENTIFIC EVIDENCE

Somewhat inconsistent evidence suggests that selenium supplements may help prevent cancer, but evidence from observational studies indicates that low intake of selenium is tied to increased risk of cancer. However, such studies are notoriously unreliable as guidelines to therapy. Only double-blind trials can truly determine whether selenium supplements can help prevent cancer.

The most important double-blind study on selenium and cancer was conducted by researchers at the University of Arizona Cancer Center. In this trial, which began in 1983, 1,312 people were divided into two groups. One group received 200 mcg of yeast-based selenium daily; the other received placebo. Participants were not deficient in selenium, although their selenium levels fell toward the bottom of the normal range. The researchers were trying to determine whether selenium could lower the incidence of skin cancers.

As it happened, no benefits for skin cancer were seen. In fact, careful analysis of the data suggests that selenium supplements actually marginally increased the risk of certain forms of skin cancer. However, researchers saw dramatic declines in the incidence of several other cancers in the selenium group. For ethical reasons, researchers felt compelled to stop the study after several years to allow all participants to take selenium.

When all the results were tabulated, it became clear that the selenium-treated group developed almost 66 percent fewer prostate cancers, 50 percent fewer colorectal cancers, and about 40 percent fewer lung cancers as compared with the placebo group. (All these results were statistically significant.) Selenium-treated persons also experienced a statistically significant (17 percent) decrease in overall mortality, a greater than 50 percent decrease in lung cancer deaths, and nearly a 50 percent decrease in total cancer deaths. A subsequent close look at the data showed that only study participants who were relatively low in selenium to begin with experienced protection from lung cancer or colon cancer; people with average or above-average levels of selenium did not benefit significantly. It has not been reported whether this limitation of benefit to low-selenium participants was true of the other forms of cancer too.

While this evidence is promising, it has one major flaw. The laws of statistics reveal that when researchers start to deviate from the question that their research was designed to answer, the results may not be trustworthy.

Combining the results of twelve placebo-controlled trials investigating the association between antioxidant supplementation and cancer, researchers found that men who took selenium experienced an overall reduction in the incidence of cancer. No similar effect, however, was observed in women. This difference cannot be explained without more research. Also, selenium supplementation appeared to modestly lower cancer mortality in both men and women.

Other evidence for the possible anticancer benefits of selenium comes from large-scale Chinese studies showing that giving selenium supplements to people who live in selenium-deficient areas reduces the incidence of cancer. In addition, animal trials have found anticancer benefits.

However, one study published in 2007 reported negative results in transplant recipients. People who undergo organ transplants are at particularly high risk of skin cancer linked to the human papilloma virus. In this double-blind study, 184 organ transplant recipients were given either placebo or selenium at a dose of 200 milligrams daily. The results in two years failed to show benefit; both the placebo and the selenium group developed precancerous and cancerous lesions at the same rate.

SAFETY ISSUES

The U.S. Institute of Medicine issues guidelines for the maximum total daily intake (in micrograms) of various nutrients, based on estimations of what should be safe for virtually all healthy persons. These tolerable upper intake levels are, thus, conservative guidelines. For selenium, they have been set as follows: infants to six months of age (45) and seven to twelve months of age (60), children one to three years of age (90) and four to eight years of age (150), children nine to thirteen years of age (280), children and adults aged fourteen years and older (400), pregnant and nursing females (400). Note that these dosages apply to combined dietary and supplemental intake of selenium. When deciding how much selenium it is safe to take, one should note that most adults already receive about 100 mcg of selenium in the daily diet.

Maximum safe doses of selenium for persons with severe liver or kidney disease have not been established. There is some evidence that supplementing selenium over the long-term in areas where selenium is already adequate in the diet may increase the risk of diabetes and perhaps hypercholesterolemia.

Highly excessive selenium intake, beginning at about 900 mcg daily, can cause selenium toxicity. Signs include depression, nervousness, emotional instability, nausea, vomiting, and, in some cases, loss of hair and fingernails.

IMPORTANT INTERACTIONS

Persons who are taking medications that reduce stomach acid, such as H_2 blockers or proton pump inhibitors, may need extra selenium.

EBSCO CAM Review Board

FURTHER READING

Bardia, A., et al. "Efficacy of Antioxidant Supplementation in Reducing Primary Cancer Incidence and Mortality." *Mayo Clinic Proceedings* 83 (2008): 23-34.

Dreno, B., et al. "Effect of Selenium Intake on the Prevention of Cutaneous Epithelial Lesions in Organ Transplant Recipients." *European Journal of Dermatology* 17 (2007): 140-145.

Gosney, M. A., et al. "Effect of Micronutrient Supplementation on Mood in Nursing Home Residents." *Gerontology* 54 (2008): 292-299.

Hurwitz, B. E., et al. "Suppression of Human Immunodeficiency Virus Type 1 Viral Load with Selenium Supplementation." *Archives of Internal Medicine* 167 (2007): 148-154.

Navas-Acien, A., J. Bleys, and E. Guallar. "Selenium Intake and Cardiovascular Risk: What Is New?" *Current Opinion in Lipidology* 19 (2008): 43-49.

Shaheen, S. O., et al. "Randomised, Double-Blind, Placebo-Controlled Trial of Selenium Supplementation in Adult Asthma." *Thorax* 62 (2007): 483-490.

Stranges, S., et al. "Effects of Long-Term Selenium Supplementation on the Incidence of Type 2 Diabetes." *Annals of Internal Medicine* 147 (2007): 217-223.

See also: Acne; Anxiety and panic attacks; Asthma; Cancer risk reduction; Cataracts; Cervical dysplasia; Depression, mild to moderate; Diabetes, complications of; Fibromyalgia: Homeopathic remedies; Gout; HIV support: Homeopathic remedies; Infertility, male; Multiple sclerosis; Osteoarthritis; Psoriasis; Rheumatoid arthritis; Ulcers; Wellness, general.

Self-care

CATEGORY: Therapies and techniques

RELATED TERMS: Self-care education, self-medication

DEFINITION: A type of therapy that can be performed by persons themselves, often aided by training from a practitioner or by educational materials.

PRINCIPAL PROPOSED USES: Arthritis, chronic low back pain, coronary artery disease, headaches, hypertension, incontinence, insomnia, postsurgical symptoms, treatment- and disease-related symptoms of cancer

OVERVIEW

A person undertakes self-care decisions and actions to address a health problem or to improve his or her health. Popular self-care therapies include relaxation, meditation, imagery, hypnosis, biofeedback, education, special diets, natural products, and nutrition supplements. Adults in the United States spend $22 billion a year on self-care classes and materials.

MECHANISM OF ACTION

It is difficult to evaluate the action of self-care therapy because in most situations, it is not feasible to use placebo controls. For example, in one of the better-documented modalities, the Arthritis Self-Management Program, retrospective analysis shows that pain reduction was maintained four years after therapy began and that physician visits decreased by 40 percent. The program used education, cognitive restructuring, relaxation, and physical activity, but it is impossible to show what treatment was responsible for what result; also, no control group was included for comparison.

USES AND APPLICATIONS

Several health care trends favor the use of self-care therapies, which have been tried by up to 50 percent of the U.S. population. Some persons see conventional health care becoming more effective but also unaffordable for many. Studies show that those who have delayed or skipped medical care for financial reasons are highly likely to try self-care, particularly self-medication.

At the other end of the spectrum are those who distrust mainstream health care and want instead a type of care that promotes empowerment and personal control. Another factor leading people to try self-care is having learned about and becoming comfortable with complementary and alternative medicine (CAM) therapies over time. In addition, CAM therapies that previously could be found only through nontraditional outlets are now widely available. Likely CAM users include the elderly, those who are well educated, and those with conditions such as severe depression and panic attacks. Studies also show that people between the ages of thirty-five and fifty years are part of a fast-growing group of CAM users.

Another recent study showed that twice as many people read self-help literature as see a CAM practitioner to learn relaxation techniques. This follows a general trend showing that the use of self-care therapies has increased at the same time that consultation with CAM providers has decreased. An analysis of persons on Medicare showed that the most frequently sought forms of CAM were those for back problems, chronic pain, general health improvement, and arthritis. Research has demonstrated the efficacy of relaxation, biofeedback therapy, cognitive strategies, and education in treating chronic pain conditions such as osteoarthritis, rheumatoid arthritis, and fibromyalgia. Persons using self-care engaged in health-affirming practices such as exercise, smoking reduction, and limiting alcohol consumption.

SCIENTIFIC EVIDENCE

Some of the studies used to measure self-care are flawed because the research questions depend on a person's ability to report CAM use accurately or to remember his or her use of CAM. Typically, information is collected once, so there is no opportunity to study CAM use over time.

Flawed methodology can occur if researchers do not spell out distinctions between complementary and alternative therapies versus more radical alternatives. Peer-reviewed studies of self-care have shown improvements in cancer-related pain, headache pain, and cardiovascular disease as a result of relaxation techniques, behavior modification, imagery, hypnosis, stress management, and health education. Clinical trials showed, for example, a 43 percent reduction in headache activity, improvement of chemotherapy-related symptoms such as nausea and vomiting, and a 41 percent reduction in cardiac deaths.

One study looked at changes in health status longitudinally and found no difference in health status when researchers compared therapies such as chiropractic, massage, acupuncture, and herbs with conventional medicine. However, the results of CAM therapies in general, and of self-care specifically, may take longer to manifest. Researchers have called for controlled clinical trials, including large-scale surveys, and in-depth studies of specific populations.

SAFETY ISSUES

A lack of relevant scientific studies makes it difficult to determine the safety and efficacy of self-care. Herbal remedies may interact with prescription medicines in harmful ways, with both the person seeking care and the prescribing physician unaware of the risks. Scientific literature on interactions is scarce. Existing information may be skewed, because many people do not tell their physicians that they are using a self-care modality of CAM.

Merrill Evans, M.A.

FURTHER READING

Astin, J. A., et al. "Complementary and Alternative Medicine Use Among Elderly Persons." *Journal of Gerontology: Medical Sciences* 55A (2000): M4-M9. A study of seniors' use of CAM and a discussion of the efficacy of CAM and of issues of communication with physicians regarding CAM therapies.

_____. "Mind-Body Medicine: State of the Science, Implications for Practice." *Journal of the American Board of Family Medicine* 16 (2003): 131-147. A meta-analysis of the efficacy of numerous CAM therapies.

Nahin, R. L., et al. "Costs of Complementary and Alternative Medicine (CAM) and Frequency of Visits to CAM Practitioners: United States, 2007." *National Health Statistics Reports* 18 (2009): 1-15. A government study of the frequency and cost of visits to CAM practitioners, using National Health Interview Survey data.

Pagán, J. A., and M. V. Pauly. "Access to Conventional Medical Care and the Use of Complementary and Alternative Medicine." *Health Affairs* 24 (2004): 255-262. Examines why people seek CAM and discusses the long-term implications for health care delivery.

Palinkas, L. A., and M. L. Kabongo. "The Use of Complementary and Alternative Medicine by Primary Care Patients." *Journal of Family Practice* 49 (2000): 1121-1130. A study of reasons why people seek CAM care while also seeking care from a physician. Also looks at the impact of combining these therapies.

Sparber, A., and J. C. Wootton. "Use of Alternative and Complementary Therapies for Psychiatric and Neurologic Diseases." *Journal of Alternative and Complementary Medicine* 8 (2002): 93-96. This study examines the role of CAM in treating patients with depression and anxiety.

See also: Autogenic training; Biofeedback; Guided imagery; Hypnotherapy; Meditation; Mind/body medicine; Relaxation therapies; Transcendental Meditation.

Senna

CATEGORY: Herbs and supplements
RELATED TERMS: *Cassia acutifolia, C. angustifolia, C. senna*
DEFINITION: Natural plant product used to treat specific health conditions.
PRINCIPAL PROPOSED USE: Constipation

OVERVIEW

Senna extract is an over-the-counter treatment, approved by the U.S. Food and Drug Administration, for occasional constipation. Because there is no controversy regarding senna's effectiveness for this purpose, the supporting evidence is not presented here. Rather, this article addresses the concerns that have been raised regarding senna's safety.

SAFETY ISSUES

Senna contains chemicals in the anthranoid family, such as anthraquinones, anthrones, and dianthrones. Related substances are found in a variety of plants used for laxative purposes, such as cascara sagrada, common buckthorn, and turkey rhubarb. The mechanism of action of anthranoids, however, is somewhat worrisome: Anthranoids seem to work primarily by damaging the cells lining the colon. In general, cell damage can be a precursor to cancer, and on this basis, concerns have been raised that senna might increase colon cancer risk.

Evaluating this possibility is more difficult than it sounds. The most obvious method is to survey a large population over time to see whether people who use senna have a higher incidence of colon cancer. However, studies of this type (observational studies) are inherently unreliable, because they do not show cause and effect. People with colon cancer or other precancerous conditions may become constipated and take senna, and this would cause a statistical association between use of senna and colon cancer, even if senna did not cause the cancer. In any case, the results of such studies have been mixed, and overall the association, if any, does not appear to be strong.

Studies in animals have generally been reassuring, but a few such trials, as well as test-tube studies, have found some evidence of possible increased risk with long-term use. Senna does have one potential safety advantage over other herbal anthranoid laxatives: Its particular anthranoids are not very absorbable. This reduces the potential risk of harm deeper in the body.

It appears reasonable to conclude that short-term use of senna is quite safe, while long-term use might or might not be safe. However, senna is not recommended for long-term use anyway. Chronic senna consumption can cause dependency, meaning that the user is unable to have a bowel movement without it. In addition, there have been sporadic reports of unusual reactions to chronic use of senna, such as hepatitis.

As is the case with all laxatives, people with significant colonic disease, such as ulcerative colitis, should not use senna. If senna is taken to the point of diarrhea, the body may become depleted of the mineral potassium. This is particularly dangerous for people using drugs in the digoxin family, which can cause dangerous cardiac arrythmias if potassium levels in the blood are inadequate. People who additionally use medications that themselves deplete the body of potassium, such as thiazide or loop diuretics, are at special risk of this complication of senna overuse.

The safety of senna during pregnancy has not been established, and pregnant women are advised to avoid senna during the first trimester. Nursing women should also avoid using senna.

IMPORTANT INTERACTIONS

Persons who are taking digoxin, thiazide diuretics, or loop diuretics should be especially careful not to overuse senna.

EBSCO CAM Review Board

FURTHER READING

Beuers, U., U. Spengler, and G. R. Pape. "Hepatitis After Chronic Abuse of Senna." *The Lancet* 337 (1991): 372-373.

De Witte, P., and L. Lemli. "The Metabolism of Anthranoid Laxatives." *Hepatogastroenterology* 37 (1990): 601-605.

Nascimbeni, R., et al. "Constipation, Anthranoid Laxatives, *Melanosis coli*, and Colon Cancer: A Risk Assessment Using Aberrant Crypt Foci." *Cancer Epidemiology, Biomarkers, and Prevention* 11 (2002): 753-757.

Nusko, G., et al. "Anthranoid Laxative Use Is Not a Risk Factor for Colorectal Neoplasia." *Gut* 46 (2000): 651-655.

Van Gorkom, B. A., et al. "Cytotoxicity of Rhein, the Active Metabolite of Sennoside Laxatives, Is Reduced by Multidrug Resistance-Associated Protein 1." *British Journal of Cancer* 86 (2002): 1494-1500.

See also: Constipation; Gastrointestinal health.

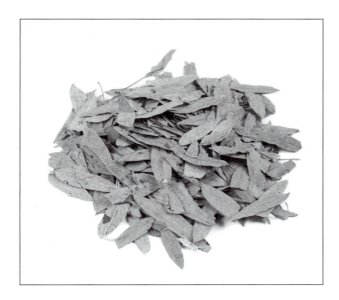

Senna leaves. (Geoff Kidd/Photo Researchers, Inc.)

Sexual dysfunction in men

CATEGORY: Condition

RELATED TERMS: Erectile dysfunction, impotence

DEFINITION: Treatment of erectile dysfunction and other male sexual disorders.

PRINCIPAL PROPOSED NATURAL TREATMENTS: Carnitine, ginseng, L-arginine

OTHER PROPOSED NATURAL TREATMENTS: Acupuncture, ashwagandha, *Avena sativa*, *Butea superba*, catuaba, *Cordyceps*, damiana, dehydroepiandrosterone, diindolylmethane, *Eleutherococcus*, ginkgo, horny goat weed (*Epimedium grandiflorum*), L-citrulline, maca (*Lepidium meyenii*), *Mucuna pruriens*, melatonin, molybdenum, muira puama (potency wood), *Polypodium vulgare*, pomegranate, pygeum, *Rhodiola rosea*, saw palmetto, schisandra, suma, traditional Chinese herbal medicine, *Tribulus terrestris*, velvet antler, zinc

HERBS AND SUPPLEMENTS TO USE ONLY WITH CAUTION: Androstenedione, licorice, soy or soy isoflavones, yohimbe

INTRODUCTION

Impotence, or erectile dysfunction, is the inability to achieve an erection. Impotence has a minimum of fifteen possible causes, including diabetes, drug side-effects, pituitary tumors, hardening of the arteries, hormonal imbalances, and psychological factors. A few of these conditions respond to specific treatment. For example, if a blood pressure drug is causing impotence, the best approach is to change drugs. If a pituitary tumor is secreting the hormone prolactin, treating that tumor may result in immediate improvement. However, in most cases, conventional treatment of impotence is nonspecific.

The drugs Viagra and Cialis have revolutionized treatment for erectile dysfunction. These medications work by increasing tissue sensitivity to the blood-vessel-dilating substance nitric oxide (NO) in the penis. Older methods include mechanical devices that utilize a vacuum to produce an erection, drugs for self-injection, and implantation of penile prostheses.

PROPOSED NATURAL TREATMENTS

Korean red ginseng. Two double-blind, placebo-controlled trials, involving about 135 people, found evidence that Korean red ginseng may improve erectile function. In the better of the two trials, 45 participants received either placebo or Korean red ginseng at a dose of 900 milligrams (mg) three times daily for eight weeks. After a one-week period of no treatment, the two groups were switched. The results indicate that while using Korean red ginseng, men experienced significantly better sexual function than while they were taking placebo.

In an analysis combining the results of six controlled trials, researchers found some evidence for the benefits of Korean red ginseng. However, the small size and generally low quality of the studies left some doubt about this conclusion.

L-arginine. Nitric oxide (NO) plays a role in the development of an erection. Drugs such as Viagra increase the body's sensitivity to the natural rise in NO that occurs with sexual stimulation. A simpler approach might be to raise NO levels, and one way to accomplish this involves the use of the amino acid L-arginine. Oral arginine supplements may increase nitric oxide levels in the penis and elsewhere. Based on this, L-arginine has been advertised as "natural Viagra." However, there is little evidence that arginine works. Drugs based on raising NO levels in the penis have not worked for pharmaceutical developers; the body seems to simply adjust to the higher levels and maintain the same level of response.

The main support for the use of arginine in erectile dysfunction comes from a small double-blind trial in which fifty men with erectile dysfunction received either 5 grams (g) of L-arginine or placebo daily for six weeks. More men in the treated group experienced improvement in sexual performance than in the placebo group.

A double-blind crossover study of thirty-two men found no benefit with 1,500 mg of arginine given daily for seventeen days; the much smaller dose and shorter course of treatment may explain the discrepancy between these two trials.

Arginine has also been evaluated with the drug yohimbine (made from the herb yohimbe). A double-blind, placebo-controlled trial of forty-five men found that one-time use of this combination therapy one or two hours before intercourse improved erectile function, especially in those with only moderate erectile dysfunction scores. Arginine and yohimbine were both taken at a dose of 6 g. One should not use the drug yohimbine (or the herb yohimbe) except under physician supervision, as it presents a number of safety risks.

Carnitine. In a six-month double-blind trial of 120 men with an average age of sixty-six, carnitine (propionyl-L-carnitine, 2 g per day, plus acetyl-L-carnitine, 2 g per day) and testosterone (testosterone undecanoate, 160 mg per day) were separately compared with placebo. The results indicated that both carnitine and testosterone improve erectile function; however, while testosterone significantly increased prostate volume, carnitine did not.

Another double-blind, placebo-controlled study found that propionyl-L-carnitine at 2 g per day enhanced the effectiveness of sildenafil (Viagra) in forty men with diabetes who had previously failed to respond to sildenafil a minimum of eight times. In another double-blind study, a combination of the propionyl and acetyl forms of carnitine enhanced the effectiveness of Viagra in men who had erectile dysfunction caused by prostate surgery. Carnitine has also shown promise for treating male infertility.

Other treatments. A proprietary combination therapy containing arginine and *Ginkgo biloba*, ginseng, and vitamins and minerals has shown some promise in an unpublished study. Also, in a three-week, double-blind, placebo-controlled trial, twenty men with erectile dysfunction received either placebo or a special form of magnet therapy called pulsed electromagnetic field therapy (PEMF). PEMF was administered by means of a small box worn near the genital area and kept in place as long as possible during the study period; neither participants nor observers knew whether the device was actually activated or not. The results showed that the use of PEMF significantly improved sexual function compared with placebo.

A double-blind, placebo-controlled study enrolled forty men with difficulty achieving or maintaining an erection who also had low measured levels of dehydroepiandrosterone (DHEA). The results showed that DHEA at a dose of 50 mg daily improved sexual performance; however, the authors failed to provide a statistical analysis of the results, making the meaningfulness of this study impossible to determine.

Severe zinc deficiency is known to negatively affect sexual function. Because marginal zinc deficiency is relatively common, it is logical to suppose that supplementation with zinc may be helpful for some men. However, this hypothesis has only been studied in men receiving kidney dialysis. The results were promising.

The herb *Butea superba* has shown some promise for erectile dysfunction, according to a three-month randomized, double-blind study performed in Thailand. In other studies, weak evidence hints at potential benefit with pomegranate juice, melatonin, and oligomeric proanthocyanidins (alone or with arginine).

Based on preliminary evidence, the herb maca (*Lepidium meyenii*) has been advertised as an "herbal Viagra." In one study in rats, the use of maca enhanced male sexual function. There is one published human trial too. In this small, twelve-week, double-blind, placebo-controlled study, the use of maca at 1,500 mg or 3,000 mg increased male libido. The study did not report benefits in male sexual function, just in desire. Because the loss of sexual function is a more common problem in men than loss of sexual desire, these results do not justify the "herbal Viagra" claim. Contrary to some reports, maca does not appear to affect testosterone levels.

Many other herbs are also reputed to improve sexual function in men, including ashwagandha, *Avena sativa* (oat straw), catuaba, *Cordyceps*, damiana, diindolylmethane, *Eleutherococcus* (Siberian ginseng), L-citrulline, *Mucuna pruriens*, molybdenum, muira puama (potency wood), pygeum, *Polypodium vulgare*, *Rhodiola rosea*, saw palmetto, schisandra, suma, traditional Chinese herbal medicine, and *Tribulus terrestris*. However, there is no real evidence that these herbs offer any benefits.

Numerous case reports and uncontrolled studies had indicated that the herb *Ginkgo biloba* offers dramatic benefits for male (and female) sexual disorders caused by antidepressants. However, double-blind, placebo-controlled studies are necessary to truly establish efficacy. When studies of this type were performed, it became clear that people had been misled about ginkgo's efficacy by the power of suggestion: Ginkgo failed to improve sexual function to any greater extent than placebo.

In a small single-blind study, acupuncture proved superior to fake acupuncture for treatment of erectile dysfunction. However, because the treating practitioners administrating the control treatment were aware that they were providing sham acupuncture, it is quite likely that they unconsciously communicated lack of confidence as they provided it; this is an inherent limitation of single-blind studies.

Deer or antelope velvet antler is a popular treatment for sexual dysfunction. However, the one double-blind study performed on the subject failed to find benefit.

HERBS AND SUPPLEMENTS TO USE WITH CAUTION

The U.S. Food and Drug Administration has warned consumers not to purchase or consume several brands of dietary supplements after samples were found adulterated with the prescription drug

Safety Concerns: Erectile Dysfunction and Dietary Supplements

Erectile dysfunction (ED) can be a difficult topic to discuss, but the discussion must occur because erection problems can be a sign of health problems, such as blocked blood vessels or nerve damage from diabetes.

Many people simply turn to dietary supplements, which are marketed to help with ED or are sold as sexual enhancement products. However, undeclared ingredients in dietary supplements may pose a threat to consumers because the interaction of the analogue with some prescription drugs (such as nitroglycerin) may lower blood pressure to dangerous levels. Consumers with diabetes, high blood pressure, high cholesterol, or heart disease often take other prescription drugs. ED is a common problem in men with these conditions, and consumers may seek these types of products to enhance sexual performance. Experts advise that persons who have experienced any adverse events from sexual enhancement products consult a health care professional.

The following list of warnings and recalls by the U.S. Food and Drug Administration (FDA) presents only a few of these types of products that are on the market:

- Expanded Recall: Via Xtreme Ultimate Sexual Enhancer Dietary Supplement for Men Recall (2011)
- Ethos Environmental Issues a Voluntary Recall of Specific Lots of the Dietary Supplement Regenerect (2011)
- Best Enhancer Recalled for Undeclared Drug Ingredient (2011)
- RockHard Weekend, Pandora: Recall—Undeclared Drug Ingredient (2010)
- FDA Warns Consumers to Avoid Man Up Now Capsules (2010)
- TimeOut Capsules Contaminated with Potentially Dangerous Ingredient (2010)
- Mr. Magic Male Enhancer: Undeclared Drug Ingredient (2010)

tadalafil (Cialis), an analogue of sildenafil (Viagra). The products named in the warning are SIGRA, STAMINA Rx, STAMINA Rx for Women, Y-Y, Spontane ES, and Uroprin (all manufactured by NVE and distributed by Hi-Tech).

The herb yohimbe is the source of the drug yohimbine, which has been shown to be modestly better than placebo for impotence. However, because of many drug interactions and other risks, yohimbine is not recommend for use except under the supervision of a physician. Because there is no agency regulating the quality and labeling of herbal products, the herb yohimbe presents even more risks, such as unpredictable yohimbine content.

Soy or soy isoflavones, and the herb licorice, may reduce testosterone levels in men. For this reason, men with impotence, infertility, or decreased libido may want to avoid these natural products.

One report claims that both tea tree oil and lavender oil have estrogenic (estrogen-like) and antiandrogenic (testosterone-blocking) effects. If this were true, men with erectile dysfunction would be advised to avoid use of these herbs. However, a literature search failed to find any other published reports that corroborate this claim.

One case report suggests that a product containing the herb *Epimedium grandiflorum* (horny goat weed) caused rapid heart rate and symptoms similar to mania. The supplement androstenedione, often taken for male sexual dysfunction in the belief that it increases testosterone levels, actually appears to increase estrogen levels in men and might, therefore, increase problems with erectile function.

EBSCO CAM Review Board

FURTHER READING

Cavallini, G., S. Caracciolo, et al. "Carnitine Versus Androgen Administration in the Treatment of Sexual Dysfunction, Depressed Mood, and Fatigue Associated with Male Aging." *Urology* 63 (2004): 641-646.

Cavallini, G., F. Modenini, et al. "Acetyl-L-Carnitine plus Propionyl-L-Carnitine Improve Efficacy of Sildenafil in Treatment of Erectile Dysfunction After Bilateral Nerve-Sparing Radical Retropubic Prostatectomy." *Urology* 66 (2005): 1080-1085.

Cherdshewasart, W., and N. Nimsakul. "Clinical Trial of *Butea superba*, an Alternative Herbal Treatment for Erectile Dysfunction." *Asian Journal of Andrology* 5 (2003): 243-246.

Conaglen, H. M., J. M. Suttie, and J. V. Conaglen. "Effect of Deer Velvet on Sexual Function in Men and Their Partners." *Archives of Sexual Behavior* 32 (2003): 271-278.

Engelhardt, P. F., et al. "Acupuncture in the Treatment of Psychogenic Erectile Dysfunction." *International Journal of Impotence Research* 15 (2003): 343-346.

Forest, C. P., H. Padma-Nathan, and H. R. Liker. "Efficacy and Safety of Pomegranate Juice on Improvement of Erectile Dysfunction in Male Patients with Mild to Moderate Erectile Dysfunction." *International Journal of Impotence Research* 19 (2007): 564-567.

Gentile, V., et al. "Preliminary Observations on the Use of Propionyl-L-Carnitine in Combination with Sildenafil in Patients with Erectile Dysfunction and Diabetes." *Current Medical Research and Opinion* 20 (2004): 1377-1384.

Henley, D. V., et al. "Prepubertal Gynecomastia Linked to Lavender and Tea Tree Oils." *New England Journal of Medicine* 356 (2007): 479-485.

Jang, D. J., et al. "Red Ginseng for Treating Erectile Dysfunction." *British Journal of Clinical Pharmacology* 66 (2008): 444-450.

See also: Carnitine; Ginseng; Infertility, male; L-arginine; Sexual dysfunction in women.

Sexual dysfunction in women

CATEGORY: Condition

RELATED TERMS: Antidepressant-induced sexual dysfunction, female sexual arousal disorder, hypoactive sexual desire disorder, low libido

DEFINITION: Treatment of sexual disorders in women.

PRINCIPAL PROPOSED NATURAL TREATMENTS: None

OTHER PROPOSED NATURAL TREATMENTS: Combination herb and supplement therapies, dehydroepiandrosterone, diindolylmethane, *Ginkgo biloba*, horny goat weed, maca, molybdenum, *Rhodiola rosea*, topical treatment containing gamma-linolenic acid, vitamin C

INTRODUCTION

Although male sexual disorders have long been the subject of intensive medical research, sexual disorders in women have received relatively little attention until recently. The tremendous commercial success of the erectile dysfunction drug Viagra has prompted pharmaceutical companies to focus on finding a comparable treatment for women.

Many women experience loss of libido, painful intercourse, or difficulty achieving orgasm. In most cases, the causes are unknown. Possible identifiable causes include side effects from drugs such as antidepressants or sedatives, hormonal insufficiency, or adrenal insufficiency. Conventional treatments for sexual dysfunction in women are limited, except when a simple treatable cause is present (such as the use of an antidepressant in the selective serotonin reuptake inhibitor, or SSRI, category).

PROPOSED NATURAL TREATMENTS

Although there is no good evidence for natural treatments for sexual dysfunction, several substances have shown promising results in preliminary trials. These substances include dehydroepiandrosterone, yohimbine, and arginine.

Dehydroepiandrosterone. Some evidence suggests that the hormone dehydroepiandrosterone (DHEA) may be helpful for improving sexual function in older women. DHEA, however, may not be helpful for younger women.

DHEA is produced by the adrenal glands. Levels of DHEA decline naturally with age and fall precipitately in cases of adrenal failure. Because both elderly people and those with adrenal insufficiency report a drop in libido, several studies have examined whether supplemental DHEA can increase libido in these groups.

A twelve-month, double-blind, placebo-controlled trial evaluated the effects of DHEA (50 milligrams [mg] daily) in 280 persons between the ages of sixty and seventy-nine. The results showed that women older than age seventy years experienced an improvement in libido and sexual satisfaction. No benefits were seen in younger women. Two other trials did not find benefit, but they enrolled much fewer people and ran for a shorter time.

Two small, double-blind, placebo-controlled studies tested whether a one-time dose of DHEA at 300 mg could increase ease of sexual arousal in pre- or postmenopausal women, respectively. The results again indicate that DHEA is effective for older women but not for younger women.

One four-month, double-blind, placebo-controlled study of twenty-four women with adrenal failure found that 50 mg per day of DHEA (with standard treatment for adrenal failure) improved libido and sexual satisfaction. DHEA is not usually prescribed to persons with adrenal failure, but this study suggests that it should be.

Combination products. A double-blind, placebo-controlled trial evaluated a combination therapy containing the amino acid arginine; the herbs ginseng, ginkgo, and damiana; and multivitamins-multiminerals. Researchers enrolled seventy-seven women between the age of twenty-two and seventy-one years and followed them for four weeks. All participants complained of poor sexual function. The results showed superior sexual satisfaction scores in the treatment group compared with the placebo group. Some of the specific benefits seen included enhanced libido, increased frequency of intercourse and orgasm, greater vaginal lubrication, and augmented clitoral sensation. A larger follow-up study performed by the same research group also reported benefits. However, confirmation by an independent research group will be necessary before these results can be taken as reliable.

Yohimbine is a drug derived from the bark of the yohimbe tree. Studies have used only the standardized drug, not the actual herb. One small, double-blind, crossover study of yohimbine combined with arginine found an increase in measured physical arousal among twenty-three women with sexual arousal disorder, compared with placebo. However, the women themselves did not report any noticeable effects. Only the combination of yohimbine and arginine produced results; neither substance was effective when taken on its own.

An open trial of yohimbine alone to treat sexual dysfunction induced by the antidepressant fluoxetine (Prozac) found improvement in eight of nine people, two of whom were women. However, in the absence of a placebo group, these results cannot be taken as reliable; in addition, concerns exist about the safety of combining yohimbe with antidepressants.

Yohimbine and the herb yohimbe are relatively dangerous substances in general. One should use them only with physician supervision. The other constituents used in these combination therapies may also present some risks.

Other treatments. One double-blind, placebo-controlled study found evidence that the use of vitamin C led to an increase in intercourse frequency in healthy women, presumably because it increased libido. A

> ## Care in Using Yohimbe Bark for Sexual Dysfunction
>
> The yohimbe tree (*Pausinystalia yohimbe*) is a tall evergreen that is native to western Africa. The bark of the tree contains a chemical called yohimbine. The amount of yohimbine in dietary supplements may vary; some yohimbe products have been found to contain very little yohimbine. Yohimbe bark has traditionally been used in Africa as an aphrodisiac (to increase sexual desire). The herb is currently used for sexual dysfunction.
>
> Yohimbe use comes with various side effects. The product has been associated with high blood pressure, increased heart rate, headache, anxiety, dizziness, nausea, vomiting, tremors, and sleeplessness. Also, yohimbe can be dangerous if taken in large doses or for long periods of time.
>
> Health experts advise that yohimbe should not be combined with MAO inhibitors, as effects may be additive. Also, yohimbe should be used with caution when taken with medicines for high blood pressure, tricyclic antidepressants, or phenothiazines (a group of medicines used mostly for mental health conditions such as schizophrenia). Finally, persons with kidney problems and persons with psychiatric conditions should not use yohimbe.

small double-blind trial reported that a proprietary topical treatment containing gamma-linolenic acid and a variety of additional supplements and herbs improved sexual function in woman with sexual arousal disorder.

A preliminary study has been used to claim that the herb ephedra is helpful for women with sexual dysfunction. However, this trial was small, enrolled women without sexual disorders, and examined only sexual responsiveness to visual stimuli. In another study, ephedrine improved sexual dysfunction caused by SSRIs, but so did placebo, and there was no significant difference between the benefits seen with the two treatments. There are serious health risks associated with ephedra. For this reason, ephedra is not recommended for use by women with sexual dysfunction.

Numerous case reports and uncontrolled studies raised hopes that the herb *Ginkgo biloba* might be an effective treatment for sexual dysfunction, particularly as a result of antidepressant medication. However, the results of a number of double-blind studies indicate that ginkgo is no more effective than placebo, whether or not subjects are taking antidepressants. Other treatments that are often proposed for treating female sexual dysfunction, but that lack any meaningful supporting evidence, include horny goat weed, maca, molybdenum, diindolylmethane, and *Rhodiola rosea*.

EBSCO CAM Review Board

FURTHER READING

Brody, S. "High-Dose Ascorbic Acid Increases Intercourse Frequency and Improves Mood." *Biological Psychiatry* 52 (2002): 371.

Ferguson, D. M., et al. "Randomized, Placebo-Controlled, Double Blind, Crossover Design Trial of the Efficacy and Safety of Zestra in Women with and Without Female Sexual Arousal Disorder." *Journal of Sex and Marital Therapy* 29, suppl. 1 (2003): 33-44.

Hackbert, L., and J. R. Heiman. "Acute Dehydroepiandrosterone (DHEA) Effects on Sexual Arousal in Postmenopausal Women." *Journal of Women's Health and Gender-Based Medicine* 11 (2002): 155-162.

Ito, T. Y., et al. "The Enhancement of Female Sexual Function with ArginMax, a Nutritional Supplement, Among Women Differing in Menopausal Status." *Journal of Sex and Marital Therapy* 32 (2006): 369-378.

Kang, B. H., et al. "A Placebo-Controlled, Double-Blind Trial of *Ginkgo biloba* for Antidepressant-Induced Sexual Dysfunction." *Human Psychopharmacology* 17 (2002): 279-284.

Meston, C. M. "A Randomized, Placebo-Controlled, Crossover Study of Ephedrine for SSRI-Induced Female Sexual Dysfunction." *Journal of Sex and Marital Therapy* 30 (2004): 57-68.

_____, and J. R. Heiman. "Acute Dehydroepiandrosterone Effects on Sexual Arousal in Premenopausal Women." *Journal of Sex and Marital Therapy* 28 (2002): 53-60.

_____, and M. Worcel. "The Effects of Yohimbine plus L-Arginine Glutamate on Sexual Arousal in Postmenopausal Women with Sexual Arousal Disorder." *Archives of Sexual Behavior* 31 (2002): 323-332.

_____, A. H. Rellini, and M. J. Telch. "Short- and Long-Term Effects of *Ginkgo biloba* Extract on Sexual Dysfunction in Women." *Archives of Sexual Behavior* 37 (2008): 530-547.

Wheatley, D. "Triple-Blind, Placebo-Controlled Trial of *Ginkgo biloba* in Sexual Dysfunction Due to Antidepressant Drugs." *Human Psychopharmacology* 19 (2004): 545-548.

See also: Adrenal extract; Dehydroepiandrosterone (DHEA); Ephedra; Infertility, female; Menopause; Sexual dysfunction in men.

Shiatsu

CATEGORY: Therapies and techniques
RELATED TERMS: Acupressure, massage, reflexology
DEFINITION: A technique in which practitioners apply pressure to specific points on the body to balance the body's flow of energy.
PRINCIPAL PROPOSED USES: Muscle pain, muscle tension, stress
OTHER PROPOSED USES: Anxiety, arthritis, carpal tunnel syndrome, constipation, depression, fatigue, fibromyalgia, headaches, hypertension, insomnia, nausea, premenstrual syndrome, repetitive strain injuries

OVERVIEW

Shiatsu, a Japanese word meaning "finger pressure," is a traditional, noninvasive healing technique in which the fingertips and especially the thumbs are used to apply pressure along the body's meridian system to unblock energy dams and reinstate optimal energy flow. This energy, called *qi* in Chinese and *ki* in Japanese, is considered the essence of life. The underlying belief is that unbalanced energy invites illness and injury.

The Chinese introduced shiatsu into Japan more than fifteen hundred years ago. In 1940, the Japan Shiatsu College was founded by Tokujiro Namikoshi to systematically train shiatsu practitioners in anatomy, physiology, and therapeutic technique. The localized deep-muscle stimulation, sometimes referred to as "acupuncture without needles," is believed to induce a healing response.

MECHANISM OF ACTION

Shiatsu is performed on a large quilted floor mat with the client lying down. No massage oil is used, and the client may remain dressed in comfortable clothing. The practitioner finds the energy points on each of the fourteen meridians along the body and

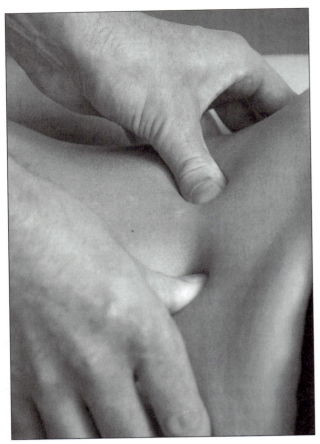

Patient receiving shiatsu massage for lower back pain.
(AJ Photo/Photo Researchers, Inc.)

works them to trigger the release of endorphins, which in turn reduce blood pressure, increase circulation, and stimulate lymphatic drainage.

Shiatsu also involves the rotating and stretching of the joints to straighten the pathways. In areas of low energy, long stretches will allow energy to flow in, as will pressure held for ten to fifteen seconds. Conversely, quick stretches and brief periods of pressure will dispel excess energy that has built up.

Shiatsu is considered a method of touch communication, as the practitioner reads the energy flow of the client and assesses overall health. By the end of a session, the client may express an emotional release, such as by crying or laughing. The caring touch of the shiatsu practitioner is thought to arouse the self-healing response within the client.

Uses and Applications

Shiatsu is used to improve body function, to release tension, and to improve circulation for relief from stress. It quiets an overstimulated sympathetic nervous system. It also stimulates the release of endorphins, natural painkillers produced by the body, and excites the immune system. These effects make shiatsu beneficial for targeting muscular, internal, and emotional pain. In addition to bringing relief from discomfort, shiatsu also imparts a calmer mind, clearer thinking, and a general sense of well-being. Self-shiatsu may be performed, often in combination with yoga breathing, meditation, and sound therapy.

In Japan, shiatsu has been recognized and regulated as a distinct health profession since the mid-twentieth century. It is indicated for nervous system disorders such as neuralgia; for stroke recovery, polio, and insomnia; for digestive system disorders such as chronic enteritis and constipation; and for metabolic disorders such as gout. It is contraindicated in cases of trauma, internal bleeding, malignancies, ulcers, active infections, acute inflammation, and blood vessel disease.

Scientific Evidence

In double-blind studies, shiatsu has been shown to improve the quality of sleep for elderly nursing home residents with sleep disturbances and to reduce agitation in elderly nursing home residents with dementia. It increased arm movement and decreased depression in persons recovering from hemiplegia stroke. The use of shiatsu was significantly correlated with increasing body weight in premature babies. It reduced chronic low back pain more effectively than physical therapy, and improvement was still evident at the six-month follow-up. However, studies have failed to show that shiatsu is any more effective than placebo at preventing nausea and vomiting in surgical patients, in emergency room patients with fractures, and in women in labor.

Choosing a Practitioner

Reputable practitioners of shiatsu in the United States should have graduated from an accredited massage therapy school and must practice in accordance with each state's respective licensing requirements. The term "Shiatsupractor" (a registered trademark of the International Shiatsu Association) is a title recognized around the world and is given to those who have completed formal education and training as a professional shiatsu practitioner.

SAFETY ISSUES

Shiatsu should not be performed on persons who are prone to blood clots because there is a risk that the localized pressure could dislodge clots. This massage technique should not be applied directly over open wounds, inflamed skin or rashes, bruises, tumors, hernias, mending bone fractures, or surgical sites. It is not recommended for pregnant women, for people with osteoporosis, or for people who have recently undergone chemotherapy or radiation therapy.

Bethany Thivierge, M.P.H.

FURTHER READING

American Organization for Bodywork Therapies of Asia. http://www.aobta.orga.

Beresford-Cooke, Carola. *Shiatsu Theory and Practice.* 3d ed. New York: Churchill Livingstone/Elsevier, 2010. This illustrated textbook includes a DVD of shiatsu techniques and routines.

Liechti, Elaine. *Shiatsu: Complete Illustrated Guide.* Rockport, Mass.: Element Books, 2002. In addition to the history of shiatsu and diagrams of techniques and pressure points, this book contains information on self-shiatsu.

Lundberg, Paul. *The Book of Shiatsu: A Complete Guide to Using Hand Pressure and Gentle Manipulation to Improve Your Health, Vitality, and Stamina.* New York: Fireside Books, 2003. Written by a master shiatsu practitioner and instructor. An authoritative guide that also presents many color drawings and photographs.

Shiatsu Diffusion Society. http://shiatsupractors.org.

Somma, Corinna. *Shiatsu.* Upper Saddle River, N.J.: Prentice Hall, 2006. This textbook includes protocols for the various client positions and study questions and chapter tests.

See also: Acupressure; Acupuncture; Biodynamic massage; Craniosacral therapy; Energy medicine; Manipulative and body-based practices; Massage therapy; Meridians; Metamorphic technique; Osteopathic manipulation; Pain management; Progressive muscle relaxation; Qigong; Reflexology; Relaxation therapies; Rolfing; Stress; Therapeutic touch.

Shiitake

CATEGORY: Herbs and supplements
RELATED TERMS: Black forest mushroom, donggu, huagu, *Lentinula edodes*, xianggu
DEFINITION: Natural plant product used to treat specific health conditions.
PRINCIPAL PROPOSED USES: Cancer prevention, cancer treatment support, genital warts, immune support

OVERVIEW

The shiitake mushroom is native to Japan, China, and other East Asian countries, where it grows naturally on fallen trees in forests, hence the common name black forest mushroom. Deliberate cultivation of shiitake, for both food and medicine, is of ancient origin.

During the Ming Dynasty (1368-1644), shiitake developed a reputation as a tonic, a substance said to increase energy, prevent disease, aid convalescence from illness, and slow bodily deterioration caused by aging. It was also used more specifically to treat respiratory illnesses, liver diseases, and intestinal infestation with worms. The soft fleshy cap (fruiting body) is the part used medicinally.

THERAPEUTIC DOSAGES

When taken orally, shiitake mushroom is most commonly used in the form of an extract: lentinus edodes mycelium extract (LEM). The typical dose of LEM is 1 to 3 grams three times daily. Purified lentinan (a constituent of shiitake) suitable for intravenous use is licensed as a pharmaceutical in Japan; it is not available in the United States.

THERAPEUTIC USES

There are no proposed uses of shiitake mushroom or shiitake mushroom extracts that are supported by reliable scientific evidence. Current investigation of shiitake focuses primarily on the potential immune-stimulating and anticancer effects of some its constituents, most prominently lentinan (LNT), a polysaccharide substance in the beta-glucan family. Limited evidence from case reports and highly preliminary human studies hints that use of intravenously injected, purified lentinan might enhance the effectiveness of chemotherapy for stomach cancer, pancreatic cancer, and ovarian cancer. Lentinan products designed for oral use should not be injected.

One study found hints that oral lentinan might reduce recurrence rates of genital warts following laser surgery. Extremely weak evidence hints that lentinan might have immune-stimulating and liver-protective effects.

In an animal study, lentinan reduced the risk of colon cancer in mice with ulcerative colitis. Another study failed to find oral shiitake extract helpful for treatment of prostate cancer.

SAFETY ISSUES

As a widely eaten food, shiitake mushroom is believed to be fairly safe. As with any food, allergic reactions can occur.

The safety of concentrated shiitake extracts, however, is less clear. Safety in pregnant or nursing women, young children, and people with severe liver or kidney disease has not been evaluated.

EBSCO CAM Review Board

FURTHER READING

Curnow, P., and M. Tam. "Contact Dermatitis to Shiitake Mushroom." *Australasian Journal of Dermatology* 44 (2003): 155-157.

DeVere White, R. W., et al. "Effects of a Mushroom Mycelium Extract on the Treatment of Prostate Cancer." *Urology* 60 (2002): 640-644.

Fujimoto, K., M. Tomonaga, and S. Goto. "A Case of Recurrent Ovarian Cancer Successfully Treated with Adoptive Immunotherapy and Lentinan." *Anticancer Research* 26 (2006): 4015-4018.

Kupfahl, C., G. Geginat, and H. Hof. "Lentinan Has a Stimulatory Effect on Innate and Adaptive Immunity Against Murine *Listeria monocytogenes* Infection." *International Immunopharmacology* 6 (2006): 686-696.

Markova, N., et al. "Protective Activity of Lentinan in Experimental Tuberculosis." *International Immunopharmacology* 3 (2003): 1557-1562.

Suzuki, K., et al. "Chronic Hypersensitivity Pneumonitis Induced by Shiitake Mushroom Spores Associated with Lung Cancer." *Internal Medicine* 40 (2001): 1132-1135.

See also: Cancer risk reduction; Cancer treatment support; Immune support; Warts.

Shingles

CATEGORY: Condition

RELATED TERMS: Chickenpox, herpes zoster, postherpetic neuralgia

DEFINITION: Treatment of a painful and acute skin infection and continuing irritation of the nerves that develops years after a person has had chickenpox.

PRINCIPAL PROPOSED NATURAL TREATMENTS: Capsaicin, proteolytic enzymes

OTHER PROPOSED NATURAL TREATMENTS: Acupuncture, adenosine monophosphate, vitamin B_{12}, vitamin E

INTRODUCTION

Shingles, or herpes zoster, is an acute, painful infection caused by the varicella zoster virus, the organism that causes chickenpox. It develops many years after the original chickenpox infection, typically in the elderly or those with compromised immune systems.

The first sign of shingles infection may be a tingling feeling, itchiness, or shooting pain on an area of skin. A rash may then appear with raised dots or blisters. When the rash is at its peak, rash symptoms can range from mild itching to extreme pain. People with shingles on the upper half of the face should seek medical attention, as the virus may cause damage to the eyes.

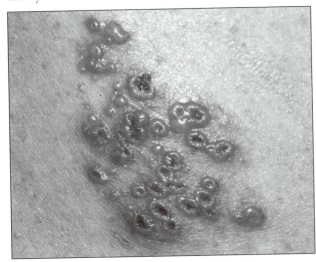

A shingles rash. (©EH Gill/Custom Medical Stock Photo)

Shingles usually resolves without complications within three to five weeks. However, in some people, especially the elderly, the pain may persist for months or years. This condition is known as postherpetic neuralgia (PHN). It is thought to be caused by a continuing irritation of the nerves after the infection is over.

Conventional medical treatment for shingles includes antiviral drugs (acyclovir, famicyclovir, valacyclovir). When used properly, these lead to faster resolution of symptoms, which include lesions and acute neuralgia, and may reduce the incidence and severity of PHN. Steroids (such as prednisone) and tricyclic antidepressants (such as amitriptyline) are also prescribed to lessen shingles symptoms, and the former might help prevent PHN. People who do develop PHN may be treated, in severe cases, with nerve blocks.

PRINCIPAL PROPOSED NATURAL TREATMENTS

For the initial attack of shingles, proteolytic enzymes may be helpful. Capsaicin cream is a treatment for PHN that is approved by the U.S. Food and Drug Administration (FDA).

Proteolytic enzymes. There is some evidence that proteolytic enzymes may be helpful for the initial attack of shingles. Proteolytic enzymes are produced by the pancreas to aid in the digestion of protein. Certain foods also contain these enzymes. Besides their use in digestion, these enzymes may have some effects in the body as a whole when taken orally.

Proteolytic enzymes are thought to benefit cases of shingles by decreasing the body's inflammatory response and regulating immune response to the virus. The most-studied proteolytic enzymes include papain (from papaya), bromelain (from pineapple), and trypsin and chymotrypsin (extracted from the pancreas of various animals).

A double-blind study of 190 people with shingles compared proteolytic enzymes to the standard antiviral drug acyclovir. Participants were treated for fourteen days and their pain was assessed at intervals. Although both groups had similar pain relief, the enzyme-treated group experienced fewer side effects. Similar results were seen in another double-blind study in which ninety people were given either an injection of acyclovir or enzymes, followed by a course of oral medication for seven days.

Capsaicin. Capsaicin, the "hot" in hot peppers, has been found effective for treating the pain related to PHN and has been approved by the FDA for that purpose. Capsaicin is thought to work by inhibiting chemicals in nerve cells that transmit pain.

Topical capsaicin cream is available in two strengths, 0.025 and 0.075 percent. Both preparations are indicated for use in neuralgia. The cream should be applied sparingly to the affected area three to four times daily. Treatment should continue for several weeks because the benefit may take a while to develop. Capsaicin creams are approved over-the-counter drugs and should be used as directed. Over-the-counter creams containing concentrated capsaicin are recognized as safe, but caution should be used near the eyes and mucous membranes. Mild to moderate burning may occur at first, but it decreases over time.

A transdermal patch containing a relatively high concentration of capsaicin (8 percent) has been developed. Compared to a low-concentration version (0.04 percent), this high-concentration patch was associated with significant improvements in pain in a trial involving 402 adults with PHN for a minimum of six months.

OTHER PROPOSED NATURAL TREATMENTS

Adenosine monophosphate (AMP), a natural byproduct of cell metabolism, has been studied as a possible treatment for initial shingles symptoms and for PHN prevention.

In a double-blind, placebo-controlled study of thirty-two people with shingles, AMP was injected three times per week for four weeks. At the end of the four-week treatment period, 88 percent of those treated with AMP were pain-free versus only 43 percent in the placebo group; all participants still in pain were then given AMP, and no recurrence of pain was reported in three to eighteen months of follow-up. However, this was a preliminary study, and more evidence is needed before AMP can be considered a proven treatment for shingles. Oral AMP has not been tried for this condition. (One should not self-inject AMP products meant for oral consumption.)

Vitamins E and B_{12} have also been suggested as possible treatments for PHN, but the evidence that they work is extremely weak. Also, a single-blind, placebo-controlled study of sixty-two people with PHN failed to find any benefit with acupuncture treatment.

EBSCO CAM Review Board

FURTHER READING

Alper, B. S., and P. R. Lewis. "Treatment of Postherpetic Neuralgia: A Systematic Review of the Literature." *Journal of Family Practice* 51 (2002): 121-128.

Backonja, M., et al. "NGX-4010, a High-Concentration Capsaicin Patch, for the Treatment of Postherpetic Neuralgia." *Lancet Neurology* 7 (2008): 1106-1112.

Billigmann, P. "Enzyme Therapy: An Alternative in Treatment of Herpes Zoster." *Fortschritte der Medizin* 113 (1995): 43-48.

Weaver, Bethany A. "Herpes Zoster Overview: Natural History and Incidence." *Journal of the American Osteopathic Association* 109 (2009): S2-S6.

See also: Aging; Cayenne; Herpes; Pain management; Proteolytic enzymes.

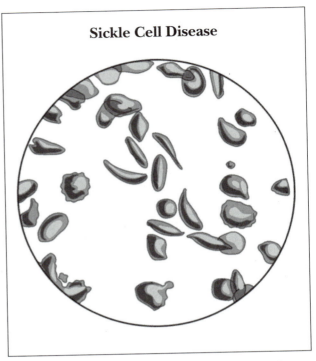

Sickle Cell Disease

The red blood cells are sickle-shaped rather than round, which causes blockage of capillaries.

Sickle cell disease

CATEGORY: Condition

RELATED TERMS: Sickle cell anemia

DEFINITION: Treatment of an inherited blood disorder characterized by anemia, clogged blood vessels, and organ and tissue damage.

PRINCIPAL PROPOSED NATURAL TREATMENT: Zinc

OTHER PROPOSED NATURAL TREATMENTS: Alpha-linolenic acid, beta-carotene, coenzyme Q_{10}, fish oil, folate, garlic, green tea, lipoic acid, magnesium, oligomeric proanthocyanidins, suma, vitamin B_2, vitamin B_6, vitamin B_{12}, vitamin C, vitamin E

INTRODUCTION

Sickle cell disease is an inherited blood disorder. Normally, red blood cells are disc-shaped and flexible. In sickle cell disease, however, hemoglobin (the chemical within red blood cells that carries oxygen around the body) is abnormal. This defect causes red blood cells to collapse into a crescent, or sickle, shape.

These abnormal blood cells are destroyed at an unusually high rate, causing a shortage of red blood cells (anemia). In addition, they can suddenly clump together and clog up small blood vessels throughout the body. This clumping causes what is called a sickle cell crisis. When blood vessels are blocked by sickle-shaped red blood cells, parts of the body are deprived of oxygen. This can cause severe pain and damage to the organs and tissues that are deprived.

The common triggers of sickle cell crisis include smoking, exercise, exposure to high altitudes, fever, infection, dehydration, and the drop in oxygen and changes in air pressure that can occur during air travel. Diagnosis of sickle cell disease and sickle cell trait (a condition in which a person has one of the two genes necessary to develop sickle cell disease) can be done through blood testing, using a technique called hemoglobin electrophoresis.

Treatment involves managing the anemia, chronic pain, and organ damage caused by sickle cell disease. In addition, the drug hydroxyurea can reduce occurrences of sickle cell crisis. It is also important to minimize exposure to conditions or situations that can trigger sickle cell crisis.

PRINCIPAL PROPOSED NATURAL TREATMENTS

Children with sickle cell disease often do not grow normally. Zinc deficiency can also cause growth retardation, and there is some evidence that people with sickle cell disease are more likely than others to be deficient in the mineral zinc. For this reason, zinc supplementation at nutritional doses has been suggested for children with sickle cell disease.

In a placebo-controlled study, forty-two children (aged four to ten years) with sickle cell disease were given either zinc supplements (10 milligrams [mg] of zinc daily) or placebo for one year. Results showed that by the end of the study, the participants given zinc showed enhanced growth compared to those given placebo. Curiously, researchers did not find any solid connection between the severity of zinc deficiency and the extent of response to treatment.

Zinc is thought to have a stabilizing effect on the cell membrane of red blood cells in people with sickle cell disease. For this reason, it has been tried as an aid for preventing sickle cell crisis. In a double-blind, placebo-controlled study of 145 people with sickle cell disease conducted in India, participants received either placebo or about 50 mg of zinc three times daily. During eighteen months of treatment, the zinc-treated subjects had an average of 2.5 crises, compared to 5.3 crises for the placebo group. However, zinc did not seem to reduce the severity of a crisis, as measured by the number of days spent in the hospital for each crisis.

Sickle cell disease can also cause skin ulcers (non-healing sores). In a twelve-week, placebo-controlled trial, the use of zinc at 88 mg three times per day enhanced the rate of ulcer healing. In another placebo-controlled trial, 25 mg of zinc three times per day for three months reduced the frequency of infections in children with sickle cell disease.

The high dosages of zinc used in the last two studies can cause dangerous toxicity and should be taken only under the supervision of a doctor. The nutritional dose described in the first study, however, is safe.

Other Proposed Natural Treatments

A year-long, double-blind, placebo-controlled, cross-over study of eighty-two people with sickle cell disease tested a combination herbal treatment made from plants indigenous to Nigeria. The results indicate that the use of the herbal mixture reduced the incidence of sickle cell crisis. A small, double-blind, placebo-controlled trial found intriguing evidence that fish oil may reduce the frequency of painful sickle cell episodes, possibly by reducing the tendency of the blood to clot.

Also suggested for people with sickle cell disease are numerous other herbs and supplements, including alpha-linolenic acid, beta-carotene, coenzyme Q_{10}, folate, garlic, green tea, lipoic acid, magnesium, oligomeric proanthocyanidins, suma, and vitamins B_2, B_6, B_{12}, C, and E, but the supporting evidence for these treatments remains far too preliminary to be relied upon.

EBSCO CAM Review Board

Further Reading

Ballas, S. K. "Hydration of Sickle Erythrocytes Using a Herbal Extract (*Pfaffia paniculata*) In Vitro." *British Journal of Haematology* 111 (2000): 359-362.

Bao, B., et al. "Zinc Supplementation Decreases Oxidative Stress, Incidence of Infection, and Generation of Inflammatory Cytokines in Sickle Cell Disease Patients." *Transl Res.* 152 (2008): 67-80.

Ohnishi, S. T., T. Ohnishi, and G. B. Ogunmola. "Sickle Cell Anemia: A Potential Nutritional Approach for a Molecular Disease." *Nutrition* 16 (2000): 330-338.

Tomer, A., et al. "Reduction of Pain Episodes and Prothrombotic Activity in Sickle Cell Disease by Dietary N-3 Fatty Acids." *Thrombosis and Haemostasis* 85 (2001): 966-974.

Zemel, B. S., et al. "Effect of Zinc Supplementation on Growth and Body Composition in Children with Sickle Cell Disease." *American Journal of Clinical Nutrition* 75 (2002): 300-307.

See also: Atherosclerosis and heart disease prevention; Iron; Zinc.

Silica hydride

Category: Herbs and supplements

Related terms: Active hydrogen, "Hunza water," microhydrin

Definition: Natural substance combination used as a dietary supplement for specific health benefits.

Principal proposed uses: Disease prevention, general well-being

Overview

Supplements labeled "silica hydride" are marketed as a kind of universal cure, said to promote wellness, to prevent disease, and to potentially cure virtually all illnesses. As a chemical term, "silica hydride" is not well defined, but supplements sold under that name appear to contain a mixture of silicon and oxygen (silica), along with hydrogen (supposedly in the form of hydrides) and various minerals. Proponents of this supplement claim that much of human illness results from the presence, in ordinary tap water, of too many positively charged hydrogen ions. Silica hydride supplements, proponents claim, remedy this by providing negatively charged hydrogen ions (hydride ions). These hydride ions are said to act as powerful antioxidants to increase cellular production of energy and provide many other benefits.

From the point of view of standard chemistry, however, the notion of enhancing health through hydride ions is highly problematic. A hydride is a hydrogen ion that carries two extra electrons, making it negatively charged. In its natural state, a hydrogen ion possesses no electrons and therefore carries a positive charge. When a hydrogen ion is forced to carry extra electrons, it becomes highly unstable and highly reactive. Hydrides are so reactive that as soon as they contact a molecule of water, they rip the water molecule

Marketing Silica Hydride

Inventor Patrick Flanagan promotes the use of his product, MegaH, containing silica hydride and touted by Flanagan as "The Most Powerful Antioxidant Known." The product, like all dietary supplements sold in the United States, has not been approved by the U.S. Food and Drug Administration, and, as Flanagan's web site makes clear, it "is not intended to diagnose, treat, cure, or prevent any disease." The MegaH advertisement is included here for illustrative purposes only.

The primordial antioxidant! As the original creators of Silica Hydride and Microcluster® technology, Phi Sciences sets the benchmark for quality and effectiveness in antioxdants [sic]. Mega H™ consists of tiny molecular cages, five nanometers in diameter, made from a silica-mineral hydride complex with embedded H- ions. Once inside the body, it releases H- ions that are the most powerful known antioxidants; increases ATP production (energy); and reduces pain, swelling, and inflammation. As a dietary supplement, Mega H™ Silica Hydride provides powerful hydrogen ions (hydrides), that scavenges free radicals, including hydroxyl, peroxide, superoxide and singlet oxygen radical species. Additionally Mega H™ has demonstrated the ability to increase internal cellular energy (ATP and NADH) and metabolic activity.

to pieces. The result: The hydride disappears, leaving behind hydrogen gas (a substance that, within the body, is relatively inert) and hydroxide ions (the essence of alkalinity, and the active ingredient in the household product Draino). Thus, if silica hydride supplements really did provide hydride ions, the ions would instantly disappear the moment they contacted anything moist, such as the mouth, the stomach, or the intestines. During its short existence, the hydride would have no time to act as an antioxidant or perform any other functions. It would simply leave behind a residue of alkalinity, a goal that could be accomplished more easily by, for example, consuming baking soda.

Silica hydride supplements were popularized by the controversial Patrick Flanagan, an American inventor who was previously responsible for the idea of "pyramid power." In brief, this is the notion (once widely popular) that it is healthy to sit in or wear pyramidal objects. Flanagan has had numerous interests, one of them being silica hydride. It is his contention that silica hydride supplements enhance health by simulating the especially healthful water naturally consumed by the Hunza.

The Hunza are a real people who live in the tribal areas of Pakistan. They have a long, complex, and often tragic history. In the mythology of the Western health-food tradition, however, the Hunza are something else entirely: an emblem of health and longevity.

Based on stories told by a few nonexpert travelers, it became a well-known "fact" that the Hunza never get cancer and commonly remain spry and healthy long past the age of one hundred years. Whole villages were said to be full of people older than 140 years of age. This cartoonish and ultimately disrespectful caricature of a real people figured prominently in the marketing campaign that made yogurt a common food in the United States. They were called the "healthy Hunza," and the source of their health was said to be the yogurt that figures prominently in their diet.

More recently, purveyors of silica hydride, "Hunza water," and "Hunza bread" claim their products as the source of the Hunza's healthiness. However, there is no factual relationship between the actual Hunza and their use as an advertising emblem. The Hunza are a real people; they get cancer as other people do, and the tales of their amazing longevity were long ago debunked. This is a phenomenon well known to anthropologists: People who say they are 130 years old on one visit might say they are 120 on the next visit and 140 when asked the question one year later. In many tribal areas, reported age is a matter of emotion as much as of years; thirty or forty years may be added to a person's actual age (if that actual age is even known) to indicate status in the community. The actual life expectancy among the Hunza appears to be unremarkable.

SCIENTIFIC EVIDENCE

There is no meaningful evidence to indicate that silica hydride offers any health benefits. Web sites promoting silica hydride cite a host of supporting studies that supposedly prove the benefits of the product. However, many of these studies remain unpublished in the archives of the manufacturer, while others are based on diagnostic techniques that also exist on a far fringe. There are a number of published and apparently reasonable articles by the inventor of the product and people associated with him, but, aside from the obvious conflict of interest, their conclusions are merely theoretical, analyzing chemical reactions rather than medicinal effects.

Only double-blind, placebo-controlled studies can actually prove a medical treatment effective. A literature search uncovered two such studies of silica hydride supplements published in medical journals. Both of these trials were inspired by the highly questionable claim that silica hydride enhances energy production through effects on adenosine triphosphate, a substance involved in the energy economy of the body. The larger of these studies examined whether a widely marketed silica hydride product could improve sports performance. These independent researchers found that silica hydride products did enhance exercise capacity, but so did a placebo, and the two were equally effective. In other words, the supplement did not work. The other study is often reported as positive, but in fact, it measured exercise capacity in too indirect a manner for its results to be meaningful.

DOSAGE

Supplements labeled "silica hydride" are commonly recommended to be taken at a dose of 250 milligrams twice daily.

SAFETY ISSUES

No serious adverse effects were reported in the two published human trials. However, because the term "silica hydride" does not have a precise chemical meaning, it is difficult to make a general statement regarding the safety of substances said to contain it.

EBSCO CAM Review Board

FURTHER READING

Glazier, L. R., T. Stellingwerff, and L. L. Spriet. "Effects of Microhydrin Supplementation on Endurance Performance and Metabolism in Well-Trained Cyclists." *International Journal of Sport Nutrition and Exercise Metabolism* 14 (2004): 560-573.

Stephanson, C. J., and G. P. Flanagan. "Antioxidant Capacity of Silica Hydride: A Combinational Photosensitization and Fluorescence Detection Assay." *Free Radical Biology and Medicine* 35 (2003): 1129-1137.

_____. "Differential Metabolic Effects on Mitochondria by Silica Hydride Using Capillary Electrophoresis." *Journal of Medicinal Food* 7 (2004): 79-83.

Stephanson, C. J., A. M. Stephanson, and G. P. Flanagan. "Antioxidant Capability and Efficacy of Mega-h Silica Hydride, an Antioxidant Dietary Supplement, by In Vitro Cellular Analysis Using Photosensitization and Fluorescence Detection." *Journal of Medicinal Food* 5 (2002): 9-16.

_____. "Evaluation of Hydroxyl Radical-scavenging Abilities of Silica Hydride, an Antioxidant Compound, by a Fe2+-EDTA-Induced 2-Hydroxyterephthalate Fluorometric Analysis." *Journal of Medicinal Food* 6 (2003): 249-253.

See also: Wellness, general.

Silicon

CATEGORY: Herbs and supplements

DEFINITION: Natural elemental substance used to treat specific health conditions.

PRINCIPAL PROPOSED USES: Aging skin, brittle hair, brittle nails

OTHER PROPOSED USES: Prevention of atherosclerosis, prevention of Alzheimer's disease, prevention of osteoporosis

OVERVIEW

Silicon is one of the most prevalent elements on earth; it makes up more than a quarter of the earth's crust, mostly as silicon dioxide. Silicon is hypothesized to play an essential role in the body, but its actual role is uncertain. Silicon supplements are currently marketed for improving the health of bone, skin, hair, and nails. The substance silicone, once used in breast implants, also contains silicon, but in an unusual synthetic form.

REQUIREMENTS AND SOURCES

Scientists have found it difficult to determine whether silicon is an essential nutrient in humans and, if it is, to identify the necessary daily intake. Silicon is found in whole grains, some root vegetables, and beer. Silicon-containing chemicals are also added to products such as salt and baking soda to prevent caking. The average intake of silicon is approximately 10 to 40 milligrams (mg) daily.

THERAPEUTIC DOSAGES

When used as a supplement, common recommended dosage levels of silicon range from 10 to 30 mg per day.

THERAPEUTIC USES

Silicon is a constituent of the enzyme prolylhydrolase, which helps the body produce collagen and glycosaminoglycans. In addition, silicon is directly found in protein complexes that include glycosaminoglycans. These substances are essential for healthy bone, nails, hair, and skin.

Animal studies hint that silicon deprivation causes bone weakness as well as slowed wound healing. Artificial bone grafts containing silicon have been used successfully in surgical repair of damaged bones. Furthermore, in a major observational study, higher intake of silicon was associated with stronger bones. Based on these findings, silicon has been proposed as a bone-strengthening substance for preventing or treating osteoporosis. However, only double-blind, placebo-controlled studies can prove a treatment effective. Only one such study has been performed on silicon as a treatment for osteoporosis, and it found equivocal results at best.

One double-blind, placebo-controlled study did find potential benefits with a proprietary silicon supplement for aging skin, brittle nails, and brittle hair. Fifty women with sun-damaged skin were given either 10 mg silicon (as choline-stabilized orthosilicic acid) or placebo daily for twenty weeks. Measurements of skin roughness and elasticity showed improvement in the silicon group compared with the placebo group. Brittleness of hair and nails also improved. However, this study, performed by the manufacturer of the product, did not meet the highest standards of design and reporting. Another study of the same product demonstrated stronger and thicker hair over a nine-month period in women with fine hair, compared with placebo.

Silicon has also been claimed to help prevent atherosclerosis, but there is no meaningful evidence to support this claim. Another potential use of silicon relates to the aluminum hypothesis of Alzheimer's disease, the theory that aluminum toxicity is a prominent contributor to the development of this condition. Some Web sites promoting silicon supplements make the claim that increased dietary silicon decreases aluminum absorption. However, whether or not silicon actually has this effect remains unclear. Furthermore, the hypothesis that aluminum is a major risk factor for Alzheimer's disease has lost ground in recent years.

SAFETY ISSUES

Silicon is thought to be a safe supplement when used at doses similar to the average daily intake. Based on conservative evaluation of data from animal studies, it has been estimated that even a much higher dose of 13 mg per kilogram of body weight should present little to no risk. (For an adult of average weight, this works out to 760 mg daily.) However, maximum safe doses in young children, pregnant or nursing women, or people with severe liver or kidney disease have not been established.

EBSCO CAM Review Board

FURTHER READING

Barel, A., et al. "Effect of Oral Intake of Choline-Stabilized Orthosilicic Acid on Skin, Nails, and Hair in Women with Photodamaged Skin." *Archives of Dermatological Research* 297 (2005): 147-153.

Jugdaohsingh, R., et al. "Dietary Silicon Intake Is Positively Associated with Bone Mineral Density in Men and Premenopausal Women of the Framingham Offspring Cohort." *Journal of Bone and Mineral Research* 19 (2004): 297-307.

Phan, P. V., et al. "The Effect of Silica-Containing Calcium-Phosphate Particles on Human Osteoblasts In Vitro." *Journal of Biomedical Materials Research A* 67 (2003): 1001-1008.

Radin, S., et al. "Osteogenic Effects of Bioactive Glass on Bone Marrow Stromal Cells." *Journal of Biomedical Materials Research A* 73A (2005): 21-29.

Seaborn, C. D., and F. H. Nielsen. "Silicon Deprivation Decreases Collagen Formation in Wounds and
Bone, and Ornithine Transaminase Enzyme Activity in Liver." *Biological Trace Element Research* 89
(2002): 251-261.

Wickett, R. R., et al. "Effect of Oral Intake of Choline-
Stabilized Orthosilicic Acid on Hair Tensile Strength
and Morphology in Women with Fine Hair." *Archives
of Dermatological Research* 299 (2007): 499-505.

See also: Alzheimer's disease; Atherosclerosis and
heart disease prevention; Osteoporosis.

Silver

CATEGORY: Herbs and supplements
RELATED TERM: Colloidal silver
DEFINITION: Natural mineral substance used to treat
specific health conditions.
PRINCIPAL PROPOSED USES: Not recommended

OVERVIEW

The mineral silver has a long history of use in
Ayurveda, the traditional medicine of India. Silver is
toxic to many microbes, and on this basis a suspension
of finely ground silver granules called colloidal silver
was once popular among physicians in the United
States as an antiseptic. Silver is now used medically in
the form of silver sulfadiazine, a cream used to prevent infection in persons with severe burns. In addition, silver is used in some water purifiers to stop the
growth of bacteria.

Oral colloidal silver is widely promoted on the
Internet and elsewhere as a treatment for hundreds
of conditions. However, there is absolutely no evidence that this form of silver provides any medical
benefits whatsoever, and it can lead to an unsightly
and permanent discoloration of the skin that is
called argyria.

REQUIREMENTS AND SOURCES

Silver is not an essential nutrient.

THERAPEUTIC DOSAGES

A typical recommended dose of colloidal silver is 1
to 4 teaspoons a day, providing 25 to 100 micrograms
of silver.

THERAPEUTIC USES

Colloidal silver kills microbes on contact, and for
this reason, it can be properly described as an antiseptic. Despite widespread claims, however, it is not an
antibiotic. The term "antibiotic," as most commonly
used, indicates a substance that is absorbed after administration and that kills germs (such as bacteria)
throughout the body. Colloidal silver does not have
this property. When taken by mouth, it may destroy
bacteria, fungi, and other organisms in the mouth
and digestive tract, but it is not absorbed in sufficient
concentrations to kill germs anywhere else. Colloidal
silver is, thus, more analogous to bleach than to penicillin. Although both bleach and silver kill the germs
that cause sinus infections, an individual cannot treat
a sinus infection by drinking either bleach or silver.

Confusion about the difference between an antibiotic and an antiseptic has led to an enormous number
of false claims regarding silver's benefits. There is no
reliable evidence that the use of colloidal silver benefits any health condition.

SAFETY ISSUES

While oral use of silver is not believed to be toxic,
it can cause a serious cosmetic problem known as
argyria: gray-black silver deposits that stain the skin
and mucous membranes. The effect is unattractive
and, to make matters worse, permanent; once it occurs, the discoloration never goes away. A growing
number of cases of argyria have been reported in the
United States as a result of the widespread marketing
of colloidal silver products. Safety of the use of silver
in young children, pregnant or nursing women, and
people with severe liver or kidney disease has not
been established.

EBSCO CAM Review Board

FURTHER READING

Gulbranson, S. H., J. A. Hud, and R. C. Hansen. "Argyria
Following the Use of Dietary Supplements Containing
Colloidal Silver Protein." *Cutis: Cutaneous Medicine
for the Practitioner* 66 (2000): 373-374, 376.

McKenna, J. K., C. M. Hull, and J. J. Zone. "Argyria Associated with Colloidal Silver Supplementation."
International Journal of Dermatology 42 (2003): 549.

White, J. M., A. M. Powell, K. Brady, and R. Russell-
Jones. "Severe Generalized Argyria Secondary to
Ingestion of Colloidal Silver Protein." *Clinical and
Experimental Dermatology* 28 (2003): 254-256.

Wickless, S. C., and T. A. Shwayder. "Medical Mystery—The Answer." *New England Journal of Medicine* 351 (2004): 2349-2350.

See also: Ayurveda.

Sjögren's syndrome

CATEGORY: Condition

RELATED TERMS: Sicca, xerostomia

DEFINITION: Treatment of the condition in which the immune system destroys moisture-producing glands.

PRINCIPAL PROPOSED NATURAL TREATMENTS: Herb-vitamin-mineral combination, N-acetylcysteine

OTHER PROPOSED NATURAL TREATMENTS: Aloe vera, bovine colostrum, citrus bioflavonoids, dandelion, dehydroepiandrosterone, echinacea, fish oil, flaxseed oil, gamma-linolenic acid, garlic, inositol, magnesium, methionine, olive leaf extract, red clover, vitamin A, vitamin C, vitamin E, zinc

INTRODUCTION

Sjögren's syndrome is an autoimmune condition in which the immune system destroys moisture-producing glands, such as tear glands and salivary glands. When Sjögren's syndrome occurs by itself, it is called primary Sjögren's syndrome. When it occurs in the context of other autoimmune conditions, such as rheumatoid arthritis or systemic lupus erythematosus (lupus), it is called secondary Sjögren's syndrome.

Sjögren's is most common in women between forty and sixty years of age. Symptoms include dry eyes (sicca), dry mouth (xerostomia), difficulty swallowing, loss of taste and smell, swollen salivary glands, severe dental cavities caused by dry mouth, oral yeast infections (thrush), and vaginal dryness. Fatigue and joint pain also may occur, ranging in intensity from mild to disabling. Sjögren's can also affect the kidneys, digestive tract, lungs, liver, pancreas, or other internal organs.

As with other autoimmune diseases, the symptoms of Sjögren's tend to wax and wane. The disease is diagnosed by blood tests and by examination of the eyes and mouth. Treatment primarily involves the use of artificial tears, artificial saliva, and vaginal lubricants to relieve dryness. In some cases, anti-inflammatory or immune-suppressant drugs may be used.

PRINCIPAL PROPOSED NATURAL TREATMENTS

N-acetylcysteine. N-acetylcysteine (NAC) is a specially modified form of the dietary amino acid cysteine. When taken orally, NAC helps the body make the important antioxidant enzyme glutathione. NAC is also thought to help loosen secretions, and for this reason it has been tried as a treatment for Sjögren's syndrome.

In a double-blind, placebo-controlled crossover trial of twenty-six people with Sjögren's syndrome, the use of NAC at a dose of 200 milligrams three times per day improved eye-related symptoms. The supplement also showed some promise for mouth-related symptoms, but the effects were less clear-cut. While these are promising results, a much larger trial is necessary to fully document the potential benefits of this treatment approach.

Herb-vitamin-mineral combination. A product containing vitamins and minerals and the herbs paprika, rosemary, peppermint, milfoil, hawthorn, and pumpkin seed has been used in Scandinavia for many years as a treatment for various mouth-related conditions. A double-blind, placebo-controlled study of forty-four people found that four months' treatment with this combination improved some signs and symptoms of Sjögren's syndrome, including the rate of salivary flow. A larger study is needed to fully explore the potential benefits of this treatment.

OTHER PROPOSED NATURAL TREATMENTS

Colostrum is the fluid that a woman's breasts produce during the first day or two after she has given birth. Preliminary evidence suggests that oral hygiene products containing bovine colostrum (colostrum from cows) may provide beneficial effects for the mouth symptoms of Sjögren's syndrome.

One small study found preliminary evidence that toothpaste containing betaine may be helpful for dry mouth symptoms of Sjögren's syndrome. Also, gamma-linolenic acid (GLA), an essential fatty acid in the omega-6 family, has been tried as a treatment for the fatigue often associated with Sjögren's. However, in a six-month, double-blind, placebo-controlled trial of ninety people, the use of GLA failed to prove more effective than placebo. One small double-blind study, however, found that a combination of GLA and the omega-6 fatty acid linoleic acid (found in many vegetable oils) may improve dry-eye symptoms in Sjögren's. Flax oil, a source of omega-3 fatty acids, has also shown some promise for this latter purpose.

A twelve-month, double-blind, placebo-controlled study failed to find benefit with the hormone dehydroepiandrosterone (DHEA), taken at a dose of 200 mg daily. The researchers noted that the belief by participants that they were being given DHEA instead of placebo "was a stronger predictor for improvement of fatigue and well-being than the actual use of DHEA." An earlier double-blind, placebo-controlled study also failed to find benefit.

Numerous other natural products are widely recommended for Sjögren's syndrome, but they lack supporting scientific evidence. These include aloe vera, citrus bioflavonoids, dandelion, echinacea, fish oil, garlic, inositol, magnesium, methionine, olive leaf extract, red clover, vitamin A, vitamin C, vitamin E, and zinc.

HERBS AND SUPPLEMENTS TO USE WITH CAUTION

One case report weakly hints that the herb echinacea might potentially trigger dangerous symptoms (specifically, critical hypokalemic renal tubular acidosis) in people with Sjögren's. Numerous herbs and supplements may interact adversely with drugs used to treat Sjögren's syndrome.

EBSCO CAM Review Board

FURTHER READING

Aragona, P., et al. "Systemic Omega-6 Essential Fatty Acid Treatment and PGE1 Tear Content in Sjögren's Syndrome Patients." *Investigative Ophthalmology and Visual Science* 46 (2005): 4474-4479.

Hartkamp, A., et al. "Effect of Dehydroepiandrosterone Administration on Fatigue, Well-Being, and Functioning in Women with Primary Sjögren's Syndrome." *Annals of the Rheumatic Diseases* 67 (2008): 91-97.

Pillemer, S. R., et al. "Pilot Clinical Trial of Dehydroepiandrosterone (DHEA) Versus Placebo for Sjögren's Syndrome." *Arthritis and Rheumatism* 51 (2004): 601-604.

Rantanen, I., et al. "Effects of a Betaine-Containing Toothpaste on Subjective Symptoms of Dry Mouth." *Journal of Contemporary Dental Practice* 4 (2003): 11-23.

Theander, E., et al. "Gammalinolenic Acid Treatment of Fatigue Associated with Primary Sjögren's Syndrome." *Scandinavian Journal of Rheumatology* 31 (2002): 72-79.

See also: Immune support; Lupus; N-acetylcysteine; Vitamins and minerals.

Skin, aging

CATEGORY: Condition

RELATED TERMS: Photoaging, sun-damaged skin

DEFINITION: Treatment of skin changes caused by aging and skin damage caused by long-term exposure to the sun.

PRINCIPAL PROPOSED NATURAL TREATMENTS: Alpha-hydroxy acids, antioxidants (carotenoids, green tea, milk thistle, oligomeric proanthocyanidin complexes, selenium, soy isoflavones, vitamin C, vitamin E)

OTHER PROPOSED NATURAL TREATMENTS: Acupuncture, aloe, *Arnica*, beta-carotene, calendula, chamomile, coriander oil, dead sea minerals, dehydroepiandrosterone, glucosamine, gotu kola, "growth hormone enhancers," IGF-1, IGF-2, TGF-A, and other growth factors, niacinamide, para-aminobenzoic acid, silicon, thuja, vitamin A, *Vitis vinifera*

HERBS AND SUPPLEMENTS TO USE WITH CAUTION: St. John's wort; vitamin A (among people using tretinoin)

INTRODUCTION

The substances collagen and elastin give skin its firmness and elasticity. With age, though, the collagen and elastin content of the skin gradually decreases. As a result, the skin becomes looser, weaker, less elastic, and drier. In addition, the fat pads under the skin begin to disappear. Wrinkles form, and the skin begins to sag.

This gradual loss of structure has several causes: genetic programming (a built-in "clock" that causes aging), cumulative sun damage (photoaging), and direct chemical effects from cigarette smoking or abrasive chemicals, or both. Sun damage also causes fine wrinkles that disappear when stretching the skin, surface roughness, mottled pigmentation, "liver" spots, and skin cancer.

In people who already have signs of aging skin and wish to reverse it, a number of treatments are available. The drug tretinoin (retinoic acid, or Retin-A), a substance related to vitamin A, has been shown effective for reversing the fine wrinkles, splotchy pigmentation, and rough skin of sun damage. The hormone estrogen is thought to help restore normal skin tone in menopausal women, but the evidence for this widely held belief remains weak.

More aggressive treatments for aging skin include injections of botulin toxin, dermabrasion, chemical peels, soft tissue augmentation, laser resurfacing, and Gore-Tex threads.

PRINCIPAL PROPOSED NATURAL TREATMENTS

Two classes of natural treatments have shown promise in the treatment of aging skin: alpha-hydroxy acids (AHAs) and antioxidants. However, the evidence that they work remains incomplete, and AHAs can cause significant side effects.

Alpha-hydroxy acids. Alpha-hydroxy acids, such as glycolic acid and lactic acid, are substances derived from fruit and dairy products. These are milder relatives of the substances used by dermatologists in chemical peels, which are designed to remove damaged layers of the skin. Cosmetics manufacturers are now adding AHAs to many skin-care products.

Meaningful evidence in support of AHAs comes from one double-blind, placebo-controlled study reported in 1996. This twenty-two-week study enrolled seventy-four women with sun-damaged skin. Participants received either 8 percent glycolic acid, 8 percent L-lactic acid, or placebo cream and applied it to the face and forearm. Although participants showed improvements in each of the three groups, superior results were achieved with each of the AHA creams than with the placebo cream. Another double-blind study compared estrogen cream, glycolic acid cream, and their combination with placebo. Both estrogen and glycolic acid improved skin aging.

AHAs are not always harmless. Possible side effects include burning, blistering, severe redness, swelling (especially in the area of the eyes), bleeding, rash, and increased sensitivity to the sun. There are also concerns that AHAs may increase the risk of skin cancer. For all these reasons, the U.S. Food and Drug Administration continues to investigate the use of AHAs in cosmetic products to determine whether they should be reclassified as drugs.

Antioxidants. The ultraviolet light from the sun creates free radicals, naturally occurring substances that can harm many tissues of the body, including the skin. Antioxidants are substances that neutralize free radicals. On this basis, various antioxidants have been investigated for their potential usefulness in treating or preventing photoaging.

A small, three-month, double-blind, placebo-controlled study found benefit with a cream containing 5 percent alpha-lipoic acid. The use of this antioxidant substance improved several measures of aging skin

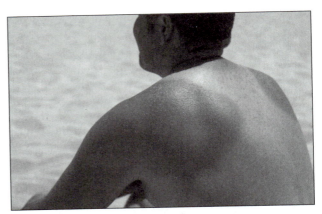

Repeated sunburn can age the skin prematurely. (Ian Hooton/ Photo Researchers, Inc.)

especially skin roughness, compared with placebo. Benefits have also been seen in preliminary studies with a cream containing vitamin C. In a small double-blind study, the use of mixed antioxidants (lycopene, beta-carotene, vitamin E, and selenium) for twelve weeks improved skin roughness and scaling.

Oligomeric proanthocyanidin complexes (OPCs) made from grape seed or pine bark are widely marketed for the treatment of aging skin. These substances, closely related to bioflavonoids, have antioxidant properties and might also protect and strengthen collagen and elastin. These effects provide theoretical reasons to believe that OPCs might be helpful for the treatment of aging skin. However, despite widespread marketing, no properly designed studies have been reported to indicate that OPCs provide any benefit.

In an eight-week, double-blind, placebo-controlled study of forty women who already had sun-damaged skin, the combined use of oral green tea and a topical green tea cream failed to prove more effective than placebo in improving the condition of sun-damaged skin. Some possible benefits were seen in microscopic evaluation of skin condition.

Studies on laboratory animals found that topical vitamin C and vitamin E helped prevent burning on exposure to ultraviolet light. A small double-blind study found that 2 grams (g) of vitamin C and 1,000 international units (IU) of vitamin E taken orally for eight days resulted in a modest decrease of sunburn induced by ultraviolet light. In addition, a fifty-day, placebo-controlled study of forty people found that higher doses of these vitamins provided a sun protection factor (SPF) of about 2.16. (The sun protection factor is 15 or higher in many sunscreens.) It appears that these vitamins must be taken together for best effect; when used alone, they do not appear to work.

The oral use of beta-carotene, lycopene, and other carotenoids has shown preventive effects in some studies. Benefits have also been seen with mixtures of various antioxidants taken together (vitamin E, zeoxanthin, lutein, beta-carotene, and others).

Oral vitamin A has shown some promise for preventing skin cancer in people at risk for it, but the doses used in studies were quite high, considerably above recommendations for the maximum safe dose. Vitamin A should not be used with the drug tretinoin.

Topical vitamin A may be helpful for treatment of aging skin. One double-blind, placebo-controlled study found that a 0.4 percent vitamin A lotion applied three times a week significantly reduced the number of "fine" wrinkles in seniors. Benefits were also seen in terms of some biochemical measures of skin health.

Because these antioxidants work in an entirely different manner from standard sunscreen, it is reasonable to believe that they could offer a synergistic effect if taken while using sunscreen. However, this hypothesis has not been studied.

Other substances with antioxidant actions that have shown some promise for treating or preventing aging skin include cocoa, *Vitis vinifera* extract, milk thistle, and zinc. However, the supporting evidence that the use of these substances (taken either orally or topically) offers any benefit for the skin remains far too preliminary to be relied upon.

Any discussion of the potential benefits of antioxidants for preventing cancer must include the startling finding of a large study that tested the effect of mixed antioxidants. This trial, enrolling 7,876 women and 5,141 men, evaluated the potential benefits of a combination of vitamin C, vitamin E, beta-carotene, selenium, and zinc for preventing cancer. According to results published in 2007, no benefits were seen among the male participants, but among women, skin cancer rates actually appeared to increase. The cause of these findings remains unclear.

OTHER PROPOSED NATURAL TREATMENTS

In a double-blind study of fifty women with signs of aging skin, the use of topical niacinamide cream significantly improved skin appearance and elasticity compared with placebo cream. A study published in 2007 tested a purified soy isoflavone product (technically, isoflavone aglycones) for treatment of aging skin. In this double-blind trial, twenty-six Japanese women in their late thirties and early forties were given either placebo or 40 milligrams (mg) daily of soy isoflavone aglycones for twelve weeks. Researchers monitored two types of wrinkles near the eye: "fine" wrinkles and "linear" wrinkles. The results indicated that the use of the soy product significantly reduced fine wrinkles compared with placebo. (Effects on linear wrinkles were not significant.) As a secondary measure, researchers also analyzed skin elasticity and found an improvement in the women given the isoflavones compared to those given placebo.

An unusual soy extract containing soybean trypsin inhibitor and Bowman-Birk protease inhibitor has also shown promise for aging skin. Sixty-five women with moderate skin damage from the sun received either soybean extract or placebo cream for twelve weeks. Compared to the women in the placebo group, treated women showed an improvement in mottled pigmentation, blotchiness, dullness, and fine lines, and an overall enhancement of texture, skin tone, and appearance.

The substance glucosamine is widely used for osteoarthritis, in part because it seems to help collagen regenerate. For this reason, it has been advocated as a treatment for aging skin. However, the only evidence that it works comes from one poorly designed study. In this single-blind trial, seventy-two women with symptoms of aging skin were divided into two unequal groups: a small group that received no treatment and a much larger one that received a proprietary mixture of glucosamine, amino acids, and minerals. The results indicated greater improvement in the treated group compared to the untreated group. However, because this was not a double-blind, placebo-controlled study, the results cannot be taken as reliable.

The mineral silicon also has been proposed as a treatment for aging skin. In the one potentially meaningful published study, fifty women with sun-damaged skin were given either 10 mg silicon daily (as orthosilicic acid) or placebo for twenty weeks. Measurements of skin roughness and elasticity showed improvement in the silicon group compared with the placebo group. However, this study, performed by the manufacturer of a silicon product, was not well designed or well reported.

A proprietary dietary supplement containing soy, fish protein polysaccharides, white tea extract, and many other ingredients has also shown promise, according to a study performed by the manufacturer. Another study provides weak evidence that the substance DHEA (dehydroepiandrosterone) might be helpful for improving skin condition in the elderly.

In a preliminary double-blind study, coriander oil applied topically was more effective than a placebo cream at reducing redness from UVB exposure. This effect may or may not translate into long-term benefit for aging sun-damaged skin.

Numerous herbs and other natural products have been advocated for the treatment of aging skin. These products include aloe, *Arnica*, calendula, chamomile, dead sea minerals, gotu kola, para-aminobenzoic acid, thuja, and vitamin A. Other products claim to contain biological substances called growth factors (with names such as IGF-1, IGF-2, TGF-A, TGF-B, EGF, and FGF) and go on to claim that these growth factors improve skin condition. Still others claim to raise levels of human growth hormone in the body and, therefore, help produce youthful skin. However, there is no meaningful evidence that any of these treatments work.

Acupuncture face lifts are widely available for treating facial wrinkles. They involve a series of treatments in which fine needles are inserted into the face. However, there is no evidence to indicate that this method produces any benefit.

Herbs and Supplements to Use with Caution

The herb St. John's wort contains a substance, hypericin, that increases the skin's sensitivity to the sun. For this reason, it is possible that the use of St. John's wort could accelerate sun damage of skin. Also, persons using the drug Retin-A should not take high doses of vitamin A, as each might increase the toxicity of the other.

EBSCO CAM Review Board

Further Reading

Bissett, D. L., et al. "Niacinamide: A B Vitamin That Improves Aging Facial Skin Appearance." *Dermatological Surgery* 31 (2005): 860-865.

Chiu, A. E., et al. "Double-Blinded, Placebo-Controlled Trial of Green Tea Extracts in the Clinical and Histologic Appearance of Photoaging Skin." *Dermatological Surgery* 31 (2005): 855-860.

Cornacchione, S., et al. "In Vivo Skin Antioxidant Effect of a New Combination Based on a Specific *Vitis vinifera* Shoot Extract and a Biotechnological Extract." *Journal of Drugs in Dermatology* 6 (2007): 8-13.

Elmets, C. A., et al. "Cutaneous Photoprotection from Ultraviolet Injury by Green Tea Polyphenols." *Journal of the American Academy of Dermatology* 44 (2001): 425-432.

Fuchs, K. O., et al. "The Effects of an Estrogen and Glycolic Acid Cream on the Facial Skin of Postmenopausal Women." *Cutis* 71 (2003): 481-488.

Greul, A. K., et al. "Photoprotection of UV-Irradiated Human Skin: An Antioxidative Combination of Vitamins E and C, Carotenoids, Selenium, and Proanthocyanidins." *Skin Pharmacology and Applied Skin Physiology* 15 (2002): 307-315.

Heinrich, U., K. Neukam, et al. "Long-Term Ingestion of High Flavanol Cocoa Provides Photoprotection Against UV-Induced Erythema and Improves Skin Condition in Women." *Journal of Nutrition* 136 (2006): 1565-1569.

Heinrich, U., H. Tronnier, et al. "Antioxidant Supplements Improve Parameters Related to Skin Structure in Humans." *Skin Pharmacology and Physiology* 19 (2006): 224-231.

Hercberg, S., et al. "Antioxidant Supplementation Increases the Risk of Skin Cancers in Women but Not in Men." *Journal of Nutrition* 137 (2007): 2098-2105.

Kafi, R., et al. "Improvement of Naturally Aged Skin with Vitamin A (Retinol)." *Archives of Dermatology* 143 (2007): 606-612.

Skovgaard, G. R., A. S. Jensen, and M. L. Sigler. "Effect of a Novel Dietary Supplement on Skin Aging in Post-menopausal Women." *European Journal of Clinical Nutrition* 60 (2006): 1201-1206.

Wallo, W., J. Nebus, and J. J. Leyden. "Efficacy of a Soy Moisturizer in Photoaging." *Journal of Drugs in Dermatology* 6 (2007): 917-922.

See also: Aging; Antioxidants; Carotenoids; Eczema; Green tea; Milk thistle; Oligomeric proanthocyanidins; Photosensitivity; Selenium; Soy; Vitamin C; Vitamin E.

Skullcap

Category: Herbs and supplements
Related term: *Scutellaria lateriflora*

DEFINITION: Natural plant product used to treat specific health conditions.

PRINCIPAL PROPOSED USES: None

OTHER PROPOSED USES: Anxiety, insomnia

OVERVIEW

Native Americans and traditional European herbalists used skullcap to induce sleep, relieve nervousness, and moderate the symptoms of epilepsy, rabies, and other diseases related to the nervous system. In other words, skullcap was believed to function as an herbal sedative.

A relative of skullcap, *Scutellaria baicalensis*, is a common Chinese herb. However, the root instead of the above-the-ground portion of the plant is used, and the overall effects appear to be far different. Only European skullcap (*S. lateriflora*) is addressed here.

THERAPEUTIC DOSAGES

When taken by itself, the usual dosage of skullcap is approximately 1 to 2 grams (g) three times a day. However, skullcap is more often taken in combination with other sedative herbs, such as valerian, passionflower, hops, and melissa, also called lemon balm. Individuals using an herbal combination should follow the label instructions for dosage. Skullcap is usually not taken on a long-term basis.

THERAPEUTIC USES

Skullcap is still popular as a sedative, but there has been virtually no scientific investigation of how well the herb really works. The only meaningful reported study was a small double-blind, placebo-controlled trial that found indications that the herb might reduce anxiety levels in healthy volunteers.

SAFETY ISSUES

Not much is known about the safety of skullcap, but it is known to cause confusion and stupor when taken in too-high amounts. There have been reports of liver damage following consumption of products labeled skullcap; however, since skullcap has been known to be adulterated with germander, an herb toxic to the liver, it may not have been the skullcap that was at fault. The safety of skullcap for use by young children, pregnant or nursing women, and those with severe liver or kidney disease has not been established.

EBSCO CAM Review Board

FURTHER READING

Newall, C. A., L. A. Anderson, and J. D. Phillipson. "Skullcap." In *Herbal Medicines: A Guide for Health-Care Professionals*. London: Pharmaceutical Press; 1996.

Wolfson, P., and D. L. Hoffmann. "An Investigation into the Efficacy of *Scutellaria lateriflora* in Healthy Volunteers." *Alternative Therapies in Health and Medicine* 9 (2003): 74-78.

See also: Anxiety; Insomnia.

Slippery elm

CATEGORY: Herbs and supplements

RELATED TERMS: *Ulmus fulva, U. rubra*

DEFINITION: Natural plant product used to treat specific health conditions.

PRINCIPAL PROPOSED USES: None

OTHER PROPOSED USES: Cough, dyspepsia, esophageal reflux, gastritis, hemorrhoids, inflammatory bowel disease, irritable bowel syndrome

OVERVIEW

The dried inner bark of the slippery elm tree was a favorite medicinal substance of many Native American tribes and was subsequently adopted by European colonists. Like marshmallow and mullein, slippery elm was used as a treatment for sore throat, coughs, dryness of the lungs, inflammation of the skin, wounds, and irritation of the digestive tract. It was also made into a kind of porridge to be taken by weaned infants and during convalescence from illness. Various heroes of the American Civil War are said to have credited slippery elm with their recovery from war wounds.

THERAPEUTIC DOSAGES

Cough lozenges made with slippery elm may be sucked as needed. For internal use, a typical dose of slippery elm is 500 to 1,000 milligrams (mg) three times daily.

THERAPEUTIC USES

Slippery elm has not been scientifically studied to any significant extent. It is primarily used today in cough lozenges that are widely available in pharmacies. Based on its soothing properties, slippery elm is

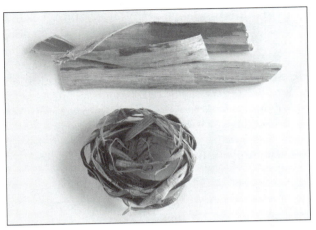
Dried slippery elm bark. (Steve Gorton/Getty Images)

also sometimes recommended for the treatment of irritable bowel syndrome, inflammatory bowel disease (such as Crohn's disease and ulcerative colitis), gastritis, esophageal reflux (heartburn), and hemorrhoids. However, there is no meaningful evidence that it is helpful for any of these conditions.

SAFETY ISSUES

Other than occasional allergic reactions, slippery elm has not been associated with any toxicity. However, its safety has never been formally studied. Safety in young children, pregnant or nursing women, and those with severe liver or kidney disease has not been established.

EBSCO CAM Review Board

FURTHER READING

Castleman, M. "Slippery Elm." In *The New Healing Herbs.* Rev. ed. Emmaus, Pa.: Rodale Press, 2001.

See also: Cough; Dyspepsia; Gastritis; Gastroesophageal reflux disease; Irritable bowel syndrome (IBS).

Smoking addiction

CATEGORY: Condition
RELATED TERMS: Addiction, nicotine, cigarette addiction, nicotine dependency, nicotine withdrawal, quitting smoking, smoking and nutrition, smoking cessation, tobacco dependency

DEFINITION: Treatment of nicotine addiction and nutritional deficiencies in smokers.
PRINCIPAL PROPOSED NATURAL TREATMENTS:
- *For addiction:* None
- *For nutrition:* Folate, multivitamin-multimineral supplements, vitamin C, vitamin E

OTHER PROPOSED NATURAL TREATMENTS: Acupuncture, alfalfa, cysticine (toxic), eucalyptus, gotu kola, hops, hypnotherapy, licorice, lobelia, melatonin, passionflower, skullcap, wild oats (*Avena sativa*)
HERBS AND SUPPLEMENTS TO AVOID: High-dose beta-carotene

INTRODUCTION

Nicotine is one of the most addictive drugs known. The combination of this chemical with the flavor of tobacco smoke and the oral satisfaction of a cigarette leads to the addiction of many smokers. Smoking is an addiction that is difficult to break.

Conventional treatment for smoking addiction focuses primarily on methods to separate nicotine addiction from the other habit-forming features of cigarettes. These treatments include the nicotine patch and the nicotine inhaler. Also, the drugs varencicline and bupropion (Zyban) have shown benefit.

Furthermore, cigarette smoking is one of the biggest risk factors for developing cancer and heart disease. The more cigarettes a person smokes and the longer it is kept up, the greater the risk of dying from cancer, heart attack, or stroke. Probably less well known is that smokers are also much more likely to catch colds and other infections.

Because cigarette smoking poses such a public health risk, many studies have attempted to discern whether the use of vitamin supplements by smokers might help avert cancer and other diseases. However, the results have not been promising, and one supplement, beta-carotene, may actually be dangerous for smokers.

PROPOSED NATURAL TREATMENTS: ADDICTION

There are no proven natural aids for treating cigarette addiction. The herb lobelia has been widely promoted for stopping smoking. The origin of this idea appears to be a long-standing misconception: that a constituent of lobelia (lobeline) closely resembles the drug nicotine. However, lobeline and nicotine are not biochemically similar, and they are not believed to have generally similar actions in the nervous system.

Nonetheless, research suggests that lobeline might have some unusual effects on the nervous system that could make it helpful for treating addiction, especially addiction to amphetamines.

The herb wild oats (*Avena sativa*) has also been suggested as a treatment for cigarette addiction, but on balance the evidence indicates that it is not effective. Weak evidence supports a role for melatonin in reducing nicotine withdrawal symptoms.

The substance cysticine is a toxic compound found in the seeds of *Laburnum anagyroides* and related plants. Weak evidence, mostly from studies in Eastern Europe, hints that the careful use of this substance might aid smoking cessation. Numerous other herbs are promoted for stopping smoking. These include alfalfa, eucalyptus, gotu kola, hops, licorice, passion-flower, and skullcap, none of which have been evaluated scientifically.

Acupuncture, especially in the form of ear acupuncture (auriculopuncture), is widely used as a treatment for cigarette addiction. However, a 1999 meta-analysis of twelve placebo-controlled trials did not find acupuncture more effective than sham (fake) acupuncture for smoking cessation. A subsequent double-blind, placebo-controlled study of 330 adolescent smokers, conducted in 2000, also found no benefit. One study found that while acupuncture may not be effective for treating cigarette addiction on its own, it might (in some unknown manner) increase the effectiveness of smoking cessation education. In this placebo-controlled study of 141 adults, acupuncture plus education was twice as effective as sham acupuncture plus education and was four times as effective as acupuncture alone. Nonetheless, these benefits were seen only in the short term; at long-term follow-up, acupuncture's advantage disappeared.

While hypnotherapy benefits some smokers, it does not appear to be superior to other methods for quitting. In a review of nine studies, researchers found no consistent evidence that hypnotherapy was better than fourteen other interventions for nicotine addiction. Another randomized trial found that, when combined with a nicotine patch, hypnotherapy was no better than cognitive-behavioral therapy.

PROPOSED NATURAL TREATMENTS: NUTRITION

People who smoke often have deficiencies in numerous nutrients, including zinc, calcium, folate, vitamin B_{12}, vitamin C, vitamin E, beta-carotene, ly-copene, and essential fatty acids in the omega-3 and omega-6 families. There are many possible causes for this depletion, including free radicals in cigarette smoke that destroy natural antioxidants. However, the most important single cause for nutrient depletion might be poor diet rather than smoking itself. (Smokers have, on average, a less well-balanced diet than nonsmokers.) In addition, some evidence suggests that folate or vitamin C supplements may improve arterial function in smokers, thereby potentially helping to prevent heart disease.

High doses of vitamin E have not proven helpful for preventing heart disease or lung cancer in smokers. However, vitamin E consumption has shown some promise for reducing the risk of prostate cancer in smokers.

For all these reasons, many smokers benefit from general nutritional support in the form of a multivitamin-multimineral tablet. However, high doses of the antioxidant vitamin beta-carotene may not be helpful for smokers and could even cause harm.

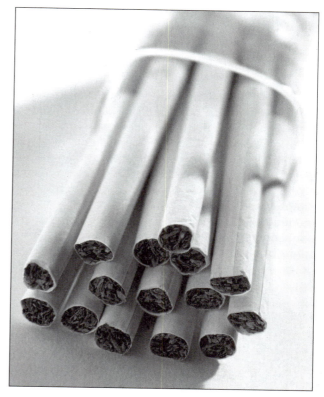

Nicotine from smoking a cigarette can create an intense craving that is very hard to resist. (PhotoDisc)

Beta-carotene: A supplement to avoid. Although nutritional doses of the antioxidant nutrient beta-carotene help to supply needed vitamin A, there is evidence that smokers should avoid high doses of beta-carotene. An enormous double-blind, placebo-controlled study called the Alpha-Tocopherol, Beta-Carotene Cancer Prevention (ATBC) trial enrolled 29,133 Finnish male smokers and examined the effects of vitamin E and beta-carotene supplements on lung cancer rates among them. The results showed that 20 milligrams (mg) of beta-carotene daily for five to eight years increased the risk of lung cancer by 18 percent.

In addition, a statistical analysis of the ATBC study, including 1,862 smokers with heart problems, found that persons taking either beta-carotene or a beta-carotene and vitamin E combination had significantly increased risk of fatal heart attack compared to those taking placebo. Another statistical review of the study analyzed the effects of beta-carotene on persons with angina pectoris, one of the first symptoms of heart disease. Results indicated that beta-carotene was associated with a slight increase in angina.

Another large, double-blind, placebo-controlled trial enrolling 18,314 smokers, former smokers, and workers exposed to asbestos studied the effects of a different combination, beta-carotene and vitamin A, on lung cancer and cardiovascular disease. Evidence from the trial suggests that 30 mg of beta-carotene and 25,000 international units of vitamin A, taken together daily, have no beneficial effects and may be harmful. Persons taking the supplements had a 28 percent higher incidence of lung cancer than the placebo group, a 17 percent higher death rate from lung cancer, and a 26 percent higher death rate from cardiovascular disease. The trial was stopped twenty-one months early based on these findings. Although nutritional dosages of beta-carotene (about 3 mg daily for adults) are probably healthful, smokers should avoid doses of beta-carotene greater than 20 to 30 mg daily.

EBSCO CAM Review Board

FURTHER READING

Abbot, N. C., L. F. Stead, and A. R. White. "Hypnotherapy for Smoking Cessation." *Cochrane Database of Systematic Reviews* (2000): CD001008. Available through *EBSCO DynaMed Systematic Literature Surveillance* at http://www.ebscohost.com/dynamed.
Bier, I. D., et al. "Auricular Acupuncture, Education, and Smoking Cessation." *American Journal of Public Health* 92 (2002): 1642-1647.
Carmody, T. P., et al. "Hypnosis for Smoking Cessation." *Nicotine and Tobacco Research* 10 (2008): 811-818.
Etter, J. F. "Cytisine for Smoking Cessation." *Archives of Internal Medicine* 166 (2006): 1553-1559.
Jia, X., et al. "A Pilot Study on the Effects of Almond Consumption on DNA Damage and Oxidative Stress in Smokers." *Nutrition and Cancer* 54 (2006): 179-183.
Mangoni, A. A., et al. "Folic Acid Enhances Endothelial Function and Reduces Blood Pressure in Smokers." *Journal of Internal Medicine* 252 (2002): 497-503.
Raitakari, O. T., et al. "Oral Vitamin C and Endothelial Function in Smokers: Short-Term Improvement, but No Sustained Beneficial Effect." *Journal of the American College of Cardiology* 35 (2000): 1616-1621.
Van den Berg, H., M. van der Gaag, and H. Hendriks. "Influence of Lifestyle on Vitamin Bioavailability." *International Journal for Vitamin and Nutrition Research* 72 (2002): 53-59.
Yiming, C., et al. "Laser Acupuncture for Adolescent Smokers." *American Journal of Chinese Medicine* 28 (2000): 443-449.

See also: Alcoholism; Chronic obstructive pulmonary disease (COPD); Eating disorders; Folate; Heart attack; Hypertension; Narcotic dependency; Obesity and excess weight; Smoking and nutrition; Vitamin C; Vitamin E.

Soft tissue pain

CATEGORY: Condition
RELATED TERMS: Musculoskeletal pain, pain, muscle, pain, soft tissue
DEFINITION: Treatment of muscle, tendon, and ligament pain.
PROPOSED NATURAL TREATMENTS: Acupuncture, biofeedback, boswellia, butterbur, chiropractic, devil's claw, hypnosis, magnet therapy, massage, D-phenylalanine, prolotherapy, proteolytic enzymes, relaxation therapy, white willow

INTRODUCTION

When specific causes of symptoms are not known, doctors sometimes refer to conditions simply by naming the symptoms. Such is the case for soft tissue pain. The term "soft tissue pain" simply refers to discomfort somewhere in the interconnected system of muscles, tendons, and ligaments, as opposed to the bones, and says nothing about the particular cause.

The most commonly used conventional treatments for soft tissue pain consist primarily of drugs that relieve pain and inflammation, such as ibuprofen and acetaminophen, in general, and muscle relaxants. Physical therapy methods are commonly recommended for selected forms of soft tissue pain, but there is little to no reliable scientific evidence that they help. Other methods, such as therapeutic exercises, may help, but most reported studies are significantly flawed by the lack of a credible placebo treatment.

A similar lack of reliable evidence exists regarding other nonsurgical, nondrug methods used to control soft tissue pain, such as injection therapy, radiofrequency denervation, and transcutaneous electrical nerve stimulation (TENS). Surgery may be useful for certain selected forms of soft tissue pain, although the supporting research evidence is generally incomplete.

PROPOSED NATURAL TREATMENTS

Natural treatments for soft tissue pain include treatments for back pain, bursitis, fibromyalgia, neck pain, rotator cuff injury, sciatic pain, sports injuries, sprains, tendonitis, and tension headache. Alternative therapies that may be useful for soft tissue pain in general include acupuncture, biofeedback, chiropractic, hypnosis, magnet therapy, massage, prolotherapy, and relaxation therapy. Herbs and supplements that may have a general pain-relieving effect include boswellia, butterbur, devil's claw, D-phenylalanine, proteolytic enzymes, and white willow.

EBSCO CAM Review Board

FURTHER READING

Bisset, L., et al. "A Systematic Review and Meta-analysis of Clinical Trials on Physical Interventions for Lateral Epicondylalgia." *British Journal of Sports Medicine* 39 (2005): 411-422.

Frost, H., et al. "Randomised Controlled Trial of Physiotherapy Compared with Advice for Low Back Pain." *British Medical Journal* 329 (2004): 708.

Hayden, J. A., et al. "Meta-analysis: Exercise Therapy for Nonspecific Low Back Pain." *Annals of Internal Medicine* 142 (2005): 765-775.

Milne, S., et al. "Transcutaneous Electrical Nerve Stimulation (TENS) for Chronic Low Back Pain." *Cochrane Database of Systematic Reviews* (2001): CD003008. Article is available through *EBSCO DynaMed Systematic Literature Surveillance* at http://www.ebscohost.com/dynamed.

Niemisto, L., et al. "Radiofrequency Denervation for Neck and Back Pain." *Cochrane Database of Systematic Reviews* (2003): CD004058. Available through *EBSCO DynaMed Systematic Literature Surveillance* at http://www.ebscohost.com/dynamed.

Robertson, V. J., and K. G. Baker. "A Review of Therapeutic Ultrasound: Effectiveness Studies." *Physical Therapy* 81 (2001): 1339-1350.

See also: Acupressure; Acupuncture; Back pain; Biofeedback; Bone and joint health; Bursitis; Carpal tunnel syndrome; Injuries, minor; Neck pain; Nonsteroidal anti-inflammatory drugs (NSAIDs); Pain management; Sports and fitness support: Enhancing recovery; Sports-related injuries: Homeopathic remedies; Temporomandibular joint syndrome (TMJ); Tendonitis.

Soy

CATEGORY: Functional foods
RELATED TERMS: Hydrolyzed soy protein, isoflavones, soybean, soy protein, soy protein extract, tofu
DEFINITION: Natural food product promoted as a dietary supplement for specific health benefits.
PRINCIPAL PROPOSED USE: High cholesterol
OTHER PROPOSED USES: Allergic rhinitis, cancer prevention, cyclic mastitis, diabetes, high blood pressure, menopausal symptoms, menstrual migraines, osteoarthritis, osteoporosis, ulcerative colitis

OVERVIEW

The soybean has been prized for centuries in Asia as a nutritious, high-protein food with myriad uses, and today it is popular in the United States not only in Asian food but also as a cholesterol-free meat and dairy substitute in traditional American foods. Soy burgers, soy yogurt, tofu (a soft soy product) hot dogs, and tofu cheese can be found in a growing number of grocery stores, alongside the traditional white blocks of tofu. Also, soy is increasingly used as a protein filler in many prepared foods, including fast-food hamburger.

Soy appears to reduce blood cholesterol levels. The U.S. Food and Drug Administration (FDA) has authorized allowing foods containing soy to carry a "heart-healthy" label.

Soybeans contain isoflavones, chemicals that are similar to estrogen. These are widely thought to be the active ingredients in soy, although there is substantial evidence that other constituents may be equally or more important.

SOURCES

It is easy to get a healthy dose of soy by eating Japanese, Chinese, Thai, or Vietnamese foods. Tofu is one of the world's most versatile foods. It can be stir-fried, steamed, or added to soup. A cake of tofu can be mashed and used in place of ricotta cheese in lasagna. Many other soy products are available, including plain soybeans, soy cheese, soy burgers, soy milk, and tempeh. Soy supplements are also available.

THERAPEUTIC DOSAGES

The FDA allows soy foods containing 6.5 grams (g) of soy to carry a heart-healthy label. Evidence suggests that a daily intake of 25 g of soy protein is adequate to noticeably reduce cholesterol. This amount is typically found in about two-and-one-half cups of soy milk or in one-half pound of tofu.

Soy is increasingly added to foods in the United States as a protein filler, and there are concerns that some people in the United States may be greatly exceeding the amount of soy eaten anywhere else in the world. Even the 25-g amount recommended for reducing cholesterol levels is relatively high. For comparison, in Asia, the average intake of soy is only about 10 g daily.

THERAPEUTIC USES

According to the combined evidence of numerous controlled studies, soy can reduce blood cholesterol levels and improve the ratio of LDL (bad) to HDL (good) cholesterol. At an average dosage of 47 g daily, total cholesterol falls by about 9 percent, LDL cholesterol falls by 13 percent, and triglycerides fall by 10 percent.

Soy's effects on HDL cholesterol itself are less impressive. There is inconsistent evidence regarding whether soy might help reduce high blood pressure. Indeed, a comprehensive and careful review of studies investigating the influence of phytoestrogens (including soy meals) on blood pressure found no meaningful effect. However, another review found that soy protein (as opposed to other soy products) could significantly reduce blood pressure.

Soy may reduce the common menopausal symptom known as hot flashes, but study results conflict. Soy has not been found helpful for improving the hot flashes that often occur in persons who have had breast cancer.

Unlike estrogen, soy appears to reduce the risk of uterine cancer. Its effect on breast cancer is not as well established, but there are reasons to believe that soy can help reduce breast cancer risk too, possibly by reducing estrogen levels and lengthening the menstrual cycle. Soy has shown inconsistent promise for helping to prevent prostate and colon cancers.

One preliminary double-blind trial found evidence that soy protein can reduce symptoms of osteoarthritis. In addition, soy might help prevent osteoporosis.

In preliminary double-blind studies, a special extract of soy sauce called Shoyu polysaccharides has shown promise as a treatment for allergic rhinitis (hay fever).

Another special extract of soy, Bowman-Birk inhibitor concentrate, has shown promise for helping to prevent cancer and also for treating ulcerative colitis.

Soy may be beneficial in diabetes. A soy extract, pinitol, may improve blood sugar control in diabetics. Also, in addition to its favorable effects on cholesterol, the long-term consumption of a diet rich in soy may reduce blood sugar and improve kidney function in diabetic persons with renal dysfunction. A small study found hints that soy isoflavones might help reduce the buildup of abdominal fat.

A product containing soy isoflavones and other herbs has shown some promise for migraine headaches associated with the menstrual cycle (menstrual migraines). Weak evidence suggests that soy protein may be helpful for cyclic breast pain. Finally, a fermented soy product called natto has shown some promise for dissolving blood clots.

SCIENTIFIC EVIDENCE

High cholesterol. Numerous controlled studies indicate that soy can reduce LDL cholesterol by about 10 percent and perhaps slightly raise HDL cholesterol. It has often been assumed that isoflavones are the active ingredients in soy responsible for improving cholesterol profile. However, studies that used purified isoflavones (as opposed to whole soy, or soy protein) have generally failed to find benefit. It is possible that non-isoflavone constituents of soy, such as proteins, fiber, and phospholipids, may be equally or perhaps even more important than the isoflavones in soy.

In a careful review of thirty studies involving almost three thousand people, researchers determined that isolated soy protein (in the range of 15 to 40 g per day) modestly reduced LDL cholesterol levels by an average of 6 percent. In another study involving two soy milk products, one made from whole soy beans and the other from isolated soy proteins, researchers found that both were more effective than cow's milk at reducing LDL cholesterol levels. In addition, the substance pinitol appears to have cholesterol-lowering properties.

However, there are other possibilities too. One study suggests that the isoflavone daidzein may be effective for reducing cholesterol only when it is converted by intestinal bacterial into a substance called equol. It appears that only about one-third of people have the "right" intestinal bacteria to make equol.

Another study found that soy products may at times have an unusual isoflavone profile, one containing high levels of the isoflavone glycitein rather than the more usual genistein and daidzein. Glycitein could be inactive regarding cholesterol reduction; in other words, variations in the proportions of specific isoflavone constituents might have made some studied soy isoflavone products inactive.

It has also been suggested that soy protein must be kept in its original state to be effective. Ordinary soy protein extracts are somewhat damaged ("denatured"). In a double-blind study of 120 people, a special soy protein extract, in which the proteins were protected from damage, proved more effective for improving cholesterol profile than did standard denatured soy protein extracts.

Hot flashes. Although study results are not entirely consistent, soy may be helpful for symptoms of menopause, especially hot flashes. For example, a double-blind, placebo-controlled study involving 104 women found that isoflavone-rich soy protein provided significant relief of hot flashes compared with placebo (milk protein). Improvements in hot flashes and other menopausal symptoms, such as vaginal dryness, were also seen in several other studies of soy or soy isoflavones. However, about as many studies have failed to find benefit with soy or concentrated isoflavones. Furthermore, in three double-blind, placebo-controlled trials, isoflavone-rich soy failed to reduce hot flashes among those who had had breast cancer.

Another double-blind study, of 241 women experiencing hot flashes, found equivalent benefits for isoflavone-free and isoflavone-rich soy products. The high rate of the placebo effect seen in many studies of menopausal symptoms may account for these discrepancies. In addition, it is possible that certain formulations of soy contain unidentified ingredients beyond isoflavones that play an important role.

Osteoporosis. In one study that evaluated the benefits of soy in osteoporosis, sixty-six postmenopausal women took either placebo (soy protein with isoflavones removed) or soy protein with 56 or 90 mg of isoflavones daily for six months. The group that took the higher dosage of isoflavones showed significant gains in spinal bone density. There was little change in the placebo or low-dose isoflavone groups. This study suggests that the soy isoflavones in soy protein may be effective for osteoporosis. Nearly the same results were seen in a similar study. This twenty-four-week, double-blind study of sixty-nine postmenopausal women found that soy can significantly reduce bone loss from the spine.

Similar benefits with soy or soy isoflavones have been seen in other human and animal trials; however, other studies have failed to find benefit. On balance, it is probably fair to say that isoflavones (either as soy, purified isoflavones, or tofu extract) are likely to have a modestly beneficial effect on bone density at most.

One small but long-term study suggests that progesterone cream (another treatment proposed for

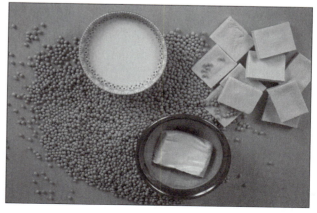

An assortment of soy products is shown here. (Francoise Sauze/Photo Researchers, Inc.)

use in preventing or treating osteoporosis) may decrease the bone-sparing effect of soy isoflavones. Estrogen and most other medications for osteoporosis work by fighting bone breakdown. It has been hypothesized that soy may also work in other ways, by helping to increase new bone formation.

SAFETY ISSUES

Studies in animals have found soy essentially nontoxic. Researchers found no evidence of ill effects when they gave healthy postmenopausal women 900 mg of soy isoflavones a day for eighty-four consecutive days. However, soy or its isoflavones could conceivably have some potentially harmful effects in certain specific situations.

Soy appears to have numerous potential effects involving the thyroid gland. When given to persons with impaired thyroid function, soy products have been observed to reduce absorption of thyroid medication. In addition, some evidence hints that soy isoflavones may directly inhibit the function of the thyroid gland, although this inhibition may be significant only in persons who are deficient in iodine. However, studies of healthy humans and animals given soy isoflavones or other soy products have generally found that soy either had no effect on thyroid hormone levels or actually increased levels.

In view of soy's complex effects regarding the thyroid, persons with impaired thyroid function should not take large amounts of soy products except under the supervision of a physician.

One study found that soy products may decrease testosterone levels in men. This could conceivably cause problems for men with infertility or erectile dysfunction.

Soy may reduce the absorption of the nutrients zinc, iron, and calcium. To avoid absorption problems, one should probably take these minerals a minimum of two hours before or after eating soy.

Other concerns relate to the estrogenic properties of soy isoflavones. For example, while soy is thought to reduce the risk of developing breast cancer, it is possible that soy might not be safe for women who have already had breast cancer. In addition, there are concerns that intensive use of soy products by pregnant women could exert a hormonal effect that impacts unborn fetuses. Finally, fears have been expressed by some experts that soy might interfere with the action of oral contraceptives. However, one study of thirty-six women found reassuring results.

One observational study raised concerns that soy might impair mental function. However, observational studies are highly unreliable by nature, and experts do not consider the results of this study a serious issue. Additionally, a number of studies looking at cognitive improvement have found that soy or soy isoflavones either have no effect on mental function or perhaps minimally improve it.

IMPORTANT INTERACTIONS

It may be best to eat soy at a different time of day to avoid problems absorbing zinc, iron, or calcium supplements. Also, persons taking a thyroid hormone should consult a physician before increasing their intake of soy products.

EBSCO CAM Review Board

FURTHER READING

Arjmandi, B. H., et al. "Soy Protein May Alleviate Osteoarthritis Symptoms." *Phytomedicine* 11 (2005): 567-575.

Fournier, L. R., et al. "The Effects of Soy Milk and Isoflavone Supplements on Cognitive Performance in Healthy, Postmenopausal Women." *Journal of Nutrition, Health, and Aging* 11 (2007): 155-164.

Hooper, L., et al. "Flavonoids, Flavonoid-Rich Foods, and Cardiovascular Risk." *American Journal of Clinical Nutrition* 88 (2008): 38-50.

Kok, L., et al. "A Randomized, Placebo-Controlled Trial on the Effects of Soy Protein Containing Isoflavones on Quality of Life in Postmenopausal Women." *Menopause* 12 (2005): 56-62.

Pawlak, R., B. Malinauskas, and A. Corbett. "Benefits, Barriers, Attitudes, and Beliefs About Soy Meat-Alternatives Among African American Parishioners Living in Eastern North Carolina." *Ethnicity and Disease* 20 (2010): 118-122.

Sites, C. K., et al. "Effect of a Daily Supplement of Soy Protein on Body Composition and Insulin Secretion in Postmenopausal Women." *Fertility and Sterility* 88 (2007): 1609-1617.

See also: Cancer risk reduction; Cholesterol, high; Diabetes; Isoflavone; Menopause; Migraines; Osteoarthritis; Osteoporosis; Ulcerative colitis.

Spirituality

Category: Issues and overviews
Related terms: Faith healing, integrative medicine, prayer, religion
Definition: The use of spirituality, one's sense of meaning in life and relationship with the transcendent, as part of healing in complementary and alternative medicine.

Overview

For many around the world, spirituality plays an integral part in complementary and alternative medicine, or CAM. Large-scale surveys conducted in the United States, Europe, and other parts of the world show that spirituality is associated with higher levels of CAM usage and with the use of a wider variety of CAM modalities to treat many illnesses, including depression, headaches, back and neck pain, gastrointestinal problems, allergies, diabetes, and cancer.

Prayer and other Modalities

Spirituality is considered by some researchers and practitioners to constitute CAM practices per se. Some CAM modalities, such as prayer, are explicitly spiritual in nature, while other modalities, particularly mind/body therapies, often have a spiritual component. The most prominent example of spirituality as CAM is that of prayer, an active process of appealing to a higher spiritual power. Prayer as CAM includes solitary and group prayer on behalf of oneself or others. Based on data from the 2002 National Health Information Survey, the National Center for Complementary and Alternative Medicine (NCCAM) reported in 2004 that prayer for oneself was the most widely used CAM modality among Americans. (It was endorsed by more than 60 percent of survey respondents.) Prayer for others was the second most commonly used modality, and prayer in groups was the fifth most commonly used modality. Older adults, women, and ethnic and racial minorities were more likely to use prayer as CAM.

The NCCAM, however, no longer considers prayer a form of CAM, a change that has led to much controversy. For example, considering prayer a form of CAM leads to increased estimates of CAM usage. Excluding prayer from the definition of CAM, however, does not reflect the true numbers of CAM users.

Another spiritually based CAM is faith healing. This includes therapeutic approaches based on religious faith. Faith healing is most commonly associated with some Christian denominations and is typically conducted in religious communal settings. The therapeutic powers of faith healers are attributed to their evocation of divine or supernatural influences, which may bring about miracles. Relatedly, other cultural and religious traditions feature spiritual healers, such as shamans and curanderos, whose healing powers are largely spiritual in nature. Many traditional cultures do not draw clear distinctions among physical, mental, and spiritual health. In addition to explicitly spiritual modalities, other CAM modalities, such as meditation, yoga, Tai Chi, qigong, and Reiki, often have a spiritual component.

Effectiveness

Evidence regarding the effectiveness of spirituality-based forms of CAM is preliminary, given the many limitations of research and the complexity of the issues. For example, the most common spiritual CAM modality, prayer, is complex and can take many forms, including conversation, intercession, contemplation, and ritual; these different types of prayer may have different effects on health and well-being. Research suggests that some types of prayer can be beneficial to the person praying and can include the alleviation of emotional distress and pain. Such effects have been attributed to increased relaxation, less distraction, an increase in positive emotions, and divine intervention. Research indicates that most people who use prayer as CAM find prayer to be helpful.

More controversial is distance or intercessory prayer, which involves the influence of praying for the health of another person independent of that person's knowledge of the prayer. Intercessory prayer has received much research attention, including attention from researchers using large, randomized control trials. In the aggregate, results are inconsistent and the interpretation of findings remains hotly debated.

Evidence of the effectiveness of faith healing, for example, is sparse. A small but growing body of literature suggests, however, that CAM modalities such as meditation and yoga are more effective in alleviating pain and improving functioning when they include an explicit spiritual component.

Although persons rarely discuss with health care providers their reliance on spirituality as part of their approach to personal health, evidence suggests that such communication may facilitate understanding and promote better care. Approaches to integrative medicine now emphasize the need to pay attention to the spiritual issues and concerns of one's patients.

Crystal L. Park, Ph.D.

FURTHER READING

Barnes, P. M., B. Bloom, and R. L. Nahin. "Complementary and Alternative Medicine Use Among Adults and Children: 2007 United States." *National Health Statistics Reports* 12 (December 10, 2008): 1-23. Results of the second nationwide health survey in the United States and explains why prayer was excluded from the survey's definitions of CAM modalities.

Barnes, P. M., et al. "Complementary and Alternative Medicine Use Among Adults: United States, 2002." *CDC Advance Data Report*, no. 343 (2004). Available at http://nccam.nih.gov/news/camstats/2002/report.pdf. Summarizes the first nationwide survey of CAM usage in the United States and reveals that praying for oneself and for others were by far the most frequently used CAM modalities.

McCaffrey, A. M., et al. "Prayer for Health Concerns: Results of a National Survey on Prevalence and Patterns of Use." *Archives of Internal Medicine* 164, no. 8 (2004): 858-862. Focuses on the frequency and predictors of prayer use as a form of CAM and the potential implications of prayer for health care.

Roberts, L., et al. "Intercessory Prayer for the Alleviation of Ill Health." *Cochrane Database of Systematic Reviews* (2009): CD000368. Reviews findings regarding intercessory prayer and describes the limitations of research on this topic. Available through *EBSCO DynaMed Systematic Literature Surveillance* at http://www.ebscohost.com/dynamed.

Tippens, K., K. Marsman, and H. Zwickey. "Is Prayer CAM?" *Journal of Alternative and Complementary Medicine* 15 (2009): 435-438. Discusses the implications of including prayer in definitions of CAM.

See also: Faith healing; Innate intelligence; Integrative medicine; Meditation; Qigong; Reiki; Tai Chi; Traditional healing; Yoga.

Spirulina

CATEGORY: Herbs and supplements
RELATED TERM: Blue-green algae

DEFINITION: Natural plant product used to treat specific health conditions.
PRINCIPAL PROPOSED USE: Nutritional support
OTHER PROPOSED USES: Cancer prevention, fibromyalgia, hay fever, herpes, high cholesterol, hives, human immunodeficiency virus support, immune support, liver protection, weight loss

OVERVIEW

The supplement known as spirulina consists of one or more members of a family of blue-green algae. The name was inspired by the spiral shapes in which these plants array themselves as they grow. Other blue-green algae products are also available on the market, and they are discussed in this article as well.

Spirulina grows in the wild in salty lakes in Mexico and on the African continent. It reproduces quickly, and because the individual plants tend to stick together, it is easy to harvest. Records of the Spanish conquistadores suggest that the Aztecs used spirulina as a food source; we also know that the Kanembu people of central Africa harvested it from what is now called Lake Chad.

This plant contains high levels of various B vitamins, beta-carotene, other carotenoids, and minerals, including calcium, iron, magnesium, manganese, potassium, and zinc. It is also a source of gamma-linolenic acid (GLA). Spirulina is a rich source of protein (dried spirulina contains up to 70 percent protein by weight) but one would have to ingest a great many spirulina capsules to obtain a significant amount of protein this way. Spirulina also contains vitamin B_{12}, a nutrient otherwise found almost exclusively in animal foods. However, the B_{12} in spirulina is not absorbable.

Spirulina has not been proven effective for any medical condition, and there are significant safety concerns involving all forms of blue-green algae.

REQUIREMENTS AND SOURCES

People other than those living within 35 degrees of the equator or on the shores of alkaline lakes will have difficulty finding spirulina anywhere but in health food stores. Most such stores carry a number of brands of spirulina that has been dried and processed into powder or tablets.

THERAPEUTIC DOSAGES

Researchers studying spirulina's effects on health have used a variety of dosages, ranging from 1 to 8.4 grams (g) daily.

THERAPEUTIC USES

There is no question that spirulina is a nutritious food, but it is not inexpensive. Protein can be obtained much more easily and inexpensively from legumes, nuts, grains, and animal foods; iron from dark greens, prunes, and meat; and carotenes and vitamins from standard fruits and vegetables.

Spirulina might have other specific therapeutic uses beyond general nutritional support, but the evidence supporting these recommendations is highly preliminary at best. Manufacturers of spirulina supplements sometimes claim that the plant can reduce appetite and thereby help overweight individuals control their food intake. However, one small double-blind study of spirulina for weight loss failed to find a significant difference between spirulina and placebo treatment. One small double-blind trial did find evidence that a blue-green alga called *Chlorella pyrenoidosa* might be useful for fibromyalgia.

It is commonly stated that spirulina and related products can enhance immunity. However, most of the evidence supporting this statement is too weak to mean much; the one meaningful trial, a double-blind study of 124 healthy adults, failed to find that chlorella supplements enhanced the immune response to influenza vaccine.

Evidence from animal studies, preliminary human trials, and one small double-blind, placebo-controlled study suggests that spirulina and other forms of algae might improve cholesterol profile. Very preliminary evidence hints that spirulina may help prevent cancer.

Test-tube and animal studies suggest that spirulina might have some activity against human immunodeficiency virus (HIV), but much more research needs to be done before it can be concluded that spirulina is helpful against HIV infection.

Highly preliminary evidence suggests that spirulina or other blue-green algae products may counter allergic reactions, such as hay fever and hives, help protect the liver from toxic chemicals, reduce blood pressure, and control symptoms of ulcerative colitis.

Despite widespread publicity regarding the use of spirulina in the treatment of attention deficit disorder, there is no evidence that spirulina is effective against the disorder.

SCIENTIFIC EVIDENCE

There are no well-documented uses of spirulina.

Fibromyalgia. Fibromyalgia is a common chronic

Combating Global Hunger and Undernourishment with Spirulina

The Intergovernmental Institution for the use of Microalgae Spirulina Against Malnutrition, a United Nations Permanent Inter-Governmental Observer, highlights the benefits of spirulina in fighting global hunger and undernourishment.

Spirulina offers remarkable health benefits to an undernourished person. It is rich in beta carotene that can overcome eye problems caused by vitamin A deficiency. The protein and B-vitamin complex makes a major nutritional improvement in an infant's diet. It is the only food source, except for mother's milk, containing substantial amounts of an essential fatty acid, GLA, that helps regulate the entire hormone system.

One tablespoon a day can eliminate iron anemia, the most common mineral deficiency. Spirulina is the most digestible protein food, especially important for malnourished people whose intestines can no longer absorb nutrients effectively. Clinical studies have shown it helps rebuild healthy intestinal flora. These health benefits have made it an excellent food for rapid recovery of children from malnutrition-related diseases in Mexico, Togo, Romania, China, Rwanda, Zaire, India, Ukraine, and Belarus. Spirulina is being produced in more than twenty-two countries and used in over seventy-seven countries.

The United Nations World Health Organization (WHO) has confirmed that spirulina represents an interesting food for multiple reasons, and it is able to be administered to children without any risk. Other proposed uses of spirulina are for cancer prevention, fibromyalgia, hay fever, herpes infection, high cholesterol, hives, HIV infection, liver protection, [and] weight loss.

Source: http://www.iimsam.org.

condition, the main symptoms of which are specific tender points on various parts of the body, widespread musculoskeletal discomfort, morning stiffness, fatigue, and disturbed sleep. The cause of fibromyalgia is not known, and current treatments are far from completely satisfactory. A recent study suggests that the nutritious algae *C. pyrenoidosa* might be helpful. In this double-blind, placebo-controlled trial, thirty-seven people with fibromyalgia were given either placebo or chlorella supplements at a dose of 10 g daily.

At the end of three months, the individuals were switched to the opposite group and then treated for an additional three months. The results showed significant improvements in symptoms when participants used chlorella compared with placebo.

Weight loss. A double-blind, placebo-controlled trial investigated the possible weight-loss effects of spirulina. However, while individuals taking 8.4 g of spirulina daily lost weight, the difference between the spirulina group and the placebo group was not statistically significant. Larger and longer studies are needed to establish whether spirulina is indeed an effective treatment for obesity.

SAFETY ISSUES

Spirulina itself appears to be nontoxic. Studies in rats showed that high spirulina intake caused no weight reduction or toxicity symptoms in rats, nor did spirulina affect the rats' ability to reproduce normally.

Nevertheless, there are areas of serious concern for consumers. Various forms of blue-green algae can be naturally contaminated with highly toxic substances called microcystins. Some states, such as Oregon, place strict limits on the concentration of microcystins allowed in blue-green algae products, but the same protections cannot be assumed to have been applied to all products on the market. Furthermore, the maximum safe intake of microcystins is not clear, and it is possible that when individuals use blue-green algae for a long time, toxic effects might build up. Long-term use by children raises particular concerns, especially in light of the widely popularized, but unsubstantiated, belief that blue-green algae is useful for attention deficit disorder. Blue-green algae can also contain a different kind of highly toxic substance called anatoxin.

In addition, when spirulina is grown with the use of fermented animal waste fertilizers, contamination with dangerous bacteria can occur. There are also concerns that spirulina might concentrate radioactive ions found in its environment. Probably of most concern is spirulina's ability to absorb and concentrate heavy metals such as lead and mercury if they are present in its environment.

One study of spirulina samples grown in a number of locations found them to contain unacceptably high levels of these toxic metals. However, a second study on this topic claimed that the first used an unreliable method of analyzing heavy-metal content and concluded that a person would have to eat more than 77 g daily of the most heavily contaminated spirulina to reach unsafe mercury and lead consumption levels. These researchers, however, went on to suggest that it is not prudent to eat more than 50 g of spirulina daily because the plant contains a high concentration of nucleic acids, substances related to DNA. When these are metabolized, they create uric acid, which could cause gout or kidney stones. This is of special concern to those who have already had uric acid stones or attacks of gout. The safety of the use of spirulina by pregnant and nursing women, young children, and individuals with kidney or liver disease has not been determined.

EBSCO CAM Review Board

FURTHER READING

Cingi, C., et al. "The Effects of Spirulina on Allergic Rhinitis." *European Archives of Oto-Rhino-Laryngology* 265 (2008): 1219-1223.

Dillon, J. C., A. P. Phuc, and J. P. Dubacq. "Nutritional Value of the Alga Spirulina." *World Review of Nutrition and Dietetics* 77 (1995): 32-46.

Halperin, S. A., et al. "Safety and Immunoenhancing Effect of a Chlorella-Derived Dietary Supplement in Healthy Adults Undergoing Influenza Vaccination." *Canadian Medical Association Journal* 169 (2003): 111-117.

Jochimsen, E. M., et al. "Liver Failure and Death After Exposure to Microcystins at a Hemodialysis Center in Brazil." *New England Journal of Medicine* 338 (2003): 873-878.

Mao, T. K., et al. "Effects of a Spirulina-Based Dietary Supplement on Cytokine Production from Allergic Rhinitis Patients." *Journal of Medicinal Food* 8 (2005): 27-30.

Merchant, R. E., and C. A. Andre. "A Review of Recent Clinical Trials of the Nutritional Supplement *Chlorella pyrenoidosa* in the Treatment of Fibromyalgia, Hypertension, and Ulcerative Colitis." *Alternative Therapies in Health and Medicine* 7 (2001): 79-80, 82-91.

Shaish, A., et al. "9-Cis Beta-Carotene-Rich Powder of the Alga *Dunaliella bardawil* Increases Plasma HDL-Cholesterol in Fibrate-Treated Patients." *Atherosclerosis* 189 (2006): 215-221.

See also: Allergies; Cancer risk reduction; Cholesterol, high; Fibromyalgia: Homeopathic remedies; Hives; HIV support.

Spleen extract

CATEGORY: Herbs and supplements

DEFINITION: Natural substance derived from nonhuman animals and used as a supplement to strengthen the immune system.

PRINCIPAL PROPOSED USE: Immune support

OVERVIEW

The spleen is an organ located under the left side of the rib cage. Its functions in the body include removing "worn-out" red blood cells and supplying certain types of white blood cells (immune cells). For use as a supplement, spleen extracts are made from the spleens of cows, pigs, or other animals.

According to a theory prevalent in some parts of alternative medicine, the consumption of spleen extracts can strengthen the function of an underperforming spleen. On this basis, spleen extracts are sometimes suggested for supporting the immune system. However, there is no meaningful scientific rationale or scientific evidence to indicate that this approach actually works.

Some manufacturers of glandular products claim that the animal version of an organ provides nutrients that support the corresponding organ in humans. However, there is no evidence that the human spleen requires any nutrients that are uniquely available in animal spleens.

It has been suggested by one manufacturer that consuming extracts of an organ might offer benefit in an indirect manner. According to this theory, some people may possess antibodies to certain of their own organs, and if they consume a similar organ, these antibodies will be diverted from their target. However, this explanation does not make a great deal of sense. Antibodies are primarily produced against proteins, and even if cow spleens had the same proteins as human spleens, which is unlikely, proteins are digested in the intestines and not absorbed whole into the bloodstream.

It may be that, on an unconscious level, those who recommend glandular extracts are being influenced by the ancient notion of "sympathetic magic"–the idea that eating a lion's heart, for example, will create courage. However, this is a prescientific form of reasoning that is difficult to take seriously in the modern era.

In any case, there is no meaningful scientific evidence to indicate that the use of spleen extracts offers any benefits. Only double-blind, placebo-controlled studies can show a treatment effective, and at present none have been reported for spleen extracts. The only published studies on oral use of spleen glandular extracts date back to the 1930s and do not remotely reach current scientific standards. More recent studies have evaluated injected extracts of spleen, but these findings are not likely to apply to the oral product.

EBSCO CAM Review Board

FURTHER READING

Gray, G. A. "The Treatment of Agranulocytic Angina with Fetal Calf Spleen." *Texas State Journal of Medicine* 29 (1933): 366-369.

Greer, A. E. "Use of Fetal Spleen in Agranulocytosis: Preliminary Report." *Texas State Journal of Medicine* 28 (1932): 338-343.

Minter, M. M. "Agranulocytic Angina: Treatment of a Case with Fetal Calf Spleen." *Texas State Journal of Medicine* 29 (1933): 338-343.

See also: Adrenal extract.

Sports and fitness support: Enhancing performance

CATEGORY: Condition

RELATED TERM: Ergogenic aids

DEFINITION: Treatment to enhance athletic performance and fitness.

PRINCIPAL PROPOSED NATURAL TREATMENTS: Creatine, hydroxymethyl butyrate

OTHER PROPOSED NATURAL TREATMENTS: Acupuncture, alanine, antioxidant vitamins, arginine, branched-chain amino acids, caffeine, carnitine, chromium, citrulline, ciwujia, coenzyme Q_{10}, *Cordyceps, Cystoseira canariensis,* deer antler, dehydroepiandrosterone, dihydroxyacetone pyruvate, galactose, gamma oryzanol, ginseng, glutamine, guarana, human growth hormone enhancers, inosine, iron, lipoic acid, low-glycemic-index diet, magnesium, ma huang (ephedra), medium-chain triglycerides, methoxyisoflavone, multivitamins, nicotinamide adenine dinucleotide, ornithine alpha-ketoglutarate, *Panax notoginseng,* pantothenic acid-pantethine, phosphate, phosphatidylserine, policosanol,

Rhodiola rosea, ribose, schisandra, suma, *Tribulus terrestris*, trimethylglycine, whey protein

HERBS AND SUPPLEMENTS TO USE ONLY WITH CAUTION: Androstenedione, boron, vanadium

INTRODUCTION

In the competitive world of sports, the smallest advantage can make an enormous difference in the outcome of a contest. A substance that improves an athlete's strength, speed, or endurance is called an ergogenic aid.

The most effective ergogenic aids (stimulants, anabolic steroids, and human growth hormone) are both dangerous and illegal. Numerous natural options are marketed as alternatives. The many supplements used in the hope of improving sports performance are discussed here.

PRINCIPAL PROPOSED NATURAL TREATMENTS

Two natural supplements have shown meaningful promise as ergogenic aids: creatine and hydroxymethyl butyrate.

Creatine. Creatine, one of the best-selling and best-documented supplements for enhancing athletic performance, is a naturally occurring substance that plays an important role in the production of energy in the body. The body converts creatine to phosphocreatine, a form of stored energy used by muscles. In theory, taking supplemental creatine will build up a reserve of phosphocreatine in the muscles to help them perform on demand. Supplemental creatine may also help the body make new phosphocreatine faster when it has been used up by intense activity. However, the balance of evidence suggests that if creatine supplements have any benefit for sports performance, it is slight and limited to highly specific forms of exercise.

Several small double-blind studies have found that creatine can improve performance in exercises that involve repeated short bursts of high-intensity activity with intervening rest periods of adequate length. A double-blind, placebo-controlled study investigated creatine and swimming performance in eighteen men and fourteen women. Men taking the supplement had significant increases in speed when doing six bouts of fifty-meter swims started at three-minute intervals, compared to men taking placebo. However, their speed did not improve when swimming ten sets of twenty-five-yard lengths started at one-minute intervals. Researchers theorize that the shorter rest time

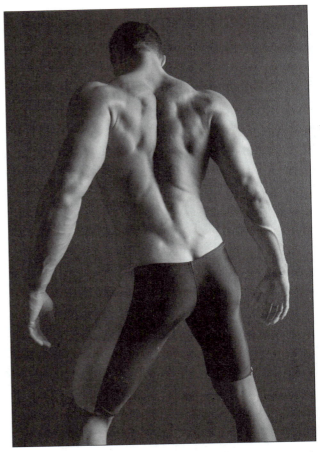

Muscular athletic male body. (© Maxfx/Dreamstime.com)

between laps was not enough for the swimmers' bodies to resynthesize phosphocreatine.

None of the women enrolled in the study showed any improvement with the creatine supplement. The authors of this study noted that women normally have more creatine in their muscle tissue than do men, so perhaps creatine supplementation (at least at this level) is not of benefit to women, as it appears to be for men. Further research is needed to fully understand the difference between the genders in response to creatine.

In an earlier double-blind study, sixteen physical education students carried out ten six-second bursts of extremely intense exercise on a stationary bicycle, separated by thirty seconds of rest. The results showed that the students who took 20 grams (g) of creatine for six days were better able to maintain cycle speed throughout the repetitions. Many other studies showed similar improvements in performance capacity involving repeated bursts of action. However, there have been negative results too; in general, minimal to no benefits have been seen in studies involving athletes engaged in normal sports rather than contrived laboratory tests.

In contrast, studies of endurance or nonrepetitive aerobic-burst exercise generally have not shown benefits from creatine supplementation. Therefore, creatine probably will not help with marathon running or single sprints.

In addition to repetitive burst exercise, creatine has also shown promise for increasing isometric exercise capacity (pushing against a fixed resistance). Also, two double-blind, placebo-controlled studies, each lasting twenty-eight days, provide some evidence that creatine and creatine plus hydroxymethyl butyrate can increase lean muscle and bone mass. However, one double-blind trial failed to find creatine helpful for enhancing general fitness, including resistance exercise performance, in elderly men. The contradictory results seen in these small trials suggest that creatine offers at most a very modest sports performance benefit.

Hydroxymethyl butyrate. Beta-hydroxy beta-methylbutyric acid (HMB) is a chemical that occurs naturally in the body when the amino acid leucine breaks down. Leucine is found in particularly high concentrations in muscles. During athletic training, damage to the muscles leads to the breakdown of leucine and to increased HMB levels. Some evidence suggests that taking HMB supplements might signal the body to slow down the destruction of muscle tissue. On this basis, HMB has been studied as a sports performance supplement for enhancing strength and muscle mass.

According to many of the small double-blind trials that have been reported, HMB appears to improve muscle-growth response to weight training. For example, in a controlled study, forty-one male volunteers age nineteen to twenty-nine years were given either 0, 1.5, or 3 g of HMB daily for three weeks. The participants also lifted weights three days per week according to a defined (and rather severe) schedule. The results suggested that HMB can enhance strength and muscle mass in direct proportion to intake.

In another controlled study reported in the same article, thirty-two male volunteers took either 3 g of HMB or placebo daily and then lifted weights for two or three hours daily, six days per week, for seven

weeks. The HMB group saw a significantly greater increase in bench-press strength than the placebo group. However, there was no significant difference in body weight or fat mass by the end of the study.

Similarly, a double-blind, placebo-controlled trial of thirty-nine men and thirty-six women found that in four weeks, HMB supplementation improved response to weight training. Two placebo-controlled studies of women found that 3 g of HMB had no effect on lean body mass and strength in sedentary women, but it did provide an additional benefit when combined with weight training. Also, a double-blind study of thirty-one men and women, all seventy years old and undergoing resistance training, found significant improvements in fat-free mass attributable to the use of HMB (3 g daily).

However, there have been negative studies too, but all were small, so their results are ultimately not reliable. Larger studies will be necessary to truly establish whether HMB is helpful for power athletes working to enhance strength and muscle mass.

OTHER PROPOSED NATURAL TREATMENTS

Numerous other supplements are marketed as ergogenic aids, said to improve speed, strength, or endurance. However, the evidence that they work is marginal at best, and in many cases the best available evidence indicates that these substances are not effective.

Ginseng. There are three different herbs commonly called ginseng: Asian or Korean ginseng (*Panax ginseng*), American ginseng (*Panax quinquefolius*), and Siberian ginseng (*Eleutherococcus senticosus*). The latter is not truly ginseng, but the Russian scientists responsible for promoting it believed that it functioned identically and named it ginseng. According to some experts, a fourth herb, ciwujia, is actually *Eleutherococcus*, while others claim it is a related but different species.

Ginseng has shown some promise as a mild ergogenic aid, but published evidence remains at best incomplete and contradictory. Other forms of ginseng generally lack any meaningful supporting evidence.

For example, an eight-week, double-blind, placebo-controlled trial evaluated the effects of *P. ginseng* with and without exercise in forty-one people. The participants were given either *P. ginseng* or placebo and then underwent exercise training or remained untrained throughout the study. The results showed that ginseng improved aerobic capacity in people who did not exercise but offered no benefit in those who did exercise.

In a nine-week, double-blind, placebo-controlled trial of thirty highly trained athletes, treatment with *P. ginseng* or *P. ginseng* plus vitamin E produced significant improvements in aerobic capacity. Another double-blind, placebo-controlled trial of thirty-seven participants also found some benefit. Also, a double-blind, placebo-controlled study of 120 people found that *P. ginseng* gradually improved reaction time and lung function in a twelve-week treatment period among participants from forty to sixty years of age. (No benefits were seen in younger people.)

However, in an eight-week double-blind trial that followed sixty healthy men in their twenties, no benefit with *P. ginseng* could be demonstrated. Many other small trials of *P. ginseng* have failed to find evidence of benefit. These mixed outcomes suggest that ginseng is only slightly effective at best.

A double-blind study of twenty endurance athletes in eight weeks failed to find evidence of benefit with a standard *Eleutherococcus* formulation. Furthermore, in a small, double-blind, placebo-controlled trial of endurance athletes, the use of *Eleutherococcus* actually increased physiologic signs of stress during intensive training. Ciwujia has not yet been studied in meaningful double-blind trials.

Medium-chain triglycerides. Medium-chain triglycerides (MCTs) are fats with an unusual chemical structure that allows the body to digest them easily. Most fats are broken down in the intestine and reassembled into a special form that can be transported in the blood. However, MCTs are absorbed intact and taken to the liver, where they are used directly for energy. In this sense, they are processed like carbohydrates. For that reason, MCTs have been proposed as an alternative to carbo-loading (consumption of a large quantity of carbohydrates before intense physical exercise) for providing a concentrated source of easily utilized energy.

A number of double-blind studies have evaluated MCTs' effects on high-intensity or endurance exercise performance, but the results have been thoroughly inconsistent. This is not surprising because all of the studies were too small to properly eliminate the effects of chance.

Iron. The majority of athletes are probably not iron-deficient, and people should not take iron supplements if they already have enough iron in their bodies. However, if a person is deficient in this essential mineral, iron supplements may enhance athletic training.

A double-blind, placebo-controlled trial of forty-two nonanemic women with evidence of slightly low iron reserves found that iron supplements significantly increased the benefits gained from exercise. Participants were put on a daily aerobic training program for the latter four weeks of this six-week trial. At the end of the trial, those receiving iron showed significantly greater gains in speed and endurance than those given placebo. In addition, a double-blind, placebo-controlled study of forty nonanemic elite athletes with mildly low iron stores found that twelve weeks of iron supplementation enhanced aerobic performance.

Benefits with iron supplementation for marginally iron-depleted athletes were observed in other double-blind trials too. However, several other studies failed to find significant improvements. These contradictory results suggest that the benefits of iron supplements for nonanemic, iron-deficient athletes is small at most.

Colostrum. Colostrum is the fluid that new mothers' breasts produce during the first day or two after birth. Colostrum contains growth factors, such as IGF-1, that could enhance muscle development, and on this basis it has been tried as a sports supplement.

An eight-week double-blind study found that the use of colostrum enhanced sprinting performance. Other double-blind studies found improvements in rowing performance and in vertical jump.

In addition, one small double-blind study found that colostrum, compared to whey protein, increased lean mass in healthy men and women undergoing aerobic and resistance training. However, no improvements in performance were seen in this trial.

Finally, in a double-blind, placebo-controlled study, the use of colostrum in an eight-week training period did not improve performance on an exercise-to-exhaustion test; however, it did improve performance on a repeat bout twenty minutes later. Research suggests that the growth factor IGF-1 in colostrum is not directly absorbed into the body, yet consumption of colostrum nonetheless increases IGF-1 levels in the blood, perhaps by stimulating its natural release.

Pyruvate. Pyruvate, also called dihydroxyacetone pyruvate, supplies the body with pyruvic acid, a natural compound that plays important roles in the manufacture and use of energy. Pyruvate supplements have become popular with bodybuilders and other athletes based on slim evidence that pyruvate can improve body composition. However, the evidence regarding pyruvate as an ergogenic aid is weak and contradictory at best. One study failed to find that pyruvate supplements improved body composition or exercise performance; furthermore, pyruvate appeared to negate the beneficial effect of exercise on cholesterol profile.

Policosanol. Policosanol is a mixture of waxy substances manufactured from sugarcane. It contains octacosanol, which is also made from wheat germ oil. Both are marketed as performance-enhancing dietary supplements said to increase muscle strength and endurance and to improve reaction time and stamina. However, the only evidence for policosanol as a performance enhancer comes from one small double-blind trial with marginal results.

Phosphatidylserine. Phosphatidylserine (PS) is a phospholipid and a major component of cell membranes. Good evidence suggests that PS can improve mental function, especially in the elderly. However, PS has also been marketed as a sports supplement, said to help bodybuilders and power athletes develop larger and stronger muscles. This claim is based on modest evidence indicating that PS slows the release of cortisol following heavy exercise.

Cortisol is a hormone that causes muscle tissue to break down. For reasons that are unclear, the body produces increased levels of cortisol after heavy exercise. Strength athletes who believe natural cortisol release works against their efforts to rapidly build muscle mass hope that PS will help them advance more quickly. However, only two double-blind, placebo-controlled studies of PS as a sports supplement have been reported, and neither found effects on cortisol levels. Of these small trials, one found a possible ergogenic benefit and the other did not.

Another study evaluated the use of phosphatidylserine for improving the performance of golfers. While improvement in perceived stress levels failed to reach statistical significance, participants who were given phosphatidylserine did tee-off successfully at a greater rate than those given placebo.

Branched-chain amino acids: leucine, isoleucine, and valine. Amino acids are molecules that form proteins when joined together. Three of them (leucine, isoleucine, and valine) are called branched-chain amino acids (BCAAs), a term that describes the shape of the molecules. Muscles have a particularly high BCAA content.

Both strength training and endurance exercise use greater amounts of BCAAs than normal daily activities, perhaps increasing an athlete's need for dietary intake of these amino acids. Sports such as mountaineering and skiing may cause even greater depletion of BCAAs because of metabolic changes that occur at higher altitudes. Athletes have tried BCAA supplements to build muscle, improve performance, postpone fatigue, and cure overtraining syndrome (prolonged fatigue and other symptoms caused by excessive exercise). However, most of the evidence suggests that BCAAs are not helpful for these purposes.

Whey protein is rich in BCAAs, and on this basis, it has also been proposed as a bodybuilding aid. However, there is little evidence that whey protein is more effective for this purpose than any other protein. One small double-blind study found evidence that both casein and whey protein were more effective than placebo at promoting muscle growth after exercise, but whey was no more effective than the far less expensive casein. Another study failed to find benefits with combined whey and soy protein supplementation. However, a single small study did find ergogenic benefits with whey compared to casein.

Other amino acids. Besides BCAAs, athletes use a number of other amino acids, sometimes individually and sometimes in combination. Amino acids believed by some to have ergogenic effects include arginine, glutamine, and ornithine (ornithine and glutamine combined form ornithine alpha-ketoglutarate), and the branched-chain amino acids leucine, isoleucine, and valine. However, evidence supporting the use of amino acids as ergogenic aids is sparse to nonexistent. The few clinical trials performed generally do not show positive results.

Carnitine. Carnitine, a substance closely related to amino acids, is used by the body to convert fat into energy. Even though the body can manufacture all it needs, supplemental carnitine could, in theory, improve the ability of certain tissues to produce energy, leading to its promotion as a sports performance enhancer. However, there is no meaningful evidence that this is the case.

Chromium. The mineral chromium has been sold as a "fat burner" and is also said to help build muscle tissue. However, studies evaluating its benefits as a performance enhancer and studies assessing its effectiveness as an aid to bodybuilding have yielded almost entirely negative results.

Yoga for Athletes

Athletes can enjoy the stress relief and deep relaxation of yoga as much as anyone. Experts on yoga claim compelling reasons for athletes to try yoga. Although there are many kinds of yoga, for simplicity's sake, four of the more popular types are discussed here. The claims made for the following types of yoga are not evidence-based but, rather, represent the opinions of yoga teachers:

Iyengar yoga. Iyengar yoga practitioners use props such as blocks and belts to aid them in performing many of the more difficult postures, and great attention is paid to a precise alignment of postures. Iyengar practitioners claim that this type of yoga improves body awareness (awareness of how you sit, stand, walk, and so forth), balance, flexibility, and endurance. They also claim that it improves circulation, aids digestion, and reduces tension.

- *Focus*: Posture, alignment, and balance. It also focuses on extension and achieving greater symmetry in the body.

- *General benefits*: This type of yoga builds strength and endurance early on.

- *Benefit to athletes*: Body awareness may improve overall performance and may help prevent injury.

- *Kundalini yoga.* Kundalini yoga involves postures, meditation, and the coordination of breath.

- *Focus*: Breath and breathing techniques (more so than the other types mentioned here). It focuses on body awareness from the inside out. It is a combination of physical work and meditation, with more of an emphasis on the latter.

- *General benefits*: Kundalini yoga is purported to make the nervous system stronger, which may enable you to better handle stress. It may also improve mental clarity, which increases your ability to concentrate more fully on a sport. Kundalini yoga tones the entire body but makes the muscles pliable rather than tight.

- *Benefit to athletes*: Learning to breathe deeply (belly breathing) may help prevent injuries because the body is more relaxed.

Power yoga. In power yoga, rooms are often heated to 90° Fahrenheit to make the muscles malleable. After a warm-up, students do a series of sun salutations (a series of poses that flow one into another without stopping). Then, they perform a series of standing poses to stretch and strengthen the legs and back. After practicing a series of floor poses, class ends with relaxation.

- *Focus*: Strength, endurance, flexibility, and balance. Because the poses are linked and flow one into another, it is more aerobic than the other types of yoga mentioned here.

- *General benefits*: This style of yoga strengthens and stabilizes the core and allows for greater freedom of movement. It may help improve stamina, flexibility, and reaction time. It also teaches you how to coordinate your breathing with physical movements.

- *Benefit to athletes*: "Power yoga takes the whole body through a full range of motion, strengthens it isometrically, and fixes imbalances caused by sports training," says Baptiste.

Kripalu yoga. Kripalu yoga is delineated into three stages: learning the postures and exploring the body's ability, holding the postures for an extended time and developing an inner awareness, and moving from one posture to another in a spontaneous movement.

- *Focus*: Releasing chronic tension and energizing the physical systems of the body. It focuses on the sensation of yoga—how your body feels.

- *General benefits*: Kripalu yoga helps release chronic muscle tension to allow for a full range of motion in joints and to relax you deeply. It brings peace of mind, strengthens your body, and teaches you how to harness energy and strength.

- *Benefit to athletes*: Kripalu yoga is a full-body exercise that can help correct imbalances created by repetitive motion.

While it is not entirely clear if yoga can enhance athletic performance, the increased flexibility and relaxation, improved core strength, and variation in exercise that yoga can bring to your routine make it a good practice for most people.

Yoga is generally considered a very safe exercise. However, as with any sport or other physical activity, approach to yoga requires professional guidance, especially if one is a beginner. Injuries are not common with yoga; however, they may happen, especially if the exercises are done haphazardly or without a proper warm-up. The best way to prevent injuries is to progress slowly, listen to your body, and remember that yoga is not about competition.

Ann E. Boehler; reviewed by Brian Randall, M.D.

Coenzyme Q_{10}. Coenzyme Q_{10} (CoQ_{10}) is a natural substance that plays a fundamental role in the mitochondria, the parts of the cell that produce energy from food. On this basis, CoQ_{10} has been proposed as a performance enhancer for athletes. However, most clinical trials have found no significant improvement with the use of CoQ_{10}.

Inosine. Inosine is an important chemical found throughout the body. It plays many roles, one of which is helping to make ATP, the body's main form of usable energy. Based primarily on this fact, inosine supplements have been proposed as an energy booster for athletes. However, most of the available evidence suggests that it does not work.

Ribose. Ribose is a carbohydrate that is also vital for the manufacture of ATP. Ribose has shown some promise for improving exercise capacity in people with certain enzyme deficiencies and other rare conditions that cause muscle pain during exertion. On this basis, it has been touted as an athletic performance enhancer; however, six small, double-blind, placebo-controlled trials in humans failed to find any benefit. In one of these studies, dextrose (a form of ordinary sugar), proved effective while ribose did not.

Gamma oryzanol. Preliminary evidence suggests that gamma oryzanol, a substance derived from rice bran oil, may increase endorphin release and aid muscle development. These findings have created interest in using gamma oryzanol as a sports supplement. However, a nine-week, double-blind, placebo-controlled trial of twenty-two weight-trained males found no difference between placebo and 500 mg daily of gamma oryzanol in terms of performance, body composition, or hormone levels.

Trimethylglycine. Trimethylglycine (TMG) is a naturally occurring compound that may help to prevent atherosclerosis. It is, therefore, sometimes taken as a supplement. In the course of its metabolism in the body, TMG is turned into another substance, dimethylglycine (DMG).

In Russia, DMG is used extensively as an athletic performance enhancer, and it has recently become popular among American athletes. TMG is less expensive, and it may have the same effects as DMG, inasmuch as it changes into DMG in the body. However, there is no evidence that DMG is effective and even some evidence that it is not.

Dehydroepiandrosterone. Athletes have used dehydroepiandrosterone (DHEA) on the belief that (like phosphatidylserine) it might limit the body's response to cortisol and thereby cause an increase in muscle tissue growth. However, study results have not established whether or not DHEA really interferes with cortisol. Furthermore, studies of DHEA as an aid to increasing muscle mass or enhancing sports performance have produced mixed results at best.

Tribulus terrestris. Tribulus terrestris is a tropical plant with a long history of medicinal use. It has been tried for low libido in both men and women, and for impotence and female infertility.

One theory regarding how *T. terrestris* might help with sexual disorders is that a component from the plant called protodioscine is converted into the hormone DHEA in the body. DHEA is used by the body as a building block for both testosterone and estrogen (and other hormones). This finding has led bodybuilders and strength athletes to try *T. terrestris* for increasing muscular development. However, the scientific evidence seems to be against it. This is not surprising, because DHEA itself has not been found effective as a sports supplement.

One study involving fifteen men compared the effects of *T. terrestris* (3.21 mg per kilogram of body weight; for example, 292 mg daily for a two-hundred-pound man) with placebo on body composition and endurance among men engaged in resistance training. At the end of the eight-week study, the only significant difference between the treatment and placebo groups was that the placebo group showed greater gains in endurance.

Another double-blind, placebo-controlled study, which enrolled twenty-two athletes and followed them for five weeks, failed to find benefit. The dose used in this trial was fixed at 450 mg daily for all participants.

Phosphate. Because phosphate plays a fundamental role in the body's energy-producing pathways, it has been suggested that taking high doses of phosphate (phosphate loading) before athletic activities might enhance performance. Phosphate-containing chemicals are also part of the process that allows oxygen release from hemoglobin, and this too has intrigued researchers looking for ergogenic aids. However, while some studies have found that phosphate loading improves maximum oxygen utilization, others have not. Flaws in study design cast doubt on the positive results.

Commercial preparations. A small double-blind study of a mixture of various herbs and supplements marketed as SPORT found no evidence that it can improve sports performance in trained athletes.

Stimulants: Ma huang and caffeine. A number of plant-derived stimulants are used by some athletes to improve their performance. These stimulants include ephedrine from the Chinese herb ma huang (also called ephedra) and caffeine from coffee, tea, maté, cola, or guarana (a plant native to South America). Both ephedrine and caffeine are central nervous system stimulants. Caffeine also appears to change the way the body burns calories, possibly allowing it to burn fats first and preserve muscle glycogen for later in an athletic performance (in a way, "saving the best for last").

Caffeine does appear to improve performance during endurance-type exercises. The International Olympic Committee has set a tolerance limit for caffeine in the urine at 12 micrograms per milliliter.

Ephedrine's value in enhancing sports performance has not been established; at the same time, there are serious safety issues associated with its use. Some sports federations have determined that specific amounts of ephedrine in an athlete's system are grounds for disqualification.

Other. One small double-blind trial found that the use of the herb *Rhodiola rosea* improved endurance exercise performance. However, another study failed to find benefit with a combination of *Cordyceps* and *Rhodiola*.

A variety of antioxidants have been proposed for enhancing recovery after heavy exercise. One study found weak evidence that a combination of vitamin E (400 mg daily) and vitamin C (1,000 mg daily) taken for three weeks can improve aerobic performance.

Heavy exercise causes increased calcium loss through sweat, and the body does not compensate for this by reducing calcium loss in the urine. The result can be a net calcium loss great enough so that it presents health concerns for menopausal women, who are already at risk for osteoporosis. One study found that the use of an inexpensive calcium supplement (calcium carbonate), taken at a dose of 400 mg twice daily, is sufficient to offset this loss.

A small study found endurance exercise benefits with the herb *Panax notoginseng*. Another small trial suggests that acupuncture may enhance peak performance capacity. Weak evidence hints that arachidonic acid supplements might enhance response to resistance training.

The use of a low-glycemic-index snack three hours before endurance running may be more helpful than a high-glycemic-index (carbohydrate) snack. However, another study failed to find benefit.

Galactose is a type of sugar that the body combines with glucose to create lactose ("milk sugar"). For various theoretical reasons, it has been hypothesized that the use of galactose might enhance endurance exercise performance. However, the one small study designed to test this hypothesis found, instead, that the consumption of galactose before endurance exercise actually proved detrimental.

A small double-blind study failed to find any performance or training-enhancing benefits with a newly marketed silicate product. Also failing to show benefit in preliminary trials are astaxanthin, fish oil, N-acetylcysteine, soy isoflavones, and tyrosine.

Numerous other natural substances have been marketed as ergogenic aids, despite an essentially absolute absence of evidence that they help. These substances include *Cordyceps*, *Cystoseira canariensis*, deer antler, ipriflavone, lipoic acid, methoxyisoflavone, nicotinamide adenine dinucleotide, and suma. One study found that L-citrulline, another purported ergogenic aid, actually decreases exercise capacity.

Many marketers sell products that they claim will act like human growth hormone, often called HGH enhancers. However, these products are entirely speculative because there are no natural treatments proven to raise human growth hormone levels. Similarly, there are no herbs or supplements known to act as "natural anabolic steroids."

One small study failed to find benefit with a liquid multivitamin-multimineral supplement. Also, the amino acid beta-alanine is said to raise levels of carnosine, which in turn is hypothesized to enhance performance in athletes undergoing resistance training. However, a double-blind study of twenty-six athletes failed to find benefit with 6 g of alanine daily.

TREATMENTS NOT RECOMMENDED

Three commonly recommended supplements are not recommended for athletes: vanadium, boron, and androstenedione. The mineral vanadium has been suggested for use by bodybuilders based on its effects on insulin, but there is no evidence that it helps. A double-blind, placebo-controlled study involving thirty-one weight-trained athletes found no benefit of supplementation at more than one thousand times the nutritional dose. Furthermore, there are serious safety concerns about taking vanadium at such high doses.

The mineral boron has been proposed as a sports supplement because it is thought to increase testosterone levels. However, studies have failed to provide meaningful evidence that it helps increase muscle mass or enhance performance. Furthermore, clinical studies suggest that boron supplementation is more likely to increase estrogen than testosterone. Increased estrogen is not likely to have a sports performance benefit in men, and in women it might increase the risk of breast cancer. Therefore, supplemental boron is not recommended as a sports supplement.

The hormone androstenedione is said to enhance athletic performance and strength by increasing testosterone production, thereby building muscle. However, in double-blind studies, when androstenedione was given to men, it neither altered total testosterone levels nor improved sports performance, strength, or lean body mass. It did, however, increase estrogen levels, an effect that would not be considered favorable. Androstenedione does appear to raise testosterone levels in women, but it is not clear whether this would produce favorable results.

EBSCO CAM Review Board

FURTHER READING

Candow, D. G., et al. "Effect of Whey and Soy Protein Supplementation Combined with Resistance Training in Young Adults." *International Journal of Sport Nutrition and Exercise Metabolism* 16 (2006): 233-244.

Chilibeck, P. D., et al. "Effect of Creatine Ingestion After Exercise on Muscle Thickness in Males and Females." *Medicine and Science in Sports and Exercise* 36 (2004): 1781-1788.

De Bock, K., et al. "Acute *Rhodiola rosea* Intake Can Improve Endurance Exercise Performance." *International Journal of Sport Nutrition and Exercise Metabolism* 14 (2004): 298-307.

Earnest, C. P., et al. "Low vs. High Glycemic Index Carbohydrate Gel Ingestion During Simulated 64-km Cycling Time Trial Performance." *Journal of Strength and Conditioning Research* 18 (2004): 466-472.

Fry, A. C., et al. "Effect of a Liquid Multivitamin/Mineral Supplement on Anaerobic Exercise Performance." *Research in Sports Medicine* 14 (2006): 53-64.

Igwebuike, A., et al. "Lack of DHEA Effect on a Combined Endurance and Resistance Exercise Program in Postmenopausal Women." *Journal of Clinical Endocrinology and Metabolism* 93 (2008): 534-538.

Kendrick, I. P., et al. "The Effects of Ten Weeks of Resistance Training Combined with Beta-Alanine Supplementation on Whole Body Strength, Force Production, Muscular Endurance, and Body Composition." *Amino Acids* 34 (2008): 547-554.

Martin, B. R., et al. "Exercise and Calcium Supplementation: Effects on Calcium Homeostasis in Sportswomen." *Medicine and Science in Sports and Exercise* 39 (2007): 1481-1486.

Rogerson, S., et al. "The Effect of Five Weeks of *Tribulus terrestris* Supplementation on Muscle Strength and Body Composition During Preseason Training in Elite Rugby League Players." *Journal of Strength and Conditioning Research* 21 (2007): 348-353.

Smith, W. A., et al. "Effect of Glycine Propionyl-L-Carnitine on Aerobic and Anaerobic Exercise Performance." *International Journal of Sport Nutrition and Exercise Metabolism* 18 (2008): 19-36.

Wu, C. L., and C. Williams. "A Low Glycemic Index Meal Before Exercise Improves Endurance Running Capacity in Men." *International Journal of Sport Nutrition and Exercise Metabolism* 16 (2006): 510-527.

See also: Androstenedione; Boron; Branched-chain amino acids; Chromium; Coenzyme Q_{10}; Colostrum; Creatine; Dehydroepiandrosterone (DHEA); *Eleutherococcus*; Ephedra; Gamma oryzanol; Ginseng; Hydroxymethyl butyrate; Inosine; Iron; Medium-chain triglycerides; Phosphatidylserine; Phosphorus; Pyruvate; Ribose; Sports and fitness support: Enhancing recovery; Sports-related injuries; *Tribulus terrestris*; Trimethylglycine; Vanadium.

Sports and fitness support: Enhancing recovery

CATEGORY: Condition

DEFINITION: Treatment to aid recovery from the side effects of intense exercise and physical training.

PRINCIPAL PROPOSED NATURAL TREATMENT: Vitamin C

OTHER PROPOSED NATURAL TREATMENTS: Beta-carotene, beta-sitosterol, branched-chain amino acids, bromelain, carotenoids (astaxanthin plus lycopene), cherry juice, collagen hydrolysate, glucosamine, glutamine, horse chestnut, oligomeric proanthocyanidins, probiotics, selenium, thymus extract, vitamin E

INTRODUCTION

In the competitive world of sports, the smallest advantage can make an enormous difference in the outcome of a contest. A dietary supplement that could improve an athlete's strength, speed, or endurance could make the difference between, say, tenth place and first place in a race.

Supplements could conceivably play another helpful role for athletes: aiding recovery from the side effects of intense exercise. While exercise of moderate intensity is almost undoubtedly a purely positive activity, high-intensity endurance exercise, such as running marathons, can cause respiratory infections. In addition, all forms of exercise, when carried to extreme, can cause severe muscle soreness, which may in turn affect training. Herbs and supplements advocated for these problems are discussed here.

PRINCIPAL PROPOSED NATURAL TREATMENTS

Extremely intense exercise, such as training for and running in a marathon, is known to lower immunity, and endurance athletes frequently get sick after maximal exertion. Vitamin C might help prevent this, although not all studies agree.

According to a double-blind, placebo-controlled study involving ninety-two runners, taking 600 milligrams of vitamin C for twenty-one days before a race made a significant difference in the incidence of sickness afterward. Within two weeks of the end of the race, 68 percent of the runners taking placebo developed symptoms of a common cold, whereas only 33 percent of those taking the vitamin C supplement developed cold symptoms. As part of the same study, nonrunners of the same gender and similar age to those running were also given vitamin C or placebo. For this group, the supplement had no apparent effect on the incidence of upper respiratory infections. Vitamin C seemed to be specifically effective in this capacity for those who exercised intensively.

Two other studies found that vitamin C could reduce the number of colds experienced by groups of people involved in rigorous exercise in extremely cold environments. One study involved 139 children attending a skiing camp in the Swiss Alps, while the other enrolled 56 military men engaged in a training exercise in Northern Canada during the winter months. In both cases, the participants took either 1 gram (g) of vitamin C or placebo daily at the time their training program began. Cold symptoms were monitored for one to two weeks following training, and significant differences in favor of vitamin C were found.

However, one very large study of 674 U.S. Marine Corps recruits found no such benefit. The results showed no difference in the number of colds between the treatment and placebo groups.

There are many possible explanations for this discrepancy. Perhaps basic training in the Marine Corps is significantly different from the other forms of exercise studied. Another point to consider is that the recruits did not start taking vitamin C at the beginning of training, but waited three weeks before doing so. The study also lasted a bit longer than the earlier positive studies. Perhaps vitamin C is more effective at preventing colds in the short term. Of course, another possibility is that vitamin C does not work.

OTHER PROPOSED NATURAL TREATMENTS

Like vitamin C, the amino acid glutamine may be helpful for preventing the infections that occur after severe exercise. Glutamine is an important fuel source for some immune system cells. Some evidence suggests that athletes who have trained very hard have lower-than-normal levels of glutamine in their blood. One double-blind clinical trial involving 151 athletes found that supplementation with 5 g of glutamine immediately after heavy exercise, followed by another 5 g two hours later, reduced the incidence of infections significantly. Only 19 percent of those taking glutamine reported infections, while 51 percent of the placebo group succumbed to illness.

Probiotics are healthy organisms found in the digestive tract. Not only can they help prevent intestinal infections, they appear also to help prevent colds. In a double-blind, controlled trial involving twenty healthy, elite distance runners, researchers found that a probiotic supplement (*Lactobacillus fermentum*) given for four months during winter training was significantly more effective at reducing the number and severity of respiratory symptoms compared with placebo. Weaker evidence suggests that beta-sitosterol might also offer some promise for this purpose. However, thymus extract, another proposed immune booster for athletes, does not seem to work, according to a double-blind, placebo-controlled trial of sixty athletes.

Exercising increases the presence of free radicals, naturally occurring substances that can damage tissue. Some researchers have theorized that such damage may in part cause the muscle soreness, and perhaps muscle deterioration, that can accompany a strenuous workout. Based on this theory, but on little direct evidence, various antioxidants have been proposed to help prevent muscle soreness or muscle damage. These antioxidants include astaxanthin plus lycopene, beta-carotene, cherry juice, coenzyme Q_{10}, oligomeric proanthocyanidins, selenium, vitamin C, and vitamin E. One double-blind trial compared vitamin C, vitamin E, and placebo for muscle soreness in twenty-four male volunteers. Vitamin C relieved muscle soreness, but E did not. Two other studies failed to find C combined with E effective. Another study failed to find benefit with the algae-derived carotenoid astaxanthin.

One small double-blind study found that the use of a mixed amino acid reduced muscle soreness caused by endurance exercising of the arm. These researchers actually performed two studies. The first involved simply taking the amino acid thirty minutes before exercising; this study failed to find benefit. The second, more effective regimen added one dose immediately after exercise and two doses daily for the next four days. In addition, a specific family of amino acids, branched-chain amino acids, have shown some promise for reducing muscle damage after long-distance running.

The proteolytic enzyme supplement bromelain, used for sports injuries, has also been proposed for reducing muscle soreness after exercise. However, a double-blind, placebo-controlled trial that compared bromelain with placebo failed to find benefit. Another study, this one using a mixed proteolytic enzyme supplement, also failed to find benefits.

Collagen hydrolysate is a nutritional supplement that may benefit cartilage tissue in joints. In a randomized, placebo-controlled study involving healthy college athletes with joint pain, 10 g daily of collagen hydrolysate appeared to effectively reduce the pain in a period of twenty-four weeks.

The supplement phosphatidylserine has also failed to prove effective for reducing muscle soreness after exercise, as have chondroitin and magnet therapy. In one study, the supplement glucosamine not only failed to prove effective for reducing exercise-induced muscle soreness; it actually increased soreness.

Athletes who train excessively may experience a condition called overtraining syndrome. Symptoms include depression, fatigue, reduced performance, and physiologic signs of stress. Numerous supplements have been suggested as treatments for this condition, including glutamine and, most prominently, antioxidants, but none have been proven effective.

EBSCO CAM Review Board

FURTHER READING

Arendt-Nielsen, L., et al. "A Double-Blind Randomized Placebo Controlled Parallel Group Study Evaluating the Effects of Ibuprofen and Glucosamine Sulfate on Exercise Induced Muscle Soreness." *Journal of Musculoskeletal Pain* 15 (2007): 21-28.

Avery, N. G., et al. "Effects of Vitamin E Supplementation on Recovery from Repeated Bouts of Resistance Exercise." *Journal of Strength and Conditioning Research* 17 (2003): 801-809.

Beck, T. W., et al. "Effects of a Protease Supplement on Eccentric Exercise-Induced Markers of Delayed-Onset Muscle Soreness and Muscle Damage." *Journal of Strength and Conditioning Research* 21 (2007): 661-667.

Bloomer, R. J., et al. "Astaxanthin Supplementation Does Not Attenuate Muscle Injury Following Eccentric Exercise in Resistance-Trained Men." *International Journal of Sport Nutrition and Exercise Metabolism* 15 (2005): 401-412.

Braun, W. A., et al. "The Effects of Chondroitin Sulfate Supplementation on Indices of Muscle Damage Induced by Eccentric Arm Exercise." *Journal of Sports Medicine and Physical Fitness* 45 (2006): 553-560.

Cox, A. J., et al. "Oral Administration of the Probiotic *Lactobacillus fermentum* VRI-003 and Mucosal Immunity in Endurance Athletes." *British Journal of Sports Medicine* 44 (2010): 222-226.

Koba, T., et al. "Branched-Chain Amino Acids Supplementation Attenuates the Accumulation of Blood Lactate Dehydrogenase During Distance Running." *Journal of Sports Medicine and Physical Fitness* 47 (2007): 316-322.

Mastaloudis, A., et al. "Antioxidants Did Not Prevent Muscle Damage in Response to an Ultramarathon Run." *Medicine and Science in Sports and Exercise* 38 (2006): 72-80.

Nosaka, K., P. Sacco, and K. Mawatari. "Effects of Amino Acid Supplementation on Muscle Soreness and Damage." *International Journal of Sport Nutrition and Exercise Metabolism* 16 (2006): 620-635.

See also: Bone and joint health; Branched-chain amino acids; Chondroitin; Glucosamine; Injuries, minor; Pain management; Soft tissue pain; Sports and fitness support: Enhancing performance; Sports-related injuries: Homeopathic remedies; Vitamin C; Vitamin E.

Sports-related injuries: Homeopathic remedies

CATEGORY: Homeopathy

DEFINITION: The use of highly diluted remedies to treat injuries from sports and exercise.

STUDIED HOMEOPATHIC REMEDIES:

- *Topical combination homeopathic remedy:* Preparation containing *Arnica montana, Calendula, Hamamelis,* aconite, belladonna, *Bellis perennis, Chamomilla, Echinacea angustifolia, E. purperea,* millefolium, *Hepar sulphuris calcareum, Mercurius solubilis, Symphytum,* and *Hypericum*
- *Oral homeopathic remedies: Arnica;* combination of *Arnica, Rhus toxicodendron,* and sarcolactic acid
- *Traditional homeopathic remedies: Arnica,* belladonna, *Hypericum, Rhus tox, Symphyrum*

INTRODUCTION

Although vigorous exercise is one of the most important steps toward good health, it can also have side effects, ranging from muscle soreness to injury. While these adverse consequences of exercise can be minimized by graduated training and careful activity, problems may develop anyway. Homeopathic treatments (especially topical creams) are quite popular for such sports-related conditions, and they have shown some promise in studies.

SCIENTIFIC EVALUATIONS OF HOMEOPATHIC REMEDIES

There is some evidence to support the use of homeopathic creams for the treatment of sports injuries. However, studies of oral homeopathic remedies for exercise-induced muscle soreness have not been promising.

Topical combination homeopathic treatments for sports injuries. Investigators performed a double-blind, placebo-controlled study of sixty-nine people with sports-related ankle sprains to test the efficacy of a combination homeopathic ointment. The particular product tested contains a combination of the following fourteen homeopathic preparations: *Arnica montana, Calendula, Hamamelis,* aconite, belladonna, *Bellis perennis, Chamomilla, Echinacea angustifolia, E. purperea,* millefolium, *Hepar sulphuris calcareum, Mercurius solubilis, Symphytum,* and *Hypericum.*

During the two-week trial, all of the participants received electrical muscle stimulation. The investigators also applied cream, either the treatment cream or placebo cream seven times during the study. The results showed that people given the real treatment recovered more rapidly than those given placebo.

In another double-blind, placebo-controlled study, researchers evaluated the effectiveness of the same homeopathic ointment and a modified version of the ointment for the treatment of various mild to moderate sports injuries, including sprains. All of the approximately one hundred participants in the trial had slight to moderate sports-induced injuries that had occurred in the past four days. The first application of ointment (and a bandage) was applied by the investigators on day one of treatment. Then the participants applied the ointment themselves, twice daily for fourteen more days. The results were promising. By the end of the trial, participants who used either form of the ointment experienced significantly superior improvement, compared with those taking placebo, according to some but not all measures.

Oral homeopathic remedies for sports-related muscle soreness. A double-blind, placebo-controlled study tested homeopathic *Arnica* (30x) in 519 long-distance runners but did not find positive results. Participants took five pills twice daily, beginning the evening before a race and continuing for four successive days. Evaluation after the race showed that *Arnica* was no more effective than placebo for reducing soreness or speeding recovery after a race. Earlier, much smaller studies had found some suggestion of benefit for long-distance runners, but the results were, in general, not statistically significant.

A double-blind, placebo-controlled study, conducted in the physiotherapy department of a homeopathic hospital in England, evaluated the efficacy of an oral homeopathic preparation in the treatment of muscle soreness caused by stepping exercise. The remedy used was a combination of *Arnica*, *Rhus tox*, and sarcolactic acid. The results showed no statistical difference between the treatment group and the control group.

TRADITIONAL HOMEOPATHIC TREATMENTS

Classical homeopathy offers many possible homeopathic treatments for sports injuries. These therapies are chosen based on various specific details of the person seeking treatment.

For injuries that are sensitive to touch and have pain that is shooting, violent, tingling, or cutting, and if the injured person feels worse at night and in the cold, then that person may match the symptom picture for homeopathic *Hypericum*. An injury with symptoms like these suggests nerve involvement, indicating an urgent need for physician examination.

If the affected person feels worse when exposed to motion, drafts, and heat, and during the afternoon, and if the person experiences spasms, shooting pains, tearing sensations, jerking, trembling, swelling, redness, and heat, possibly with cold extremities, then he or she may fit the classic symptom picture for homeopathic belladonna. If one has a sprain with a great deal of swelling and inflammation of the soft tissue around a joint, the homeopathic remedy *Arnica* might be recommended. *Arnica* is also commonly used as a remedy for exercise-induced muscle soreness.

A person with an injury to a bone, cartilage, or tendon that is aggravated by touch, motion, and pressure (while warmth helps) may fit the symptom picture for homeopathic *Symphytum*. Many homeopathic practitioners use *Symphytum* after *Arnica* if deep pain or soreness remains after the initial soreness has cleared. A person with stiff, painful muscles brought on by straining, overlifting, or getting wet when already hot and perspiring, and a person whose muscles seize up with rest but loosen with exercise and heat, may fit the traditional homeopathic indications for *Rhus tox*.

EBSCO CAM Review Board

FURTHER READING

Plezbert, J. A., and J. R. Burke. "Effects of the Homeopathic Remedy *Arnica* on Attenuating Symptoms of Exercise-Induced Muscle Soreness." *Journal of Chiropractic Medicine* 4 (2005): 152-161.

Tveiten, D., and S. Bruset. "Effect of *Arnica* D30 in Marathon Runners." *Homeopathy* 92 (2003): 187-189.

Vickers, A. J., P. Fisher, C. Smith, S. E. Wyllie, and R. Rees. "Homeopathic *Arnica* 30x Is Ineffective for Muscle Soreness After Long-Distance Running." *Clinical Journal of Pain* 14 (1998): 227-231.

Vickers, A. J., P. Fisher, C. Smith, S. E. Wyllie, and G. T. Lewith. "Homeopathy for Delayed Onset Muscle Soreness." *British Journal of Sports Medicine* 31 (1997): 304-307.

See also: Exercise; Homeopathy; Pain management; Sports and fitness support: Enhancing performance; Sports and fitness support: Enhancing recovery.

SSRIs

CATEGORY: Drug interactions

DEFINITION: Medications used for severe and mild to moderate depression and for a variety of other conditions.

INTERACTIONS: Ephedra, fish oil, 5-HTP, folate, ginkgo, St. John's wort, SAMe (S-adenosylmethionine)

DRUGS IN THIS FAMILY: Citalopram (Celexa), fluoxetine (Prozac), fluvoxamine (Luvox), paroxetine (Paxil), sertraline (Zoloft)

5-HYDROXYTRYPTOPHAN (5-HTP) AND S-ADENOSYLMETHIONINE (SAMe)

Effect: Possible Harmful Interaction

The body uses the natural substance 5-HTP to manufacture serotonin, and supplemental forms have been used for treating depression and migraine headaches. SAMe is a naturally occurring compound derived from the amino acid methionine and the energy molecule adenosine triphosphate. SAMe is widely used as a supplement for treating osteoarthritis and depression.

Based on one case report and the latest knowledge about how they work, SAMe and 5-HTP should not be taken with SSRIs, as they might increase the risk of serotonin syndrome. This syndrome is a toxic reaction brought on by too much serotonin activity. The condition requires immediate medical attention, with symptoms including anxiety, restlessness, confusion, weakness, tremor, muscle twitching or spasm, high fever, profuse sweating, and rapid heartbeat.

The report describes a case of apparent serotonin syndrome in a person taking SAMe with clomipramine, a tricyclic antidepressant that increases serotonin activity.

Although SAMe is not currently known to affect serotonin, it does appear to have antidepressant effects and may in some way increase serotonin activity. Because SSRIs increase serotonin activity even more than clomipramine, a similar problem might occur if one combines SAMe with an SSRI. The supplement 5-HTP is used by the body to manufacture serotonin, so it could also increase the risk of serotonin syndrome when combined with an SSRI.

St. John's Wort
Effect: Possible Harmful Interaction

The herb St. John's wort (*Hypericum perforatum*) is primarily used to treat mild to moderate depression. One of its actions appears to be increasing the activity of serotonin in the brain.

Persons taking an SSRI medication should not take the herb St. John's wort at the same time. It is possible that serotonin levels might be raised too high, causing a dangerous condition called serotonin syndrome.

Several case reports appear to bear this out. Serotonin syndrome was reported in five elderly persons who began using St. John's wort while taking sertraline (four reports) or nefazodone (one report). One

person had symptoms resembling serotonin syndrome after combining paroxetine (50 milligrams [mg] daily) and St. John's wort (600 mg daily). Another person taking St. John's wort with two other serotonin-enhancing drugs was reported to experience serotonin syndrome.

Furthermore, persons wishing to switch from an SSRI to St. John's wort may need to wait a few weeks for the SSRI to be cleansed from the body before it is safe to start taking the herb. The waiting time required depends on which SSRI is being taken.

Folate
Effect: Possible Helpful Interaction

Folate is a B vitamin that offers many important health benefits. It helps prevent birth defects and disorders and possibly reduces the risk of heart disease. A recent study suggests that folate can also help SSRI antidepressants work better. In this double-blind, placebo-controlled trial, 127 persons with severe depression were given either Prozac plus folate (500 micrograms [mcg] daily) or Prozac alone. Researchers wanted to see whether the vitamin would increase the medication's effectiveness.

The results were different for men and women. Female participants definitely benefited from receiving folate along with the medication. While just under 50 percent of the women taking Prozac alone fully recovered from their depression, combination treatment produced a recovery rate of nearly 75 percent. This is a marked difference, and one that makes a strong case for combining folate with antidepressant therapy.

Men, however, did not do any better on combination treatment than on Prozac alone. Researchers found evidence that a higher dose would have been necessary for male participants, perhaps 800 to 1,000 mcg daily. However, for dosages this high, medical supervision is necessary.

Fish Oil
Effect: Supplementation Probably Not Helpful

Fish oil contains essential fatty acids in the omega-3 family. Fish oil, its constituents, and a slightly modified fish oil constituent called ethyl-EPA have all been tested for treatment of depression. While a few small studies have suggested that these substances might enhance the effectiveness of antidepressant drugs, the results of larger and better-designed studies have been mostly negative.

Serotonin Syndrome

Serotonin syndrome is a rare, but serious, drug reaction. Serotonin is a chemical produced by nerve cells. Some antidepressants, such as SSRIs, can raise the amount of serotonin in the brain. Up to a point, this increase can be good, but too much serotonin can cause serotonin syndrome. Common symptoms include confusion, hallucinations, loss of coordination, fever, rapid heart rate, and vomiting.

Serotonin syndrome happens most often when a person takes, at the same time, two drugs (or drugs and dietary or herbal supplements) that raise serotonin in the brain. Products other than SSRIs that raise serotonin include the following:

- Migraine headache medicines
- Supplemental L-tryptophan
- Herbal products, such as St. John's wort
- Over-the-counter cough medicines that contain dextromethorphan
- Prescription pain killers, such as meperidine

GINKGO

Effect: Supplementation Probably Not Helpful

SSRIs can cause many sexual side effects, including inability to achieve orgasm (in women) and impotence (in men). Case reports and open studies raised hopes that the herb ginkgo could help reverse these problems. However, only double-blind, placebo-controlled studies can truly establish efficacy of a treatment, and when studies of this type were finally performed to evaluate ginkgo's potential effectiveness for this purpose, no benefits were seen.

EPHEDRA

Effect: Supplementation Probably Not Helpful

Like ginkgo, ephedrine (extracted from the herb ephedra) does not appear any more effective than placebo for treatment of female sexual dysfunction caused by SSRIs.

EBSCO CAM Medical Review Board

FURTHER READING

Frangou, S., et al. "Efficacy of Ethyl-Eicosapentaenoic Acid in Bipolar Depression." *British Journal of Psychiatry* 188 (2006): 46-50.

Grenyer, B. F., et al. "Fish Oil Supplementation in the Treatment of Major Depression." *Progress in Neuro-Psychopharmacology and Biological Psychiatry* 1, no. 31 (2007): 1393-1396.

Hallahan, B., et al. "Omega-3 Fatty Acid Supplementation in Patients with Recurrent Self-Harm." *British Journal of Psychiatry* 190 (2007): 118-122.

Jazayeri, S., et al. "Comparison of Therapeutic Effects of Omega-3 Fatty Acid Eicosapentaenoic Acid and Fluoxetine, Separately and in Combination, in Major Depressive Disorder." *Australian and New Zealand Journal of Psychiatry* 42 (2008): 192-198.

Kang, B. H., et al. "A Placebo-Controlled, Double-Blind Trial of *Ginkgo biloba* for Antidepressant-Induced Sexual Dysfunction." *Human Psychopharmacology: Clinical and Experimental* 17 (2002): 279-284.

Lin, P. Y., and K. P. Su. "A Meta-analytic Review of Double-Blind, Placebo-Controlled Trials of Antidepressant Efficacy of Omega-3 Fatty Acids." *Journal of Clinical Psychiatry* 68 (2007): 1056-1061.

Marangell, L. B., et al. "A Double-Blind, Placebo-Controlled Study of the Omega-3 Fatty Acid Docosahexaenoic Acid in the Treatment of Major Depression." *American Journal of Psychiatry* 160 (2003): 996-998.

Meston, C. M. "A Randomized, Placebo-Controlled, Crossover Study of Ephedrine for SSR-Induced Female Sexual Dysfunction." *Journal of Sex and Marital Therapy* 30 (2004): 57-68.

Rogers, P. J., et al. "No Effect of N-3 Long-Chain Polyunsaturated Fatty Acid (EPA and DHA) Supplementation on Depressed Mood and Cognitive Function." *British Journal of Nutrition* 99, no. 2 (2008): 421-431.

Wheatley, D. "Triple-Blind, Placebo-Controlled Trial of *Ginkgo biloba* in Sexual Dysfunction Due to Antidepressant Drugs." *Human Psychopharmacology* 19, no. 8 (2004): 545-548.

See also: Depression, mild to moderate; Ephedra; Fish oil; 5-Hydroxytryptophan; Folate; Food and Drug Administration; Ginkgo; St. John's wort; SAMe; Supplements: Overview; Tricyclic antidepressants.

Stanols and sterols

CATEGORY: Herbs and supplements
RELATED TERMS: Campestanol, 5-alpha-stanols, phytostanols, phytosterols, sitostanol, stanol esters, sterol esters, stigmastanol
DEFINITION: Natural substances promoted as dietary supplements for specific health benefits.
PRINCIPAL PROPOSED USE: Lowering cholesterol

OVERVIEW

Stanols are substances that occur naturally in various plants. Their cholesterol-lowering effects were first observed in animals in the 1950s. Since then, a substantial amount of research suggests that plant stanols (usually modified into stanol esters) can help to lower cholesterol in persons with normal or mildly to moderately elevated levels. Stanols are available in margarine spreads, salad dressings, and dietary supplement tablets. Related substances called sterols or phytosterols (such as beta-sitosterol) and sterol esters appear to lower cholesterol in much the same manner as stanols.

SOURCES

Sterols are found in most plant foods and occur naturally in wood pulp, tall oil (a by-product of paper manufacturing), and soybean oil. Stanols can also be manufactured from the sterols found in many foods. Stanol and sterol esters are manufactured by processing stanols or sterols with fatty acids from vegetable oils. Stanol-sterols and their esters are added to margarine spreads and salad dressings and are also available as dietary supplement tablets.

THERAPEUTIC DOSAGES

Typical dosages of stanol-sterols and their esters to improve cholesterol profile range from 2.7 to 5.1 grams (g) per day. One study suggests that using stanol products once a day may be as effective as dividing up the intake throughout the day. It may take up to three months to show a substantial decrease in total cholesterol values.

THERAPEUTIC USES

Strong evidence suggests that stanol-sterols and their ester forms can significantly improve cholesterol profile. There are no other known medicinal uses of stanols or stanol esters. Phytosterols do offer additional potential benefits.

SCIENTIFIC EVIDENCE

Because they are structurally similar to cholesterol, stanols (and sterols) can displace cholesterol from the "packages" that deliver cholesterol for absorption from the intestines to the bloodstream. This displaced cholesterol is then excreted from the body. This action not only interferes with the absorption of cholesterol from food; it also has the additional (and probably more important) effect of removing cholesterol from substances made in the liver that are recycled through the digestive tract.

Numerous double-blind, placebo-controlled studies, ranging in length from thirty days to twelve months and involving more than one thousand people, have found that sterol-stanols and their esters are effective for improving cholesterol profile. The combined results suggest that these substances can reduce total cholesterol and LDL (bad) cholesterol by about 10 to 15 percent. They do not, however, have much of an effect on HDL (good) cholesterol or on triglycerides.

For example, in a double-blind, placebo-controlled study, 153 people with mildly elevated cholesterol were given sitostanol esters in margarine (at 1.8 or 2.6 g of sitostanol per day) or margarine without sitostanol ester for one year. The results in the treated group receiving 2.6 g per day showed improvements in total cholesterol by 10.2 percent and LDL cholesterol by 14.1 percent, significantly better than the results in the control group. Neither triglycerides nor HDL cholesterol levels were affected.

Fish oil too has been shown to have a favorable effect on fats in the blood, in particular triglycerides. A study investigating the possible benefit of combining sterols with fish oil found that together they significantly lowered total cholesterol, LDL cholesterol, and triglycerides and also raised HDL cholesterol in persons with undesirable cholesterol profiles.

Even people already taking standard medications to improve cholesterol profile (specifically, drugs in the statin family) appear to benefit when they use stanols-sterols as well. According to one study, persons who are on statins and who start taking sterol ester margarine too will improve to the same extent as if those persons doubled the statin dose. Stanols and sterols also appear to be safe and effective for improving cholesterol profile in people with type 2 diabetes.

SAFETY ISSUES

Sterols are presumed safe because they are found in many foods. Stanols are also considered safe, but for a different reason: They are not absorbed. No adverse effects have been reported in any of the studies on lowering cholesterol, with the exception of one study that reported mild gastrointestinal complaints in a few preschool children. In addition, no toxic signs were observed in rats given stanol esters for thirteen weeks at levels comparable to or exceeding those recommended for lowering cholesterol.

Although concerns have been expressed that stanol esters might impair absorption of the fat-soluble vitamins A, D, and E, this does not seem to occur at the dosages required to lower cholesterol. Stanol esters might interfere with the absorption of alpha-carotene and beta-carotene, although some studies have found no such effect. It is also not clear whether sterols or sterol esters impair nutrient absorption. Until more is learned, it may be reasonable for people using stanol or sterol products to also take multivitamin-multimineral tablets.

EBSCO CAM Review Board

FURTHER READING

Allen, R. R., et al. "Daily Consumption of a Dark Chocolate Containing Flavanols and Added Sterol

Esters Affects Cardiovascular Risk Factors in a Nor-motensive Population with Elevated Cholesterol." *Journal of Nutrition* 138 (2008): 725-731.

Castro Cabezas, M., et al. "Effects of a Stanol-Enriched Diet on Plasma Cholesterol and Triglycerides in Patients Treated with Statins." *Journal of the American Dietetic Association* 106 (2006): 1564-1569.

Hendriks, H. F., et al. "Safety of Long-Term Consumption of Plant Sterol Esters-Enriched Spread." *European Journal of Clinical Nutrition* 57 (2003): 681-692.

Katan, M. B., et al. "Efficacy and Safety of Plant Stanols and Sterols in the Management of Blood Cholesterol Levels." *Mayo Clinic Proceedings* 78 (2003): 965-980.

O'Neill, F. H., et al. "Comparison of Efficacy of Plant Stanol Ester and Sterol Ester." *American Journal of Cardiology* 96 (2005): 29-36.

Plana, N., et al. "Plant Sterol-Enriched Fermented Milk Enhances the Attainment of LDL-Cholesterol Goal in Hypercholesterolemic Subjects." *European Journal of Nutrition* 47 (2008): 32-39.

Woodgate, D., C. H. Chan, and J. A. Conquer. "Cholesterol-Lowering Ability of a Phytostanol Softgel Supplement in Adults with Mild to Moderate Hypercholesterolemia." *Lipids* 41 (2006): 127-132.

See also: Beta-sitosterol; Cholesterol, high; Triglycerides, high.

Statin drugs

RELATED TERM: HMG-CoA reductase inhibitors

CATEGORY: Drug interactions

DEFINITION: Medications used to improve cholesterol profile.

INTERACTIONS: Chaparral, Chinese skullcap, coenzyme Q_{10}, coltsfoot, comfrey, fish oil, grapefruit juice, pomegranate, red yeast rice, St. John's wort, vitamin B_3

DRUGS IN THIS FAMILY: Atorvastatin calcium (Lipitor), fluvastatin (Lescol), lovastatin (Mevacor), pravastatin (Pravachol), simvastatin (Zocor), rosuvastatin (Crestor)

CHAPARRAL, COMFREY, AND COLTSFOOT

Effect: Possible Harmful Interaction

The herb chaparral (*Larrea tridentate* or *L. mexicana*) has been promoted for use in arthritis, cancer, and various other conditions, but there is insufficient evidence supporting its effectiveness. There are, however, concerns about its apparent liver toxicity.

Several cases of chaparral-induced liver damage have been reported, some of them severe enough to require liver transplantation. Based on these reports, combining chaparral with other agents that are harmful to the liver, such as statin drugs, may amplify the risk of potential liver problems. Other herbs that are toxic to the liver include comfrey (*Symphytum officinale*) and coltsfoot (*Tussilago farfara*).

CHINESE SKULLCAP

Effect: Possible Harmful Interaction

The herb Chinese skullcap (*Scutellaria baicalensis*) contains the substance baicalin as one of its presumed major active ingredients. One study found evidence that consumption of baicalin might lower blood levels of statin drugs.

ST. JOHN'S WORT

Effect: Possible Harmful Interaction

The herb St. John's wort, used to treat depression, may decrease blood levels of various drugs in the statin family, including simvastatin, lovastatin, and atorvastatin (but possibly not pravastatin). One study documented that when people taking atorvastatin for high cholesterol additionally took St. John's wort, cholesterol levels promptly rose.

GRAPEFRUIT JUICE

Effect: Possible Harmful Interaction

Grapefruit juice impairs the body's normal breakdown of several drugs, including statins, allowing them to build up to potentially excessive levels in the blood. One study indicates that this effect can last for three days or more following the last glass of grapefruit juice.

Because grapefruit juice can increase the risk of serious drug side effects, persons taking interacting statins should avoid grapefruit juice altogether. Grapefruit juice may not affect fluvastatin or pravastatin because these drugs are broken down differently than other statins.

VITAMIN B_3

Effect: Possible Benefits and Risks

Niacin (nicotinic acid) is vitamin B_3. In high doses (often 1,500 milligrams [mg] daily or more), niacin is effective in lowering cholesterol levels. Its other form, niacinamide (nicotinamide), does not affect cholesterol.

Combining high-dose niacin with statin drugs further improves cholesterol profile by raising HDL (good) cholesterol. However, there are real concerns that this combination therapy could cause a potentially fatal condition of muscle breakdown called rhabdomyolysis.

A growing body of evidence, however, suggests that the risk is relatively slight in persons with healthy kidneys. Furthermore, even much lower doses of niacin than the usual dose given to improve cholesterol levels (100 mg versus 1,000 mg or more) may provide a similar benefit. At this dose, the risk of rhabdomyolysis should be decreased. Nonetheless, it is not safe to try this combination except under close physician supervision.

POMEGRANATE
Effect: Possible Harmful Interaction

One case report suggests that the consumption of pomegranate juice might increase the risk of rhabdomyolosis with the use of rosuvastatin (Crestor).

RED YEAST RICE
Effect: Possible Harmful Interaction

Red yeast rice is an herbal cholesterol-lowering therapy. It contains a mixture of statins; its primary statin ingredient is lovastatin, making it most closely resemble the prescription drug Mevacor. Based on the similarity of red yeast rice to statin drugs, the two should not be combined without medical supervision.

COENZYME Q_{10} (CoQ_{10})
Effect: Supplementation Possibly Helpful

CoQ_{10} is a vitamin-like substance that plays a fundamental role in the body's energy production and appears to be important for normal heart function. Statin drugs inhibit the enzyme necessary for the body's synthesis of both cholesterol and CoQ_{10} and, as an inevitable part of their mechanism of action, reduce CoQ_{10} levels in the body. Because these drugs are used to protect the heart, and because CoQ_{10} deficiency could in theory impair heart function, it has been suggested that this side effect may work against the intended purpose of taking statins. Furthermore, one might naturally hypothesize that some of the side effects of statins could be caused by this induced CoQ_{10} deficiency.

Taking CoQ_{10} supplements does prevent the lowering of CoQ_{10} levels caused by statin drugs and accomplishes this without interfering with their therapeutic effects. However, studies designed to determine whether the use of CoQ_{10} supplements actually offers any benefit to people taking statins have returned inconsistent results at best. The most recent of these studies, for example, a relatively large double-blind, placebo-controlled trial of forty-four people, failed to find that the use of CoQ_{10} at a dose of 200 mg daily reduced the side effects of simvastatin.

FISH OIL
Effect: Supplementation Probably Helpful

Three double-blind, placebo-controlled studies suggest that combining fish oil (or its constituent docosahexaenoic acid, or DHA) with statin drugs may result in additional improvement in lipid profile.

EBSCO CAM Review Board

FURTHER READING

Andrén, L., A. Andreasson, and R. Eggertsen. "Interaction Between a Commercially Available St. John's Wort Product (Movina) and Atorvastatin in Patients with Hypercholesterolemia." *European Journal of Clinical Pharmacology* 63 (2007): 913-916.

Jim, L. K., and J. P. Gee. "Adverse Effects of Drugs on the Liver." In *Applied Therapeutics: The Clinical Use of Drugs*, edited by M. A. Koda-Kimble et al. 9th ed. Philadelphia: Wolters Kluwer/Lippincott Williams & Wilkins, 2009.

Marcoff, L., and P. D. Thompson. "The Role of Coenzyme Q10 in Statin-Associated Myopathy." *Journal of the American College of Cardiology* 49 (2007): 2231-2237.

Sorokin, A. V., et al. "Rhabdomyolysis Associated with Pomegranate Juice Consumption." *American Journal of Cardiology* 98 (2006): 705-706.

Strey, C. H., et al. "Endothelium-ameliorating Effects of Statin Therapy and Coenzyme Q(10) Reductions in Chronic Heart Failure." *Atherosclerosis* 179 (2005): 201-206.

Young, J. M., et al. "Effect of Coenzyme Q(10) Supplementation on Simvastatin-Induced Myalgia." *American Journal of Cardiology* 100 (2007): 1400-1403.

See also: Cholesterol, high; Coenzyme Q_{10}; Fish oil; Food and Drug Administration; Herbal medicine; Liver disease; Red yeast rice; Supplements: Introduction; Vitamin B$_3$.

Stevia

CATEGORY: Herbs and supplements

RELATED TERM: *Stevia rebaudiana*

DEFINITION: Natural plant product used to sweeten foods and beverages and to treat specific health conditions.

PRINCIPAL PROPOSED USE: Food and beverage sweetener

OTHER PROPOSED USES: Diabetes, hypertension

OVERVIEW

Stevia, a member of the Aster family, has a long history of native use in Paraguay as a sweetener for teas and foods. It contains a substance known as stevioside that is one hundred to three hundred times sweeter than sugar but provides no calories.

In the early 1970s, a consortium of Japanese food manufacturers developed stevia extracts for use as a zero-calorie sugar substitute. Subsequently, stevia extracts became common ingredients in Asian soft drinks, desserts, chewing gum, and many other food products. Extensive Japanese research has found stevia to be extremely safe. However, there have not been enough studies in the United States for the Food and Drug Administration to approve stevia as a sugar substitute. Without its being identified as such, stevia is nonetheless widely used by savvy manufacturers to sweeten commercial beverage teas and other products.

Although stevia is best known as a sweetener, stevia extracts also can be taken in very high doses to possibly reduce blood pressure, according to two large Chinese studies.

THERAPEUTIC DOSAGES

Stevia is sold as a powder to be added to foods as needed for appropriate sweetening effects. It tastes slightly bitter if placed directly in the mouth. In liquids, however, bitterness is generally not noticeable, and most people find the taste delightfully unique.

In the studies of stevia that have shown an effect on blood pressure, stevia was given as a standardized extract supplying 250 to 500 milligrams (mg) of stevioside three times daily (a dose considerably higher than any reasonable use of stevia as a sweetener).

THERAPEUTIC USES

Stevia is primarily useful as a sweetening agent. In addition, two double-blind studies suggest that it may also offer potential benefits for hypertension. Weak evidence hints at potential benefits for diabetes.

SCIENTIFIC EVIDENCE

A one-year double-blind, placebo-controlled study of 106 persons with high blood pressure evaluated the potential benefits of stevia for reducing blood pressure. In the treated group, the average blood pressure at the beginning of the study was about 166/102. Participants were given either placebo or stevioside (stevia extract) at a dose of 250 mg three times daily. By the end of the study, the average blood pressure had fallen to 153/90, a substantial if not quite adequate improvement. Note that this is a high dose of steviosides, the sweetness equivalent of more than one-third of a pound of sugar daily. However, this study is notable for finding no benefits at all in the placebo group. This is unusual and tends to cast doubt on the results.

Benefits were also seen in a two-year double-blind, placebo-controlled study of 174 people with mild hypertension (average initial blood pressure of approximately 150/95). This study, performed by some of the same researchers who worked on the study just described, used twice the dose of the previous study: 500 mg three times daily. A reduction in blood pressure of approximately 6 to 7 percent was seen in the treatment group compared with the placebo group, beginning within one week and enduring throughout the entire two years. At the end of the study, 34 percent of those in the placebo group showed heart damage from high blood pressure (left ventricular hypertrophy), while only 11.5 percent of the stevioside

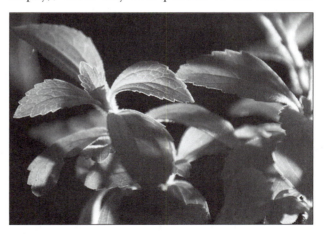

Leaves of the stevia plant. (Getty Images)

group did, a difference that was statistically significant. No significant adverse effects were seen.

However, once again, no benefits at all were seen in the placebo group. This result means the that study design had problems. Both studies were performed in China, a country that has a documented history of questionable medical study results.

Furthermore, a study by an independent set of researchers failed to replicate these findings. In this study, stevioside was given according to body weight, at a dose of 3.75 milligrams per kilogram (mg/kg) per day, 7.5 mg/kg per day, or 15 mg/kg per day. Compared with placebo, none of these doses affected the blood pressure of the study participants, all of whom had mild high blood pressure. These finding do not entirely refute those described above, however, as the dosage of stevia used was somewhat on the low side. For example, for a man weighing 60 kg (132 pounds), the highest dose would be 300 mg three times a day.

Another study involving diabetics as well as healthy subjects found that stevia, at a dose of 250 mg three times daily, had no significant effect on blood pressure after three months of treatment.

SAFETY ISSUES

Animal tests and the extensive Japanese experience with stevia suggest that this is a safe herb. Based primarily on the apparently incorrect belief that stevia has been used traditionally to prevent pregnancy, some researchers have expressed concern that stevia might have an antifertility effect in men or women. However, evidence from most (though not all) animal studies suggests that this is not a concern at normal doses.

The two studies described above in which use of very high dosages of a stevia extract led to reductions in blood pressure raise at least theoretical concerns about stevia's safety. In theory, the herb could excessively reduce blood pressure in some people. Furthermore, if stevia can reduce blood pressure, that means that it is, in some fashion, acting on the cardiovascular system.

Because sugar substitutes are meant to be consumed in essentially unlimited quantities by a very wide variety of people, the highest levels of safety standards are appropriate, and unknown effects on the heart and blood circulation are potentially worrisome. This concern is somewhat mitigated by the fact that the daily dose of stevioside used in those studies was considerably higher than is likely to be consumed if whole stevia is used for sweetening purposes. Reassurance also comes from the study that found no effect with a dose of 15 mg/kg per day.

Safety of stevia use in young children, pregnant or nursing women, and those with severe liver or kidney disease has not been conclusively established. Because of the concerns noted above, individuals with cardiovascular disease should use high doses of stevia extracts only under physician supervision.

EBSCO CAM Review Board

FURTHER READING

Barriocanal, L. A., et al. "Apparent Lack of Pharmacological Effect of Steviol Glycosides Used as Sweeteners in Humans: A Pilot Study of Repeated Exposures in Some Normotensive and Hypotensive Individuals and in Type 1 and Type 2 Diabetics." *Regulatory Toxicology and Pharmacology* 51 (2008): 37-41.

Chan, P., et al. "A Double-Blind Placebo-Controlled Study of the Effectiveness and Tolerability of Oral Stevioside in Human Hypertension." *British Journal of Clinical Pharmacology* 50 (2000): 215-220.

See also: Diabetes; Hypertension.

St. John's wort

CATEGORY: Herbs and supplements

RELATED TERM: *Hypericum perforatum*

DEFINITION: Natural plant product used to treat specific health conditions.

PRINCIPAL PROPOSED USE: Mild to moderate depression

OTHER PROPOSED USES: Anxiety, attention deficit disorder, burning mouth syndrome, diabetic neuropathy and other forms of neuropathy, eczema, insomnia, menopause, obsessive-compulsive disorder, premenstrual syndrome, seasonal affective disorder, viral infections

OVERVIEW

St. John's wort is a common perennial herb of many branches and bright yellow flowers that grows wild in much of the world. Its name derives from the herb's tendency to flower around the time of the feast of St. John. ("Wort" simply means "plant" in Old English.) The species name *perforatum* derives from the watermarking of translucent dots that can be seen when the leaf is held up to light.

St. John's wort has a long history of use in treating emotional disorders. During the Middle Ages, St. John's wort was popular for "casting out demons." In the nineteenth century, the herb was classified as a nervine, or a treatment for so-called nervous disorders. When pharmaceutical antidepressants were invented, German researchers began to look for similar properties in St. John's wort.

THERAPEUTIC DOSAGES

The typical dosage of St. John's wort is 300 milligrams (mg) three times a day of an extract standardized to contain 0.3 percent hypericin. Some products are standardized to hyperforin content (usually 2 percent to 3 percent) instead of hypericin. These are usually taken at the same dosage. Two studies found benefits with a single daily dose of 900 mg.

Another form of St. John's wort has shown effectiveness in double-blind studies. This form contains little hyperforin and is taken at a dose of 250 mg twice daily. There is some evidence that this form of St. John's wort may be less likely than other forms to interact with medications.

THERAPEUTIC USES

In Germany, other parts of Europe, and the United States, St. John's wort is now a widely used treatment for depression. The evidence base for its use approaches that of many modern prescription drugs at the time of their first approval.

Most studies of St. John's wort have evaluated individuals with major depression of mild to moderate intensity. This contradictory-sounding language indicates that the level of depression rises to greater severity than simply feeling "blue." However, it is not as severe as the most severe forms of depression. Typical symptoms include depressed mood, lack of energy, sleep problems, anxiety, appetite disturbance, difficulty concentrating, and poor stress tolerance. Irritability can also be a sign of depression.

Taken as a whole, research suggests that St. John's wort is more effective than placebo and approximately as effective as standard drugs. Furthermore, St. John's wort appears to cause fewer side effects than many antidepressants. However, the herb does present one significant safety risk: It interacts harmfully with a great many standard medications.

St. John's wort has also shown promise for treatment of severe major depression. St. John's wort alone should never be relied on for the treatment of severe depression. Persons who are feeling suicidal or who are unable to cope with daily life or who are paralyzed by anxiety, incapable of getting out of bed, unable to sleep, or uninterested in eating should consult a physician or other health practitioner.

St. John's wort has been tried in the treatment of many other conditions in which prescription antidepressants are thought useful, such as attention deficit disorder, anxiety, insomnia, menopausal symptoms, premenstrual syndrome (PMS), seasonal affective disorder (SAD), and social phobia. However, there is no convincing evidence that it offers any benefit for these conditions. One substantial double-blind study did find St. John's wort potentially helpful for somatoform disorders (commonly called psychosomatic illnesses).

Standard antidepressants are also often used for diabetic neuropathy and other forms of neuropathy (nerve pain). However, a small double-blind, placebo-controlled trial failed to find St. John's wort effective for this purpose. Another study failed to find St. John's wort helpful for obsessive-compulsive disorder.

St. John's wort contains, among other ingredients, the substances hypericin and hyperforin. Early reports suggested that St. John's wort or synthetic hypericin might be useful against viruses such as HIV (human immunodeficiency virus), but these have not panned out. However, there is some evidence that hyperforin may be able to fight certain bacteria, including some that are resistant to antibiotics. This evidence is far too preliminary for any conclusions to be drawn regarding the effectiveness of St. John's wort as an antibiotic. Based on weak evidence that hypericin might have anti-inflammatory properties, St. John's wort cream has been tried as a treatment for eczema, with some promising results.

One interesting double-blind study evaluated a combination therapy containing St. John's wort and black cohosh in 301 women with general menopausal symptoms as well as depression. The results showed that use of the combination treatment was significantly more effective than placebo for both problems.

In a small placebo-controlled trial, hypericin extract showed no benefit for burning mouth syndrome, a poorly understood condition in which a person experiences ongoing moderate to severe pain in the tongue or mouth, or both.

SCIENTIFIC EVIDENCE

Depression. Two main kinds of studies have examined the use of St. John's wort for depression: those that compared St. John's wort to placebo and others that compared it to prescription antidepressants. A 2008 detailed review of twenty-nine randomized, placebo-controlled trials found that St. John's wort was consistently more effective than placebo and just as effective as standard antidepressants.

St. John's wort versus placebo. Studies of St. John's wort (and other antidepressants) use a set of questions called the Hamilton Depression Index (HAM-D). This scale rates the extent of depression, with higher numbers indicating more serious symptoms.

Double-blind, placebo-controlled trials involving a total of more than fifteen hundred participants with major depression of mild to moderate severity have generally found that use of St. John's wort can significantly reduce HAM-D scores compared with placebo. In addition, continued treatment with St. Johns wort over six months may be effective at preventing a relapse of moderate depression in patients who recover from an initial acute episode. For example, in a six-week trial, 375 persons with average seventeen-item HAM-D scores of about 22 (indicating major depression of moderate severity) were given either St. John's wort or placebo. Persons taking St. John's wort showed significantly greater improvement than those taking placebo.

Three double-blind, placebo-controlled trials evaluating individuals with a similar level of depression failed to find St. John's wort more effective than placebo. However, three studies cannot overturn a body of positive research. It should be noted that 35 percent of double-blind studies involving pharmaceutical antidepressants have also failed to find the active agent significantly more effective than placebo. As if to illustrate this, in two of the three studies in which St. John's wort failed to prove effective, a conventional drug (Zoloft in one case, Prozac in the other) also failed to prove effective. The reason for these negative outcomes is not that Zoloft or Prozac does not work. Rather, statistical effects can easily hide the benefits of a drug, especially in a condition such as depression, where there is as a high placebo effect and no really precise method of measuring symptoms. Thus, unless a whole series of studies find St. John's wort ineffective, especially trials in which a comparison drug treatment does prove effective, St. John's

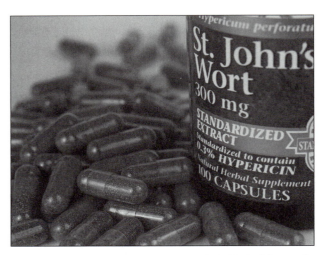

In Germany, other parts of Europe, and the United States, St. John's wort is now a widely used treatment for depression. (Cordelia Molloy/Photo Researchers, Inc.)

wort should still be regarded as probably effective for major depression of mild to moderate severity.

St. John's wort versus medications. At least eight double-blind trials enrolling a total of more than twelve hundred people have compared St. John's wort with fluoxetine (Prozac), citalopram (Celexa), paroxetine (Paxil), or sertraline (Zoloft). In all of these studies, the herb proved as effective as the drug and generally caused fewer side effects.

In the largest of these trials, a six-week study of 388 people with major depression of mild to moderate severity, St. John's wort proved just as effective as the drug citalopram (Celexa) and more effective than placebo. Additionally, Celexa caused a significantly higher rate of side effects than St. John's wort. There were also significantly more side effects in the placebo group than in the St. John's wort group, presumably because treatment of depression reduces physical symptoms of psychological origin. St. John's wort also has been compared with older antidepressants, with generally favorable results.

How does St. John's wort work for depression? Like pharmaceutical antidepressants, St. John's wort is thought to raise levels of neurotransmitters in the brain, such as serotonin, norepinephrine, and dopamine. The active ingredient of St. John's wort is not known. Extracts of St. John's wort are most often standardized to the substance hypericin, which has led to the widespread misconception that hypericin is the active ingredient. However, there is no evidence that hypericin itself is an antidepressant.

Another ingredient of St. John's wort, hyperforin, has shown considerable promise as the most important ingredient. Hyperforin was first identified as a constituent of *Hypericum perforatum* in 1971 by Russian researchers, but it was incorrectly believed to be too unstable to play a major role in the herb's action. However, subsequent evidence corrected this view. It now appears that standard St. John's wort extract contains about 1 percent to 6 percent hyperforin. Evidence from animal and human studies suggests that it is the hyperforin in St. John's wort that raises the levels of neurotransmitters. Nonetheless, there may be other active ingredients in St. John's wort also at work. In fact, two double-blind trials using a form of St. John's wort with low hyperforin content found it effective. More research is necessary to discover just how St. John's wort acts against depression.

Polyneuropathy. A double-blind, placebo-controlled trial of fifty-four people with diabetic neuropathy or other forms of neuropathy (pain, numbness, or tingling caused by injury to nerves) did not find St. John's wort effective for this purpose.

SAFETY ISSUES

St. John's wort taken alone usually does not cause immediate side effects. In a study designed to look for side effects, 3,250 people took St. John's wort for four weeks. Overall, about 2.4 percent reported problems. The most common complaints were mild stomach discomfort (0.6 percent); allergic reactions, primarily rash, (0.5 percent); tiredness (0.4 percent); and restlessness (0.3 percent). Another study followed 313 individuals treated with St. John's wort for one year. The results showed a similarly low incidence of adverse effects.

In the extensive German experience with St. John's wort as a treatment for depression, there have been no published reports of serious adverse consequences from taking the herb alone. Animal studies involving enormous doses of St. John's wort extracts for twenty-six weeks have not shown any serious effects.

However, there are a number of potential safety risks with St. John's wort that should be considered. These are outlined in the following sections.

Photosensitivity. Cows and sheep grazing on St. John's wort have sometimes developed severe and even fatal sensitivity to the sun. In one study, highly sun-sensitive people were given twice the normal dose of the herb. The results showed a mild but measurable increase in reaction to ultraviolet (UV) radiation. Another trial found that a one-time dose of St. John's wort containing two or six times the normal daily dose did not cause an increased tendency to burn, nor did seven days of treatment at the normal dose. However, there is a case report of severe and unexpected burning in an individual who used St. John's wort and then received UV therapy for psoriasis. In addition, two individuals using topical St. John's wort experienced severe reactions to sun exposure.

Persons who are especially sensitive to the sun should not exceed the recommended dose of St. John's wort and should continue to take the usual precautions against burning. Individuals receiving UV treatment should not use St. John's wort at all, and those who apply St. John's wort to the skin should keep those parts of their bodies shielded from the sun.

In addition, combining St. John's wort with other medications that cause increased sun sensitivity, such as sulfa drugs and the anti-inflammatory medication piroxicam (Feldene), may lead to problems. The medications omeprazole (Prilosec) and lansoprazole (Prevacid) may also increase the tendency of St. John's wort to cause photosensitivity.

Finally, a report suggests that regular use of St. John's wort might also increase the risk of sun-induced cataracts. Although this information is preliminary, it would be prudent for persons taking the herb on a long-term basis to wear sunglasses when outdoors.

Drug interactions. Herbal experts have warned for some time that combining St. John's wort with drugs in the Prozac family (SSRIs) might raise serotonin too much and cause a number of serious problems. Recently, case reports of such events have begun to trickle in. This is a potentially serious risk. St. John's wort should not be combined with prescription antidepressants except on the specific advice of a physician. Because some antidepressants, such as Prozac, linger in the blood for quite some time, persons who have been taking such drugs should exercise caution when switching from these to St. John's wort. Antimigraine drugs in the triptan family (such as sumatriptan, or Imitrex) and the pain-killing drug tramadol also raise serotonin levels and might interact similarly with St. John's wort.

However, perhaps the biggest concern with St. John's wort is that it appears to decrease the effectiveness of numerous medications, including protease inhibitors and reverse transcriptase inhibitors (for HIV infection), cyclosporine and tacrolimus (for organ transplants), digoxin (for heart disease), statin drugs (used for high cholesterol), warfarin (Coumadin, a blood thinner), chemotherapy drugs, oral contraceptives, tricyclic antidepressants, protein pump inhibitors (such as Prilosec), atypical antipsychotics such as olanzapine or clozapine (for schizophrenia), anesthetics, and the new heart disease drug ivabradine. In fact, there are theoretical reasons to believe that this herb might reduce the effectiveness of, or otherwise interact with, about 50 percent of all medications. Problems could arise, for instance, if a person is taking St. John's wort while also working with a physician to adjust the dosage of a particular medication to obtain an optimum balance of efficacy and side effects. If the person subsequently stops taking the herb, blood levels of the drug may then rise, with potentially dangerous consequences.

Note that these proposed interactions are not purely academic; they could lead to catastrophic consequences. Indeed, St. John's wort appears to have caused several cases of heart, kidney, and liver transplant rejection by interfering with the action of cyclosporine. The herb also appears to decrease the effectiveness of oral contraceptives and by doing so is thought to have led to unwanted pregnancies.

On a less dramatic level, one study showed that among people taking a cholesterol-lowering medication in the statin family, use of St. John's wort caused cholesterol levels to rise. (The same would be expected to occur if a person were using red yeast rice to treat high cholesterol, as red yeast rice supplies naturally occurring statin drugs.)

Finally, some people with HIV take St. John's wort in the false belief that the herb will fight AIDS. The unintended result may be to reduce the potency of standard anti-HIV drugs.

There is some evidence that low-hyperforin St. John's wort may have less potential for drug interactions than other forms of St. John's wort. Nonetheless, it is recommended that people taking any oral or injected medication that is critical to their health or well-being entirely avoid using any form of St. John's wort until more is known; those who are already taking the herb should not stop taking it until they

can simultaneously have their drug levels monitored. It is also recommended that persons who are soon to undergo general anesthesia avoid use of the herb.

Safety in special circumstances. One animal study found no ill effects of St. John's wort on the offspring of pregnant mice. However, these findings alone are not sufficient to establish the herb as safe for use during pregnancy. Furthermore, the St. John's wort constituent hypericin can accumulate in the nucleus of cells and directly bind to DNA. For this reason, pregnant or nursing women should avoid St. John's wort. Furthermore, safety for use by young children or people with severe liver or kidney disease has not been established.

Case reports suggest that, like other antidepressants, St. John's wort can cause episodes of mania in individuals with bipolar disorder (manic-depressive disease). There is also one report of St. John's wort causing temporary psychosis in a person with Alzheimer's disease.

Other concerns. Certain foods contain a substance called tyramine. These foods include aged cheeses, aged or cured meats, sauerkraut, soy sauce, other soy condiments, beer (especially beer on tap), and wine. Drugs in the MAO inhibitor family interact adversely with tyramine, causing severe side effects such as high blood pressure, rapid heart rate, and delirium. One case report suggests that St. John's might present this risk as well. However, other studies suggest that normal doses of the herb should not cause MAO-like effects. Until this issue is sorted out, it is recommended that individuals taking St. John's wort avoid tyramine-containing foods. Since MAO inhibitors react adversely with stimulant drugs such as Ritalin, ephedrine (found in the herb ephedra), and caffeine, St. John's wort should not be combined with these.

One small study suggests that high doses of St. John's wort might slightly impair mental function. Another case report associates use of St. John's wort with hair loss; the authors note that standard antidepressants may also cause hair loss at times.

One study raised questions about possible antifertility effects of St. John's wort. When high concentrations of St. John's wort were placed in a test tube with hamster sperm and ova, the sperm were damaged and less able to penetrate the ova. However, since it is unlikely that such a large amount of St. John's wort can actually come in contact with sperm and ova when they are in the body rather than in a test tube, these results may not be meaningful in real life.

In one reported case, St. John's wort may have interacted with the menopause drug tibolone to produce severe liver damage.

Transitioning from medications to St. John's wort. For persons who are taking a prescription drug for mild to moderate depression, switching to St. John's wort may be a reasonable idea if they prefer taking an herb. To avoid overlapping treatments, the safest approach is for an individual to stop taking the drug and allow it to wash out of his or her system before starting St. John's wort. The individual should consult with his or her doctor regarding how much time is necessary.

For persons taking medication for severe depression, however, switching over to St. John's wort is not a good idea. The herb is unlikely to work well enough for such a use, and depression could worsen to a dangerous level.

IMPORTANT INTERACTIONS

Persons who are taking antidepressant drugs, including MAO inhibitors, SSRIs, and tricyclics, or possibly the drugs tramadol or sumatriptan (Imitrex), should not take St. John's wort at the same time. To switch from such medications to St. John's wort, individuals should let the medications flush out of their systems for a while (perhaps weeks, depending on the drug) before they start taking the herb.

Individuals who are taking digoxin, cyclosporine and tacrolimus, protease inhibitors or reverse transcriptase inhibitors, oral contraceptives, tricyclic antidepressants, warfarin (Coumadin), statin drugs, theophylline, chemotherapy drugs, newer antipsychotic medications (such as olanzapine and clozapine), anesthetics, or, indeed, any critical medication should be aware that St. John's wort might cause such drugs to be less effective. Those who have been taking St. John's wort while adjusting medication dosages to achieve proper blood levels should not suddenly stop St. John's wort, as this could cause the drugs in the body to rebound to dangerously high levels.

Persons who are taking medications that cause sun sensitivity, such as sulfa drugs and the anti-inflammatory medication piroxicam (Feldene), as well as omeprazole (Prilosec) or lansoprazole (Prevacid), should keep in mind that St. John's wort might have an additive effect. Those who are taking stimulant drugs or herbs such as Ritalin, caffeine, or ephedrine

(ephedra) should be aware that St. John's wort might interact adversely with these substances.

EBSCO CAM Review Board

FURTHER READING

Bjerkenstedt, L., et al. "Hypericum Extract LI 160 and Fluoxetine in Mild to Moderate Depression: A Randomized, Placebo-Controlled Multi-center Study in Outpatients." *European Archives of Psychiatry and Clinical Neuroscience* 255 (2005): 40-47.

Fava, M., et al. "A Double-Blind, Randomized Trial of St. John's Wort, Fluoxetine, and Placebo in Major Depressive Disorder." *Journal of Clinical Psychopharmacology* 25 (2005): 441-447.

Hebert, M. F., et al. "Effects of St. John's Wort *Hypericum perforatum* on Tacrolimus Pharmacokinetics in Healthy Volunteers." *Journal of Clinical Pharmacology* 44 (2004): 89-94.

Kasper, S., et al. "Continuation and Long-Term Maintenance Treatment with Hypericum Extract WS 5570 After Recovery from an Acute Episode of Moderate Depression." *European Neuropsychopharmacology* 18 (2008): 803-813.

Sardella, A., et al. "*Hypericum perforatum* Extract in Burning Mouth Syndrome." *Journal of Oral Pathology and Medicine* 37 (2008): 395-401.

Uebelhack, R., J. U. Blohmer, et al. "Black Cohosh and St. John's Wort for Climacteric Complaints." *Obstetrics and Gynecology* 107 (2006): 247-255.

Uebelhack, R., J. Gruenwald, et al. "Efficacy and Tolerability of Hypericum Extract STW 3-VI in Patients with Moderate Depression." *Advances in Therapy* 21 (2004): 265-275.

See also: Depression, mild to moderate; Mental health.

Strep throat

CATEGORY: Condition
RELATED TERMS: Pharyngitis, streptococcal, rheumatic fever, streptococcal pharyngitis
DEFINITION: Treatment of a throat infection caused by the bacterium *Streptococcus*.
PRINCIPAL PROPOSED NATURAL TREATMENTS: None
OTHER PROPOSED NATURAL TREATMENTS: Throat Coat tea (symptoms only), *Pelargonium sidoides* (for less serious forms of sore throat only)

INTRODUCTION

Most cases of sore throat are caused by viruses, generally the same viruses that cause the common cold. One familiar type of sore throat, however, streptococcal pharyngitis, commonly known as strep throat, is caused by bacteria in the *Streptococcus* family. Strep throat is relatively common in children.

Symptoms of strep throat include intense throat pain (generally developing suddenly), difficulty swallowing, and fever ranging from 101° to 104° Fahrenheit. In children, headache, abdominal pain, nausea, and vomiting may also occur. The back of the throat generally (but not always) becomes beefy red in color, possibly with white or red dots. However, none of these signs or symptoms is absolutely characteristic of strep throat. In some cases, there are no symptoms. Ultimately, diagnosis of strep throat must be made through a laboratory examination of material swabbed from the back of the throat.

The primary significance of strep throat is not the throat infection itself, but rather a delayed complication called rheumatic fever. Strep throat itself will disappear in three to five days even without treatment. However, the involvement of a certain group of streptococcal bacteria, called group A beta-hemolytic streptococci, puts the infected person at risk of a severe, dangerous complication developing about one to five weeks later, when all seems to be well. This is the feared second effect of strep throat known as rheumatic fever.

The initial attack of rheumatic fever involves five major signs and symptoms: carditis (inflammation of the heart, often causing a heart murmur); chorea (rapid, purposeless, nonrepetitive movements that are not under conscious control); migratory polyarthritis (severe joint pain, redness, and swelling that move from joint to joint); subcutaneous nodules (nodules under the skin); and erythema marginatum (a serpentine, flat rash). These symptoms will eventually subside. However, when they are gone, the valves of the heart may be permanently damaged, necessitating open-heart surgery.

About 3 percent of untreated group A beta-hemolytic strep throat cases lead to rheumatic fever. Children aged four to fifteen years are most at risk. Adults with strep throat may develop rheumatic fever, but the chance is extremely low. Rheumatic fever is rare in the United States because of prompt treatment of strep throat, but it is common in developing countries, where it is one of the leading causes of heart disease.

The cause of rheumatic fever is interesting. It is thought that certain strains of strep bacteria contain glycoproteins that, from the perspective of the immune system, resemble glycoproteins found in the heart, joints, or nerve tissue. When the body makes antibodies to attack the strep bacteria, those antibodies also damage the body.

The only known way to prevent rheumatic fever in people with strep throat involves using antibiotics at relatively high doses and for a prolonged time. The goal is to eradicate the invading bacteria so that the body does not make antibodies against it.

PROPOSED NATURAL TREATMENTS

The unique relationship of rheumatic fever and strep throat is confusing and may lead a person to use alternative treatments for it in ways that are not helpful. For most diseases, the risk is over when symptoms abate. Based on this natural understanding of illness, many people use herbs or other natural treatments for strep throat and then feel safe when throat pain and fever disappear.

However, with strep throat, the situation is different. Symptoms of strep throat disappear on their own, without treatment, in three to five days. The big risk comes one to five weeks later, when rheumatic fever may strike. Antibiotic treatment for strep throat is not primarily intended to treat the strep throat itself (although it does that), but rather to prevent rheumatic fever. There are no herbs or supplements known to prevent rheumatic fever.

Some people try to treat strep throat with herbs, such as echinacea, believed to stimulate the immune system. However, this approach has a serious problem: If echinacea did manage to increase the immune system's activity, the result would be to increase the intensity of rheumatic fever, not decrease it, because rheumatic fever is caused, in a sense, by an overactive immune system, not an underactive one.

Strep throat caused by group A beta-hemolytic streptococci cannot be treated with alternative medicine. Conventional diagnosis and treatment are necessary to ensure safety. However, if tests are done and a case of strep throat does not appear to be caused by group A beta-hemolytic strep, other forms of treatment may be appropriate.

According to a double-blind, placebo-controlled study of 143 children, the herb *Pelargonium sidoides* might actually shorten the duration of infections that are not group A strep. Whether it is helpful as supplementary treatment to antibiotics for children undergoing treatment for group A strep remains unknown.

The popular herb tea Throat Coat might help sooth sore throat discomfort. Throat Coat contains herbs traditionally thought to soothe inflamed mucous membranes. One small double-blind study did indeed find that Throat Coat was superior to a placebo for this purpose. It seems reasonable to use Throat Coat along with conventional treatment even for group A strep infections. However, this tea contains licorice, which can be toxic if taken to excess.

EBSCO CAM Review Board

FURTHER READING

Bereznoy, V. V., et al. "Efficacy of Extract of *Pelargonium sidoides* in Children with Acute Non-Group A Beta-Hemolytic *Streptococcus* Tonsillopharyngitis." *Alternative Therapies in Health and Medicine* 9 (2003): 68-79.

Brinckmann, J., H. Sigwart, and L. van Houten Taylor. "Safety and Efficacy of a Traditional Herbal Medicine (Throat Coat) in Symptomatic Temporary Relief of Pain in Patients with Acute Pharyngitis." *Journal of Alternative and Complementary Medicine* 9 (2003): 285-298.

Gerber M. "*Streptococcus pyogenes* (Group A *Streptococcus*)." In *Principles and Practice of Pediatric Infectious Diseases*, edited by Sarah S. Long, Larry K. Pickering, and Charles G. Prober. 3d ed. Philadelphia: Churchill Livingstone/Elsevier, 2008.

See also: Colds and flu; Herbal medicine; *Pelargonium sidoides.*

Stress

CATEGORY: Condition
DEFINITION: Treatment of conditions associated with emotional, mental, and physical stress.
PRINCIPAL PROPOSED NATURAL TREATMENT: *Panax ginseng*

OTHER PROPOSED NATURAL TREATMENTS: Adrenal extracts, alternative therapies (such as biofeedback, guided imagery, hypnotherapy, massage, relaxation therapy, Tai Chi, and yoga), ashwagandha, astragalus, bach flower remedies, *Eleutherococcus senticosus*, gamma-aminobutyric acid, kava, lysine plus arginine, maitake, multivitamin-multimineral supplements, phosphatidylserine, reishi, rhodiola, schisandra, shiitake, suma, theanine from black tea, tyrosine, valerian

INTRODUCTION

The effects of stress on health can be far-reaching. Some of the conditions often associated with stress include insomnia, high blood pressure, tension headaches, anxiety, depression, decreased mental function, and drug or alcohol abuse. Stress is known to cause changes in the body's chemistry, altering the balance of hormones in our systems in ways that can lower our resistance to disease. As a result, people can become more susceptible to colds and flu and other types of illness. Too much stress sometimes brings on outbreaks of cold sores or genital herpes for people who carry these viruses in their systems. Other chronic diseases such as irritable bowel syndrome, asthma, inflammatory bowel disease, and rheumatoid arthritis may also flare up during times of stress.

Avoiding situations that cause one to feel tense, unhappy, or worn down is beneficial. However, it is not always possible to live a stress-free existence. Work deadlines, family demands, relationship problems, traffic jams, missed appointments, forgotten birthdays, personality conflicts, college exams–all of these things, and many more, can be sources of stress. Furthermore, though most people associate stress with unpleasant events, even wonderful events, such as weddings, vacations, and holidays, can be genuinely stressful.

Not everyone responds to these situations with stress. For some persons, their pulse rate would not even go up during an earthquake, and then there are those for whom being five minutes late to an event causes panic. How one manages stress can determine its impact.

There are many different methods of dealing with stress. The basics for good health that are well known (but often forgotten) help in coping with stress: Eating a balanced diet and getting adequate rest helps the body adapt and respond to life events. Ironically, stress can interfere with one's ability to take care of oneself in this way. When a person worries so much that he or she cannot sleep, getting adequate rest becomes impossible. Stress can affect eating habits too. Widely accepted stress management tools that can help a person break from a stress-induced downward spiral include exercise, meditation, and biofeedback.

For some people, stressful circumstances can trigger symptoms severe enough to warrant seeking medical attention. Conditions associated with stress, such as insomnia, anxiety, depression, and panic attacks, may become severe enough to require medication.

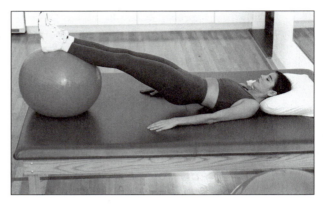

Exercise may help some people reduce stress. (PhotoDisc)

PRINCIPAL PROPOSED NATURAL TREATMENTS

One proposed natural approach to treating the physical consequences of stress involves the use of adaptogens. The term "adaptogen" refers to a hypothetical treatment described as follows: An adaptogen helps the body adapt to stresses of various kinds, whether heat, cold, exertion, trauma, sleep deprivation, toxic exposure, radiation, infection, or psychological stress. Furthermore, an adaptogen should cause no side effects, be effective in treating a wide variety of illnesses, and help return an organism toward balance no matter what may have gone wrong.

However, physical exercise is the only indubitable example of an adaptogen. There is no solid evidence that any substance functions in this way. However, there is some suggestive evidence for the herb *Panax ginseng.*

Panax ginseng. Most of the evidence cited to indicate that *Panax ginseng* has adaptogenic effects comes from animal studies involving ginseng extracts injected into the abdomen. Such studies are of questionable relevance to the oral use of ginseng by humans; furthermore, the majority of these studies were performed in the former Soviet Union and failed to reach acceptable scientific standards. However, a few potentially meaningful studies in humans have found effects that are at least consistent with the possibility of benefits in stressful situations.

Animal studies. According to a number of animal studies, most of which were poorly designed and reported, *P. ginseng* injections into the bloodstream or abdomen can increase stamina; improve mental function; protect against radiation, infections, toxins, exhaustion, and stress; and activate white blood cells. However, when ginseng is injected into the abdomen or bloodstream, it enters the body directly without going through the digestive tract. This mode of administration is strikingly different from taking ginseng by mouth.

A smaller number of animal studies (again, most of them poorly designed) have looked at the potential benefits of ginseng administered orally and have often reported benefit. In addition, studies in mice found that consuming ginseng before exposure to a virus significantly increased the survival rate and number of antibodies produced.

Human studies. Human studies of *P. ginseng* have only indirectly examined its potential benefits as an adaptogen. For example, a double-blind, placebo-controlled study found evidence that *P. ginseng* may improve immune system response. This trial enrolled 227 participants at three medical offices in Italy. One-half were given ginseng at a dosage of 100 milligrams (mg) daily, and the other one-half received placebo. Four weeks into the study, all participants received influenza vaccine.

The results showed a significant decline in the frequency of colds and flu in the treated group, compared with the placebo group (fifteen versus forty-two cases). Also, antibody levels in response to the vaccination rose higher in the treated group than in the placebo group.

These findings have been taken by some researchers to support their belief that ginseng has an adaptogenic effect. However, the study might instead simply indicate a general form of immune support unrelated to stress.

Other studies have looked at *P. ginseng*'s effects on overall mental function, general well-being, and sports performance. While it is true that positive results in such studies might tend to hint at an adaptogenic effect, the results were, in general, too mixed to provide conclusive evidence for benefit. It is not clear that *P. ginseng* offers general benefits for stress.

OTHER PROPOSED NATURAL TREATMENTS

Multivitamins plus minerals. A treatment as simple as multivitamin-multimineral tablets may be helpful for stress. In a double-blind, placebo-controlled study, three hundred men and women were given either a multivitamin-multimineral tablet or placebo for thirty days. The results showed that people taking the nutritional supplement experienced less anxiety overall and an enhanced ability to cope with stressful circumstances. The supplement used in this study supplied the following nutrients and dosages: vitamin B_1 (10 mg), vitamin B_2 (15 mg), vitamin B_6 (10 mg), vitamin B_{12} (10 micrograms), vitamin C (1,000 mg), calcium (100 mg), and magnesium (100 mg).

Benefits were seen in another double-blind, placebo-controlled trial that enrolled eighty healthy male volunteers. The supplement used in this trial was similar but not identical.

It is not clear how these nutrients help stress. However, considering that many people would benefit from general nutritional supplementation in any case, it might be worth trying.

Eleutherococcus senticosus. In the 1940s, the same scientist who first dubbed *P. ginseng* an adaptogen decided that a much less expensive herb, *Eleutherococcus senticosus*, is also an adaptogen. A thorny bush that grows much more rapidly than true ginseng, this plant later received the misleading name of "Siberian ginseng" or "Russian ginseng." Its chemical makeup, however, is unrelated to that of *P. ginseng*.

As with *P. ginseng*, many animal studies finding adaptogenic benefits with *Eleutherococcus* have been reported, but most were relatively poorly designed and used injections rather than oral administration of the herb, making the results not particularly relevant to the normal human usage of the herb.

Numerous human trials of *Eleutherococcus* have been reported as well, some involving enormous numbers of participants. However, most of these were not double-blind and many were not even controlled, making the results nearly meaningless.

Again, as with *P. ginseng*, a few reasonably well-designed studies in humans have been reported that may have indirect bearing on the herb's potential adaptogenic properties. For example, in one double-blind trial, participants took either 10 milliliters of extract of *Eleutherococcus* or placebo three times daily for four weeks. Blood samples were analyzed to determine changes in immune cells. A statistically significant increase in numbers of cells important to immune functions was observed in the treatment group compared with the placebo group.

This study has been widely advertised as proving the *Eleutherococcus* strengthens immunity. However, mere changes in immune cell profile do not automatically translate into enhanced immunity. More meaningful data were obtained in a double-blind, placebo-controlled study involving ninety-three people who experience recurrent flare-ups of herpes. The use of *Eleutherococcus* significantly reduced the severity, frequency, and duration of herpes outbreaks relative to placebo during the six-month trial. This study does suggest a possible immune-strengthening effect.

Like *P. ginseng*, *Eleutherococcus* has been studied for enhancing sports performance, but published studies have not been encouraging. One small, double-blind, placebo-controlled trial of endurance athletes found that the use of *Eleutherococcus* actually may increase physiologic signs of stress during intensive training.

Other possible adaptogens. Three small double-blind trials suggest that the herb rhodiola (*Rhodiola rosea*) may improve mental alertness in people undergoing sleep deprivation or other stressful circumstances. Numerous other herbs are said to be adaptogens too. These include ashwagandha, astragalus, maitake, reishi, shiitake, suma, and schisandra. However, there is little evidence that they have adaptogenic effects. One study failed to find greater adaptogenic effects with fish oil compared with placebo.

Other options. Preliminary evidence, including small double-blind trials, suggests that the amino acid tyrosine may improve memory and mental function under conditions of sleep deprivation or other forms of stress. Another double-blind study found that the use of vitamin C at doses of 3,000 mg daily (slow release) reduced both physical and emotional responses to stress.

In small double-blind studies, theanine, a constituent of black tea, appeared to reduce the body's reaction to acute physical or psychological stress. Benefits have also been seen with a combination of lysine (2.64 grams per day) and arginine (2.64 grams per day).

One double-blind study found evidence that a processed form of casein (a protein found in milk) may reduce a variety of stress-related symptoms. According to another small double-blind trial, a mixture of soy phosphatidylserine and lecithin may decrease the physiological response to mental stress. Another study evaluated the use of phosphatidylserine for reducing stress in golfers, but the benefits seen failed to reach statistical significance.

A proprietary Ayurvedic herbal formula containing *Bacopa monniera* and almost thirty other ingredients has shown some promise for treating symptoms of stress. In a three-month, double-blind, placebo-controlled trial of forty-two people in high-stress jobs who complained of fatigue, participants using the herbal formula reported fewer stress-related problems. Also, in a three-month, double-blind, placebo-controlled study of fifty adult students, this formula appeared to improve memory and attention and to reduce other signs of stress.

In naturopathic medicine, adrenal extract is often recommended for the treatment of stress, but there is no evidence that this treatment is effective. Equivocal evidence hints that valerian, alone or with lemon balm, might reduce anxiety symptoms during stressful situations.

Many people report that they experience stress relief through the use of alternative therapies such as biofeedback, guided imagery, hypnotherapy, massage, relaxation therapy, Tai Chi, and yoga. One study failed to find regular massage more effective for controlling stress than the use of a relaxation tape. Another study failed to find either cognitive behavioral therapy or increased physical activity helpful for stress-related illnesses. Three studies failed to find Bach flower remedies helpful for situational anxiety (anxiety caused by stressful situations).

EBSCO CAM Review Board

FURTHER READING

Ellis, J. M., and P. Reddy. "Effects of *Panax ginseng* on Quality of Life." *Annals of Pharmacotherapy* 36 (2002): 375-379.

Halberstein, R., et al. "Healing with Bach Flower Essences: Testing a Complementary Therapy." *Complementary Health Practice Review* 12 (2007): 3-14.

Heiden, M., et al. "Evaluation of Cognitive Behavioural Training and Physical Activity for Patients with Stress-Related Illnesses." *Journal of Rehabilitative Medicine* 39 (2007): 366-373.

Jager, R., et al. "The Effect of Phosphatidylserine on Golf Performance." *Journal of the International Society of Sports Nutrition* 4 (2007): 23.

Kim, J. H., et al. "Efficacy of Alpha-S1-Casein Hydrolysate on Stress-Related Symptoms in Women." *European Journal of Clinical Nutrition* 61 (2007): 536-541.

Kraemer, W. J., et al. "Cortitrol Supplementation Reduces Serum Cortisol Responses to Physical Stress." *Metabolism* 54 (2005): 657-668.

See also: Adrenal extract; Anxiety and panic attacks; *Eleutherococcus*; Ginseng; Immune support; Insomnia; Mental health; Relaxation therapies.

Strokes

CATEGORY: Condition

RELATED TERMS: Cerebral vascular accident, transient ischemic attack

DEFINITION: Treatment of cell death in the brain caused by a sudden loss of blood supply.

PRINCIPAL PROPOSED NATURAL TREATMENTS

- *For prevention:* Policosanol; all herbs and supplements used for high cholesterol, high blood pressure, or atherosclerosis
- *For treatment:* Glycine, vinpocetine

OTHER PROPOSED NATURAL TREATMENTS: Acupuncture, aromatherapy, bilberry, beta-carotene, feverfew, fish oil, folate, garlic, ginger, ginkgo, music therapy, quercetin, vitamin E, white willow

HERBS AND SUPPLEMENTS TO USE ONLY WITH CAUTION: Ephedra, iron

OTHER NATURAL TREATMENT TO AVOID: Chelation therapy

INTRODUCTION

Strokes occur when part of the brain suddenly loses its blood supply and dies. The underlying cause is generally atherosclerosis, a condition in which the walls of blood vessels become thickened and irregular. As atherosclerosis progresses, blood flow through important arteries becomes restricted to a much smaller passage than is normal. This narrow passage can then suddenly become blocked, often by a blood clot. When this happens, brain cells downstream of the blockage are suddenly deprived of oxygen (cerebral ischemia). Brain cells require a constant supply of oxygen to survive. Within seconds, they begin to malfunction, and within minutes they die.

In what are called transient ischemic attacks (TIAs), the blockage to blood flow is temporary, and symptoms rapidly disappear. However, in a true stroke, called a cerebral vascular accident (CVA), the blockage lasts long enough to cause cell death in a significant section of the brain. Less commonly, strokes are caused by bleeding into the brain, which is known as a hemorrhagic stroke.

The symptoms of a stroke depend on the area of the brain affected. Paralysis of one limb or one side of the face is common. Loss of speech or sensation may also occur. Much of the loss that occurs in a stroke is permanent, but some recovery usually does occur in time. There are two main causes of this recovery. The first involves the body's ability to grow new blood vessels. Nerve cells on the margins of the dead area may cling to survival, functioning imperfectly on whatever oxygen drifts to them. Eventually, new blood vessel growth enables the nerve cells to recover perfectly.

The second cause of recovery involves the brain's remarkable ability to adapt to difficult circumstances: To a lesser or greater extent, surviving parts of the brain can take over tasks once performed by brain cells that have died.

Conventional treatment for a stroke has several phases, but the most important is prevention. Stopping smoking, losing weight, reducing cholesterol levels, and controlling blood pressure prevent atherosclerosis and thereby reduce the risk of stroke. Also, physicians may recommend the use of blood-thinning drugs, such as aspirin, to prevent the blood clots that so frequently are the final step to a stroke. Furthermore, if there is evidence that the main blood vessels leading to the brain are seriously narrowed, surgery or angioplasty may be considered to widen those vessels.

Treatment of a stroke that has just occurred involves maintaining life during the immediate recovery period and limiting the spread of brain damage (if possible). Finally, physical and occupational therapists help the stroke survivor to adapt.

PRINCIPAL PROPOSED NATURAL TREATMENTS

There are a number of alternative options that may be useful for preventing or even possibly treating

Ephedra Ban

In 2004, the U.S. Food and Drug Administration (FDA) warned consumers about the dangers of ephedra and advised them to stop using dietary supplements containing ephedra. To protect consumers, the FDA published a final rule on April 12, 2004, that banned the sale of dietary supplements containing ephedrine alkaloids.

After a careful review of the available evidence about the risks and benefits of ephedra in supplements, the FDA found that these supplements presented an unreasonable risk of illness or injury to consumers. The data showed little evidence of ephedra's effectiveness, except for short-term weight loss, while confirming that the substance raises blood pressure and stresses the heart. The increased risk of heart problems and strokes negates any benefits of weight loss.

Essentially all marketed dietary supplements that contain a source of ephedrine alkaloids, such as ephedra, ma huang, *Sida cordifolia*, and pinellia, were affected by this rule. The rule did not pertain to traditional Chinese herbal remedies. It generally did not apply to products such as herbal teas that are regulated as conventional foods. In addition, products regulated as drugs that contain chemically synthesized ephedrine are not dietary supplements and thus are not covered by this rule.

strokes. The best documented are those that fight atherosclerosis.

Stroke prevention. Meaningful evidence indicates that numerous herbs and supplements are helpful for improving the cholesterol profile, which in turn should decrease atherosclerosis and help prevent strokes. Weaker evidence supports the use of other herbs and supplements for lowering blood pressure or for treating atherosclerosis in general.

Policosanol. Various herbs and supplements with blood-thinning properties have been suggested for use instead of or with aspirin to prevent blood clots. The best evidence regards the supplement policosanol.

Several double-blind, placebo-controlled trials indicate policosanol significantly reduces the blood's tendency to clot. In one such study of forty-three people, the use of policosanol at 20 milligrams (mg) per day proved approximately as effective as 100 mg of aspirin; in addition, when the two treatments were taken in combination, the effect was greater than with either treatment alone. Furthermore, this supplement appears to reduce cholesterol levels, making it potentially an all-around stroke-preventing treatment. However, while the long-term use of aspirin has been shown to reduce stroke risk, no equivalent studies of policosanol have been done. In addition, combined treatment with policosanol and aspirin (or related drugs) could conceivably thin the blood too much, resulting in dangerous bleeding events.

Stroke treatment. Cells at the margin of a stroke may cling to life until new blood vessels form to supply them with full circulation. Certain herbs and supplements might facilitate this by increasing blood flow or,

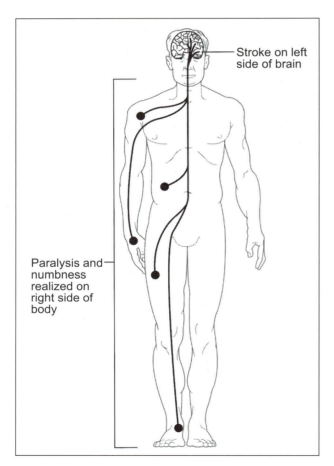

A major stroke to one hemisphere of the brain generally results in impairment of motor functions on the opposite side of the body.

alternatively, by reducing brain-cell oxygen requirements. Although the evidence remains preliminary, two supplements have shown some promise for this purpose: vinpocetine and glycine.

Vinpocetine. In a single-blind, placebo-controlled trial, thirty persons who had just experienced a stroke received either placebo or vinpocetine with conventional treatment for thirty days. Three months later, evaluation showed that participants in the vinpocetine group were significantly less disabled.

A few other studies, some of poor design, also provide suggestive evidence that vinpocetine may be helpful for strokes. However, this body of evidence remains far from conclusive. A review combining two relatively high-quality studies involving sixty-three persons could not determine whether or not vinpocetine provided any benefit for persons who had a stroke. Also, there are concerns that vinpocetine could interact harmfully with standard drugs used to thin the blood.

Glycine. The supplement glycine also has been proposed as a treatment for limiting permanent stroke damage. However, the supporting evidence is largely limited to one moderate-sized Russian trial. In this double-blind, placebo-controlled study, two hundred people received glycine within six hours of an acute stroke. The results indicate that the use of glycine at 1 gram daily for five days led to less long-term disability than placebo treatment.

However, paradoxically, there are potential concerns that high-dose glycine could actually increase harm caused by strokes, and drugs that block glycine have been investigated as treatments to limit stroke damage. The authors of the Russian study on strokes made an argument that the overall effect of supplemental glycine is protective; nonetheless, until this controversy is settled, one should not take glycine following a stroke except on a physician's advice.

OTHER PROPOSED NATURAL TREATMENTS

Evidence suggests that high consumption of fish or fish oil reduces stroke incidence. This is believed to occur as a result of a number of effects, including impairment of blood clots, improvement of cholesterol profile, and other unidentified means.

Many other herbs and supplements may also reduce the blood's tendency to clot and, thereby, help prevent strokes. These herbs and supplements include bilberry, feverfew, garlic, ginger, ginkgo, quercetin, vitamin E, and white willow. However, the supporting evidence for these supplements remains weak at best, and the mere fact that they thin the blood does not prove that they will reduce stroke risk. For example, while vitamin E is known to reduce blood clotting and is also a strong antioxidant, several large studies have failed to find vitamin E helpful for stroke prevention.

Similarly, the herb white willow has been advocated as a substitute for aspirin because it contains salicin, a substance very much like aspirin. However, willow, taken in usual doses, does not appear to impair blood coagulation to the same extent as aspirin, and for that reason, it is probably not equally effective. The supplement folate has shown some promise for preventing strokes. Also, besides vitamin E, other antioxidants, such as beta-carotene, have been proposed for stroke prevention, but there is no evidence that they are effective.

Acupuncture is widely used in China for enhancing recovery from strokes. However, while some studies have suggested benefits, the best-designed and largest studies have not been promising. For example, in a single-blind, placebo-controlled trial of 104 people who had just experienced strokes, ten weeks of twice-weekly acupuncture did not prove more effective than fake acupuncture. Similarly negative results were seen in a single-blind, controlled study of 150 people recovering from stroke, which compared acupuncture (including electro-acupuncture), high-intensity muscle stimulation, and sham treatment. All participants received twenty treatments in a ten-week period. Neither acupuncture nor muscle stimulation produced any benefits. In addition, a ten-week study of 106 people, which provided a total of thirty-five traditional acupuncture sessions to each participant, also failed to find benefit. Finally, ninety-two persons who randomly received either twelve acupuncture treatments or comparable sham treatment for four weeks demonstrated the same level of improvement up to one year later. The few studies that did report improvements from acupuncture were small, and some did not use a placebo group. In a review of fifty-six trials (mostly written in Chinese), researchers found that 80 percent showed positive results. However, the small size and variable quality of these studies make it difficult to draw reliable conclusions about the benefits of acupuncture in the setting of a stroke. In one study, acupressure combined with lavender, rosemary, and peppermint aromatherapy was more effective than acupressure alone for treating the shoulder pain caused by hemiplegic strokes. However, this study lacked a proper placebo group and therefore means little. A review of nine trials found limited evidence in support of moxibustion (the application of heat to acupuncture points) in addition to standard care for stroke rehabilitation. Also, the semisynthetic substance citicholine (closely related to the nutrient choline) has shown some promise for aiding recovery from strokes.

In a study investigating the effects of music therapy, stroke patients who listened to music of their own choosing in the early stages of their recovery demonstrated more improvement in memory and attention than those patients who listened to language (that is, books on tape). Music listeners were also less depressed and confused than subjects who listened neither to music nor to language.

HERBS AND SUPPLEMENTS TO USE WITH CAUTION

If one is at risk for a stroke, it might be advisable to avoid excessive intake of iron. Some evidence suggests that high iron levels may increase stroke risk and worsen strokes that do occur.

People susceptible to stroke should exercise great caution regarding the herb ephedra. Ephedra contains ephedrine, a drug that raises blood pressure and stimulates the heart, and it has caused heart attacks and strokes. Certain preparations of ephedra may present an additional risk beyond ephedrine's effects on the circulatory system: direct toxicity to nerves.

Finally, numerous herbs and supplements may interact adversely with drugs used to prevent or treat strokes, so persons should be cautious when considering the use of herbs and supplements.

EBSCO CAM Review Board

FURTHER READING

Bereczki, D., and I. Fekete. "Vinpocetine for Acute Ischaemic Stroke." *Cochrane Database of Systematic Reviews* (2008): CD000480. Available through *EBSCO DynaMed Systematic Literature Surveillance* at http://www.ebscohost.com/dynamed.

Hopwood, V., et al. "Evaluating the Efficacy of Acupuncture in Defined Aspects of Stroke Recovery." *Journal of Neurology* 255 (2008): 858-866.

Iso, H., et al. "Intake of Fish and Omega-3 Fatty Acids and Risk of Stroke in Women." *Journal of the American Medical Association* 285 (2001): 304-312.

Lee, M. S., B. C. Shin, and J. I. Kim. "Moxibustion for Stroke Rehabilitation." *Stroke* 41 (2010): 817-820.

Sarkamo, T., et al. "Music Listening Enhances Cognitive Recovery and Mood After Middle Cerebral Artery Stroke." *Brain* 131 (2008): 866-876.

Shin, B. C., and M. S. Lee. "Effects of Aromatherapy Acupressure on Hemiplegic Shoulder Pain and Motor Power in Stroke Patients." *Journal of Alternative and Complementary Medicine* 13 (2007): 247-252.

Wang, X., et al. "Efficacy of Folic Acid Supplementation in Stroke Prevention." *The Lancet* 369 (2007): 1876-1882.

Wayne, P. M., et al. "Acupuncture for Upper-Extremity Rehabilitation in Chronic Stroke." *Archives of Physical Medicine and Rehabilitation* 86 (2005): 2248-2255.

Wu, P., et al. "Acupuncture in Poststroke Rehabilitation." *Stroke* 41 (2010): e171-179.

See also: Cardiomyopathy; Chelation therapy; Cholesterol, high; Epilepsy; Glycine; Hypertension; Policosanol; Strokes: Homeopathic remedies; Vinpocetine.

Strokes: Homeopathic remedies

CATEGORY: Homeopathy

RELATED TERM: Cerebral vascular accident

DEFINITION: The use of highly diluted remedies to treat cell death in the brain caused by a sudden loss of blood supply.

STUDIED HOMEOPATHIC REMEDIES: *Arnica*, belladonna, *Gelsemium*

SCIENTIFIC EVALUATIONS OF HOMEOPATHIC REMEDIES

Homeopathic treatment has been proposed as a cost-effective method of aiding recovery from stroke. However, two reported double-blind, placebo-controlled studies of homeopathic *Arnica* did not yield promising results.

The first study enrolled forty people who had suffered a significant stroke within the prior seven days. Participants were given either *Arnica* 30c (centesimal) or placebo in a dosage of one tablet every two hours, for six doses. Participants were then followed for three months to see if the *Arnica* group would recover more fully. The results showed no significant difference between the participants receiving *Arnica* and those who received placebo.

In the second trial, researchers administered *Arnica* 1m (an extreme dilution of one part in 102,000) to forty people. Again, no statistically significant improvements were seen in the treatment group compared with the placebo group.

TRADITIONAL HOMEOPATHIC TREATMENTS

Classical homeopathy offers possible homeopathic treatments for stroke. These therapies are chosen based on various specific details of the person seeking treatment. *Arnica* was chosen for the foregoing studies because of its traditional use for the treatment of acute traumatic conditions. It is typically given as an emergency treatment right after a stroke and for weeks or months into the recovery period.

Belladonna is also sometimes used for stroke "first aid," especially when the victim's face is flushed, the eyes are fixed wide open, and he or she has a headache, nosebleed, and fever and is sensitive to sound and light. The loss of ability to speak after a stroke is a traditional indication for *Gelsemium*. Other aspects of this remedy's symptom picture include a sensation of mental dullness, weakness, pain along the spine, dizziness, and headache in the forehead and at the base of the skull.

EBSCO CAM Review Board

FURTHER READING

Bell, I. R. "Adjunctive Care with Nutritional, Herbal, and Homeopathic Complementary and Alternative Medicine Modalities in Stroke Treatment and Rehabilitation." *Topics in Stroke Rehabilitation* 14 (2007): 30-39.

Kraft, K. "Complementary/Alternative Medicine in the Context of Prevention of Disease and Maintenance of Health." *Preventive Medicine* 49 (2009): 88-92.

Savage, R. H., and P. F. Roe. "A Double Blind Trial to Assess the Benefit of *Arnica montana* in Acute Stroke Illness." *British Homeopathic Journal* 66 (1977): 207-220.

_____. "A Further Double Blind Trial to Access the Benefit of *Arnica montana* in Acute Stroke Illness." *British Homeopathic Journal* 67 (1978): 210-222.

See also: Homeopathy.

Strontium

CATEGORY: Herbs and supplements

DEFINITION: Natural substance used to treat specific health conditions.

PRINCIPAL PROPOSED USE: Osteoporosis

OTHER PROPOSED USE: Cavities (caries)

OVERVIEW

Strontium is a trace element widely found in nature. It became famous in the 1960s when a radioactive form of strontium produced by atomic bomb testing, strontium 90, became prevalent in the environment. Nonradioactive strontium has recently undergone study as a treatment for osteoporosis, with some promising results. The major human studies of strontium for osteoporosis have involved a special form of the mineral called strontium ranelate.

REQUIREMENTS AND SOURCES

There is no known daily requirement for strontium.

THERAPEUTIC DOSAGES

Based on current evidence, strontium ranelate can be taken at a dose of 500 milligrams (mg) to 1 gram (g) daily to prevent osteoporosis and at a higher dose of 2 g daily to treat existing osteoporosis. It is not clear whether combining strontium with standard treatments for osteoporosis will enhance or diminish the ultimate benefits.

THERAPEUTIC USES

Strontium has fundamental chemical similarities to calcium. When dietary intake of strontium is raised, strontium begins to take the place of calcium in developing bone. This replacement appears to be beneficial (at least with low doses of strontium), leading to an increase in bone formation, a decrease in bone breakdown, and an overall rise in bone density. The net result is a reduced incidence of fractures due to osteoporosis, according to two very large studies. In addition, highly preliminary evidence hints that strontium might help prevent cavities by strengthening dental enamel.

SCIENTIFIC EVIDENCE

As noted, the major human studies of strontium for osteoporosis involved strontium ranelate. In a three-year double-blind, placebo-controlled study of 5,091 women with osteoporosis, use of strontium at a dose of 2 g daily significantly improved bone density and reduced incidence of all fractures compared with placebo.

Additionally, in a three-year double-blind, placebo-controlled study of 1,649 postmenopausal women with osteoporosis and a history of at least one vertebral fracture, use of strontium ranelate at a dose of 2 g daily reduced the incidence of new vertebral fractures by 49 percent in the first year and 41 percent in the full three-year period (compared with placebo). Use of strontium also significantly increased measured bone density. No significant side effects were seen.

A fourth study tested strontium ranelate for preventing osteoporosis in postmenopausal women who had not developed it. In this two-year double-blind, placebo-controlled study, 160 women received either placebo or strontium ranelate at a dose of 125 mg, 500 mg, or 1 g daily. The results showed that the more strontium taken, the greater the gains in bone density.

While some treatments for osteoporosis act to increase bone formation and others decrease bone breakdown, some evidence suggests that strontium ranelate has a dual effect, providing both these benefits at once.

Other forms of strontium aside from strontium ranelate, such as strontium chloride, have shown potential benefits in animal studies but have not undergone significant testing in people.

SAFETY ISSUES

When taken in recommended doses, strontium supplements appear to be safe and usually free of side effects other than occasional mild gastrointestinal upset, including diarrhea. There is some weak evidence that long-term use of strontium ranelate could, rarely, cause memory loss or seizures. Similarly weak evidence hints that strontium could raise risk of blood clots; however, one small study was somewhat reassuring on this score.

Excessive intake of strontium can actually weaken bone by replacing too much of the bone's calcium with strontium.

Maximum safe doses of strontium in young children, pregnant or nursing women, or people with severe liver or kidney disease have not been established. For persons who are taking standard treatment for osteoporosis, it is not clear whether the addition of strontium will enhance or diminish the benefits.

EBSCO CAM Review Board

FURTHER READING

Halil, M., et al. "Short-Term Hemostatic Safety of Strontium Ranelate Treatment in Elderly Women with Osteoporosis." *Annals of Pharmacotherapy* 41 (2007): 41-45.

Marie, P. J. "Strontium Ranelate: A Dual Mode of Action Rebalancing Bone Turnover in Favour of Bone Formation." *Current Opinion in Rheumatology* 18, suppl. 1 (2006): S11-S15.

Meunier, P. J., C. Roux, et al. "The Effects of Strontium Ranelate on the Risk of Vertebral Fracture in Women with Postmenopausal Osteoporosis." *New England Journal of Medicine* 350 (2004): 459-468.

Meunier, P. J., D. O. Slosman, et al. "Strontium Ranelate: Dose-Dependent Effects in Established Postmenopausal Vertebral Osteoporosis." *Journal of Clinical Endocrinology and Metabolism* 87 (2002): 2060-2066.

Reginster, J. Y., R. Deroisy, and I. Jupsin. "Strontium Ranelate: A New Paradigm in the Treatment of Osteoporosis." *Drugs of Today* (Barcelona) 39 (2003): 89-101.

Reginster, J. Y., R. Deroisy, M. Dougados, et al. "Prevention of Early Postmenopausal Bone Loss by Strontium Ranelate: The Randomized, Two-Year, Double-Masked, Dose-Ranging, Placebo-Controlled PREVOS Trial." *Osteoporosis International* 13 (2002): 925-931.

Reginster, J. Y., E. Seeman, et al. "Strontium Ranelate Reduces the Risk of Nonvertebral Fractures in Postmenopausal Women with Osteoporosis: Treatment of Peripheral Osteoporosis (TROPOS) Study." *Journal of Clinical Endocrinology and Metabolism* 90 (2005): 2816-2822.

See also: Cavity prevention; Osteoporosis.

Sublingual immunotherapy

CATEGORY: Therapies and techniques

DEFINITION: Treatment of allergies by placing an allergen solution, such as pollen extract, under the tongue.

PRINCIPAL PROPOSED USE: Allergic rhinitis

OTHER PROPOSED USES: Asthma, latex allergy, other forms of allergy

OVERVIEW

Sublingual immunotherapy (SLIT) is a method of treating allergies that closely resembles conventional "allergy shots." In both of these methods, small amounts of allergenic substances are administered periodically and over time, through a route different from that in which the body ordinarily encounters them. For example, plant pollens ordinarily cause their allergic reactions by being inhaled. With allergy shots, pollen extracts are injected under the skin, while in SLIT, they are placed under the tongue.

The immune system has many components, and only one of them, the IgE/eosinophil system, produces typical allergic reactions. The intended effect of the alternate routes of administration is to "train" other branches of the immune system to neutralize allergens before the IgE/eosinophil system can react to their presence.

The great potential advantage of SLIT over allergy shots is that SLIT does not involve needles; this makes it less unpleasant and also capable of being done at home rather than at a doctor's office. The absence of needles may also explain why SLIT has long been categorized as a form of alternative rather than conventional medicine.

There are no universally accepted criteria by which a treatment is classified as part of alternative rather than conventional medicine. Some treatments, such as acupuncture, fall in the alternative category because they belong to a system of medicine considerably unlike that of the modern conventional system; others, like traditional herbology, fall in the alternative category because they involve unprocessed "natural" substances rather than drugs; still others are considered alternative simply because they have been rejected for one reason or another by conventional medicine or have been adopted by practitioners of other forms of alternative medicine.

SLIT is primarily in the last camp. Until approximately the year 2000, SLIT was most commonly the province of practitioners who identified themselves as holistic or alternative, and the therapy was looked on with skepticism by mainstream medicine. In recent years, however, numerous well-designed studies of SLIT have been reported, causing the method to gain increasing acceptance among conventional allergists.

SCIENTIFIC EVIDENCE

Perhaps the best evidence for the effectiveness of SLIT involves treatment of allergic rhinitis (hay fever). In a double-blind study of 855 adults with grass allergies, SLIT using grass pollen tablets for approximately eighteen weeks markedly reduced allergy symptoms, including nasal congestion and itchy eyes. Marked

Research Spotlight: Peanut Allergy in Children

A new treatment may be a safe and effective form of immunotherapy for children with peanut allergy, according to researchers at Duke University Medical Center and Massachusetts General Hospital. Currently, there are no treatments available for people with peanut allergy. The double-blind, placebo-controlled study, funded in part by National Center for Complementary and Alternative Medicine and published in the *Journal of Allergy and Clinical Immunology*, investigated the safety, clinical effectiveness, and immunologic changes with sublingual immunotherapy—a treatment that involves administering very small amounts of the allergen extract under a person's tongue.

Researchers randomly assigned eighteen children (aged one to eleven years) with known peanut allergy to receive either peanut sublingual immunotherapy or placebo. Participants in the peanut group received increased doses of peanut extract every two weeks for six months. Following each dose increase, participants continued the same daily dose at home. Once a maximum dose of 2,000 micrograms of peanut protein was reached, participants continued to take this daily maintenance dose at home for approximately six more months.

After a total of twelve months of sublingual immunotherapy, participants underwent a food challenge, which involved taking increasing doses of peanut protein in the form of peanut flour mixed with food. The food-challenge placebo consisted of oat flour mixed with food given in the same increments. Allergy skin-prick tests were performed, and participants' blood samples were taken at different points throughout the study.

The researchers found that the participants who had received peanut sublingual immunotherapy could safely consume twenty times more peanut protein than those who had received the placebo (1710 milligrams [mg] versus 85 mg). This level of desensitization is clinically significant because it represents protection from accidental ingestion of peanut, which is often less than 100 mg (or one peanut). In addition, allergy skin-prick tests showed a decreased allergic response to peanut in the treatment group. The blood tests showed immunologic changes in the treatment group, suggesting a significant change in allergic response.

benefits for most common hay fever symptoms were also seen in another double-blind study enrolling 634 people. In a third double-blind study involving 105 persons, SLIT led to a significant improvement over placebo in symptoms of rhinitis and conjunctivitis from grass and rye pollen allergies. Skin reactivity to these allergens, a more objective sign of allergy, also showed a more substantial reduction in persons using SLIT. Other studies have also shown benefit for hay fever caused by grass pollen or other allergens, including dust mites and tree pollen.

However, in a 2008 comprehensive review of studies investigating SLIT for grass pollen and house dust-mite allergies, researchers were unable to substantiate claims of effectiveness, largely because of the variable quality of the studies they uncovered.

As with conventional allergy shots for hay fever, it appears that if SLIT is in fact effective, it must be used for a long time for best results. Three years of treatment may be better than two, and two years better than one. To provide benefits for grass allergy season, SLIT must begin a minimum of eight weeks before the onset of the grass allergy season; even longer lead times produce even better results. Putting all this evidence together, it appears that SLIT may work best if used every year and year-round.

One study suggests that SLIT not only is effective for treating allergy; it also may be useful in preventing the development of new allergies or mild persistent asthma in children with allergic rhinitis or intermittent asthma. SLIT has also shown promise for latex allergy and other forms of allergy.

SAFETY ISSUES

SLIT appears to be safer than conventional allergy shots. The most frequently reported adverse effects include oral itching or swelling and gastrointestinal upset; in the majority of cases, these side effects are mild and short-lived. In one study, 12 percent of persons with allergic rhinitis or asthma experienced worsening of symptoms at some point in their treatment. Severe allergic reactions appear to occur rarely. However, SLIT has not been tested in person with high-risk asthma. Another problem is that no allergy extracts for use in SLIT have been officially approved for use in the United States, so the products available remain incompletely regulated.

EBSCO CAM Review Board

FURTHER READING

Cox, L. S., et al. "Sublingual Immunotherapy: A Comprehensive Review." *Journal of Allergy and Clinical Immunology* 117 (2006): 1021-1035.

Dahl, R., et al. "Sublingual Grass Allergen Tablet Immunotherapy Provides Sustained Clinical Benefit with Progressive Immunologic Changes over Two Years." *Journal of Allergy and Clinical Immunology* 121 (2008): 512-518.

Marogna, M., et al. "Preventive Effects of Sublingual Immunotherapy in Childhood." *Annals of Allergy, Asthma, and Immunology* 101 (2008): 206-211.

Nettis, E., et al. "Double-Blind, Placebo-Controlled Study of Sublingual Immunotherapy in Patients with Latex-Induced Urticaria." *British Journal of Dermatology* 156 (2007): 674-681.

Pfaar, O., and L. Klimek. "Efficacy and Safety of Specific Immunotherapy with a High-Dose Sublingual Grass Pollen Preparation." *Annals of Allergy, Asthma, and Immunology* 100 (2008): 256-263.

Rodriguez-Perez, N., et al. "Frequency of Acute Systemic Reactions in Patients with Allergic Rhinitis and Asthma Treated with Sublingual Immunotherapy." *Annals of Allergy, Asthma, and Immunology* 101 (2008): 304-310.

See also: Allergies; Asthma; Grass pollen extract; Immune support.

Sulforaphane

CATEGORY: Herbs and supplements
DEFINITION: Natural plant product used to treat specific health conditions.
PRINCIPAL PROPOSED USE: Cancer prevention

OVERVIEW

Sulforaphane is a chemical found in broccoli sprouts, as well as in other cabbage-family vegetables such as broccoli, Brussels sprouts, cabbage, cauliflower, and kale. Some evidence hints that sulforaphane might help prevent cancer.

REQUIREMENTS AND SOURCES

Sulforaphane is not an essential nutrient. It is found in especially high levels in broccoli sprouts.

THERAPEUTIC DOSAGES

The proper daily intake (if there is any) of sulforaphane is not known. Typical recommendations range from 200 to 400 micrograms (mcg) daily.

THERAPEUTIC USES

Numerous observational studies have found that a high consumption of vegetables in the cabbage family is associated with a reduced risk of cancer, especially breast, prostate, lung, stomach, colon, and rectal cancer. On this basis, scientists have looked for anticancer substances in these foods. Sulforaphane is one such candidate substance (indole-3-carbinol, or I3C, is another). In test-tube and animal studies, sulforaphane exhibits properties that suggest it could indeed help prevent many forms of cancer.

However, it is a long way from such studies to reliable evidence of benefit. Observational studies are notoriously poor guides to treatment, sometimes leading to conclusions that are the reverse of what is ultimately found to be correct. The problem is that they cannot show cause and effect; they can show only association. It is possible, for example, that people who consume more cabbage-family vegetables share other traits that are responsible for reduced cancer rates. Consider the history of hormone replacement therapy. In the 1990s, scientists had concluded that estrogen prevents heart disease, based largely on observational studies that showed menopausal women who use hormone replacement have lower rates of heart disease than women who do not. When double-blind, placebo-controlled studies were performed, however, the results showed that hormone replacement therapy actually increases heart disease risk. For all anyone currently knows, scientists could be making a similar mistake with cabbage-family vegetables.

Certainly, it is too great a leap to single out one constituent of such vegetables and advocate that substance for preventing cancer. Thousands of substances show anticancer properties in the test tube and fail to pan out in real life. The beta-carotene story is another instructive example. Not only did observational studies show that people who consume foods high in beta-carotene have less lung cancer, test-tube studies found that beta-carotene has anticancer properties. However, subsequent large double-blind studies found that beta-carotene supplements do not help prevent lung cancer and might even increase risk. The use of sulforaphane for preventing cancer is not recommended.

SAFETY ISSUES

No major adverse effects have been reported with sulforaphane supplements, but comprehensive studies have not been performed. Maximum safe doses in young children, pregnant or nursing women, or people with severe liver or kidney disease are not known.

Sulforaphane has shown the potential for interacting with numerous medications. For this reason, it is recommended that individuals taking any oral or injected medication that is critical to their health or well-being avoid using sulforaphane supplements until more is known. Persons who are taking any medication that is critical to their health should not take sulforaphane supplements except under physician supervision.

EBSCO CAM Review Board

FURTHER READING

Brooks, J. D., V. G. Paton, and G. Vidanes. "Potent Induction of Phase 2 Enzymes in Human Prostate Cells by Sulforaphane." *Cancer Epidemiology, Biomarkers, and Prevention* 10 (2001): 949-954.

Chiao, J. W., et al. "Sulforaphane and Its Metabolite Mediate Growth Arrest and Apoptosis in Human Prostate Cancer Cells." *International Journal of Oncology* 20 (2002): 631-636.

Frydoonfar, H. R., D. R. McGrath, and A. D. Spigelman. "The Effect of Indole-3-Carbinol and Sulforaphane on a Prostate Cancer Cell Line." *ANZ Journal of Surgery* 73 (2003): 154-156.

Johnston, N. "Sulforaphane Halts Breast Cancer Cell Growth." *Drug Discovery Today* 9 (2004): 908.

Joseph, M. A., et al. "Cruciferous Vegetables, Genetic Polymorphisms in Glutathione S-Transferases M1 and T1, and Prostate Cancer Risk." *Nutrition and Cancer* 50 (2004): 206-213.

Myzak, M. C., et al. "A Novel Mechanism of Chemoprotection by Sulforaphane: Inhibition of Histone Deacetylase." *Cancer Research* 64 (2004): 5767-5774.

Solowiej, E., et al. "Chemoprevention of Cancerogenesis: The Role of Sulforaphane." *Acta Poloniae Pharmaceutica* 60 (2003): 97-100.

See also: Cancer risk reduction.

Suma

CATEGORY: Herbs and supplements

RELATED TERMS: *Para toda, Pfaffia paniculata*

DEFINITION: Natural plant product used to treat specific health conditions.

PRINCIPAL PROPOSED USES: None

OTHER PROPOSED USES: Adaptogen (improve resistance to stress), anxiety, chronic fatigue syndrome, immune support, menopausal symptoms, menstrual problems, sexual dysfunction in men, sexual dysfunction in women, sickle cell disease, sports performance enhancement, ulcers

OVERVIEW

Suma is a large ground vine native to Central America and South America; it is sometimes called Brazilian ginseng. Indigenous peoples have long used suma to promote robust health and to treat practically all illnesses. They have called suma *para toda*, which means "for all things."

THERAPEUTIC DOSAGES

A typical dosage of suma is 500 milligrams (mg) twice daily. It is usually taken for an extended period of time.

THERAPEUTIC USES

Suma's ancient reputation has generated worldwide interest. However, to date there has been little formal scientific investigation of the herb.

According to most contemporary herbalists, suma is best understood as an adaptogen, a substance that supposedly helps the body adapt to stress and fight infection. Russian Olympic athletes have reportedly used suma (and other adaptogens) in the belief that it will enhance sports performance. In the United States, suma is often recommended as a general strengthener of the body and for the treatment of chronic fatigue syndrome, menopausal symptoms and problems, ulcers, anxiety, and impotence, and for immune support. The herb also has a considerable reputation as an aphrodisiac. However, there is no reliable scientific evidence that suma offers any benefits for these conditions. Finally, one test-tube study suggests that suma might be helpful for sickle cell disease, but it is a long way from such preliminary investigations to evidence of efficacy.

SAFETY ISSUES

Suma has not been associated with any serious adverse reactions. However, comprehensive safety studies have not been undertaken. Safety of the use of suma by young children, pregnant or nursing women, and those with severe liver or kidney disease has not been established.

EBSCO CAM Review Board

FURTHER READING

Ballas, S. K. "Short Report: Hydration of Sickle Erythrocytes Using a Herbal Extract (*Pfaffia paniculata*) In Vitro." *British Journal of Haematology* 111 (2000): 359-362.

De Oliveira, F. "*Pfaffia paniculata* (Martius) Kuntze-Brazilian Ginseng." *Revista Brasileira de Farmacognosia* 1 (1986): 86-92.

See also: Fatigue; Ginseng; Immune support.

Sunburn

CATEGORY: Condition

DEFINITION: Treatment of burns to the skin caused by overexposure to the sun.

PRINCIPAL PROPOSED NATURAL TREATMENTS: Epigallocatechin gallate (bioflavonoid in green tea), vitamin C, vitamin E

OTHER PROPOSED NATURAL TREATMENTS: Aloe vera, beta-carotene and other carotenoids, chocolate, coriander oil, jojoba, oligomeric proanthocyanidins, poplar bud, sage, *Vitis vinifera*

INTRODUCTION

Everyone is familiar with sunburn, the short-term skin inflammation caused by overexposure to the sun. Besides the familiar redness, pain, blistering, and flaking, overexposure to sunlight can lead to long-term skin damage, including premature aging and an increased risk of skin cancer.

The chief culprit in sunburn is not the sun's heat but its ultraviolet radiation, which occurs in the forms UVA and UVB. This radiation acts on substances in the skin to form chemicals called free radicals. These free radicals appear to be partly responsible for the short-term damage of sunburn and perhaps for long-term damage from the sun.

Conventional approaches to sunburn focus on prevention: staying out of the sun (especially when the sun is strongest), wearing protective clothing, and using sunscreen. Sunscreen blocks much of the radiation from the skin and helps prevent inflammation. A study of 1,383 Australians suggests that regular sunscreen use may also diminish the number of tumors caused by one form of skin cancer, squamous cell carcinoma.

Many drugs and herbs may increase one's sensitivity to the sun. Some of the drugs that increase sun sensitivity are sulfa drugs, tetracycline, phenothiazines, and piroxicam. Herbs that might increase sensitivity to the sun include St. John's wort and dong quai. Particular care should be taken when combining any of these substances, because they could amplify each other's effects.

PRINCIPAL PROPOSED NATURAL TREATMENTS

Several studies have found that vitamin C, vitamin E, and EGCG (a bioflavonoid present in green tea) may help to prevent sunburn when used either topically or orally. Many manufacturers already add vitamin E to sunscreens.

Vitamins C and E. Antioxidants such as vitamins C and E neutralize free radicals in the blood and in other parts of the body. Test-tube and animal studies suggest that antioxidants perform the same job in the skin. Levels of these antioxidants in skin cells decrease after exposure to ultraviolet radiation, suggesting they may be temporarily depleted.

In several animal studies, vitamins C and E applied topically to the skin helped to protect against ultraviolet damage. One study found that topical vitamin E seemed to work best against UVB, topical vitamin C protected more against UVA, and the two vitamins together worked better than either one by itself. Vitamin E was effective even when applied to mouse skin eight hours after ultraviolet exposure had occurred. Combining the vitamins with sunscreen yielded the best result, adding to the UV-protection offered by sunscreen alone. In addition, preliminary evidence from a small, double-blind, placebo-controlled trial suggests that a face cream containing vitamin C could improve the appearance of sun-damaged skin.

The oral use of combined vitamins C and E may offer modest benefit. One double-blind study of ten people found that 2 grams (g) of vitamin C and 1,000 international units (IU) of vitamin E taken for eight

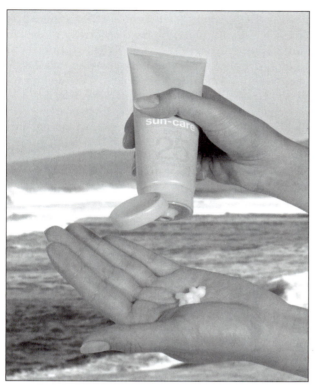

Sunscreens work by absorbing, reflecting, or scattering UVA and UVB from the sun. (© Stephen Coburn/Dreamstime.com)

days resulted in a modest decrease in skin reddening induced by ultraviolet light. A fifty-day, placebo-controlled study of forty people found that high doses of these vitamins in combination provided a minimal, but statistically significant, sun protection factor of about 2.13 (The sun protection factor of many sunscreens is 15 to 45.)

One study found benefits with a combination of vitamins E and C, selenium, oligomeric proanthocyanidins (OPCs), and carotenoids. However, research has not found that vitamin E and C, taken separately, are any more helpful than placebo.

Epigallocatechin gallate. Green tea contains a potent antioxidant known as epigallocatechin gallate, or EGCG. According to several studies, mice given green tea to drink or topical applications of green tea were protected against skin inflammation and carcinogenesis caused by exposure to UVB. Benefits were also seen in two preliminary human trials. The typical proposed dose of EGCG is 3 milligrams (mg) per square inch of skin.

OTHER PROPOSED NATURAL TREATMENTS

Beta-carotene and mixed carotenoids. Beta-carotene belongs to a large family of natural chemicals known as carotenoids. Other members of this family include lutein, lycopene, and zeaxanthin. Widely found in plants, carotenoids are a major source of the red, orange, and yellow hues seen in many fruits and vegetables. Beta-carotene is important nutritionally because the body uses it to produce vitamin A.

Beta-carotene, alone or with lutein and other carotenoids, may be able to reduce the effects of sunburn, but study results are mixed. In a double-blind study, twenty young women took 30 mg daily of beta-carotene or placebo for ten weeks before a thirteen-day stretch of controlled sun exposure at a sea-level vacation spot. Those who had taken the beta-carotene before and during the sun exposure experienced less skin redness than those taking placebo, even when both groups used sunscreen.

A twelve-week, double-blind, placebo-controlled study found beta-carotene (at 24 mg daily) and a mixture of beta-carotene, lutein, and lycopene (at 8 mg each daily) equally protective against sun-induced skin redness. Another small double-blind trial found that a mixture of lutein and the related carotenoid zeaxanthin provided benefits when taken orally, applied topically, or, even better, taken orally and applied topically at the same time.

Two open studies of mixed carotenoids found similar results. These trials, one of twenty and one of twenty-two people, found that after taking mixed carotenoids for twelve to twenty-four weeks, participants could tolerate more ultraviolet radiation before developing skin redness. Vitamin E (500 IU per day) taken with beta-carotene in one of the studies did not significantly affect the results. Another study found benefits with tomato paste (rich in lycopene). However, because these studies were not double-blind, the results are not reliable.

Not every study has found beta-carotene or mixed carotenoids to be helpful. In a double-blind trial of sixteen older women, high doses of beta-carotene taken for twenty-three days did not provide any more protection than placebo against simulated sun exposure. Another ten-week study found that high doses of beta-carotene provided greater protection against natural sunshine than placebo, but the benefits, though statistically significant, were too minor to matter. Completely negative results were seen in a four-week uncontrolled study of high doses of mixed carotenoids.

Other natural treatments. The substances collectively called OPCs, found in pine bark and grape seed, have shown some promise for sunburn protection. Also, chocolate contains polyphenol flavonols similar to those in green tea. A special form of chocolate enriched in flavonol content might, like green tea extracts, modestly protect the skin from sun damage.

Weak evidence hints at benefit with an extract of the shoots of the *Vitis vinifera* plant (the common grape vine) and with an extract of sage. Although research information is lacking, topical jojoba, poplar bud (*Populi gemma*), and aloe vera are sometimes recommended for soothing sunburn pain and itch. However, one small study found that applying aloe vera gel after UVB exposure had no effect on skin redness. In a preliminary double-blind study, coriander oil applied topically was more effective than a placebo cream at reducing redness caused by UVB exposure.

EBSCO CAM Review Board

FURTHER READING

Cornacchione, S., et al. "In Vivo Skin Antioxidant Effect of a New Combination Based on a Specific *Vitis vinifera* Shoot Extract and a Biotechnological Extract." *Journal of Drugs in Dermatology* 6 (2007): 8-13.

Elmets, C. A., et al. "Cutaneous Photoprotection from Ultraviolet Injury by Green Tea Polyphenols." *Journal of the American Academy of Dermatology* 44 (2001): 425-432.

Greul, A. K., et al. "Photoprotection of UV-Irradiated Human Skin: An Antioxidative Combination of Vitamins E and C, Carotenoids, Selenium, and Proanthocyanidins." *Skin Pharmacology and Applied Skin Physiology* 15 (2002): 307-315.

Heinrich, U., and C. Gartner et al. "Supplementation with Beta-carotene or a Similar Amount of Mixed Carotenoids Protects Humans from UV-Induced Erythema." *Journal of Nutrition* 133 (2003): 98-101.

Heinrich, U., and K. Neukam et al. "Long-Term Ingestion of High Flavanol Cocoa Provides Photoprotection Against UV-Induced Erythema and Improves Skin Condition in Women." *Journal of Nutrition* 136 (2006): 1565-1569.

Katiyar, S. K., N. Ahmad, and H. Mukhtar. "Green Tea and Skin." *Archives of Dermatology* 136 (2000): 989-994.

Palombo, P., et al. "Beneficial Long-Term Effects of Combined Oral/Topical Antioxidant Treatment with the Carotenoids Lutein and Zeaxanthin on Human Skin." *Skin Pharmacology and Physiology* 20 (2007): 199-210.

Reuter, J., et al. "Anti-inflammatory Potential of a Lipolotion Containing Coriander Oil in the Ultraviolet Erythema Test." *Journal of the German Society of Dermatology* 10 (2008): 847-851.

Stahl, W., et al. "Dietary Tomato Paste Protects Against Ultraviolet Light-Induced Erythema in Humans." *Journal of Nutrition* 131 (2001): 1449-1451.

See also: Green tea; Photosensitivity; Skin, aging; Vitamin C; Vitamin E.

Superoxide dismutase

CATEGORY: Herbs and supplements
DEFINITION: Natural substance of the human body used as a supplement to treat specific health conditions.
PRINCIPAL PROPOSED USES: None
OTHER PROPOSED USES: Antiaging, radiation therapy support, wound healing

OVERVIEW

In the body, dangerous naturally occurring substances called free radicals pose a risk of harm to many tissues. The body deploys an antioxidant defense system to hold free radicals in check. Superoxide dismutase (SOD) is one of the most important elements of this system. It controls levels of a chemical called superoxide. The body manufactures superoxide to kill bacteria and for other uses, but excess levels of superoxide can injure healthy cells. SOD converts superoxide to hydrogen peroxide, and then another enzyme, catalase, neutralizes hydrogen peroxide.

Nutrients such as vitamin C and vitamin E also help neutralize free radicals. In the 1990s, such antioxidant supplements were widely promoted for preventing a variety of diseases, including cancer and heart disease, and during this period oral SOD became popular as a supplemental antioxidant. The results of several large studies tended to dash these hopes. Compared with ordinary antioxidants, SOD suffers from the additional disadvantages of being expensive and poorly absorbed when taken by mouth.

REQUIREMENTS AND SOURCES

SOD is not an essential nutrient, and it is not obtained through food.

THERAPEUTIC DOSAGES

When SOD is taken orally, little to none of it is absorbed by the body. Some manufacturers market sublingual (under the tongue) forms of SOD that are purported to get around this problem. However, there does not appear to be any meaningful evidence that SOD can be absorbed any better this way.

Weak evidence hints that a form of SOD in which the substance is encapsulated in structures called liposomes may be absorbable. The optimum dose, if any, is not known.

THERAPEUTIC USES

Various Web sites promote SOD for a wide range of health problems, from preventing aging to enhancing sports performance. However, as noted above, oral SOD supplements may be ineffective because of poor absorption.

A bit of evidence hints that SOD injections may reduce scarring caused by radiation therapy and may also decrease symptoms of osteoarthritis. SOD applied directly to wounds may enhance wound healing, according to experiments in animals.

In test-tube and animal studies, genetic manipulation has been used to increase SOD levels in the hope of finding antiaging effects, but the results have been mixed.

Inhaled SOD appears to be useful for premature infants, helping to prevent a condition called respiratory distress syndrome. However, the only evidence for benefits with any oral form of SOD is a study in animals involving the special liposome form of the supplement mentioned above. It found possible anti-inflammatory effects.

SAFETY ISSUES

Oral SOD is presumably quite safe, since it is apparently not absorbable. The safety of other forms of SOD (including the possibly absorbable encapsulated form) has not been established.

EBSCO CAM Review Board

FURTHER READING

Davis, J. M., S. E. Richter, et al. "Long-Term Follow-Up of Premature Infants Treated with Prophylactic, In-tratracheal Recombinant Human CuZn Superoxide Dismutase." *Journal of Perinatology* 4 (2000): 213-216.

Davis, J. M., W. N. Rosenfeld, et al. "The Effects of Multiple Doses of Recombinant Human CuZn Superoxide Dismutase (rhSOD) in Premature Infants with Respiratory Distress Syndrome (RDS)." *Pediatric Research* 45 (1999): 193A.

Delanian, S., et al. "Cu/Zn Superoxide Dismutase Modulates Phenotypic Changes in Cultured Fibroblasts from Human Skin with Chronic Radiotherapy Damage." *Radiotherapy and Oncology* 58 (2001): 325-331.

Flanagan, S. W., et al. "Overexpression of Manganese Superoxide Dismutase Attenuates Neuronal Death in Human Cells Expressing Mutant (G37R) Cu/Zn-Superoxide Dismutase." *Journal of Neurochemistry* 81 (2002): 170-177.

See also: Aging; Cancer chemotherapy support: Homeopathic remedies; Cancer treatment support; Wounds, minor.

Supplements: Introduction

CATEGORY: Issues and overviews
RELATED TERMS: Micronutrients, minerals, non-nutrient supplements, vitamins
DEFINITION: Dietary supplements used to promote health.

OVERVIEW

One of the great medical discoveries of the twentieth century was the identification of the nutritional substances necessary for life. Along with the macronutrients (fat, carbohydrate, and protein), these nutritional supplements, or micronutrients, make up the essential ingredients of a healthful diet.

Vitamins and minerals have been available as supplements since the 1930s. In the 1960s, however, a new way of using supplements came into vogue: megadose therapy. The megadose approach involves taking supplements at doses far above nutrition needs in hopes of producing a specific medical benefit. Essentially, megadose therapy means using nutrients as natural drugs.

The original (and still important) method of using nutrients involves taking them at around the level of nutrition needs. This method may be considered

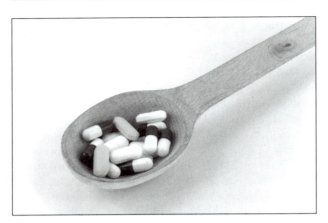

Vitamins and minerals have been available as supplements since the 1930s. (©Dreamstime.com)

nutrition insurance for the majority of people who do not get all the nutrients they need from foods.

Finally, there are a number of substances that are sold as supplements but are not nutritional in nature. While these substances might offer health benefits, one does not need them to stay alive. Examples include isoflavones, which are chemicals found in soy that may reduce the risk of cancer and some forms of heart disease; glucosamine, which is a substance found in gristle that is useful for osteoarthritis; and melatonin, a hormone that is not found to any great extent in foods but is helpful for sleep.

EBSCO CAM Review Board

FURTHER READING

American Dietetic Association et al. "American College of Sports Medicine Position Stand: Nutrition and Athletic Performance." *Medicine and Science in Sports and Exercise* 41 (2009): 709-731.

Bratman, S., and A. Girman. *Mosby's Handbook of Herbs and Supplements and Their Therapeutic Uses.* St. Louis, Mo.: Mosby, 2003.

Glisson, J. K., and L. A. Walker. "How Physicians Should Evaluate Dietary Supplements." *American Journal of Medicine* 123 (2010): 577-582.

Jerome-Morais, A., A. M. Diamond, M. E. Wright. "Dietary Supplements and Human Health: For Better or for Worse?" *Molecular Nutrition and Food Research,* December 1, 2010.

Lakhan, S. E., and K. F. Vieira. "Nutritional and Herbal Supplements for Anxiety and Anxiety-Related Disorders." *Nutrition Journal* 9 (2010): 42.

Ströhle, A., K. Zänker, and A. Hahn. "Nutrition in Oncology: The Case of Micronutrients (Review)." *Oncology Reports* 24 (2010): 815-828.

Zlotkin, S., et al. "The Role of the Codex Alimentarius Process in Support of New Products to Enhance the Nutritional Health of Infants and Young Children." *Food and Nutrition Bulletin* 31, suppl. 2 (2010): S128-S133.

See also: Herbal medicine; Supplements: Introduction; Vitamins and minerals.

Surgery support

CATEGORY: Condition

RELATED TERMS: Anesthesia, lymphedema, operation, postoperative recovery

DEFINITION: Treatment to aid in postoperative healing.

PRINCIPAL PROPOSED NATURAL TREATMENTS: Acupuncture-acupressure, bioflavonoids, oxerutins and other oligomeric proanthocyanidins, proteolytic enzymes

OTHER PROPOSED NATURAL TREATMENTS: *Arnica,* bee propolis, cayenne (capsaicin), ginger, fish oil, horse chestnut, hypnotherapy, lavender aromatherapy, magnet therapy, multivitamin-multimineral supplements, music therapy, peppermint, relaxation and guided imagery

HERBS AND SUPPLEMENTS TO USE ONLY WITH CAUTION: Garlic, ginkgo, St. John's wort, vitamin E

INTRODUCTION

Surgery, even relatively minor surgery, is a significant trauma to the body. The surgical incision itself can cause swelling (edema), pain, and bruising; anesthesia frequently causes nausea and bloating. Certain surgeries that damage the body's lymphatic system, such as radical mastectomy, can cause a specific form of long-lasting swelling called lymphedema.

Modern surgery involves numerous sophisticated nondrug techniques to help wounds heal rapidly and completely. Various medications can be used to help offset the side effects of anesthesia.

PRINCIPAL PROPOSED NATURAL TREATMENTS

A variety of herbs, supplements, and other alternative therapies show promise in alleviating problems encountered following surgery. However, many such substances have shown the potential to increase the risk of bleeding during or after surgery. Furthermore, it is not possible to determine all the potential interactions between herbs and drugs used for anesthesia. For this reason, herbs and supplements should be used for surgical support only under the supervision of a physician.

Proteolytic enzymes. According to most studies, proteolytic enzymes may help reduce pain, bruising, and swelling after surgery. A double-blind, placebo-controlled trial of eighty people undergoing knee surgery found that treatment with mixed proteolytic enzymes after surgery significantly improved rate of recovery, as measured by mobility and swelling.

Another double-blind, placebo-controlled trial evaluated the effects of a similar mixed proteolytic enzyme product in eighty persons undergoing oral surgery. The results showed reduced pain, inflammation, and swelling in the treated group compared with the placebo group. Benefits were also seen in another trial of mixed proteolytic enzymes for dental surgery and in one study involving only bromelain.

Other double-blind, placebo-controlled studies have found bromelain helpful in nasal surgery, cataract removal, and foot surgery. However, a study of 154 persons undergoing facial plastic surgery found no benefit.

Bromelain thins the blood and could increase risk of bleeding during or after surgery. For this reason, physician supervision is essential.

Oxerutins and other bioflavonoids. Oxerutins have been widely used in Europe since the mid-1960s, primarily as a treatment for varicose veins. Derived from a naturally occurring bioflavonoid called rutin, oxerutins were specifically developed to treat varicose veins and related venous problems. However, they may also be helpful for treating swelling following surgery. Closely related bioflavonoids from citrus fruit also may be helpful.

Women who have undergone surgery for breast cancer may experience a lasting and troublesome side effect: swelling in the arm caused by damage to the lymph system. With the veins, the lymphatic system is responsible for returning fluid to the heart. When this system is damaged by breast cancer surgery, fluid accumulates in the arm. Three small, double-blind, placebo-controlled studies enrolling more than one hundred people have examined the effectiveness of oxerutins in lymphedema following breast cancer surgery, with generally good results.

In a small, six-month, double-blind study, oxerutins reduced swelling and improved comfort and mobility compared with placebo. Another study found benefit with a combination formula containing oxerutins, ginkgo, and the drug heptaminol. The citrus bioflavonoids diosmin and hesperidin have also shown promise for lymphedema following breast cancer surgery, as has a product containing hesperidin plus a bioflavonoid-rich extract of the herb butcher's broom. One should not use bioflavonoid combinations containing tangeretin if also taking tamoxifen for breast cancer.

Oxerutins might also be helpful for the ordinary swelling that occurs after any type of surgery. In one double-blind trial, researchers gave oxerutins or placebo for five days to forty people recovering from minor surgery or other minor injuries and found oxerutins significantly helpful in reducing swelling and discomfort.

Oligomeric proanthocyanidins. Oligomeric proanthocyanidins (OPCs), substances found in grape seed and pine bark, may also be helpful for recovery from surgery. Like oxerutins, to which they are chemically related, OPCs are thought to work by reducing leakage from capillaries.

A double-blind, placebo-controlled study of sixty-three women with breast cancer found that 600 milligrams (mg) of OPCs daily for six months reduced postoperative symptoms of lymphedema. Additionally, in a double-blind, placebo-controlled study of thirty-two people who were followed for ten days after having a face-lift, swelling disappeared much faster in the treated group.

Acupuncture and acupressure. Acupuncture and acupressure are two related forms of treatment that involve stimulating certain locations on the body known as acupuncture points. Numerous studies have evaluated treatment on a single acupuncture point, P6, for the relief of nausea following anesthesia. This point is located on the inside of the forearm, about two inches above the wrist crease.

Many controlled studies involving more than two thousand people have tested the potential benefits of stimulation at P6 in people undergoing surgery. In most of these trials, treatment was carried out through the surgery itself, as well as afterwards. The results of these trials, involving various types of surgery and diverse forms of acupuncture and acupressure, tend to contradict one another. On balance, however, it appears that acupuncture and acupressure may reduce intraoperative (during surgery) and postoperative nausea to some extent beyond that of the placebo effect.

Acupuncture has also been explored as a means of reducing pain after surgery, with inconsistent results. In a 2008 review of fifteen randomized, controlled trials, however, researchers determined that acupuncture is capable of reducing pain and the need for opioid medications (morphine and related agents) immediately following surgery, compared with sham (fake) acupuncture. A small randomized trial of seventy persons found that acupuncture may decrease dry mouth and pain after removal of lymph nodes in the neck for cancer treatment. Contrary to popular belief, acupuncture does not appear to be helpful for providing or enhancing anesthesia itself.

OTHER PROPOSED NATURAL TREATMENTS

The herb ginger is thought to have antinausea effects. In studies, ginger has been given before surgery to prevent the nausea that many people experience when they awaken from anesthesia. However, despite some early positive results, the preponderance of evidence indicates that ginger is not helpful for this purpose.

One should not use ginger either before or immediately after surgery or labor and delivery without a physician's approval. There are theoretical concerns that ginger may affect bleeding.

Preliminary evidence suggests that peppermint oil may be helpful for postoperative flatulence and nausea. Also, a preliminary controlled study found that the honeybee product propolis mouthwash following oral surgery significantly speeded healing time compared with placebo.

One small, double-blind, placebo-controlled study found that magnet therapy patches of the "unipolar" variety reduced pain and swelling after suction lipectomy. However, a study of 165 people undergoing various forms of surgery failed to find that the use of static magnets over the surgical incision reduced postsurgical pain. Furthermore, the positioning of static magnets at the acupuncture-acupressure point P6 in persons undergoing ear, nose, and throat or gynecological surgeries reduced nausea and vomiting no better than placebo in a randomized trial. A small

pilot study involving eighty women undergoing breast augmentation procedures found that daily pulsed electromagnetic field therapy reduced postoperative discomfort significantly more than placebo therapy within three days of surgery.

A double-blind, placebo-controlled study examined thirty-seven people undergoing surgery for carpal tunnel syndrome. The use by these persons of an ointment made from the herb *Arnica* (combined with homeopathic *Arnica* tablets) appeared to slightly reduce postsurgical pain.

Horse chestnut has effects similar to OPCs and has also shown promise for reducing postoperative swelling. A preliminary study suggests that topically administered capsaicin provides short-term pain relief immediately following hernia repair surgery. In two studies, the sports supplement creatine has been tried as an aid to strengthen recovery after knee surgery, but no benefits were seen.

Good nutrition is essential to recovery from any physical trauma. For this reason, the use of a multivitamin-multimineral supplement in the weeks before surgery, and for some time afterward, might be advisable.

A placebo-controlled study failed to find that onion extract could help reduce skin scarring following surgery. Another study found that massage therapy reduced postoperative pain. The use of a fish oil product as part of a total parenteral nutrition regimen (intravenous feeding) may help speed recovery after major abdominal surgery.

Treatment via inhalation of essential oils is called aromatherapy. One controlled trial found that lavender oil, administered through an oxygen face mask, reduced the need for pain medications following gastric banding surgery.

At least twenty controlled studies, enrolling more than fifteen hundred people, have evaluated the potential benefit of hypnosis for people undergoing surgery. Their combined results suggest that hypnosis may provide benefits both during and after surgery, including reducing anxiety, pain, and nausea; normalizing blood pressure and heart rate; minimizing blood loss; and speeding recovery and shortening hospitalization. Many of these studies were of very poor quality, however.

Relaxation therapy techniques, such as meditation, guided imagery, and self-hypnosis, have also shown promise for relieving some of the discomforts of surgery. One study found minimal benefits with music therapy, however.

HERBS AND SUPPLEMENTS TO USE WITH CAUTION

Numerous herbs and supplements have the potential to cause problems during or after surgery, including some of those discussed here. For this reason, one should not use any herb or supplement in the week before surgery, except under a physician's supervision.

For example, the herb garlic significantly thins the blood, and case reports suggest that garlic can increase bleeding during or after surgery. It is probably advisable to avoid garlic supplements before surgery and not to restart the supplements after surgery until all risk of bleeding is past. However, raw garlic consumed in food may not present the same risk. A placebo-controlled study found that one-time consumption of raw garlic consumed in food at the fairly high dose of 4.2 mg did not impair platelet function. Also, volunteers who continued to consume the dietary garlic for one week did not show any change in their normal platelet function.

The use of the herb ginkgo has also been associated with serious bleeding complications related to surgery. Many other herbs and supplements have also shown potential for increasing risk of bleeding. Most prominent among these are high-dose vitamin E and policosanol. Others include bromelain, chamomile, devil's claw, dong quai, feverfew, fish oil, ginger, horse chestnut, ipriflavone, mesoglycan, papaya, phosphatidylserine, red clover, reishi, vitamin A, and white willow. In addition, one report suggests that the use of St. John's wort may interact with anesthetic drugs.

EBSCO CAM Review Board

FURTHER READING

Aasvang, E. K., et al. "The Effect of Wound Instillation of a Novel Purified Capsaicin Formulation on Postherniotomy Pain." *Anesthesia and Analgesia* 107 (2008): 282-291.

Allen, T. K., and A. S. Habib. "P6 Stimulation for the Prevention of Nausea and Vomiting Associated with Cesarean Delivery Under Neuraxial Anesthesia." *Anesthesia and Analgesia* 107 (2008): 1308-1312.

Bechtold, M. L., et al. "Effect of Music on Patients Undergoing Outpatient Colonoscopy." *World Journal of Gastroenterology* 12 (2006): 7309-7312.

Cepeda, M. S., et al. "Static Magnetic Therapy Does Not Decrease Pain or Opioid Requirements." *Anesthesia and Analgesia* 104 (2007): 290-294.

Chung, V. Q., et al. "Onion Extract Gel Versus Petrolatum Emollient on New Surgical Scars." *Dermatological Surgery* 32 (2006): 193-198.

Habib, A. S., et al. "Transcutaneous Acupoint Electrical Stimulation with the ReliefBand for the Prevention of Nausea and Vomiting During and After Cesarean Delivery Under Spinal Anesthesia." *Anesthesia and Analgesia* 102 (2006): 581-584.

Hedén, P., and A. A. Pilla. "Effects of Pulsed Electromagnetic Fields on Postoperative Pain: A Double-Blind Randomized Pilot Study in Breast Augmentation Patients." *Aesthetic Plastic Surgery* 32 (2008): 660-666.

Kim, J. T., et al. "Treatment with Lavender Aromatherapy in the Post-Anesthesia Care Unit Reduces Opioid Requirements of Morbidly Obese Patients Undergoing Laparoscopic Adjustable Gastric Banding." *Obesity Surgery* 17 (2007): 920-925.

Klaiman, P., et al. "Magnetic Acupressure for Management of Postoperative Nausea and Vomiting." *Minerva Anestesiologica* 74 (2008): 635-642.

Lang, E. V., et al. "Beneficial Effects of Hypnosis and Adverse Effects of Empathic Attention During Percutaneous Tumor Treatment." *Journal of Vascular and Interventional Radiology* 19 (2008): 897-905.

Lee, H., and E. Ernst. "Acupuncture Analgesia During Surgery." *Pain* 114 (2005): 511-517.

Pfister, D. G., et al. "Acupuncture for Pain and Dysfunction After Neck Dissection." *Journal of Clinical Oncology* 28 (2010): 2565-2570.

Scharbert, G., et al. "Garlic at Dietary Doses Does Not Impair Platelet Function." *Anesthesia and Analgesia* 105 (2007): 1214-1218.

Tyler, T. F., et al. "The Effect of Creatine Supplementation on Strength Recovery After Anterior Cruciate Ligament (ACL) Reconstruction." *American Journal of Sports Medicine* 32 (2004): 383-388.

Usichenko, T. I., et al. "Auricular Acupuncture for Pain Relief After Ambulatory Knee Surgery." *CMAJ: Canadian Medical Association Journal* 176 (2007): 179-183.

Wang, S. M., et al. "Extra-1 Acupressure for Children Undergoing Anesthesia." *Anesthesia and Analgesia* 107 (2008): 811-816.

See also: Acupuncture; Bromelain; Citrus bioflavonoids; Proteolytic enzymes; Oligomeric proanthocyanidins; Oxerutins.

Surgery support: Homeopathic remedies

CATEGORY: Homeopathy

DEFINITION: The use of highly diluted remedies to treat surgical wound pain and to treat side effects from anesthesia.

STUDIED HOMEOPATHIC REMEDIES: Acetic acid; aconite; *Aconitum napellus*; *Arnica*; *Bellis perennis*; *Calendula*; *Carbo vegetabilis*; homeopathic remedies given in succession: opium, *Arnica*, and *Raphanus*; homeopathic remedy containing *China regia*, *Raphanus sativus niger*, and *Arnica*; *Hypericum*; *Ledum*; phosphorus; *Plantago*; staphysagria

INTRODUCTION

Surgery is an unpleasant process that leads to surgical wound pain and to side effects from anesthesia. Homeopathic treatments have been studied for possible benefits in the period around surgery, with some promising results. Even though these treatments have not been proved effective, one thing can be offered in their favor: Unlike herbs, which might be dangerous during or after surgery, homeopathic tablets should be entirely safe under all circumstances.

SCIENTIFIC EVALUATIONS OF HOMEOPATHIC REMEDIES

Preliminary double-blind trials suggest that homeopathic remedies may help the digestive tract to recover after surgery. Weaker evidence suggests benefits for surgical pain and anxiety. However, a study of homeopathy for reducing bruising after surgery found no benefit.

Recovery of digestive function. After major surgery, especially to the abdomen, the digestive tract will shut down for several days. Until it starts working again, the affected person cannot eat or drink and must remain hospitalized. Passing gas is the first sign of recovery; once it occurs, the return of digestive function is imminent.

The results of several double-blind studies suggest that homeopathic remedies may reduce the time it takes for the digestive tract to recover. For example, a double-blind, placebo-controlled study of two hundred people who had undergone abdominal or chest surgery evaluated the effectiveness of the three homeopathic remedies opium, *Arnica*, and *Raphanus* given in succession every two hours. Bowel function returned more rapidly in the active treatment group than in the placebo group.

Another double-blind, placebo-controlled study of eighty people undergoing abdominal surgery evaluated the effects on bowel function of a homeopathic remedy containing *China regia*, *Raphanus sativus niger*, and *Arnica*. Again, benefits were seen in the homeopathy group compared with the placebo group. Similar results were seen in several other studies.

A meta-analysis mathematically combined the results of six published trials on homeopathy for speeding the return of bowel function. About 750 people were enrolled in these trials. The combined results indicate that the time to first signs of bowel recovery among those taking the homeopathic treatment was on average 7.4 hours less than their placebo counterparts. This difference was statistically significant.

Reducing pain. Pain following surgery is a common, if not nearly universal, experience. The homeopathic remedy *Arnica* is traditionally used as a treatment for trauma and, therefore, has been proposed for reducing surgical pain. The results from preliminary studies have been somewhat promising but far from definitive.

A study of 190 people undergoing tonsillectomy compared with placebo the use of *Arnica* 30c (centesimal) at two tablets six times daily the first day after surgery, then two tablets twice a day for the next seven days. The results showed a mathematically significant but clinically slight benefit in favor of *Arnica*.

Another double-blind, placebo-controlled study involved fifty-nine participants undergoing oral surgery. The group that received homeopathic *Arnica* at 30c potency experienced significantly less pain than the control group.

In another double-blind, placebo-controlled trial, the use of homeopathic *Arnica* D6 tablets for two weeks following surgery for carpal tunnel syndrome led to decreased pain compared with placebo treatment.

However, other double-blind studies failed to find benefit. In a study comparing *Arnica* D4 and 50 milligrams of diclofenac sodium, a common analgesic medication, *Arnica* was less effective for postoperative pain following bunion surgery among eighty-eight participants. Nevertheless, *Arnica* was equivalent to diclofenac for postoperative irritation, toe mobility, and the use of other analgesics. Because no control group was included in the study, it is unknown whether any treatment was better than placebo.

In a placebo-controlled trial, researchers tested *Arnica* 30c in the postoperative recovery of ninety-three women who had undergone total abdominal hysterectomy. In terms of pain and its relief, infection, and medication use, no statistical difference was observed between the two groups.

Another double-blind, placebo-controlled, cross-over study also failed to find benefit. In this trial, homeopathic practitioners selected one of six different remedies to be administered to each participant, according to classical homeopathic principles. The remedies were *Arnica, Hypericum, Ledum,* phosphorus, *Plantago,* or staphysagria, all at D30 potency. No significant benefits were seen.

In another controlled trial, persons recovering from knee surgery who were given a homeopathic complex (*Arnica montana* 5 CH, *Bryonia alba* 5 CH, *Hypericum perforatum* 5 CH, and *Ruta graveolens* 3 DH) were no more or less likely to adjust their morphine dose one to three days postoperatively compared with persons given placebo.

Restlessness and agitation. In addition to pain, many people experience restlessness and agitation after surgery, perhaps caused, in part, by the effects of general anesthesia. One double-blind, placebo-controlled study evaluated the potential benefits of homeopathic aconite for children who had undergone various surgeries. Fifty children who had recently undergone surgery were included in the study. Either aconite (potency not described) or placebo was administered to the children in the recovery room. The homeopathic treatment was reported to provide a statistically significant benefit compared with placebo.

Bruising. Because homeopathic *Arnica* is a popular home remedy for bruising, investigators have studied it as a possible treatment for reducing bruising after surgery. However, overall, the evidence for benefit with *Arnica* is inconclusive.

In a double-blind trial of 130 people undergoing surgery for varicose veins, researchers found no benefit with homeopathic *Arnica* at 5x (decimal-scale) potency compared with placebo. A second study of *Arnica* for varicose vein surgery also failed to find statistically significant benefits. Another double-blind trial, this one with sixty-four participants, failed to find *Arnica* helpful for reducing pain and bruising after hand surgery. A later study, involving face-lift surgery, found equivocal benefits at best.

Traditional Homeopathic Treatments

Classical homeopathy offers many possible homeopathic treatments for surgery support. These therapies are chosen based on various specific details of the person seeking treatment.

A person who experiences fear and a feeling of panic before surgery might fit the symptom picture of homeopathic *Aconitum napellus.* This remedy is said to be especially indicated for people who are afraid that they will die and for those who are easily startled by light and noise. Other aspects of the classic symptom picture include dry mouth and excessive thirst. Persons who experience bruising, swelling, or soreness after surgery may fit the classical symptom picture for *Arnica.*

Depending on the type of surgery, the homeopath might recommend other remedies believed to have particular affinities for different organs or circumstances, such as *Bellis perennis* for breast and abdominal surgeries; *Calendula, Hypericum, Arnica,* or staphysagria for dental surgeries; and *Carbo vegetabilis* when there is great weakness and loss of fluids. Homeopathic acetic acid might be used to help effect a quick recovery from the aftereffects (such as nausea and wooziness) of general anesthesia.

EBSCO CAM Review Board

Further Reading

Jeffrey, S., and J. Belcher. "Use of *Arnica* to Relieve Pain After Carpal-Tunnel Release Surgery." *Alternative Therapies in Health and Medicine* 8 (2002): 66-68.

Karow, J. H., et al. "Efficacy of *Arnica montana* D4 for Healing of Wounds After Hallux Valgus Surgery Compared to Diclofenac." *Journal of Alternative and Complementary Medicine* 14 (2008): 17-25.

Ludtke, R., and D. Hacke. "On the Effectiveness of the Homeopathic Remedy *Arnica montana.*" *Wiener Medizinische Wochenschrift* 155 (2006): 482-490.

Paris, A., et al. "Effect of Homeopathy on Analgesic Intake Following Knee Ligament Reconstruction." *British Journal of Clinical Pharmacology* 65 (2008): 180-187.

Robertson, A., R. Suryanarayanan, and A. Banerjee. "Homeopathic *Arnica montana* for Post-tonsillectomy Analgesia." *Homeopathy* 96 (2007): 17-21.

Seeley, B. M., et al. "Effect of Homeopathic *Arnica montana* on Bruising in Face-Lifts." *Archives of Facial and Plastic Surgery* 8 (2006): 54-59.

See also: Bruises; Bruises: Homeopathic remedies; Homeopathy; Pain management; Phosphorus; Surgery support; Wounds, minor.

Sweet clover

CATEGORY: Herbs and supplements
RELATED TERMS: Melilot, *Melilotus* species
DEFINITION: Natural plant product used to treat specific health conditions.
PRINCIPAL PROPOSED USES: None
OTHER PROPOSED USES: Dyspepsia, hemorrhoids, minor injuries, phlebitis, varicose veins

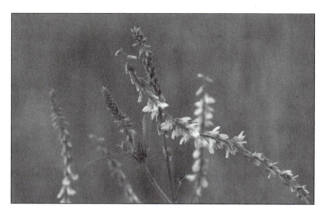

Sweet clover. (Gail Jankus/Photo Researchers, Inc.)

OVERVIEW

Sweet clover, long popular as food for grazing animals, is used medicinally as well. It contains various substances in the coumarin family. These chemicals are thought to help strengthen the walls of blood and lymph vessels. However, there is no more than preliminary evidence that sweet clover is effective for any medical condition. In addition, the use of sweet clover presents some safety concerns.

The genus name *Melilotus* originates from the Greek word for honey, *meli*, and from a term for cloverlike plants, *lotos*. Four common species make up this genus of Eurasian origins: *M. alba, M. indica, M. officinalis,* and *M. altissimus.* The fresh or dried leaves and flowering stems of sweet clover have traditionally been used as a diuretic.

THERAPEUTIC DOSAGES

Sweet clover products are standardized to their coumarin content. For treating symptoms of venous insufficiency/varicose veins, a daily dosage of a sweet clover preparation or extract providing 3 to 30 milligrams (mg) of coumarin is taken internally.

THERAPEUTIC USES

Germany's Commission E has authorized use of sweet clover extract for symptoms of venous insufficiency (a condition closely related to varicose veins), as well as for the treatment of phlebitis and hemorrhoids. When used for this purpose, however, sweet clover is generally combined with bioflavonoids such as oxerutin. There is no meaningful evidence as yet that sweet clover taken alone is effective for these conditions.

Sweet clover contains coumarins, substances related to the prescription blood thinner warfarin (Coumadin). Most scientific study relevant to sweet clover involves prescription drugs that combine coumarins and bioflavonoids. These medications have also been used to treat venous insufficiency, as well as numerous other conditions, including elephantiasis, hemorrhoids, mild digestive disturbances, and various forms of edema. However, it is not clear whether sweet clover extracts containing coumarins would work in the same way as the coumarin portion of these pharmaceutical products.

Topical treatments made from sweet clover are sometimes recommended for the treatment of hemorrhoids and minor injuries, but there is no real scientific evidence to support these proposed uses.

SAFETY ISSUES

The safety of any medicinal use of sweet clover has not been established in humans. Because sweet clover contains various substances in the coumarin family, and many (but not all) of these substances thin the blood, use of sweet clover might cause excessive bleeding in some individuals. In particular, sweet clover should not be combined with blood-thinning drugs such as warfarin, heparin, or drugs in the aspirin family.

The safety of sweet clover for pregnant or nursing women, young children, and individuals with severe liver or kidney disease has not been established. Persons who are taking blood-thinning drugs such as warfarin (Coumadin), heparin, clopidogrel (Plavix), pentoxifylline (Trental), or drugs in the aspirin family should not use sweet clover.

EBSCO CAM Review Board

FURTHER READING

Blumenthal, M., et al., eds. *The Complete German Commission E Monographs: Therapeutic Guide to Herbal Medicines.* Austin, Tex.: American Botanical Council, 1999.

Bruneton, J. *Pharmacognosy, Phytochemistry, Medicinal Plants.* 2d ed. Paris: Lavoisier, 2001.

Casley-Smith, J. R. "Benzo-Pyrones in the Treatment of Lymphoedema." *International Angiology* 18 (1999): 31-41.

See also: Dyspepsia; Injuries, minor; Phlebitis and deep vein thrombosis; Varicose veins; Warfarin.

Swimmer's ear

CATEGORY: Condition

RELATED TERMS: Acute external otitis, otitis externa

DEFINITION: Treatment for an inflammatory condition of the external ear canal commonly caused by a bacterial infection.

OVERVIEW

Swimmer's ear, or acute external otitis, is a painful condition of the external ear canal. Although not always caused by swimming, the condition is usually related to excessive moisture in the ear canal that causes a favorable environment for bacteria to multiply. In North America, 98 percent of swimmer's ear infections are caused by bacterial cellulitis involving the skin and subdermis of the ear canal.

The most common pathogens are *Pseudomonas aeruginosa, Staphylococcus aureus,* and polymicrobial infections. Swimmer's ear is a common infection with a reported yearly incidence between 1:100 and 1:250 in the general population. The chances of having swimmers ear during a lifetime may be as high as 10 percent. People who live in warmer, more humid climates and people with diabetes are at increased risk.

Treatment of swimmer's ear may require cleaning of the ear by a medical professional. Antimicrobial, steroidal, and acidifying ear drops are the mainstays of conventional medical treatment. Over-the-counter ear drops and complementary and alternative treatments of swimmer's ear may be effective for early, uncomplicated cases.

CAUSES AND SYMPTOMS

The most common cause of swimmer's ear is increased moisture that gets trapped in the ear canal. This moisture may come from bathing, showering, humidity, or swimming. Moisture itself may create an environment for bacteria already present in the ear canal to multiply, or the bacteria may be introduced into the ear canal from contaminated water sources. Causative bacteria may be present in places such as swimming pools, hot tubs, and ponds.

Other factors that may contribute to swimmer's ear include frequent cleaning of the ear canals, trauma to the skin of the ear canals, the wearing of a hearing aid, eczema of the ear canals, and obstruction of the ear canals by wax accumulation. Wax serves a protective function in the ear canal. It acts as a barrier to moisture and infection and may inhibit the growth of bacteria because of its slightly acidic pH.

Symptoms of swimmer's ear usually develop rapidly in about a forty-eight hour period. Intense itching is a common initial symptom, followed by gradual onset of pain, a sense of fullness, and decreased hearing. The pain can be quite severe and can radiate to the jaw or side of the head. In most cases, swimmer's ear is unilateral. The classic sign of swimmer's ear is pain that is elicited by pulling or pressing on the outer ear. The opening of the ear canal may also appear red and swollen. Drainage from the ear canal, fever, and swollen lymph nodes may also be present.

COMPLEMENTARY AND ALTERNATIVE TREATMENTS

There are no studies that compare complementary and alternative therapies to conventional medical treatment of swimmer's ear. However, there is a long history of using home remedies that has stood the test of time long enough to have some validity. The most common and effective home remedy is the use of ear drops made from rubbing alcohol and white vinegar.

A mixture of equal parts alcohol and vinegar will help dry the ear, and the acidity of the vinegar will inhibit bacterial growth. If there is any chance that the eardrum is perforated, these drops should not be used. People who have a history of ear surgery or ear trauma, or who have been diagnosed with a perforated eardrum, should not use any ear drop without medical clearance.

Tea tree oil is another ear drop treatment that has had some success. Studies show that this oil can inhibit the growth of about 70 percent of the bacteria that cause swimmer's ear but may not be effective against most *Pseudomonas* bacteria. Other home remedies that may be effective include using a hair dryer to reduce moisture in the ear and using hot compresses to reduce pain and swelling.

One home remedy that is not effective and may be quite dangerous is the use of ear candles. The U.S. Food and Drug Administration has issued a warning against the use of ear candles. These devices have no evidence to support their use and can cause injuries to the face and the ear canal. Serious facial burns and perforations of the eardrum have been reported.

Swimmer's ear may be effectively prevented using home remedies. These include using alcohol and vinegar drops before and after swimming, using a hair dryer after swimming to dry the ear, and using ear plugs and a bathing cap during swimming. Malignant external otitis is a serious complication of swimmer's ear, in which an untreated external ear infection spreads to the skull and the brain. Swimmer's ear symptoms that do not respond to complementary and alternative treatments should be evaluated by a medical professional.

Christopher Iliades, M.D.

FURTHER READING

American Academy of Otolaryngology: Head and Neck Surgery. "Swimmer's Ear." Available at http://www.entnet.org/healthinformation/swimmersear.cfm.

Burton, M. J., et al. "Extracts from *The Cochrane Library*: Interventions for Acute Otitis Externa." *Otolaryngology–Head and Neck Surgery* 143 (2010): 8-11.

National Center for Complementary and Alternative Medicine. http://nccam.nih.gov.

Rosenfeld, R., et al. "Clinical Practice Guideline: Acute Otitis Externa." *Otolaryngology: Head and Neck Surgery* 134 (2006): S4-S23.

See also: Candling; Ear infections; Ear infections: Homeopathic remedies; Hearing loss; Home health; Sports and fitness support: Enhancing recovery.

T

Tai Chi

CATEGORY: Therapies and techniques

RELATED TERMS: Tai Chi Chuan, Taijiquan

DEFINITION: Technique that uses gentle movements to strengthen and balance the body's energy.

PRINCIPAL PROPOSED USES: Improving balance and preventing falls in the elderly

OTHER PROPOSED USES: Cancer treatment support, fibromyalgia, high blood pressure, improving overall health, osteoarthritis, osteoporosis, enhancing immunity

OVERVIEW

Tai Chi is a traditional form of martial art used to promote health. Its gentle, dancelike moves are said to strengthen and balance the body's energy. The net results, according to tradition, include increased physical stamina, enhanced sense of well-being and comfort, and improved resistance to illness.

Tai Chi is said to have been developed by the Daoist monk Chang San-Feng sometime in the Middle Ages. (The exact dates and even the existence of this monk are disputed.) Various schools of Tai Chi developed over subsequent centuries, each with its own particular movements and postures, but all conforming to the same underlying principles.

In the 1950s, the Chinese government began to develop a series of standardized Tai Chi forms. One of these has become the most popular form of Tai Chi in the West, a thirty-seven-posture form abbreviated from a traditional approach to Tai Chi called the Yang style.

USES AND APPLICATIONS

Tai Chi is an extremely popular form of exercise among older Asians in China and other Asian countries. In the United States, it is gaining widespread use as a method of improving balance and preventing falls among the elderly. The slow movements of Tai Chi provide a gentle framework for enhancing physical control and improving balance. Tai Chi is also thought to improve overall health and enhance immunity, but

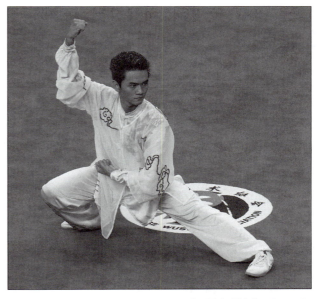

Thanh Tung Nguyen competes in the Tai Chi finals at the Asian Games in 2010. (Getty Images)

this has not been evaluated scientifically to any significant extent.

SCIENTIFIC EVIDENCE

Although there is some evidence that Tai Chi may offer medical benefits, in general this evidence is not strong. There are several reasons for this (including funding obstacles), but one is fundamental: Even with the best of intentions, it is difficult to properly ascertain the effectiveness of an exercise therapy like Tai Chi.

Only one form of study can truly prove that a treatment is effective: the double-blind, placebo-controlled trial. However, it is not possible to fit Tai Chi into a study design of this type. While it might be possible to design a placebo form of Tai Chi, it would be quite difficult to keep participants and researchers "blinded" regarding who is practicing real Tai Chi and who is practicing fake Tai Chi.

Therefore, some compromise with the highest research standards is inevitable. The compromise used in most studies, however, is less than optimal. In these trials, Tai Chi was compared to no treatment. The problem with such studies is that a treatment, any treatment, frequently appears to be better than no treatment, due to a host of factors. It would be better to compare Tai Chi to generic forms of exercise, such as daily walking, but thus far this method has not seen much use. Given these caveats, the following is a summary of what science knows about Tai Chi.

Most controlled trials of Tai Chi published in English have evaluated its potential benefits for improving balance in the elderly. Falling is one of the most common causes of injury in older people, leading to fractures, head injuries, and even death. Recovery from fall-related injuries may involve extensive immobilization in bed, which in turn increases the risk of osteoporosis, pneumonia, and depression. According to most studies, Tai Chi can improve balance and decrease the risk of falling.

For example, in a ten-week study, twenty-four older persons practiced Tai Chi (one class weekly, plus daily home practice), while a control group of twenty-two volunteers did not change their activity. The results showed that people practicing Tai Chi experienced substantially improved balance (measured by the ability to stand on one leg) compared to the control group. Some studies failed to find benefit; however, this is typical of treatments for which all studies have been small in size. For statistical reasons, small studies commonly fail to identify benefit even when there is one.

Although there is some evidence that Tai Chi can improve balance and reduce the risk of falling, researchers conducting a 2008 review of nine randomized-controlled trials were unable to conclude that Tai Chi or Tai Chi-inspired exercises can effectively prevent fall-related harm in the elderly. The trials were too inconsistent in their methods and quality.

In addition to balance, Tai Chi may mildly improve flexibility and cardiovascular health, presumably because it is a form of moderate exercise. However, one fairly large (207-participant) and long-term (one-year) study that compared Tai Chi to resistance exercise (weight lifting) found that while resistance exercises measurably improved one measure of cardiovascular risk (insulin sensitivity), Tai Chi did not affect any measures of cardiovascular risk. In a review of twenty-six published studies examining the effectiveness of Tai Chi for high blood pressure, 85 percent demonstrated a reduction in blood pressure. However, only five of these twenty-six studies were of acceptable quality.

One study found that persons with congestive heart failure can benefit from Tai Chi, but the study had no adequate control group. In two controlled studies, Tai Chi produced some benefit in bone density, suggesting the possibility that it might be helpful for preventing osteoporosis. A few studies provide inconsistent evidence for the usefulness of Tai Chi as a treatment for osteoarthritis, and a preliminary study suggests it may be beneficial for mild to moderate rheumatoid arthritis.

In a small, randomized-controlled trial of sixty-six persons, Tai Chi appeared to improve symptoms, function, and quality of life for those with fibromyalgia. In one randomized study, a certain form of Tai Chi was more effective than health education after twenty-five weeks in persons with moderate insomnia. A review of seven studies found insufficient evidence to conclude whether or not Tai Chi improves quality of life or psychological or physical outcomes in persons with breast cancer.

WHAT TO EXPECT DURING A CLASS

A Tai Chi class consists of progressive training in the movements of a Tai Chi form. Each subsequent class adds more moves to the repertoire, until finally one knows how to perform the entire series. The Tai Chi instructor will gently correct the student's movements, helping to make stances and transitions between them more precise, graceful, and balanced.

EBSCO CAM Review Board

FURTHER READING

Irwin, M. R., R. Olmstead, and S. J. Motivala. "Improving Sleep Quality in Older Adults with Moderate Sleep Complaints." *Sleep* 31 (2008): 1001-1008.

Lee, M. S., T. Y. Choi, and E. Ernst. "Tai Chi for Breast Cancer Patients." *Breast Cancer Research and Treatment* 120 (2010): 309-316.

Lee, M. S., M. H. Pittler, and E. Ernst. "Tai Chi for Osteoarthritis." *Clinical Rheumatology* 27 (2008): 211-218.

Low, S., et al. "A Systematic Review of the Effectiveness of Tai Chi on Fall Reduction Among the Elderly." *Archives of Gerontology and Geriatrics* 48 (2009): 325-331.

Wang, C. "Tai Chi Improves Pain and Functional

Status in Adults with Rheumatoid Arthritis." *Medicine and Sport Science* 52 (2008): 218-229.

Wang, C., et al. "A Randomized Trial of Tai Chi for Fibromyalgia." *New England Journal of Medicine* 363 (2010): 743-754.

Wayne, P. M., et al. "The Effects of Tai Chi on Bone Mineral Density in Postmenopausal Women." *Archives of Physical Medicine and Rehabilitation* 88 (2007): 673-680.

Yeh, G. Y., P. M. Wayne, and R. S. Phillips. "T'ai Chi Exercise in Patients with Chronic Heart Failure." *Medicine and Sport Science* 52 (2008): 195-208.

Yeh, G. Y., et al. "The Effect of Tai Chi Exercise on Blood Pressure." *Preventive Cardiology* 11 (2008): 82-89.

See also: Elder health; Integrative medicine; Manipulative and body-based therapies; Meditation; Pain management; Qigong; Reiki; Traditional healing; Yoga.

Tamoxifen

CATEGORY: Drug interactions

DEFINITION: A drug that blocks the actions of estrogen and produces some estrogen-like actions, used for the prevention and treatment of breast cancer.

INTERACTIONS: Soy isoflavones, tangeretin

TRADE NAME: Nolvadex

TANGERETIN

Effect: Possible Harmful Interaction

Tangeretin is a bioflavonoid found in citrus fruit and some citrus bioflavonoid supplements. Animal studies suggest that high intake of tangeretin reduces the effectiveness of tamoxifen. For this reason, people using tamoxifen should avoid supplements containing tangeretin, and they should also probably avoid excessive intake of citrus fruit.

SOY ISOFLAVONES

Effect: Mixed Interaction

Like tamoxifen, soy isoflavones have both estrogen-like and anti-estrogen actions. Test-tube and animal studies suggest that relatively low doses of soy isoflavones interfere with the ability of tamoxifen to inhibit breast cancer growth, but high doses of isoflavones augment the effectiveness of tamoxifen.

EBSCO CAM Review Board

FURTHER READING

Liu, B., et al. "Low-Dose Dietary Phytoestrogen Abrogates Tamoxifen-Associated Mammary Tumor Prevention." *Cancer Research* 65 (2005): 879-886.

See also: Cancer risk reduction; Cancer treatment support; Citrus bioflavonoids; Estrogen; Food and Drug Administration; Isoflavones; Supplements: Introduction; Women's health.

Tardive dyskinesia

CATEGORY: Condition

RELATED TERM: Tardive dyskinesis

DEFINITION: Treatment of the mostly uncontrollable bodily movements caused by side effects of drugs used to control schizophrenia and other psychoses.

PRINCIPAL PROPOSED NATURAL TREATMENT: Vitamin E

OTHER PROPOSED NATURAL TREATMENTS: Branched-chain amino acids, choline, 2-dimethylaminoethanol, gamma-linolenic acid, lecithin, manganese, melatonin, niacin, vitamin B_6, vitamin C

HERBS AND SUPPLEMENTS TO USE ONLY WITH CAUTION: Phenylalanine

INTRODUCTION

Tardive dyskinesia (TD) is a potentially permanent side effect of drugs used to control schizophrenia and other psychoses. This late-developing (tardy, or tardive) complication consists of annoying, mostly uncontrollable movements (dyskinesias). Typical symptoms include repetitive sucking or blinking, slow twisting of the hands, or other movements of the face and limbs. TD can cause tremendous social embarrassment to particularly vulnerable persons.

Several different theories have been proposed for the development of TD. According to one theory, long-term treatment with antipsychotic drugs causes the brain to become overly sensitive to the neurotransmitter dopamine, resulting in abnormal movements. According to another theory, imbalances among different neurotransmitters can cause or aggravate symptoms. In a third theory, TD may arise in part from damage to the brain caused by free radicals generated by schizophrenia treatments. All of these theories may contain some truth.

Vitamin E for Tardive Dyskinesia

Vitamin E is the collective name for a group of fat-soluble compounds with distinctive antioxidant activities. Antioxidants protect cells from the damaging effects of free radicals, which are molecules that contain an unshared electron. Unshared electrons are highly energetic and react rapidly with oxygen to form reactive oxygen species (ROS). The body forms ROS endogenously when it converts food into energy, and antioxidants might protect cells from the damaging effects of ROS. Vitamin E is a fat-soluble antioxidant that stops the production of ROS that is formed when fat undergoes oxidation.

Also, the brain has a high oxygen consumption rate and abundant polyunsaturated fatty acids in the neuronal cell membranes. Researchers hypothesize that if cumulative free-radical damage to neurons over time contributes to cognitive decline and neurodegenerative diseases, then ingestion of sufficient or supplemental antioxidants (such as vitamin E) might provide some protection.

Discontinuing medication that caused TD usually does not help, and it may even worsen the dyskinesia and the underlying schizophrenia. Drugs such as L-dopa and oxypertine may improve TD but present their own significant risk of side effects. Newer medications for schizophrenia that are less likely to cause TD have been developed.

PRINCIPAL PROPOSED NATURAL TREATMENTS

Vitamin E. Vitamin E is an antioxidant, a substance that works to neutralize free radicals in the body. As noted, it has been suggested that free radicals may play a role in TD. If this is true, it makes sense that vitamin E might help prevent or treat the condition.

Between 1987 and 1998, a minimum of five double-blind studies were published that indicated that vitamin E was beneficial in treating TD. Although most of these studies were small and lasted only four to twelve weeks, one thirty-six-week study enrolled forty people. Three small double-blind studies reported that vitamin E was not helpful. Nonetheless, a statistical analysis of the double-blind studies done before 1999 found good evidence that vitamin E was more effective than placebo. Most studies found that vitamin E worked best for TD of more recent onset.

However, in 1999, opinions on vitamin E changed with the publication of one more study, the largest and longest to date. This double-blind study included 107 participants from nine different research sites who took 1,600 international units of vitamin E or placebo daily for a minimum of one year. In contrast to most of the previous studies, this trial failed to find vitamin E effective for decreasing TD symptoms.

Why the discrepancy between this study and the earlier ones? The researchers, some of whom had worked on the earlier, positive studies of vitamin E, worked to develop an answer. They proposed a number of possible explanations. One was that the earlier studies were too small or too short to be accurate and that vitamin E really did not help. Another was the most complicated: that vitamin E might help only a subgroup of people who had TD–those with milder TD symptoms of more recent onset–and that fewer of these people had participated in the latest study. They also pointed to changes in schizophrenia treatment since the last study was done, including the growing use of antipsychotic medications that do not cause TD.

The effectiveness of vitamin E for a given person is simply not known. Given the lack of other good treatments for TD, and the general safety of the vitamin, it may be worth discussing with one's physician.

OTHER PROPOSED NATURAL TREATMENTS

Choline and related substances. According to one theory, TD symptoms may be caused or aggravated by an imbalance between two neurotransmitters, dopamine and acetylcholine. The nutrient choline and several related substances (lecithin, CDP-choline, and DMAE) have been suggested as possible treatments, with the goal of increasing the amount of acetylcholine that the body produces. Lecithin and CDP-choline are broken down by the body to produce choline, and choline provides one of the building blocks for acetylcholine. DMAE (2-dimethylaminoethanol, sometimes called deanol) may also increase production of acetylcholine, although this has been questioned.

Although a variety of small studies have been conducted on these substances, evidence for their effectiveness is mixed at best. Three small double-blind studies of lecithin had conflicting results: One found lecithin more helpful than placebo, one found it to be barely superior, and one found it no better than placebo. In two small double-blind trials of choline itself, some people experienced decreased TD symptoms on choline compared with placebo, but other people did not, and several people grew worse.

CDP-choline, a natural substance closely related to choline, has also been the subject of small studies with mixed results. An open study of ten people found it helpful for TD, but a small double-blind study did not find any evidence of benefit.

The substance DMAE is better studied than these other cholinergic treatments for TD, but the preponderance of evidence suggests it is not effective. Of twelve double-blind studies reviewed, only one found DMAE to be significantly effective when compared with placebo. A meta-analysis of proposed treatments for TD found DMAE to be no more effective than placebo.

Other natural treatments. A six-week, double-blind, placebo-controlled study of twenty-two people with schizophrenia and TD found that melatonin at a dose of 10 mg per day significantly improved TD symptoms. One small pilot study suggested that vitamin B_6 may be helpful for the treatment of TD. In this four-week, double-blind, crossover trial of fifteen people, treatment with vitamin B_6 significantly improved TD symptoms compared with placebo. Benefits were seen beginning at one week of treatment. A follow-up study tested the benefits of vitamin B_6 used for twenty-six weeks in fifty people with tardive dyskinesia, and, once again, the supplement proved more effective than placebo.

Preliminary evidence suggests that BCAAs (branched-chain amino acids) might decrease TD symptoms. Other proposed treatments include niacin and manganese, but evidence for their effectiveness is weak at best. Two double-blind trials of evening primrose oil, which contains large amounts of the essential fatty acid gamma-linolenic acid, found that it was not significantly more effective than placebo at reducing TD.

Prevention: High-dose vitamins? An informal twenty-year study of more than sixty thousand people treated with antipsychotic drugs plus high doses of vitamins found that only thirty-four of them (0.5 percent) developed TD. This is far fewer than might be expected: The estimated rate of TD among people treated with traditional antipsychotic medications is 20 to 25 percent. These results were based on reports from eighty psychiatrists who routinely used high-dose vitamins along with drugs to treat people with schizophrenia. Vitamins typically included C, niacin, B_6, and E in varying dosages. However, because the study design was informal, it is not possible to draw firm conclusions from its results.

HERBS AND SUPPLEMENTS TO USE ONLY WITH CAUTION

There is some concern that the amino acid phenylalanine, present in many protein-rich foods, may worsen TD. In a double-blind study of eighteen people with schizophrenia, those who took phenylalanine supplements had more TD symptoms than those who took placebo. Other herbs and supplements may interact adversely with drugs used to treat schizophrenia.

EBSCO CAM Review Board

FURTHER READING

Elkashef, A. M., and R. J. Wyatt. "Tardive Dyskinesia: Possible Involvement of Free Radicals and Treatment with Vitamin E." *Schizophrenia Bulletin* 25 (1999): 731-740.

Lerner, V., et al. "Vitamin B6 Treatment for Tardive Dyskinesia." *Journal of Clinical Psychiatry* 68 (2007): 1648-1654.

Shamir, E., et al. "Melatonin Treatment for Tardive Dyskinesia." *Archives of General Psychiatry* 58 (2001): 1049-1052.

See also: Melatonin; Schizophrenia; Vitamin B_6; Vitamin E.

Taurine

CATEGORY: Herbs and supplements
RELATED TERM: L-taurine
DEFINITION: Natural substance of the human body used as a supplement to treat specific health conditions.
PRINCIPAL PROPOSED USES: Congestive heart failure, viral hepatitis
OTHER PROPOSED USES: Alcoholism, cataracts, diabetes, epilepsy, gallbladder disease, hypertension (high blood pressure), multiple sclerosis, psoriasis, stroke

OVERVIEW

Taurine is an amino acid, one of the building blocks of proteins. Found in the nervous system and muscles, taurine is one of the most abundant amino acids in the body. It is thought to help regulate heartbeat, maintain cell membranes, and affect the release of neurotransmitters (chemicals that carry signals between nerve cells) in the brain.

REQUIREMENTS AND SOURCES

There is no dietary requirement for taurine, since the body can make it out of vitamin B_6 and the amino acids methionine and cysteine. Deficiencies occasionally occur in vegetarians, whose diets may not provide the building blocks for making taurine. People with diabetes have lower-than-average blood levels of taurine, but whether this means they should take extra taurine is unclear.

Meat, poultry, eggs, dairy products, and fish are good sources of taurine. Legumes and nuts do not contain taurine, but they do contain methionine and cysteine.

THERAPEUTIC DOSAGES

A typical therapeutic dosage of taurine is 2 grams (g) three times daily.

THERAPEUTIC USES

Preliminary evidence suggests that taurine might be helpful for treatment of congestive heart failure (CHF), a condition in which the heart has trouble pumping blood, which leads to fluid accumulating in the legs and lungs. Because CHF is too serious a condition for self-treatment, persons who are interested in trying taurine or any other supplement for CHF should first consult with their doctors.

There is also some evidence that taurine may be helpful for acute viral hepatitis. Taurine has additionally been proposed as a treatment for numerous other conditions, including alcoholism, cataracts, diabetes, epilepsy, gallbladder disease, hypertension, multiple sclerosis, psoriasis, and stroke, but the evidence for these uses is weak and, in some cases, contradictory. Taurine is also sometimes combined in an "amino acid cocktail" with other amino acids for treatment of attention deficit disorder, but there is no evidence that it works for this purpose.

SCIENTIFIC EVIDENCE

Congestive heart failure. Several studies (primarily by one research group) suggest that taurine may be useful for congestive heart failure. For example, in one double-blind, placebo-controlled trial, 58 people with CHF took either placebo or 2 g of taurine three times daily for four weeks; the groups were then switched. During taurine treatment, the study participants showed highly significant improvement in breathlessness, heart palpitations, fluid buildup, and heart X ray, as well as standard scales of heart failure severity. Animal research as well as small blinded or open studies in humans have also found positive effects. Interestingly, one very small study compared taurine with another supplement commonly used for CHF, coenzyme Q_{10}. The results suggest that taurine is more effective.

Viral hepatitis. Several viruses can cause acute viral hepatitis, a disabling and sometimes dangerous infection of the liver. The most common of these are hepatitis A and B, although there are others (hepatitis C and D).

One double-blind study suggests that taurine supplements might be useful for acute viral hepatitis. In this double-blind, placebo-controlled study, 63 people with hepatitis were given either 12 g of taurine daily or placebo. (The report does not state what type of viral hepatitis they had.) According to blood tests, the taurine group experienced significant improvements in liver function compared with the placebo group.

Acute hepatitis can also develop into a long-lasting or permanent condition known as chronic hepatitis. One small double-blind study suggests that taurine does not help chronic hepatitis. For this purpose, the herb milk thistle may be better.

SAFETY ISSUES

As an amino acid found in food, taurine is thought to be quite safe. There is strong evidence that taurine is safe at levels up to 3 g per day, although higher dosages have been tested without apparent adverse effects. However, maximum safe dosages of taurine supplements for children, pregnant or nursing women, and those with severe liver or kidney disease have not been determined.

As with any supplement taken in multigram doses, it is important that users of taurine purchase reputable products, because a contaminant present even in small percentages could add up to a real problem.

EBSCO CAM Review Board

FURTHER READING

Shao, A., and J. N. Hathcock. "Risk Assessment for the Amino Acids Taurine, L-Glutamine, and

L-Arginine." *Regulatory Toxicology and Pharmacology* 50 (2008): 376-399.

See also: Congestive heart failure; Hepatitis, viral.

Tea tree

CATEGORY: Herbs and supplements

RELATED TERMS: *Melaleuca alternifolia*, tea tree oil

DEFINITION: Natural plant product used to treat specific health conditions.

PRINCIPAL PROPOSED USES: Dandruff, tinea pedis (athlete's foot)

OTHER PROPOSED USES: Acne, oral herpes, periodontal disease, thrush, vaginal infections

OVERVIEW

Captain James Cook named this tree after finding that its aromatic, resinous leaves made a satisfying substitute for proper tea. One hundred fifty years later, an Australian government chemist, A. R. Penfold, studied tea tree leaves and discovered their antiseptic properties. Tea tree oil subsequently became a standard treatment in Australia for the prevention and treatment of wound infections. During World War II, the Australian government classified tea tree oil as an essential commodity and exempted producers of the oil from military service. However, the use of tea tree oil fell out of favor when antibiotics became widely available.

THERAPEUTIC DOSAGES

Tea tree preparations contain various percentages of tea tree oil. For treating acne, the typical strength is 5 to 15 percent; for fungal infections, 70 to 100 percent; and for use as a vaginal douche (with medical supervision), 1 to 40 percent concentrations. Tea tree oil is usually applied two to three times daily, until symptoms resolve. However, tea tree oil can be irritating to the skin, so experts recommend that users start with low concentrations until they know their tolerance.

The best tea tree products contain oil from the *alternifolia* species of *Melaleuca* only, standardized to contain not more than 10 percent cineole (an irritant) and a minimum of 30 percent terpinen-4-ol. Oil

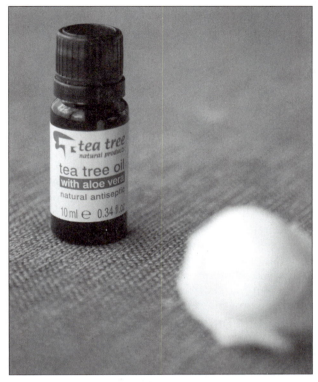

Bottle of tea tree oil. (Claudia Dulak/Photo Researchers, Inc.)

from a specially bred variant of tea tree may have increased activity against microorganisms, while irritating the skin less than the oil from other varieties.

THERAPEUTIC USES

Tea tree oil can kill many types of bacteria, viruses, and fungi on contact. This makes it an antiseptic, such as betadine, hydrogen peroxide, and many other essential oils. It is not an antibiotic in the common sense, because an antibiotic is absorbed throughout the body.

Preliminary double-blind studies suggest that tea tree oil might be useful for athlete's foot and other fungal infections of the skin and nails. One double-blind study found tea tree oil helpful for acne; another found that tea tree oil gel may reduce gum inflammation in people with periodontal disease. A single-blind study found evidence that tea tree oil may be helpful for dandruff.

Tea tree oil may be as effective as standard antiseptics for removing resistant strains of *Staphylococcus* bacteria from the skin of hospitalized persons. This does not mean tea tree oil is effective as an antibiotic for staph bacteria. It is an antiseptic. Antiseptics work on the surface of the body, while antibiotics work from within.

Additionally, tea tree oil has been proposed as a treatment for vaginal infections, thrush, and oral herpes (cold sores). However, there is no reliable evidence to indicate that it is effective for these purposes.

SCIENTIFIC EVIDENCE

Athlete's foot. In a double-blind, placebo-controlled trial, 158 people with athlete's foot were treated with placebo, with 25 percent tea tree oil solution, or with 50 percent tea tree oil solution, applied twice daily for four weeks. The results showed that the two tea tree oil solutions were more effective than placebo at eradicating infection. In the 50 percent tea tree oil group, 64 percent were cured; in the 25 percent tea tree oil group, 55 percent were cured; in the placebo group, 31 percent were cured. These differences were statistically significant. A few participants developed dermatitis in response to the tea tree oil and had to drop out of the study, but most did not experience any significant side effects.

Another double-blind, placebo-controlled trial followed 104 people with athlete's foot who were given either a 10 percent tea tree oil cream, the standard drug tolnaftate, or placebo. The results showed that tea tree oil reduced the symptoms of athlete's foot more effectively than placebo but less effectively than tolnaftate. Neither treatment cured the infection in 100 percent of the cases, but each treatment cured many cases.

A third double-blind study followed 112 people with fungal infections of the toenails, comparing 100 percent tea tree oil to a standard topical antifungal treatment, clotrimazole. The results showed equivalent benefits; however, because topical clotrimazole is not regarded as a particularly effective treatment for this condition, the results mean little.

Dandruff. In a four-week placebo-controlled study of 126 people with mild to moderate dandruff, the use of 5 percent tea tree oil shampoo significantly reduced dandruff symptoms. However, this study was not double-blind: The researchers knew which participants were receiving tea tree oil and which were receiving placebo. For this reason, the study's results cannot be taken as completely reliable.

Acne. The best evidence for benefits with tea tree oil as a treatment for acne comes from a randomized, double-blind, clinical trial of sixty people with mild to moderate acne symptoms. In this study, participants were divided into two groups and treated with placebo or with 5 percent tea tree oil gel. During the forty-five-day study period, researchers evaluated acne severity in two ways: by counting the total number of acne lesions and by rating acne severity on a standardized index. The results showed that tea tree oil gel was significantly more effective than placebo both at reducing the number of acne lesions and at reducing their severity.

SAFETY ISSUES

When used topically, tea tree oil is thought to be safe. However, it can cause allergic inflammation of the skin. In addition, one report suggests that a combination of lavender oil and tea tree oil applied topically caused gynecomastia (male breast enlargement) in three young boys. The researchers who published this report also noted that testing of tea tree oil revealed estrogenic (estrogen-like) and antiandrogenic (testosterone-blocking) effects. However, a literature search failed to find any other published reports that corroborate this claim.

Like other essential oils, tea tree oil can be toxic if taken orally in excessive doses. The safety of tea tree oil use for young children, pregnant or nursing women, and those with severe liver or kidney disease has not been established.

EBSCO CAM Review Board

FURTHER READING

Caelli, M., et al. "Tea Tree Oil as an Alternative Topical Decolonization Agent for Methicillin-Resistant *Staphylococcus aureus.*" *Journal of Hospital Infection* 46 (2000): 236-237.

Carson, C. F., et al. "*Melaleuca alternifolia* (Tea Tree) Oil Gel (6 Percent) for the Treatment of Recurrent Herpes Labialis." *Journal of Antimicrobial Chemotherapy* 48 (2001): 450-451.

Flaxman, D., and P. Griffiths. "Is Tea Tree Oil Effective at Eradicating MRSA Colonization?" *British Journal of Community Nursing* 10 (2005): 123-126.

Henley, D. V., et al. "Prepubertal Gynecomastia Linked to Lavender and Tea Tree Oils." *New England Journal of Medicine* 356 (2007): 479-485.

Satchell, A. C., et al. "Treatment of Dandruff with 5

Percent Tea Tree Oil Shampoo." *Journal of the American Academy of Dermatology* 47 (2002): 852-855.

Soukoulis, S., and R. Hirsch. "The Effects of a Tea Tree Oil-Containing Gel on Plaque and Chronic Gingivitis." *Australian Dental Journal* 49 (2004): 78-83.

See also: Acne; Athlete's foot; Periodontal disease; Vaginal infection.

Temporomandibular joint syndrome (TMJ)

CATEGORY: Condition

DEFINITION: Treatment of chronically painful and inflamed joints of the lower jaw.

PRINCIPAL PROPOSED NATURAL TREATMENTS: None

OTHER PROPOSED NATURAL TREATMENTS: Acupuncture, capsaicin cream, chiropractic, chondroitin, electromyograph biofeedback, glucosamine, massage, prolotherapy

INTRODUCTION

Temporomandibular joint (TMJ) syndrome is a disorder involving the two joints (one on each side) that attach the lower jaw to the skull. These two joints open and close the mouth and are located directly in front of each of the ears. In TMJ syndrome, the area around the temporomandibular joints becomes chronically tender and inflamed. Symptoms include pain in the temporomandibular joint; popping, clicking, or grating in the temporomandibular joint while eating and drinking; a sensation of the jaw "catching" or "locking" briefly, while attempting to open or close the mouth or while chewing; difficulty opening the mouth completely; pain in the jaw; facial pain; muscle pain or spasm in the area of the temporomandibular joint; headache; ear pain; and neck and shoulder pain.

TMJ syndrome often occurs in people who have had accidents or injuries involving the jaw, but many others have had no such incident. It is believed that grinding the teeth or clenching the jaw in response to stress may trigger the condition in many cases. Other possible causes include arthritis of the temporomandibular joint, facial bone defects or disorders, and misalignments of the jaw or of the bite.

The underlying cause of TMJ syndrome is not known. In most cases, the joint appears to be healthy, suggesting that it is the soft tissue around the joint rather than the joint itself that has the problem. However, some cases of TMJ syndrome may be caused by TMJ arthritis, TMJ dislocation, or other forms of true joint injury.

Treatment of TMJ includes stress management, avoidance of certain foods that trigger discomfort (such as gum or beef jerky), and anti-inflammatory medications. The older antidepressant drug amitriptyline, taken in low doses, and the muscle relaxant cyclobenzaprine also may help.

According to a few controlled trials, some people with more severe forms of TMJ may benefit from the use of a dental appliance. On rare occasions, surgery may be necessary.

PROPOSED NATURAL TREATMENTS

The supplement glucosamine, taken alone or with chondroitin, has shown considerable promise for the treatment of osteoarthritis. Because osteoarthritis of the temporomandibular joint can play a role in some cases of TMJ syndrome, researchers have begun to investigate the potential role of these supplements in treating the condition. Promising results were seen in a double-blind study that compared glucosamine to ibuprofen in the treatment of forty-five people with TMJ arthritis. During the three-month study, the supplement proved equal in effectiveness to the drug. However, because this study lacked a placebo group, it cannot be taken as fully reliable. Another double-blind study, this one involving glucosamine without chondroitin, did have a placebo group, but too many participants dropped out to allow meaningful conclusions to be drawn.

Electromyograph (EMG) biofeedback is a form of biofeedback therapy that involves teaching a person to gain conscious control of muscle tension. A meta-analysis (formal statistical review) of published studies suggests that EMG biofeedback might be helpful for TMJ pain. However, the reviewers noted that the evidence is incomplete and that more (and better quality) research is needed.

Similarly, while preliminary controlled trials suggest that acupuncture may be helpful for TMJ syndrome, more research is needed. A preliminary study compared traditional Chinese medicine (TCM), which incorporates acupuncture among other treatments, and naturopathic medicine (NM) with care given by clinic staffed by TMJ specialists. Researchers found that both TCM and NM provided greater benefit among 128 women. Although subjects were randomized into the different groups, the study was not blinded, and practitioners were permitted to treat each subject in any way they saw fit.

A cream made from cayenne and other hot peppers (capsaicin cream) has shown promise for many painful conditions. However, one study failed to find capsaicin cream more effective than placebo cream for TMJ syndrome. Other treatments that are sometimes recommended for TMJ, but that lack reliable scientific support, include chiropractic, massage, and prolotherapy.

EBSCO CAM Review Board

FURTHER READING

Herman, C. R., et al. "The Effectiveness of Adding Pharmacologic Treatment with Clonazepam or Cyclobenzaprine to Patient Education and Self-Care for the Treatment of Jaw Pain upon Awakening." *Journal of Orofacial Pain* 16 (2002): 64-70.

Kuttila, M., et al. "Efficiency of Occlusal Appliance Therapy in Secondary Otalgia and Temporomandibular Disorders." *Acta Odontologica Scandinavica* 60 (2002): 248-254.

La Touche, R., et al. "Effectiveness of Acupuncture in the Treatment of Temporomandibular Disorders of Muscular Origin." *Journal of Alternative and Complementary Medicine* 16 (2010): 107-112.

Raphael, K. G., and J. J. Marbach. "Widespread Pain and the Effectiveness of Oral Splints in Myofascial Face Pain." *Journal of the American Dental Association* 132 (2001): 305-316.

Ritenbaugh, C., et al. "A Pilot Whole Systems Clinical Trial of Traditional Chinese Medicine and Naturopathic Medicine for the Treatment of Temporomandibular Disorders." *Journal of Alternative and Complementary Medicine* 14 (2008): 475-487.

Smith, P., et al. "The Efficacy of Acupuncture in the Treatment of Temporomandibular Joint Myofascial Pain." *Journal of Dentistry* 35 (2007): 259-267.

See also: Bone and joint health; Fibromyalgia: Homeopathic remedies; Massage therapy; Pain management; Soft tissue pain.

Tendonitis

CATEGORY: Condition

RELATED TERMS: Achilles' tendonitis, golfer's elbow, iliotibial band tendonitis, lateral epicondylitis, medial epicondylitis, peripatellar tendonitis, rotator cuff tendonitis, tendonitis, tennis elbow

DEFINITION: Treatment of tendon inflammation.

PRINCIPAL PROPOSED NATURAL TREATMENT: Acupuncture

OTHER PROPOSED NATURAL TREATMENTS: *Arnica,* boswellia, bromelain, chondroitin, citrus bioflavonoids, creatine, devil's claw, glucosamine, horse chestnut, manganese, massage, oligomeric proanthocyanidin complexes, osteopathic manipulation, oxerutins, prolotherapy, proteolytic enzymes, vitamin C, white willow

INTRODUCTION

The tendons are some of the body's weakest links. While muscle and bone heal well after injury, the fibrous tissue that connects muscle to bone has a relatively poor blood supply, so it recovers only slowly.

Inflammation in the tendon or its sheath is called tendonitis. Symptoms include tenderness, redness, swelling, and pain on exertion, and they may last for months or years. Tendonitis occurs most commonly in the elbow (lateral or medial epicondylitis, also known as tennis elbow and golfer's elbow), knee (peripatellar tendonitis), hip (iliotibial band tendonitis), shoulder (rotator cuff tendonitis), lower calf (Achilles' tendonitis), forearm, and thumb.

Overuse of a tendon (repetitive strain injury) is the most common cause of tendonitis. This form of injury frequently occurs in computer keyboard users, people who perform manual labor, and athletes (such as tennis players and golfers). Acute injury to a tendon, such as an excessive stretch, can also cause tendonitis.

Conventional treatment consists primarily of avoiding the movement that caused the injury and allowing the body to heal on its own. Nonsteroidal anti-inflammatory drugs (such as ibuprofen) may help reduce pain but have not been shown to speed recovery. Steroid injection into the affected tendon is thought to help in certain cases, but the scientific basis for this commonly used method remains weak at best. The role of physical therapy in recovery from tendonitis also has not been well evaluated from a scientific perspective. A technique called extracorporeal shockwave therapy does not appear to work.

PRINCIPAL PROPOSED NATURAL TREATMENTS

Although the evidence remains incomplete and somewhat inconsistent, acupuncture treatment has shown considerable promise for the treatment of tendonitis. Most studies have evaluated the effect of acupuncture on tennis elbow (lateral epicondylitis).

For example, a placebo-controlled, single-blind trial of forty-five people with tennis elbow compared the effectiveness of real and sham acupuncture given twice weekly for ten weeks. The results showed significant improvement in pain intensity and ability to use the elbow among those who received real acupuncture. Good results were also seen in a placebo-controlled study of forty-eight people with tennis elbow.

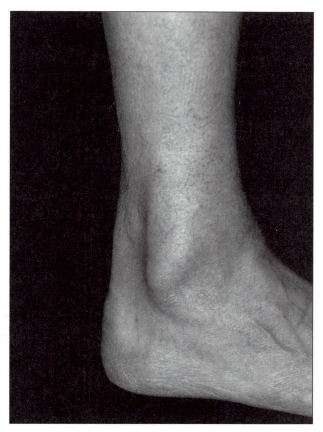

Swollen achilles tendon. (Dr. P. Marazzi/Photo Researchers, Inc.)

Another study compared superficial insertion of acupuncture needles (sham treatment insertion) with normal deep insertion in eighty-two people with tennis elbow. The results showed greater improvement among the participants treated with deep acupuncture, in the short-term. However, the difference was only temporary; by the three-month follow-up, both groups had pain to the same extent.

Benefits have also been seen in studies of people with tendonitis in the shoulder. A trial of fifty-two people with rotator cuff (shoulder) tendonitis found acupuncture more effective than sham acupuncture. Another study compared superficial to deep-insertion acupuncture in forty-four participants with shoulder pain and also found relative benefits. In this trial, the results of deep acupuncture endured for a minimum of three months.

Laser acupuncture is a widely used substitute for needle acupuncture, but it may not be effective. A double-blind study of forty-nine people with tennis elbow failed to find ten treatments with laser acupuncture more effective than the same number of treatments using fake laser acupuncture. Another study of fifty-eight persons with the same condition found laser acupuncture to be no more effective than ultrasound treatments or wearing a brace.

OTHER PROPOSED NATURAL TREATMENTS

A form of massage called deep transverse friction massage has shown some promise for tendonitis, but the research record is too weak to draw conclusions. Similarly, oscillating-energy manual therapy, an osteopathic technique based on the principle of craniosacral therapy, may be beneficial for tennis elbow (tennis elbow or lateral epicondylitis), but more research is required to be sure.

The supplements glucosamine and chondroitin are widely used for the treatment of osteoarthritis. Evidence suggests that they may work by enhancing the production of substances that keep cartilage healthy and flexible. On this basis, they have also been recommended for treating or preventing tendonitis. However, there is no direct evidence that they work.

The herb white willow contains a substance called salicin, which is quite similar to aspirin. It seems likely that appropriate doses of the herb might offer some symptomatic relief for tendonitis.

Other natural treatments sometimes recommended for tendonitis, but which lack scientific substantiation for that purpose, include prolotherapy and the following herbs and supplements: *Arnica*, boswellia, bromelain, citrus bioflavonoids, creatine, devil's claw, horse chestnut, manganese, oligomeric proanthocyanidin complexes, oxerutins, proteolytic enzymes, and vitamin C.

EBSCO CAM Review Board

FURTHER READING

Bisset, L., et al. "A Systematic Review and Meta-analysis of Clinical Trials on Physical Interventions for Lateral Epicondylalgia." *British Journal of Sports Medicine* 39 (2005): 411-422.

Ceecherelli, F., et al. "Comparison Between Superficial and Deep Acupuncture in the Treatment of the Shoulder's Myofascial Pain." *Acupuncture and Electro-therapeutics Research* 26 (2001): 229-238.

Fink, M., et al. "Acupuncture in Chronic Epicondylitis." *Rheumatology* 41 (2002): 205-209.

Nourbakhsh, M. R., and F. J. Fearon. "The Effect of Oscillating-Energy Manual Therapy on Lateral Epicondylitis." *Journal of Hand Therapy* 21 (2008): 4-14.

Oken, O., et al. "The Short-Term Efficacy of Laser, Brace, and Ultrasound Treatment in Lateral Epicondylitis." *Journal of Hand Therapy* 21 (2008): 63-68.

Trinh, K. V., et al. "Acupuncture for the Alleviation of Lateral Epicondyle Pain." *Rheumatology* 43 (2004): 1085-1090.

See also: Acupressure; Acupuncture; Back pain; Bone and joint health; Bursitis; Carpal tunnel syndrome; Injuries, minor; Neck pain; Nonsteroidal anti-inflammatory drugs (NSAIDs); Pain management; Soft tissue pain; Sports and fitness support: Enhancing recovery; Sports-related injuries: Homeopathic remedies; Temporomandibular joint syndrome.

Tetracyclines

CATEGORY: Drug interactions

DEFINITION: Antibiotics used to treat certain infections such as chlamydia and for long-term treatment of acne.

INTERACTIONS: Citrate, dong quai, minerals, St. John's wort

DRUGS IN THIS FAMILY: Demeclocycline hydrochloride (Declomycin), doxycycline (Bio-Tab, Doryx, Doxy-Caps, Doxychel, Monodox, Periostat, Vibramycin, Vibra-Tabs), minocycline hydrochloride (Dynacin, Minocin, Vectrin), oxytetracycline hydrochloride (Terramycin, Uri-Tet), tetracycline hydrochloride (Achromycin V, Panmycin, Robitet, Sumycin, Teline, Tetracap, Tetracyn, Tetralan)

MINERALS

Effect: Take at a Different Time of Day

Numerous minerals, including aluminum (found in many antacids), bismuth (in Pepto-Bismol), calcium, iron, magnesium, and zinc, interfere with the absorption of medications in the tetracycline family (and vice versa). The minerals and the drugs attach to each other and form insoluble chemicals that simply pass out of the digestive tract. The best solution is to avoid taking supplements that contain these minerals within the two hours before or after taking a tetracycline medication.

DONG QUAI, ST. JOHN'S WORT

Effect: Possible Harmful Interaction

Tetracycline antibiotics have been reported to cause increased sensitivity to the sun, amplifying the risk of sunburn or skin rash. Because St. John's wort and dong quai may also cause this problem, taking these herbal supplements during tetracycline treatment might add to this risk. People should use sunscreen or wear protective clothing during sun exposure if they are taking one of these herbs with a tetracycline antibiotic.

CITRATE

Effect: Possible Harmful Interaction

Potassium citrate, sodium citrate, and potassium-magnesium citrate are sometimes used to prevent kidney stones. These supplements reduce urinary acidity and can therefore lead to decreased blood levels and effectiveness of tetracycline antibiotics.

EBSCO CAM Review Board

FURTHER READING

Campbell, N. R., and B. B. Hasinoff. "Iron Supplements: A Common Cause of Drug Interactions." *British Journal of Clinical Pharmacology* 31 (1991): 251-255.

Neuvonen, P. J. "Interactions with the Absorption of Tetracyclines." *Drugs* 11 (1976): 45-54.

Ohnishi, M., et al. "Effect of a Kampo Preparation,

Byakkokaninjinto, on Pharmacokinetics of Cipro-floxacin and Tetracycline." *Biological and Pharmaceutical Bulletin* 32 (2009): 1080-1084.

Thappa, D. M., and J. Dogra. "Nodulocystic Acne: Oral Gugulipid Versus Tetracycline." *Journal of Dermatology* 21 (1994): 729-731.

See also: Acne; Antibiotics, general; Calcium; Dong quai; Food and Drug Administration; Iron; Magnesium; Potassium; St. John's wort; Supplements: Introduction; Vitamins and minerals; Zinc.

Theophylline

CATEGORY: Drug interactions

DEFINITION: Once among the most common treatments for asthma, theophylline is no longer widely used, having been replaced by drugs that cause fewer side effects.

INTERACTIONS: Cayenne, ipriflavone, St. John's wort, vitamin B_6

TRADE NAMES: Accurbron, Aerolate, Aquaphyllin, Asmalix, Elixomin, Elixophyllin, Lanophyllin, Quibron-T, Quibron-T-SR, Slo-bid, Slo-Phyllin, T-Phyl, Theo-24, Theo-Dur, Theo-Sav, Theo-X, Theobid, Theochron, Theoclear L.A., Theoclear-80, Theolair, Theolair-SR, Theospan-SR, Theostat 80, Theovent, Uni-Dur, Uniphyl

DRUGS IN THIS FAMILY: Aminophylline (Phyllocontin, Somophyllin, Somophyllin-DF, Truphylline), choline theophyllinate (Choledyl, Choledyl-SA, Oxtriphylline), dyphylline (Dilor, Lufyllin)

VITAMIN B_6

Effect: Supplementation Possibly Helpful

Theophylline appears to impair the normal conversion of vitamin B_6 into the more active substance pyridoxal 5'-phosphate (PLP). These findings have led some researchers to suspect that some of the many side effects of theophylline could be caused, in part, by interference with B_6 activity. Indeed, one study found that B_6 supplements might help reduce theophylline-induced tremors.

ST. JOHN'S WORT

Effect: Possible Interference with Action of Drug

Evidence suggests that the herb St. John's wort can lower blood levels of theophylline, making it less effective.

CAYENNE

Effect: Possible Increased Risk of Toxicity

Oral cayenne might increase the absorption of theophylline, which could lead to an increased risk of theophylline toxicity.

IPRIFLAVONE

Effect: Possible Increased Risk of Toxicity

Like cayenne, the supplement ipriflavone may increase levels of theophylline in the body, possibly increasing the risk of toxicity.

FURTHER READING

Bartel, P. R., et al. "Vitamin B6 Supplementation and Theophylline-Related Effects in Humans." *American Journal of Clinical Nutrition* 60 (1994): 93-99.

Jobst, K. A., et al. "Safety of St. John's Wort (*Hypericum perforatum*)." *The Lancet* 355 (2000): 575.

Nebel, A., R. K. Baker, and D. J. Kroll. "Potential Metabolic Interaction Between Theophylline and St. John's Wort." *Annals of Pharmacotherapy* 33, no. 4 (1999): 502.

Shimizu, T., et al. "Theophylline Attenuates Circulating Vitamin B6 Levels in Children with Asthma." *Pharmacology* 49 (1994): 392-397.

EBSCO CAM Review Board

See also: Asthma; Food and Drug Administration; Supplements: Introduction.

Therapeutic touch

RELATED TERMS: Distance healing, energy healing, healing touch, noncontact therapeutic touch

CATEGORY: Therapies and techniques

DEFINITION: Technique in which the placement of hands just above a person's body is used for healing.

PRINCIPAL PROPOSED USES: None

OTHER PROPOSED USES: Anxiety, human immunodeficiency virus infection support, osteoarthritis, pregnancy support, promoting general wellness, sports injuries, stress, surgery support, tension headaches, wound healing

OVERVIEW

Therapeutic touch (TT) is a form of energy healing popular in nursing in the United States. In the words of its official organization, "Therapeutic Touch is an intentionally directed process of energy exchange during which the practitioner uses the hands as a focus to facilitate the healing process." TT is used by nurses in a variety of settings, from the medical office to the intensive care unit (ICU). However, there is no meaningful evidence that it is effective.

TT was developed in the early 1970s by two people: Dolores Krieger and a self-professed healer, Dora Van Gelder Kunz. Initially, TT involved setting the hands lightly on the body of the patient, but the method rapidly evolved into a noncontact energy healing method. Certified practitioners can be found in virtually all parts of the United States and in much of the world. TT is available in mainstream health-care facilities including hospices, hospital-based alternative health programs, and even ICUs.

TT is sometimes described as a scientific version of "laying on of hands," a technique practiced by faith healers. However, there is more spirituality than science to this method; it makes use of beliefs and principles common in spiritual healing traditions but unknown to current science.

According to TT, the body has an energy field, and without physical contact, the energy field of one person can substantially affect the energy field of another. The practitioner is said to heal, balance, replenish, and improve the flow of a person's energy field, thereby leading to enhanced overall wellness. However, there is no meaningful scientific evidence for any of these beliefs.

SCIENTIFIC EVIDENCE

There has been considerable research interest in TT. However, the evidence for benefit is no more than weakly positive at best. A 1999 review of all published studies concluded that many of the studies had serious design flaws that could bias the results; in addition, the manner in which they were reported did not meet adequate scientific standards. A similar review in 2008 focusing on pain concluded that TT (along with healing touch and Reiki) may have modest effects on pain relief, particularly in the hands of more experienced practitioners, but the evidence was still fairly weak.

To be fair, proper study of TT presents researchers with some serious obstacles. The only truly meaningful way to determine whether a medical therapy works is to perform a double-blind, placebo-controlled trial. For hands-on therapies such as TT, however, a truly double-blind study is not possible, as the TT practitioner will inevitably know whether he or she is administering real TT or fake TT.

The best type of study that can be performed on TT is a single-blind study with "blinded" observers. In such studies, participants do not know whether they received real or fake TT, and an observer who also is blinded evaluates their medical outcome. However, such a study still has potential bias; practitioners could communicate a kind of cynicism when they use fake TT, and this problem appears to be insurmountable.

Further problems are involved in the choice of fake treatment. In most of the studies described here, sham TT involved practitioners counting backward in their heads by subtracting 7 serially from 100. The intent of this method was to avoid any possibility of projecting a healing concentration. It has been pointed out that this somewhat stressful effort would cause the practitioner to communicate tension rather than relaxation to study participants, and this too could bias results. However, it is difficult to suggest what should have been used instead as a placebo.

Some studies compared TT with no treatment. However, it has been well established that any therapy whatsoever will seem to produce benefit compared to no treatment for various nonspecific reasons; because of this, such studies say little to nothing about the specific benefits of TT. Finally, numerous trials have simply involved enrolling people with a medical problem, applying TT, and seeing whether they improve. Trials of this type prove nothing. Given these caveats, a summary of the research available thus far is presented here.

At the time of the 1999 review already noted, many published studies of TT were of unacceptably low quality and the results were quite inconsistent. For example, in one trial, thirty-one inpatients in a Veteran's Administration psychiatric facility received TT, relaxation therapy, or sham TT. The study was designed to evaluate the effectiveness of TT for reducing anxiety and stress. The results appear to indicate that TT was more effective for this purpose than the sham form. However, there are some serious design problems in this study that make the results difficult to trust. The real TT was administered by a woman in "street" clothes and the placebo treatment by a woman in a

The Process of Therapeutic Touch

According to the Therapeutic Touch International Association, therapeutic touch involves the following "dynamic and interactive phases":

Centering
Bringing the body and mind to a quiet, focused state of consciousness. Centering is using the breath, imagery, meditation and/or visualizations to open one's self to find an inner sense of equilibrium to connect with the inner core of wholeness and stillness.

Assessing
Holding the hands two to six inches away from the individual's energy field while moving the hands from the head to the feet in a rhythmical, symmetrical manner. Sensory cues such as warmth, coolness, static, blockage, pulling, and tingling are described by some practitioners.

Intervention

- *Clearing* (also called unruffling). Facilitating the symmetrical flow of energy through the field. Unruffling is achieved by using hand movements from the midline while continuing to move in a rhythmical and symmetrical manner from the head to the feet.

- *Balancing, rebalancing.* Projecting, directing, and modulating energy based on the nature of the living field; assisting to reestablish the order in the system. Treatment is accomplished by moving the hands to the areas that seem to need attention—energy may be transferred where there is a deficit or energy may be mobilized or repatterned from areas of congestion.

Evaluation/closure
Finishing the treatment using professional, informed, and intuitive judgment to determine when to end the session. Reassessing the field continuously during the treatment to determine balance and eliciting feedback from the individual are cues as to when to end the TT treatment.

Source: http://www.therapeutic-touch.org.

others found no significant effect, and still others found placebo more effective than real treatment. These results suggest that the effects seen were caused by chance.

Subsequent to the 1999 review, several better-quality trials were published. One such study compared real TT and sham TT in ninety-nine men and women recovering from severe burns. Researchers hypothesized that the use of TT would decrease pain and anxiety during that arduous and traumatic process, and indeed some evidence of benefit was seen.

In a smaller study (twenty-five participants), real TT appeared to reduce the pain of knee osteoarthritis compared to sham TT. Furthermore, in a study of twenty children with human immunodeficiency virus infection, the use of TT improved anxiety while sham touch did not. Another study found that an actor pretending to perform treatment similar to TT produced significant improvements in well-being in people with advanced cancer.

Taking all these studies together, it appears that real TT may be more effective than sham TT (using the serial subtraction technique). However, whether these apparent benefits are caused by the energy-healing effects claimed by practitioners or, more simply, through emotional communication, remains unclear.

Some studies provide preliminary evidence that TT does not work in the manner practitioners believe it does. For example, in one well-designed study, TT produced no effect when conducted without eye contact. The researcher, an influential person in the history of TT, had hypothesized that TT involved a kind of energy transfer that would not need eye contact. The fact that no effects were seen without the addition of eye contact suggests that it might be focused attention that makes the difference, not energy transmitted through the hands.

Furthermore, if TT actually involves contact with a person's "energy field," it would seem that the

nursing uniform; to make matters more complex, the relaxation therapy was administered by a man dressed as a clergyman. These large differences in appearance could only be expected to considerably influence the results in ways that cannot be predicted.

In a better study, sixty people with tension headaches were randomly assigned to receive either TT or placebo touch. TT proved to be significantly more effective than placebo touch. However, in a reasonably well-designed study published in 1993, the use of TT in 108 people undergoing surgery failed to reduce postoperative pain to a greater extent than sham TT.

A series of studies evaluated TT for aiding wound healing. Some found TT more effective than placebo, practitioners would be able to sense the presence of such a field. However, in a widely publicized study, twenty-one practitioners who had practiced TT for one to twenty-seven years proved unable to do this. In this trial, TT practitioners placed their hands face up through holes in a barrier. The experimenter (a nine-year-old student) held a hand above one of the practitioner's hands, and the practitioner was asked to sense its presence. The practitioners' guesses proved to be no more accurate than chance would allow. This study has been strongly criticized by proponents of TT. Some said that the experimenter was in the throes of puberty, and for that reason her energy field was too disturbed to detect; others complained about the disturbing presence of video cameras. While these criticisms are potentially valid, the burden is actually on proponents of TT to prove that there really is such a thing as a human energy field.

Nonetheless, the studies already performed do indicate that, at minimum, concentrated, positive attention provided by one human being to another is consoling and calming. This is a wonderful fact, even if there is no special energy field involved.

WHAT TO EXPECT DURING TREATMENT

Therapeutic touch is generally administered in a session that lasts about twenty minutes. The patient will be asked to lie still, relax, and remain quiet. The practitioner will place his or her hands a few inches above the person's body and move them slowly and rhythmically.

Some people experience a variety of subjective sensations while receiving TT, such as heat and moving energy. Most people find TT generally relaxing, but some undergo cathartic emotional experiences.

CHOOSING A PRACTITIONER

The original and most well-established TT organization is Therapeutic Touch International Association. This organization certifies training programs in TT.

SAFETY ISSUES

There are no known or suspected safety risks with TT.

EBSCO CAM Review Board

FURTHER READING

Coakley, A. B., and M. E. Duffy. "The Effect of Therapeutic Touch on Postoperative Patients." *Journal of Holistic Nursing* 28 (2010): 193-200.

Peters, R. M. "The Effectiveness of Therapeutic Touch." *Nursing Science Quarterly* 12 (1999): 52-61.

Pohl, G., et al. "'Laying on of Hands' Improves Well-Being in Patients with Advanced Cancer." *Supportive Care in Cancer* 15 (2007): 143-151.

Rosa, L., et al. "A Close Look at Therapeutic Touch." *Journal of the American Medical Association* 279 (1998): 1005-1010.

So, P. S., Y. Jiang, and Y. Qin. "Touch Therapies for Pain Relief in Adults." *Cochrane Database of Systematic Reviews* (2008): CD006535. Available through *EBSCO DynaMed Systematic Literature Surveillance* at http://www.ebscohost.com/dynamed.

See also: Energy medicine; Manipulative and body-based practices; Massage therapy; Metamorphic technique; Pain management; Reiki; Qigong.

Thiazide diuretics

CATEGORY: Drug interactions

DEFINITION: Thiazide diuretics are commonly used to treat hypertension.

INTERACTIONS: Calcium, coenzyme Q_{10}, licorice, magnesium, potassium, zinc

DRUGS IN THIS FAMILY: Bendroflumethiazide (Naturetin), benzthiazide (Exna), chlorothiazide (Diurigen, Diuril), chlorthalidone (Hygroton, Thalitone), hydrochlorothiazide (Esidrix, Ezide, HydroDIURIL, Hydro-Par, Microzide, Oretic), hydroflumethiazide (Diucardin, Saluron), indapamide (Lozol), methyclothiazide (Aquatensen, Enduron), metolazone (Mykrox, Zaroxolyn), polythiazide (Renese), quinethazone (Hydromox), trichlormethiazide (Diurese, Metahydrin, Naqua)

POTASSIUM

Effect: Probable Need for Supplementation

Thiazide diuretics cause a constant and significant loss of potassium. The classic treatment for this is to eat bananas and drink orange juice. Potassium supplements are also frequently prescribed.

Medications that combine thiazides and potassium-sparing diuretics might produce an unpredictable effect on potassium levels in the body. No one taking such medications should increase potassium intake except on the advice of a physician.

MAGNESIUM

Effect: Supplementation Possibly Helpful

Long-term use (use for more than six months) of thiazide diuretics might lead to magnesium deficiency. In turn, this loss of magnesium could increase the depletion of potassium. Because magnesium deficiency is common in any case, if one takes thiazide diuretics it would certainly make sense to take magnesium supplements at the U.S. Dietary Reference Intake dosage.

CALCIUM

Effect: Possible Dangerous Interaction

When taken over the long term, thiazide diuretics tend to increase levels of calcium by decreasing the amount excreted by the body and, indirectly, by affecting vitamin D. It is not likely that this will cause a problem. However, since greatly increased calcium levels in the body can cause side effects such as calcium deposits, if one is using thiazide diuretics, one should consult with a physician on the proper dose of calcium and vitamin D.

COENZYME Q_{10} (CoQ_{10})

Effect: Supplementation Possibly Helpful

Preliminary evidence suggests that thiazide diuretics might impair the body's ability to synthesize CoQ_{10}, a substance important for normal heart function. Although it is not known for sure that taking CoQ_{10} supplements will provide any specific benefit, supplementing with CoQ_{10} on general principle might be a good idea.

ZINC

Effect: Supplementation Possibly Helpful

Reportedly, thiazide diuretics can cause loss of zinc in the urine. Since zinc deficiency is relatively common, one should make sure that one gets enough zinc when using these drugs.

LICORICE

Effect: Possible Dangerous Interaction

If one is using thiazide diuretics, one should not take licorice root. Licorice root could exacerbate the potassium depletion caused by thiazides. However, the special form of licorice known as DGL (deglycyrrhizinated licorice) should not cause this problem.

EBSCO CAM Review Board

FURTHER READING

Al-Ghamdi, S. M., et al. "Magnesium Deficiency: Pathophysiologic and Clinical Overview." *American Journal of Kidney Diseases* 24 (1994): 737-752.

Crowe, M., et al. "Hypercalcaemia Following Vitamin D and Thiazide Therapy in the Elderly." *Practitioner* 228 (1984): 312-313.

Dorup, I. "Magnesium and Potassium Deficiency. Its Diagnosis, Occurrence, and Treatment in Diuretic Therapy and Its Consequences for Growth, Protein Synthesis, and Growth Factors." *Acta physiologica Scandinavica Supplementum* 618 (1994): 1-55.

Gora, M. L., et al. "Milk-Alkali Syndrome Associated with Use of Chlorothiazide and Calcium Carbonate." *Clinical Pharmacy* 8 (1989): 227-229.

Lemann, J., et al. "Hydrochlorothiazide Inhibits Bone Resorption in Men Despite Experimentally Elevated Serum 1,25-Dihydroxy Vitamin D Concentrations." *Kidney International* 28 (1985): 951-958.

Martin, B. J., and K. Millian. "Diuretic-Associated Hypomagnesemia in the Elderly." *Archives of Internal Medicine* 147 (1987): 1768-1771.

Reyes, A. J., et al. "Diuretics and Zinc." *South African Medical Journal* 62 (1982): 373-375.

Riis, B., and C. Christiansen. "Actions of Thiazide on Vitamin D Metabolism: A Controlled Therapeutic Trial in Normal Women Early in the Postmenopause." *Metabolism* 34 (1985): 421-424.

Shintani, S., et al. "Glycyrrhizin (Licorice)-Induced Hypokalemic Myopathy: Report of Two Cases and Review of the Literature." *European Neurology* 32 (1992): 44-51.

Whang, R., et al. "Refractory Potassium Repletion: A Consequence of Magnesium Deficiency." *Archives of Internal Medicine* 152 (1192): 40-45.

See also: Food and Drug Administration; Potassium-sparing diuretics; Supplements: Introduction.

Thomson, Samuel

CATEGORY: Biography

IDENTIFICATION: American herbalist and founder of a method to remove toxins from the body

BORN: February 9, 1769; Alstead, New Hampshire

DIED: October 4, 1843; Boston, Massachusetts

OVERVIEW

Samuel Thomson was an American herbalist who founded the alternative medicine system that came to be called Thomsonian medicine. This system, which involves the removal of toxins from the body through various purging methods, reached its peak in popularity in the United States in the nineteenth century. It has been suggested that Thomson was the foremost contributor to herbal science in the United States, in spite of the fact that he was not formally trained in medicine.

Thomson was born and raised in rural New Hampshire, during which time he nurtured an interest in the outdoors and in various plants and other wildlife. As a child, he reportedly consulted regularly with a local woman who had a reputation as a healer and herbalist. Thomson was discouraged from entering a life in academia, and he continued working as a farming attendant until he was seriously injured at the age of nineteen years. He reportedly healed his own wound with comfrey root and turpentine plaster, after the wound failed to heal with treatment from a formal physician. He also was said to have used another concoction of herbs to cure his case of measles.

Later in life, Thomson retained herbalists to treat his wife when she had become ill after childbirth; she had an ailment that was not healed by the efforts of several traditional doctors. Building on the methods used by the herbalists who successfully treated his wife, Thomson eventually developed his medicine system.

Thomson also discovered a use for the flowering herbal plant *Lobelia*, which became one of the key ingredients of his system of medicine. He later patented this use and promoted it as a cure for various ailments. However, its use was followed by troubling reports of serious side effects and even deaths. At one point, Thomson was brought to court to defend his herbal remedies after accusations were made by a physician who treated a patient who had used Thomson's approach.

Thomson also claimed that exposure to cold temperature causes illness, which could be cured, he believed, by reestablishing the body's original temperature. This temperature increase was often induced with steam baths, laxatives, vomiting, and such spicy foods as hot peppers.

Brandy Weidow, M.S.

FURTHER READING

Bergner, Paul. "*Lobelia* Toxicity: A Literature Review." *Medicinal Herbalism* 10 (2001): 15-26. Available online at http://medherb.com/materia_medica/lobelia_-_is_lobelia_toxic_.htm.

Lloyd, John Uri. "Life and Medical Discoveries of Samuel Thomson." *Bulletin of the Lloyd Library of Botany, Pharmacy, and Materia Medica*, no. 11 (1909). Available online at http://www.swsbm.com/ManualsOther/Samuel_Thomson-Lloyd.pdf.

See also: Cayenne; Herbal medicine; Popular health movement; Popular practitioners; Traditional Chinese herbal medicine.

Thymus extract

CATEGORY: Herbs and supplements

RELATED TERMS: Calf thymus extract, thymic extract, thymomodulin, thymus gland

DEFINITION: Natural substance from nonhuman animals that is used as a supplement to treat specific health conditions.

PRINCIPAL PROPOSED USES: None

OTHER PROPOSED USES: Asthma, eczema, food allergies, general immune support, hay fever

OVERVIEW

The thymus gland is found behind the sternum in the middle of the chest. It plays a significant role in the immune system, especially in fetuses and in very young children. The theory behind the use of thymus extracts is that they might stimulate or normalize immunity. However, there is no reliable real evidence that any thymus extracts are effective for any health condition. Furthermore, there are significant safety concerns related to the use of thymus products.

REQUIREMENTS AND SOURCES

Thymus extract is produced primarily from the thymus gland of cows. This has led to concerns regarding "mad cow disease" (bovine spongiform encephalopathy). All the studies described below used a pharmaceutical-grade form of thymus called Thymomodulin. It is not known whether the thymus dietary supplements available would have the same effect.

Therapeutic Dosages

The dosage of thymus extract used in studies has varied widely, depending on the particular thymus product used.

Therapeutic Uses

Two double-blind, placebo-controlled trials enrolling children with frequent respiratory infections, such as colds, found that treatment with thymus extract reduced the rate of infection. In theory, this might indicate an immune-boosting effect. However, small studies cannot provide reliable proof that a treatment is effective. Weak evidence from a rather convoluted trial hints that thymus extract may also be helpful for preventing respiratory infections in adults.

Intensive athletic training can suppress immune function and lead to colds as well. However, a double-blind, placebo-controlled trial of sixty athletes failed to find any significant evidence of benefit with thymus extract.

Preliminary evidence hints that thymus extracts may be helpful for food allergies, asthma, hay fever, and eczema. If thymus extract really does help these conditions, it may do so not by boosting the immune system but rather by calming it down and causing it to behave more normally. Small double-blind trials of thymus extract for hepatitis B and C found marginal benefits at most.

Injectable forms of whole thymus extract or chemicals contained in it have been studied as treatments for numerous other conditions, including cancer, cold sores, dermatomyositis, eczema, genital warts, hepatitis, human immunodeficiency virus infection, leukopenia (low white cell count), multiple sclerosis, psoriasis, respiratory infections, rheumatoid arthritis, scleroderma, and shingles (herpes zoster). The results of these studies have been mixed. In any case, the results of trials involving injected thymus cannot be considered applicable to oral thymus products.

Safety Issues

Thymus extracts have not been definitely associated with any side effects. However, there are real concerns that any glandular extract might contain the virus that causes mad cow disease. There is relatively little governmental regulation of thymus products sold as dietary supplements in the United States. Even when a ban is placed on importation of cow glands from a country where mad cow disease has been found, the ban does not apply to dietary supplements. For this reason, experts recommend that people not use thymus products sold as dietary supplements unless they are certified as free from risk of infection.

EBSCO CAM Review Board

Further Reading

Norton, S. "Raw Animal Tissues and Dietary Supplements." *New England Journal of Medicine* 343 (2000): 304-305.

See also: Allergies; Asthma; Eczema.

Thyroid hormone

Category: Drug interactions
Definition: Supplements used to treat hypothyroidism, a condition caused by deficient secretion of thyroid hormone by the thyroid gland.
Interactions: Calcium, carnitine, iron, soy
Drugs in this family: Dextrothyroxine (Choloxin), levothyroxine (Levoid, Levothroid, Levoxine, Levoxyl, Synthroid), liothyronine (Cytomel, Triostat), liotrix (Euthroid, Thyrolar), thyroglobulin (Proloid), thyroid (Armour Thyroid)

Calcium

Effect: Take at a Different Time of Day

Two case reports suggest that calcium carbonate interferes with the body's absorption of thyroid hormone when both are taken at the same time.

A prospective cohort study has validated these case reports. Twenty persons with hypothyroidism stabilized on long-term levothyroxine therapy were included in the trial. Participants were given calcium carbonate, 1,200 milligrams (mg) daily of elemental calcium, for three months. During the period the calcium supplement was taken, thyroid hormone levels in the blood declined. However, after calcium supplementation was stopped, thyroid levels climbed back up, slightly surpassing the levels measured at the beginning of the study. It is thought that calcium combines with thyroid hormone, thus reducing its absorption. To prevent this interaction, one should take thyroid hormone and calcium supplements as far apart as possible.

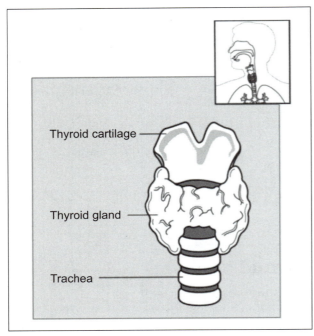

The thyroid is an important gland that produces thyroid hormone, the proper level of which is crucial to health. The inset shows the location of the thyroid gland.

IRON

Effect: Take at a Different Time of Day

Iron salts (including ferrous fumarate, ferrous gluconate, ferrous sulfate, and iron polysaccharide) may impair the effect of the thyroid hormone levothyroxine, probably by forming a complex with it and decreasing its absorption. To prevent a problem, one should take iron supplements and thyroid hormones as far apart as possible.

SOY

Effect: Possible Harmful Interaction

Soy formula may interfere with the absorption of thyroid medication in infants. In addition, soy may directly interfere with thyroid function. The result may be a need to increase the infant's dosage of thyroid medication. However, if one stops giving an infant soy formula, the thyroid dosage may need to be decreased. Of course, all changes related to thyroid treatment should be managed by a physician. Based on these findings, persons with impaired thyroid function should use soy (such as soybeans, soy milk, and tofu) with caution.

The Thyroid and Hypothyroidism

The thyroid is a two-inch-long, butterfly-shaped gland weighing less than one ounce. It is located in the front of the neck below the larynx, or voice box, and comprises two lobes, one on either side of the windpipe. The thyroid is one of a group of glands that are part of the endocrine system. The endocrine glands produce, store, and release hormones into the bloodstream that travel through the body and direct the activity of the body's cells. Thyroid hormones regulate metabolism, which is the way the body uses energy, and affect nearly every organ in the body.

Hypothyroidism occurs when the thyroid gland does not produce enough thyroid hormone to meet the body's needs. Without enough thyroid hormone, many of the body's functions slow down. About 5 percent of the U.S. population has hypothyroidism. Women are much more likely than men to develop hypothyroidism.

The thyroid gland makes two thyroid hormones, both of which affect metabolism, brain development, breathing, heart and nervous system functions, body temperature, muscle strength, skin dryness, menstrual cycles, weight, and cholesterol levels. A third hormone produced by specialized cells in the thyroid gland affects calcium levels in the blood and the buildup of calcium in the bones.

CARNITINE

Effect: Supplementation Possibly Helpful

Persons with an enlarged thyroid gland are sometimes given high doses of thyroid medication to shrink it. However, this treatment can cause unpleasant side effects, including bone loss, heart palpitations, and a feeling of malaise. A double-blind trial suggests that the supplement L-carnitine may safely reduce the adverse effects of this treatment.

EBSCO CAM Review Board

FURTHER READING

Benvenga, S., et al. "Usefulness of L-carnitine, a Naturally Occurring Peripheral Antagonist of Thyroid Hormone Action, in Iatrogenic Hyperthyroidism." *Journal of Clinical Endocrinology and Metabolism* 86 (2001): 3579-3594.

Butner, L. E., et al. "Calcium Carbonate-Induced Hypothyroidism." *Annals of Internal Medicine* 132 (2000): 595.

Singh, N., et al. "Effect of Calcium Carbonate on the

Absorption of Levothyroxine." *Journal of the American Medical Association* 283 (2000): 2822-2825.

See also: Food and Drug Administration; Supplements: Introduction.

Tiller, William A.

Category: Biography
Identification: Canadian proponent of crystal therapy and pioneer of psychoenergetics
Born: September 18, 1929; Toronto, Ontario, Canada

Overview

William A. Tiller, a proponent of crystal therapy, is most notably the pioneer of what is called psychoenergetics. Tiller claims to have discovered novel natural phenomena generated through what he calls subtle energies. He believes that certain healers and other paranormal practitioners are able to manifest these energies, which can be used to treat ailments. He defines "psychoenergetics" as the study of the interrelationship between these energies and human consciousness. Tiller outlines his ideas on this topic in *Science and Human Transformation: Subtle Energies, Intentionality, and Consciousness,* which was published in 1997. He also appeared in the 2004 independent film *What the Bleep Do We Know!?*, which explores the linkages among quantum physics, spirituality, and consciousness.

Tiller has both a master's degree and a doctoral degree from the University of Toronto. He worked for nine years as a consulting physicist at the Westinghouse Research Laboratories, where he undertook both experimental and theoretical investigations of the physics involved in freezing various materials such as water, metals, and semiconductors. In addition, he researched the relationships between the process of crystallization and the resultant properties of a given solid. Using the knowledge he gained during these efforts, he introduced new methods for growing crystals, purifying various materials, and casting certain types of metal. He also worked for more than thirty years in academia.

Tiller's credentials include professor emeritus of materials science and engineering at Stanford University and Fellow of the American Academy for the Advancement of Science. In addition, he has been chair and chief scientist of the William A. Tiller Founda-

tion, an organization devoted to researching and promoting Tiller's work on psychoenergetics. The foundation also distributes his books and other items (such as crystals) related to psychoenergetics. Also of note, Tiller was the founding director of the Academy of Parapsychology and Medicine, a short-lived organization dedicated to the advancement of psychoenergetics and to the healing principles of the body, mind, and spirit. In addition to several books, Tiller has published more than 350 articles about psychoenergetics and on other topics in widely accepted traditional fields. He also has several patents.

Some skeptics of pseudoscience have been critical of Tiller's ideas. In 1979, he received the Pigasus Award, an annual designation by skeptic James Randi, for comments Tiller made about parapsychology.

Brandy Weidow, M.S.

Further Reading

Tiller, William A. *Psychoenergetic Science: A Second Copernican-Scale Revolution.* Walnut Creek, Calif.: Pavior, 2007.
_____. *Science and Human Transformation: Subtle Energies, Intentionality, and Consciousness.* Walnut Creek, Calif.: Pavior, 1997.

See also: Bioenergetics; Crystal healing; Energy medicine; Mind/body medicine; Popular practitioners; Pseudoscience.

Time to Talk campaign

Category: Organizations and legislation
Definition: A U.S. government educational campaign promoting patient and practitioner dialogue about the use of complementary and alternative medicine.

History

The National Center for Complementary and Alternative Medicine (NCCAM), part of the National Institutes of Health, introduced the Time to Talk campaign in 2008. This educational initiative aims to open the lines of communication between patients and health care providers regarding the use of complementary and alternative medicine (CAM) practices such as chiropractic, acupuncture, meditation, and herbal supplements.

NCCAM's primary goal for the Time to Talk campaign is to integrate the safe use of CAM with conventional medicine. The campaign is aimed primarily at persons who are age fifty and older because they are the most common CAM users. Joint research between NCCAM and the American Association of Retired Persons (AARP) found that while a majority (50 to 65 percent) of Americans use CAM, only one-third share this information with their health care providers. Those surveyed, especially men and younger adults, stated they were unaware that they should share this information with their practitioner. Conversely, doctors reported not routinely asking patients whether they used CAM.

This failure to communicate may pose potential health risks, especially to those persons who take several daily prescribed medications. Also, noncommunication can lead a person to instead seek answers from unreliable sources, including publications with inaccurate or misleading health information. Through discussion, doctors can minimize the potential interaction risks with conventional medicine treatment, and health consumers can make sound, informed decisions to direct their own health care.

The Time to Talk campaign recommends listing all utilized CAM therapies and medications, including over-the-counter, dietary, and herbal supplements, when completing a medical history questionnaire before visiting with a doctor. As well, the campaign recommends being proactive about CAM by asking questions and discussing concerns during a doctor appointment. For doctors, key points in the discussion include informing the patient of the effectiveness and safety of a specific CAM therapy by providing facts from scientific, evidenced-based research, discussing how a CAM therapy may interact with a conventionally prescribed therapy, and recommending whether a CAM therapy should be pursued.

NCCAM provides free toolkits and information in English and Spanish for the Time to Talk campaign, and also wallet cards that list all CAM and conventional prescriptions and treatments. The literature and media campaigns have shown initial success. A 2009 NCCAM study assessed the provided materials and found that when patients were provided with the wallet card and fact sheets, 83 to 97 percent would use the card or discuss the matters involved with their primary physician.

Janet Ober Berman, M.S., C.G.C.

FURTHER READING

American Association of Retired Persons and National Center for Complementary and Alternative Medicine. "Complementary and Alternative Medicine: What People Fifty and Older Are Using and Discussing with Their Physicians." *Consumer Survey Report,* January 18, 2007.

Barnes, Patricia M., et al. "Complementary and Alternative Medicine Use Among Adults: United States, 2002." *CDC Advance Data Report,* no. 343 (2004).

National Center for Complementary and Alternative Medicine. "Time to Talk." Available at http://nccam.nih.gov/timetotalk.

See also: Integrative medicine; National Center for Complementary and Alternative Medicine; Popular practitioners.

Tinnitus

CATEGORY: Condition
RELATED TERMS: Ringing in the ears, tinnitus aurium
DEFINITION: Treatment of chronic ringing or other sounds in the ear.
PRINCIPAL PROPOSED NATURAL TREATMENTS: None
OTHER PROPOSED NATURAL TREATMENTS: Acupuncture, biofeedback, coenzyme Q_{10}, *Ginkgo biloba*, glutamic acid, hypnosis, ipriflavone, massage, melatonin, oxerutins, periwinkle, vitamin A with vitamin E, vitamin B_{12}, zinc

INTRODUCTION

Tinnitus aurium is the technical term for ringing in the ear, although the condition may actually involve sounds better described as buzzing, roaring, or hissing. The noise can be intermittent or continuous and can vary in pitch and loudness. Most people have experienced tinnitus occasionally for one minute or two. However, some people have tinnitus continuously, and it can range from a minor annoyance to a serious and nearly intolerable condition.

Exposure to loud noise can lead to tinnitus, as can ear obstructions, ear infections, otosclerosis (abnormal bone growth in the ear), head injuries, or heart and blood vessel disorders. In some cases, treating the underlying disorder will relieve the tinnitus. However, in many cases, the cause can be neither found nor treated.

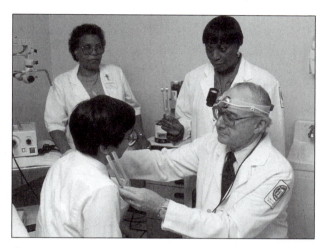

A patient is being evaluated in a tinnitus clinic. (Hank Morgan/Photo Researchers, Inc.)

One approach involves covering up the noise to make it more tolerable. This includes using hearing aids or tinnitus maskers (devices worn in the ear that emit pleasant sounds) or simply playing music to cover the noise. Avoiding loud noises and nicotine, aspirin, caffeine, and alcohol may help, because these often aggravate tinnitus. Drugs such as carbamazepine, benzodiazepines, and tricyclic antidepressants may be tried, although none of these has been proven effective for tinnitus.

Proposed Natural Treatments

There are no well-documented natural treatments for tinnitus. Several studies have evaluated *Ginkgo biloba* extract for treating tinnitus, but the results have been conflicting. While some small studies found benefit, the largest and best designed of these trials found no benefit. In this double-blind, placebo-controlled trial, 1,121 persons with tinnitus were given twelve weeks of treatment with standardized ginkgo at a dose of 50 milligrams (mg) three times daily. The results showed no difference between the treated group and the placebo group.

A separate set of researchers performed an additional study on ginkgo for tinnitus and then also conducted a meta-analysis (a statistically rigorous review) of the published data. Their conclusion: The evidence is strong enough to state that ginkgo does not benefit tinnitus.

One double-blind, placebo-controlled study found

that zinc deficiency was common in people with tinnitus. Zinc supplements appeared to help, but the study was too small to provide statistically meaningful results. In contrast, another small, double-blind, placebo-controlled study of people with tinnitus did not discover frequent zinc deficiency and failed to find any benefit with zinc supplements.

Vitamins A and E in combination, vitamin B_{12}, glutamic acid, ipriflavone, oxerutins, and periwinkle have also been suggested for the treatment of tinnitus, but the supporting evidence for their use remains far too weak to rely upon.

Melatonin may improve sleep in people with tinnitus; however, it does not appear to have any effect on the tinnitus itself. Very weak evidence, far too weak to rely upon, hints that the supplement CoQ_{10} might be useful in some cases of tinnitus. Several studies of acupuncture for tinnitus failed to find benefit. Biofeedback, massage therapy, and hypnosis have also been tried, but the results have been mixed at best.

EBSCO CAM Review Board

Further Reading

Arda, H. N., et al. "The Role of Zinc in the Treatment of Tinnitus." *Otology and Neurotology* 24 (2003): 86-89.

Khan, M., et al. "A Pilot Clinical Trial of the Effects of Coenzyme Q10 on Chronic Tinnitus Aurium." *Otolaryngology–Head Neck Surgery* 136 (2007): 72-77.

Morgenstern, C., and E. Biermann. "The Efficacy of Ginkgo Special Extract EGb 761 in Patients with Tinnitus." *International Journal of Clinical Pharmacology and Therapeutics* 40 (2002): 188-197.

Rejali, D., A. Sivakumar, and N. Balaji. "*Ginkgo biloba* Does Not Benefit Patients with Tinnitus." *Clinical Otolaryngology* 29 (2004): 226-231.

Rosenberg, S. I., et al. "Effect of Melatonin on Tinnitus." *Laryngoscope* 108 (1998): 305-310.

See also: Ear infections; Hearing loss.

Tinnitus: Homeopathic remedies

Category: Homeopathy
Related terms: Ringing in the ears, tinnitus aurium
Definition: The use of highly diluted remedies to treat chronic ringing or other sounds in the ear.

STUDIED HOMEOPATHIC REMEDIES: *Carbo vegetabilis*; *Chininum sulphuricum*; combination homeopathic remedy containing sodium salicylate, ascaridole (*Chenopodium*), coniine (*Conium*), and quinine; graphites

SCIENTIFIC EVALUATIONS OF HOMEOPATHIC REMEDIES

A twelve-week, double-blind, placebo-controlled, crossover trial with twenty-one participants tested the effectiveness of a homeopathic remedy containing sodium salicylate, ascaridole (*Chenopodium*), coniine (*Conium*), and quinine as a treatment for tinnitus. The results were negative in all measures of the condition.

TRADITIONAL HOMEOPATHIC TREATMENTS

Classical homeopathy offers many possible homeopathic treatments for tinnitus. These therapies are chosen based on various specific details of the person seeking treatment. The remedy *Carbo vegetabilis* is sometimes used for tinnitus accompanied by vertigo and nausea, especially when symptoms are most severe at night. *Chininum sulphuricum* might be recommended for use by people whose tinnitus is extremely loud (to them).

When tinnitus is associated with hearing loss, graphites is often considered. The type of tinnitus associated with this remedy is described as involving hissing or clicking sounds and loud reports (like gunshots).

EBSCO CAM Review Board

FURTHER READING

Altunc, U., M. H. Pittler, and E. Ernst. "Homeopathy for Childhood and Adolescence Ailments." *Mayo Clinic Proceedings* 82 (2007): 69-75.

Goldstein, B., A. Shulman, and M. J. Avitable. "Clear Tinnitus, Middle-Ear Pressure, and Tinnitus Relief." *International Tinnitus Journal* 13 (2007): 29-39.

Simpson, J. J., I. Donaldson, and W. E. Davies. "Use of Homeopathy in the Treatment of Tinnitus." *British Journal of Audiology* 32 (1998): 227-233.

See also: Adolescent and teenage health; Children's health; Ear infections; Ear infections: Homeopathic remedies; Homeopathy; Swimmer's ear; Tinnitus.

Tinospora cordifolia

CATEGORY: Herbs and supplements
RELATED TERMS: Amrita, guduchii
DEFINITION: Natural plant product used as a dietary supplement for specific health benefits.
PRINCIPAL PROPOSED USE: Allergic rhinitis
OTHER PROPOSED USES: Adaptogen, cancer prevention, cancer treatment support, diabetes, high cholesterol, liver protection

OVERVIEW

The herb *Tinospora cordifolia* has a long history of use in Ayurvedic medicine (the traditional medicine of India). It has been used to treat convalescence from severe illness, liver disease, arthritis, urinary problems, eye diseases, cancer, anemia, diabetes, and diarrhea. It is said to help remove toxins from the body, and on this basis it is often added to herbal formulas claimed to improve general health. Both the stem and the root are used medicinally.

THERAPEUTIC USES

According to some herbalists, tinospora has adaptogenic effects, meaning that it helps the body adapt to stress. However, there is no meaningful evidence to support this claim. Only double-blind, placebo-controlled studies can prove a treatment effective, and the only such study performed on tinospora tested other effects.

SCIENTIFIC EVIDENCE

In one study, seventy-five people with allergic rhinitis (hay fever) were given either tinospora or placebo for eight weeks. According to the investigators, the use of tinospora significantly decreased every measured symptom of allergic rhinitis in the majority of participants. In comparison, the use of placebo provided almost no benefit.

These results may sound promising, but they are so excessively dramatic as to raise doubts about the study's overall validity. It is unusual for so few benefits to be seen in the placebo group of a study on treating allergic rhinitis and for almost universal benefits to be reported in the treatment group.

In addition to having anti allergy effects, weak evidence hints that tinospora may be effective against cancer, diabetes, and high cholesterol, and that it may

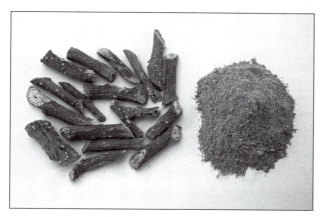

Dried and powered Tinospora cordifolia. (Dinodia Photos/Getty Images)

stimulate the immune system, protect nerve cells, and protect the liver. Tinospora also has shown some promise for decreasing the tissue damage caused by radiation and the side effects of some forms of chemotherapy and for speeding the healing of diabetic foot ulcers. However, all these findings are far too preliminary to be relied upon.

SAFETY ISSUES

The use of tinospora has not been associated with significant side effects. However, comprehensive safety testing has not been conducted. One animal study found evidence that the use of tinospora might decrease male fertility. Safety for pregnant or nursing women, young children, and persons with severe liver or kidney disease has not been established.

EBSCO CAM Review Board

FURTHER READING

Badar, V. A., et al. "Efficacy of *Tinospora cordifolia* in Allergic Rhinitis." *Journal of Ethnopharmacology* 96 (2004): 445-449.

Nair, P. K., et al. "Immune Stimulating Properties of a Novel Polysaccharide from the Medicinal Plant *Tinospora cordifolia*." *International Immunopharmacology* 4 (2004): 1645-1659.

Purandare, H., and A. Supe. "Immunomodulatory Role of *Tinospora cordifolia* as an Adjuvant in Surgical Treatment of Diabetic Foot Ulcers." *Indian Journal of Medical Sciences* 61 (2007): 347-355.

Singh, N., et al. "Effect of *Tinospora cordifolia* on the Antitumor Activity of Tumor-Associated Macrophages-Derived Dendritic Cells." *Immunopharmacology and Immunotoxicology* 27 (2005): 1-14.

See also: Allergies; Ayurveda; Cancer risk reduction; Cancer treatment support; Cholesterol, high; Diabetes; Herbal medicine; Immune support; Liver disease.

Tocotrienols

CATEGORY: Herbs and supplements
DEFINITION: Natural plant substances used to treat specific health conditions.
PRINCIPAL PROPOSED USES: None
OTHER PROPOSED USES: Cancer prevention, heart disease prevention, high cholesterol

OVERVIEW

Tocotrienols are fat-soluble substances closely related to vitamin E. Like vitamin E, they have antioxidant properties, and they help protect fatty substances in the body from being damaged by free radicals. In the 1990s, antioxidant supplements were thought to offer great potential for preventing a variety of diseases, including cancer and heart disease, and on this basis tocotrienols were offered on the market as healthful supplements. Tocotrienols have also been proposed for reducing cholesterol. However, subsequent studies have tended to discourage all these hopes. At present, there is no reliable evidence that tocotrienols offer any meaningful health benefits.

REQUIREMENTS AND SOURCES

Tocotrienols are not essential nutrients. They occur naturally in the oil extract of barley, palm fruit, rice bran, and wheat germ. Most commercially available supplements are made from rice bran oil or palm oil.

THERAPEUTIC DOSAGES

A typical recommended dose of tocotrienols is 200 milligrams daily.

THERAPEUTIC USES

While test-tube studies, animal studies, and open human trials seemed to suggest that tocotrienols can correct high cholesterol, properly designed studies failed to find benefit.

Test-tube and animal studies, as well as one double-blind human trial, have found promising hints that tocotrienols may help prevent cancer. The double-blind study among these specifically found that tocotrienols might help prevent deoxyribonucleic acid (DNA) damage, which could, in theory, help prevent many diseases associated with aging, not just cancer. However, none of this evidence rises above the level of "highly preliminary."

The hypothesis that tocotrienols can prevent heart disease simply by virtue of their antioxidant actions has lost favor, since the same hypothesis proved incorrect with vitamin E and beta-carotene. The health benefits of tocotrienols, if there are any, remain to be established.

SAFETY ISSUES

Tocotrienols are thought to be safe substances. However, maximum safe doses have not been determined.

EBSCO CAM Review Board

FURTHER READING

Ajuluchukwu, J. N., et al. "Comparative Study of the Effect of Tocotrienols and Tocopherol on Fasting Serum Lipid Profiles in Patients with Mild Hypercholesterolaemia." *Nigerian Postgraduate Medical Journal* 14 (2007): 30-33.

Chin, S. F., et al. "Reduction of DNA Damage in Older Healthy Adults by Tri E Tocotrienol Supplementation." *Nutrition* 24, no. 1 (2008): 1-10.

Qureshi, A. A., et al. "Isolation and Identification of Novel Tocotrienols from Rice Bran with Hypocholesterolemic, Antioxidant, and Antitumor Properties." *Journal of Agricultural and Food Chemistry* 48 (2000): 3130-3140.

Qureshi, A. A., et al. "Synergistic Effect of Tocotrienol-Rich Fraction (TRF 25) of Rice Bran and Lovastatin on Lipid Parameters in Hypercholesterolemic Humans." *Journal of Nutritional Biochemistry* 12 (2001): 318-329.

Szapary, P. O., and M. D. Cirigliano. "Tocotrienols in the Management of Hypercholesterolemia and Atherosclerosis." *Alternative Medicine Alert* 3 (2000): 101-105.

Theriault, A., et al. "Tocotrienol: A Review of Its Therapeutic Potential." *Clinical Biochemistry* 32, no. 5 (1999): 309-319.

Yu, W., et al. "Induction of Apoptosis in Human Breast Cancer Cells by Tocopherols and Tocotrienols." *Nutrition and Cancer* 33 (1999): 26-32.

See also: Cancer risk reduction; Cholesterol, high; Hypertension.

Tongue diagnosis

CATEGORY: Therapies and techniques
RELATED TERM: Tongue examination
DEFINITION: A diagnostic technique involving a visual inspection of the tongue.
PRINCIPAL PROPOSED USE: Diagnosis
OTHER PROPOSED USE: Diagnosis confirmation

OVERVIEW

Specific areas of the tongue are thought to reflect the health of different internal organs. The condition of the tongue changes with shifting patterns of health. In general, these changes in health appear on the tongue slowly. One exception is during a cold or flu, when a high fever may produce a very red tongue fairly quickly.

MECHANISM OF ACTION

The tongue is assessed for overall coating, shape, and color. The tongue's shape and size are thought to reflect the status of fluids in the body. For example, a very large, puffy tongue may indicate poor metabolism of fluids. The color of the tongue indicates the overall nature of the medical condition and the state of blood or qi (energy) in the body. For example, a red tongue indicates an excess of heat in the body, whereas a pale tongue indicates a deficiency of qi and blood or the presence of a cold. The coating on the tongue is an indicator of the severity of a condition and also reflects the condition of fluids in the body.

Different areas of the tongue reflect the health of the different organ systems. For example, a tongue that is red at the tip indicates heat in the heart, because the tip of the tongue correlates with conditions of the heart.

USES AND APPLICATIONS

Tongue diagnosis is generally used in conjunction with pulse diagnosis to assess a person's medical condition.

SCIENTIFIC EVIDENCE

There is no reliable scientific evidence that tongue diagnosis is an accurate indicator of medical conditions or disease. Double-blind, controlled studies are difficult to perform because diagnostic variables and disease subcategories (outcome measures) are subjective and qualitative and can vary widely depending on the experience of the practitioner. Investigators are studying new ways of imaging and analyses to determine an objective diagnostic standard for visual tongue inspections (such as optical topography imaging, computerized tongue inspection methods, and pixel-wise or RGB-color-space classification of a tongue image).

CHOOSING A PRACTITIONER

Although modern medical doctors also examine the tongue during a physical, this is not equivalent to tongue diagnoses in complementary and alternative medicine practices. Tongue diagnosis is used by practitioners in traditional Asian medicine. One should choose a practitioner who is certified by the National Certification Commission for Acupuncture and Oriental Medicine.

SAFETY ISSUES

This technique is noninvasive and has no known side effects.

Anita P. Kuan, Ph.D.

FURTHER READING

American Association of Acupuncture and Oriental Medicine. http://www.aaaomonline.org.

National Certification Commission for Acupuncture and Oriental Medicine. http://www.nccaom.org.

Wainapel, Stanley F., and Avital Fast, eds. *Alternative Medicine and Rehabilitation: A Guide for Practitioners.* New York: Demos Medical, 2003.

See also: Burning mouth syndrome; Leukoplakia; Pulse diagnosis.

Traditional Chinese herbal medicine

CATEGORY: Therapies and techniques
RELATED TERMS: *Aristolochia clematis, Astragalus mem-* *branaceus,* Banxia Houpo Tang, Biminne, Bing Gan Tang, Chinese herbs, Chinese patent remedies, Coptis formula, Daio-kanzo-to, Fuzheng Jiedu Tang, Hange Koboku-to, Hochu-ekki-to, Jianpi Wenshen recipe, Kampo, Magnolia and Pinelliae formula, PC-SPES, Saiboku-to, Saiko-keishi-to, Shakuyaku-kanzo-to, Shenshao, Shosaiko-to, Shoseiryu-to, Shuang Huang Lian, Toki-shakuyakusan, Xuezhikang, Yi Zhu decoction, Zemaphyte

DEFINITION: A holistic healing method using herbal combinations tailored to the individual person according to complex principles.

PRINCIPAL PROPOSED USE: Liver conditions

OTHER PROPOSED USES: Allergies, angina, asthma, cancer treatment support, cardiovascular disease, chronic fatigue syndrome, constipation, colds and flus, cough, dementia, diabetes, eczema, epilepsy, human immunodeficiency virus support, infertility in women, insomnia, irregular menstruation, irritable bowel syndrome, menopause, menstrual pain, muscle spasms, osteoarthritis, respiratory infections, sexual dysfunction in men, stress, stroke rehabilitation, tension headache, weight loss

OVERVIEW

The system of herbal medicine that developed in China differs in several significant ways from European herbal medicine. The most obvious difference is that Western herbal medicine focuses on simples, or herbs taken by themselves. In contrast, traditional Chinese herbal medicine (TCHM) makes almost exclusive use of herbal combinations. Also, TCHM formulas are not designed to treat symptoms of a specific illness; rather, they are tailored specifically to the individual according to the complex principles of traditional Chinese medicine (TCM). For this reason, TCHM is potentially a deeply holistic healing approach. However, it is both more difficult to use and harder to study than its Western counterpart.

TCHM is widely used in Asian countries, both in its traditional holistic form and in a simplified disease-oriented version. There have been a few properly designed scientific trials of TCHM, but the evidence base remains highly inadequate. In addition to questions regarding effectiveness, serious safety concerns need to be resolved.

History. Chinese herbal medicine has a long historical tradition, although it is not quite as ancient as popularly believed. Ancient herbology in China focused on potions whose functions were part medicinal and part magical, and it lacked a substantial theoretical base. Sometime between the second century B.C.E. and the second century C.E., the theoretical foundations of TCM were laid, but the focus was more on acupuncture than on herbs. Only by about the twelfth century were the deeper principles of Chinese medicine fully applied to herbal treatment, forming the method known as TCHM. This was further refined and elaborated during various periods of active theorizing in the fourteenth through the nineteenth centuries. Western disease concepts entered the picture in the twentieth century, leading to further changes.

In China today, TCHM is used alongside conventional pharmaceutical treatment. Considerable attempts have been made to subject TCHM to scientific evaluation; however, most of the published Chinese studies on the subject fall far short of current scientific standards. (For example, they generally lack a placebo group.)

In neighboring Japan, a variation of the TCHM system known as Kampo has become popular, and the Japanese health ministry has approved many Kampo remedies for medical use. The scientific basis for these remedies remains incomplete, but several studies of minimally acceptable quality have been reported.

Principles of traditional Chinese herbal medicine. According to the principles of all Chinese medicine, health exists when the body is balanced and its energy is freely flowing. The term "energy" refers to qi, the life energy that is said to animate the body. The term "balance" refers to the relative factors of yin and yang, the classic Daoist opposing forces of the universe. Yin and yang find their expression in various subsidiary antagonists such as cold versus heat and dampness versus dryness.

In an ideal state, yin and yang in all their forms are perfectly balanced in every part of the body. However, external or internal factors can upset this balance, leading to disease. Chinese medical diagnosis and treatment involve identifying the factors that are out of balance and attempting to bring them back into harmony. Diagnosis is carried out by means of "listening" to the pulse (in other words, taking the pulse with extraordinary care and sensitivity), observing and palpating various parts of the body, and asking a long series of questions.

It is important to realize that diagnosis according to TCHM differs greatly from Western diagnosis. Consider

---

Herbal Medicine: Safety Concerns

There are serious safety concerns regarding traditional Chinese herbal therapy. Chinese herbal medicine traditionally uses treatments, such as mercury, arsenic, lead, licorice, and the herb *Aristolochia*, that are now recognized as potentially dangerous. In Hong Kong, poisoning caused by the herb aconite (used in numerous Chinese herbal formulas) was sufficiently widespread that public health authorities launched an information campaign to combat the problem.

Besides toxicity caused by Chinese herbs, other problems have been caused by adulteration of herbal products with unlisted ingredients. For example, the Chinese herbal formula PC-SPES, used for prostate cancer, turned out to contain three pharmaceutical drugs—diethylstilbestrol (DES), warfarin (Coumadin), and indomethacin. In another episode, eight of eleven Chinese herbal creams sold in the United Kingdom for the treatment of eczema were found to contain strong pharmaceutical steroids. For all these reasons, considerable caution is advisable when using traditional Chinese herbs.

---

two hypothetical patients with the single Western diagnosis of migraine headaches. The first might be said to have "dryness in the liver and ascending qi," while the other might be diagnosed with "exogenous wind-cold." Based on these differing diagnoses, entirely different remedies might be applied. In other words, there is no such thing as a TCHM remedy for migraines per se; rather, treatment must be individualized to the imbalance determined by traditional theory.

The herbal formulas used in TCHM consist of four categories of herbs: ministerial, deputy, assistant, and envoy. The ministerial herb addresses the principal pattern of the disease. Deputy herbs assist the ministerial herb or address coexisting conditions. Assistant herbs are designed to reduce the side effects of the first two classes of herbs, and envoy herbs direct the therapy to a particular part of the body. For example, in the case of "dryness in the liver and ascending qi," an herbalist might employ a ministerial herb to reverse ascending qi, a deputy herb to exert a moistening effect, an assistant herb to prevent the stagnation of qi (qi stagnation is said to be a side effect of moistening herbs), and an envoy to carry these effects to the liver.

TCHM remedies can also be designed to fit all common causes of migraines simultaneously, mostly by multiplying the number of ingredients. Practitioners of TCHM frown upon this "one-size-fits-all" approach, but it is often popular among consumers and is easier to test scientifically.

Types of Chinese herbal remedies. To use Chinese herbal medicine in the most traditional fashion, one must visit an herbalist's shop. There, experienced herb preparers will chop, grind, fry, and slice dried herbs according to the prescription given by an experienced herbalist. The herbalist will provide a packet of dried herbs that need to be prepared according to the instructions, which typically involve adding water, boiling for several hours in a ceramic pot, pouring off the liquid, adding more water, and repeating the process twice more. Certain herbs are supposed to be added at the end of the process, while others require extra-long preparation.

If one does not wish to carry out such a complex process, or if a classic herbal shop is not available, one may wish to move one step away from tradition and purchase a prepared Kampo formula. There are several hundred such formulas designed to match the most commonly seen forms of imbalance. Available in powder, capsule, or tablet form, they can be used much more conveniently than fully traditional herbs. Many Kampo combinations are licensed in Japan and are manufactured there on a large scale by reputable manufacturers.

The lowest level of TCHM, scarcely deserving the name, involves Chinese patent remedies, which consist most commonly of tiny brown spheres in small brown bottles. They are marketed for both classical imbalances and Western disease categories. Patent remedies are inexpensive and widely available. However, there have been so many scandals involving dangerous contaminants not listed on the label that people should avoid this form of treatment entirely.

In the West, herbal medicine is part of folk medicine. However, in China, there is a distinct tradition of Chinese folk medicine that is separate from the orthodox, rather academic TCHM approach. In this Chinese folk medicine, herbs are used more simply, somewhat in the manner of Western herbal medicine. Herbs most commonly used in this manner include *Astragalus*, dong quai, ginger, kudzu (*Pueraria lobata*), licorice, *Lycium*, *Panax ginseng*, and *Schisandra*.

In addition to herbs, substances that are often considered supplements are utilized in TCHM. These substances include extract of human placenta, glandular extracts, and a variety of minerals.

Uses and applications. In the traditional system of Chinese herbal medicine, herbal formulas can be used to treat virtually any condition. Some of the most common uses in China include liver disease (hepatitis and cirrhosis), sexual dysfunction in men, infertility in women, insomnia, colds and flus, menstrual pain, irregular menstruation, and menopause.

Acupuncture is often used with herbs as a supplemental treatment; in addition, extraordinarily detailed lifestyle suggestions are common. It is not unusual for a traditional practitioner to "prescribe" dinner and to counsel changes in living situation (for example, move from the basement to the first floor or face the bed south rather than north). Exercise systems such as Tai Chi and qigong may also be recommended.

Chronic hepatitis. Hepatitis is a serious problem in many Asian countries, and conventional care is lacking. For this reason, herbal remedies are widely used.

The herbal combination Shosaiko-to (Minor Bupleurum) has been approved as a treatment for chronic hepatitis by the Japanese health ministry, and it enjoys wide use in that country and elsewhere. However, a search of the literature uncovered only one large-scale, double-blind, placebo-controlled study supporting its effectiveness. In this twenty-four-week trial, the efficacy of Shosaiko-to was tested in 222 people with chronic active hepatitis using a double-blind, placebo-controlled, crossover design. Results showed that the use of Shosaiko-to significantly improved liver function measurements compared with placebo. Although these results are promising, an absence of long-term evaluation limits their meaningfulness. (Researchers followed participants for three months only.)

Other Chinese herbal remedies have been tested as adjuncts to conventional interferon treatment with promising results. However, published trials are of generally poor quality. Persons undergoing interferon therapy should not use Chinese herbal formulas (or any herbs or supplements) except under the supervision of a physician.

Combination Chinese herbal therapies have also shown some promise for the treatment of chronic hepatitis; tested formulas include Bing Gan Tang, Yi Zhu decoction, Fuzheng Jiedu Tang, and Jianpi Wenshen recipe. However, the quality of most of these studies was quite poor. The results are mixed, and overall, the evidence for these remedies remains far too weak to rely upon. Two studies failed to find Chinese herbal treatment helpful for hepatitis C. Also note that there have been numerous cases of hepatitis and other forms of liver injury caused by Chinese herbs.

Liver cirrhosis. Shosaiko-to has also shown some promise for preventing liver cancer and liver fibrosis in people with liver cirrhosis or chronic hepatitis. However, the evidence remains marginal. For example, in a double-blind, placebo-controlled study, 260 people with cirrhosis were randomly assigned to take Shosaiko-to or placebo, along with conventional treatment. In five years of evaluation, people taking the herb appeared to be less likely to develop cancer or die, but the results just missed the ordinary cutoff for statistical significance. For the subgroup of participants without hepatitis B infection, the benefits were statistically significant at the usual cutoff point.

Irritable bowel syndrome. In a double-blind, placebo-controlled trial, 116 people with irritable bowel syndrome (IBS) were randomly assigned to receive individualized Chinese herbal formulations, a one-size-fits-all Chinese herbal formulation, or placebo. Treatment consisted of five capsules three times daily, taken for sixteen weeks. The results showed that both forms of active treatment were superior to placebo, significantly reducing IBS symptoms. However, the individualized treatment was no more effective than the generic treatment. Similar results also were seen in another study.

Constipation. The Kampo formula known as Daio-kanzo-to is a mixture of rhubarb and licorice. In a two-week, double-blind, placebo-controlled trial, 132 people with constipation were randomly assigned to one of three groups: placebo, low-dose Daio-kanzo-to, or high-dose Daio-kanzo-to. The results indicate that the higher-dose group, but not the lower-dose group, experienced statistically significant improvements in constipation compared with placebo.

Allergies. In a double-blind, placebo-controlled trial, 220 people with allergic rhinitis were given either placebo or the Kampo remedy Sho-seiryu-to for two weeks. The results showed that the use of the herbal formula significantly relieved all major symptoms of allergic rhinitis compared with placebo. Based on this and other more preliminary studies, Sho-seiryu-to has been approved by the Japanese health ministry for the treatment of allergic rhinitis and allergic conjunctivitis.

Another combination herbal therapy has shown promise for allergic rhinitis. In a twelve-week, double-blind, placebo-controlled trial, fifty-eight people with allergic rhinitis were given either placebo or an eleven-herb combination remedy called Biminne. This combination therapy contains the following herbs: *Rehmannia glutinosa, Scutellaria baicalensis, Polygonatum sibiricum, Ginkgo biloba, Epimedium sagittatum, Psoralea corylifolia, Schisandra chinensis, Prunus mume, Ledebouriella divaricata, Angelica dahurica,* and *Astragalus membranaceus.*

The use of Biminne produced significant improvements in some symptoms of allergic rhinitis, while other symptoms showed a trend toward improvement that was not statistically significant. A follow-up evaluation suggested that the results persisted for one year after treatment was stopped.

Benefits also have been seen in small studies of other formulations. However, one study failed to find that the use of herbal treatments augmented the effectiveness of acupuncture for allergic rhinitis.

Osteoarthritis. A double-blind, placebo-controlled study of ninety-six people with osteoarthritis of the knee tested the effectiveness of a mixture of three Chinese herbs (*Clematis mandshurica, Trichosanthes kirilowii,* and *Prunella vulgaris*). Participants were randomly assigned to a placebo group or one of three other groups: given either 200 milligrams (mg), 400 mg, or 600 mg of the herbal formula three times daily. After four weeks of treatment, significant improvement in arthritis symptoms was seen in all three treatment groups compared with placebo. No dose appeared conclusively superior to the others.

Muscle spasms. The Kampo remedy Shakuyaku-kanzo-to is a combination of peony root and licorice, commonly used for the treatment of muscle spasms in general. In a double-blind, placebo-controlled study, 101 people with liver cirrhosis who also suffered from severe muscular spasms at least twice per week were given either Shakuyaku-kanzo-to or placebo three times daily for two weeks. (The herb combination is not specifically aimed at liver cirrhosis. However, people with liver cirrhosis often have muscle spasms, so it made sense to try an anti-muscle-spasm formula.) The results showed significant reduction in frequency and severity of spasms among the participants using the herb, compared with those taking placebo. However, some participants using the herb developed edema (swelling caused by excess fluid) and weight gain. Researchers attributed this side effect to the licorice constituent.

Menstrual pain. In a double-blind trial of forty women with menstrual pain, the Kampo formula Toki-shakuyaku-san was compared with placebo with good results. The design of this study was interesting because researchers preselected women who, according to the principles of TCM, would be expected to respond to this Kampo treatment. Through six menstrual cycles, women using the real herbal formula experienced significantly less menstrual pain compared with those in the placebo group. Benefits took three menstrual cycles to develop.

In a 2008 review of thirty-nine randomized controlled trials involving a total of 3,475 women, researchers concluded that the use of traditional Chinese herbs shows some promise in treating menstrual pain. However, firm conclusions were not possible because of the wide variability of study design and herbs used and because of the poor quality of many of the studies.

Diabetes. A double-blind study of more than two hundred people evaluated the effectiveness of Coptis formula (a traditional combination therapy) with or without the drug glibenclamide for the treatment of diabetes. Coptis formula appeared to significantly enhance the effectiveness of the drug; however, the herbs produced marginal benefits at best when taken alone.

Asthma. The Kampo remedy Saiboku-to has been approved by the Japanese health ministry for the treatment of asthma. However, meaningful supporting evidence appears to be limited to one small trial. In this double-blind, placebo-controlled, crossover study, thirty-three people with mild to moderate asthma received Saiboku-to or placebo three times daily for four weeks. Treatment with the herbal remedy improved symptoms of asthma to a greater extent than placebo. Additional measurements suggested that Saiboku-to works by reducing asthmatic inflammation (technically, eosinophilia). A Chinese study using a proprietary formulation also reported benefits.

Eczema. A Chinese herbal mixture sold under the name Zemaphyte has shown promise as a treatment for eczema. This formula, based on herbs traditionally used for skin conditions, contains the following: *Ledebouriella seseloides, Potentilla chinensis, Akebia clem-*

atidis, Rehmannia glutinosa, Paeonia lactiflora, Lophatherum gracile, Dictamnus dasycarpus, Tribulus terrestris, Glycyrrhiza uralensis, and *Schizonepeta tenuifolia.*

In paired double-blind, placebo-controlled trials carried out by one research group, Zemaphyte produced significantly better effects than placebo for both adults and children. Each study enrolled approximately forty people and used a crossover design in which all participants received the real treatment and placebo for eight weeks each. The use of the herb significantly reduced eczema symptoms compared with placebo. However, a subsequent study of similar design performed by a different research group failed to find significant benefit with Zemaphyte. The reason for this discrepancy is not clear. In a twelve-week, double-blind study, a different traditional Chinese herbal formula also failed to prove more effective than placebo for treatment of eczema.

Tension headache. A topical ointment known as Tiger Balm is a popular treatment for headaches and other conditions. Tiger Balm contains camphor, menthol, cajaput, and clove oil. A double-blind study enrolling fifty-seven people with acute tension headache compared the application of Tiger Balm to the forehead with placebo ointment and with the drug acetaminophen (Tylenol). The placebo ointment contained mint essence to make it smell similar to Tiger Balm. Real Tiger Balm proved more effective than placebo and just as effective as acetaminophen. It also acted more rapidly.

Human immunodeficiency virus infection. Chinese herbal therapies have been investigated for the treatment of human immunodeficiency virus (HIV) infection, but the results have not been very promising. In a twelve-week, double-blind, placebo-controlled trial, thirty persons with HIV who had CD4 counts of 200 to 500 were given a Chinese herbal formula containing thirty-one herbs. The results hint that the use of the herbal combination might have improved various symptoms compared with placebo, but none of the differences were statistically significant. Participants who believed they were taking the real treatment showed significant benefit regardless of whether they were in the placebo group or the real treatment group.

In another double-blind, placebo-controlled trial, sixty-eight persons with HIV were given either placebo or a preparation of thirty-five Chinese herbs for six months. The results indicate that the use of Chinese herbs did not improve symptoms or objective measurements of HIV severity. In fact, people using the herbs reported more digestive problems than those given placebo.

Prostate cancer. For several years, the Chinese herbal combination PC-SPES underwent significant investigation as a treatment for prostate cancer, with apparently impressive results. However, subsequent investigation revealed that PC-SPES contained undisclosed pharmaceutical ingredients (principally, a form of estrogen and the strong blood thinner Coumadin) and that these ingredients were probably responsible for its benefits. The treatment has since been withdrawn.

Other uses. A large double-blind study conducted in China reported that the use of the traditional remedy Xuezhikang by people with a previous history of a heart attack could reduce the risk that they would have a subsequent severe cardiovascular problem, such as a stroke or another heart attack. Chinese herbal medicine may also be helpful for people with angina. In a small, randomized trial of sixty-six adults with stable angina, Shenshao tablets (containing ginsenosides and white peony) reduced the frequency of angina attacks.

In a small, double-blind, placebo-controlled trial, the use of the herbal combination Banxia Houpo Tang (also called Hange Koboku-to or Magnolia and Pinelliae formula) was tested for the treatment of impaired cough reflex in people who had suffered a stroke. The results indicated that the herbal combination was more effective than placebo treatment for improving the coughing response.

In a review of twenty-one studies involving almost three thousand persons, researchers concluded that Chinese herbs were as effective as commonly prescribed medications for drug withdrawal symptoms in heroin addicts. They could not draw any conclusions, however, regarding what specific herbs were most beneficial.

Various Chinese herbal formulas have been evaluated for the treatment of respiratory infections. The results of published studies appear to indicate that these formulas are more effective than standard antibiotics, but the poor design of most of these trials precludes placing much faith in their outcomes. One combination therapy called Shuang Huang Lian has better supporting evidence than most.

A double-blind study performed in Hong Kong evaluated the potential benefits in cancer chemotherapy of personalized herbal formulas designed according to the principles of TCHM. In this study, 120 people undergoing chemotherapy for early-stage breast or colon cancer were given either a personalized formula or a placebo. Researchers evaluated numerous possible effects of the treatment but found benefits in only one: the reduction of nausea. Note that even this single result is less meaningful than it may seem; it is statistically questionable to use a multiplicity of outcome measures. A review of fifteen mostly poor-quality trials with 862 participants suggested that Chinese herbal medicine might improve quality of life in persons with non-small-cell lung cancer who are undergoing chemotherapy.

One study evaluated the effectiveness of an herbal combination containing herbs commonly used for the treatment of cough, but it failed to find the treatment effective. This study has been incorrectly reported as finding the tested treatment effective; indeed, the use of the treatment did help suppress coughing, but so did the placebo treatment, and there were no significant differences between the groups.

Numerous studies have evaluated TCHM for treatment of liver cancer with generally positive results. However, study design and reporting were markedly substandard.

A double-blind, placebo-controlled study of twenty-nine people with chronic fatigue syndrome found indications that the use of the Kampo remedy Hochu-ekki-to significantly improved symptoms compared with placebo. Also, the Kampo remedies Saiko-keishi-to and Shosaiko-to have been suggested for the treatment of epilepsy, but the supporting evidence is too preliminary to be relied upon. Both of these combination treatments consist of bupleurum, peony root, pinellia root, cassia bark, ginger root, jujube fruit, Asian ginseng root, Asian scullcap root, and licorice root, but the proportions are different.

Other traditional herbal combinations with some supporting evidence (often from studies of questionable quality) include Xiao-yao-san (Free and Easy Wanderer) for depression and bipolar syndrome, Mai-men-dong-tang for allergic asthma, Yi-Gan San for dementia, Bofu-tsusho-san for weight loss and diabetes, Chang Ji Tai for irritable bowel syndrome, Ondamtanggamibang (a Korean formulation) for reducing symptoms of stress, Qinzhu Liangxue for psoriasis, and red peony root for acute pancreatitis.

In one study, the herbal formula Duhuo Jisheng Wan, widely used for osteoarthritis, proved to be as effective as the standard anti-inflammatory drug diclofenac. However, the herb caused as many side effects as the drug, and it was slower to act. (It was so slow that its benefits could have been caused solely by the placebo effect.) This study did not use a placebo control group.

One double-blind, placebo-controlled study tested the remedy Hochu-ekki-to for enhancing immune response to influenza vaccine but failed to find benefit. One study quoted as showing that a Chinese herbal formula can reduce blood pressure actually failed to find any effect on blood pressure. A review of seventeen trials found that there is limited evidence to support the use of traditional Chinese herbal preparations for the common cold.

SCIENTIFIC EVIDENCE

To establish the effectiveness of a treatment, it must be put through a double-blind, placebo-controlled trial. However, there are a few issues that make it difficult to study TCHM in this way.

The first problem involves diagnosis. There is no such thing as a TCHM remedy for migraine headaches, for example. Each person with migraines receives individualized treatment. This introduces an extra problem for experimenters. The best way to address this issue is as follows. People are chosen to participate in a study based on a Western diagnosis. Next, all participants are diagnosed by a classic herbal practitioner and prescribed a formula specific to their individual constitutions according to the principles of TCHM. Finally, another party provides participants with either the real formula or a placebo formula, under conditions whereby neither practitioners nor participants know which is which.

Other studies utilize a fixed remedy for all participants, in hopes that it will still prove effective on average. Such an approach does not really test the effectiveness of true TCHM; rather, it tests a much-simplified form of it. Still, trials of this type are valid as far as they go.

Numerous other studies simply involve enrolling people with a certain condition and giving each participant an herbal remedy. Researchers then record the extent of improvement. Such "open-label" trials, however, prove virtually nothing because even phony treatments will appear to cause benefits.

Finally, many of these studies were performed in China. Research on Chinese medicine conducted in China generally falls far short of modern scientific standards of rigor.

CHOOSING A PRACTITIONER

There is no general certification for the practice of TCHM. Many people who are certified in acupuncture, however, also have significant training in herbal medicine. (In general, five hundred hours of specific training is considered necessary.) Some states offer the license of O.M.D. (doctor of Oriental medicine); licensed O.M.D.'s are generally well versed in TCHM.

SAFETY ISSUES

There are several serious safety concerns with the use of TCHM. One concern involves the use of multiple herbs typical in this approach. In general, conventional medicine makes a point of using as few medications as possible (in theory, at least) because the greater the number of medications, the greater the risk of harm. Also, when medications are used together and harm does result, it is difficult to know what drug was at fault. From this perspective, formulas consisting of five, ten, or thirty herbs are quite worrisome.

Such combinations are actually designed for the purpose of reducing risks. According to TCHM theory, the various herbs in a formula balance and moderate each other. This theory, however, has never been put to the test, and there are reasons not to trust it. Simply put, it is very difficult to get an accurate picture of the risks of a treatment if one does not keep systematic records of adverse effects; the ancient Chinese government had no such system in place. In any case, the individualized nature of treatment would make it almost impossible to track harm. Herbalists would be expected to notice immediate, dramatic reactions to herbal formulas, and one can assume with some confidence that treatments used for thousands of years are unlikely to cause such problems in very many people who take them.

However, certain types of harm could be expected to easily elude the detection of traditional herbalists. These include safety problems that are delayed, occur relatively rarely, or are difficult to detect without scientific instruments. How would a traditional herbalist ever know, for example, if a treatment caused liver failure in 1 of every 100,000 people who used it, especially if such failure took two or more years to develop? If such a death did occur in the herbalist's patient population, it would probably be attributed to hepatitis or some other common cause.

These factors may explain why Chinese herbal medicine traditionally uses treatments that are now recognized as potentially dangerous, such as mercury, arsenic, lead, licorice, coltsfoot, and *Aristolochia clematis*. Mercury, arsenic, and lead accumulate slowly in the body, and for many years their harm can only be detected by laboratory tests. Licorice (used in many herb formulas to "harmonize" the ingredients) can raise blood pressure and disturb blood chemistry. These effects were presumably undetectable to traditional practitioners unless the effects became quite severe. The herb *Aristolochia* can cause severe kidney damage and kidney cancer, but only rarely. Modern medical surveillance has uncovered quite a few such cases, but traditional herbology considered the herb worth using. *Aristolochia* contains aristolochic acid, a substance shown in animal studies to damage the kidney when taken in high enough doses. Chinese herbal products generally list *Aristolochia* on the label when it is present, but in some cases, *Aristolochia* was apparently added accidentally (it is similar in appearance to a much safer herb).

Coltsfoot (*Tussilago farfara*), used in Chinese cough syrups and other formulations, contains pyrrolizidine alkaloids, substances that can, over time, damage the liver. This also does not appear to have been noticed by traditional herbalists. Under modern conditions of medical surveillance, many incidents have been reported in which the use of Chinese herbs appears to have caused various forms of liver injury, including acute hepatitis, chronic hepatitis, hepatic fibrosis, and acute liver failure. Ancient herbal practitioners might not have been able to distinguish these herb-induced illnesses from the effects of infectious hepatitis, a widely prevalent condition, and thereby failed to make the connection. Even today, it appears that many cases of liver failure attributed to hepatitis have been caused by the Chinese herbs used to treat hepatitis. Other reported complications of Chinese herbal treatments include movement disorders and ovarian failure.

Another set of potential problems arises from Chinese herbal medicine not restricting itself to plant products with subtle effects. Many traditional Chinese herbal remedies are, simply put, poisons. When taken in proper doses, they may be safe for use, but dosage miscalculation or use in a particularly susceptible person may lead to serious consequences, including death. For example, in Hong Kong, poisoning caused by the herb aconite (used in numerous Chinese herbal formulas) was sufficiently widespread that public health authorities launched an information campaign to combat the problem.

Besides toxicity caused by Chinese herbs, other problems have been caused by adulteration of herbal products with unlisted ingredients. For example, the Chinese herbal formula PC-SPES, used for prostate cancer, turned out to contain three pharmaceutical drugs: diethylstilbestrol, warfarin (Coumadin), and indomethacin. This appears to have been an intentional adulteration designed somewhat along the lines of a traditional Chinese formula, with one pharmaceutical adulterant that treated prostate cancer balanced by two others to offset the side effects of the first. The combination is dangerous and has caused at least one case of severe bleeding.

In another episode, eight of eleven Chinese herbal creams sold in the United Kingdom for the treatment of eczema were found to contain strong pharmaceutical steroids. Other studies have also found steroids in eczema preparations. In addition, Chinese herbal weight-loss aids have been found to contain an unlisted chemical related to the appetite-suppressant drugs fenfluramine and phentermine (Fen-Phen).

Herbal products approved by the Japanese government have undergone meaningful safety testing and are unlikely to contain known toxins or unlisted drugs. However, this does not mean they are completely safe. For example, several case reports suggest that therapy for chronic hepatitis combining an approved herbal formula with the standard drug interferon can cause severe inflammation of the lungs. The herbal formulas Takeda Kampo Ichoyaku K-matsu, Taisho Kampo Ichoyaku, and Kanebo Kampo Ichoyaku Hused, all used to treat upset stomach, might reduce the effectiveness of the Parkinson's disease medication levodopa.

EBSCO CAM Review Board

FURTHER READING

Chen, S., et al. "Oral Chinese Herbal Medicine (CHM) as an Adjuvant Treatment During Chemotherapy for Non-Small Cell Lung Cancer." *Lung Cancer* 68 (2010): 137-145.

Ernst, E. "Adulteration of Chinese Herbal Medicines with Synthetic Drugs." *Journal of Internal Medicine* 252 (2002): 107-113.

Lee, M. S., et al. "Effects of a Korean Traditional Herbal Remedy on Psychoneuroendocrine Responses to Examination Stress in Medical Students." *Human Psychopharmacology* 19 (2004): 537-543.

Leung, W. K., et al. "Treatment of Diarrhea-Predominant Irritable Bowel Syndrome with Traditional Chinese Herbal Medicine." *American Journal of Gastroenterology* 101 (2006): 1574-1580.

Liu, T. T., et al. "A Meta-analysis of Chinese Herbal Medicine in Treatment of Managed Withdrawal from Heroin." *Cellular and Molecular Neurobiology* 29 (2009): 17-25.

Matkovic, Z., V. Zivkovic, and M. Korica. "Efficacy and Safety of *Astragalus membranaceus* in the Treatment of Patients with Seasonal Allergic Rhinitis." *Phytotherapy Research* 24 (2010): 175-181.

Mok, T., et al. "A Double-Blind Placebo-Controlled Randomized Study of Chinese Herbal Medicine as Complementary Therapy for Reduction of Chemotherapy-Induced Toxicity." *Annals of Oncology* 18 (2007): 768-774.

Wang, J., Q. Y. He, and Y. L. Zhang. "Effect of Shenshao Tablet on the Quality of Life for Coronary Heart Disease Patients with Stable Angina Pectoris." *Chinese Journal of Integrative Medicine* 15 (2009): 328-332.

Zhang, X., et al. "Chinese Medicinal Herbs for the Common Cold." *Cochrane Database of Systematic Reviews* (2007): CD004782. Available through *EBSCO DynaMed Systematic Literature Surveillance* at http://www.ebscohost.com/dynamed.

See also: Alternative versus traditional medicine; Ayurveda; Chinese medicine; Folk medicine; Herbal medicine; Home health; Naturopathy; Traditional healing.

Traditional healing

CATEGORY: Issues and overviews
RELATED TERMS: Curandero, energy healing, herbal medicine, holistic medicine, shamanism
DEFINITION: Holistic indigenous practices for the prevention of disease and illness and for health and healing.

OVERVIEW

Traditional healing methods are holistic because they focus on disease prevention and on healing the body, mind, and spirit. In contrast, modern Western medicine treats specific symptoms. Traditional healing methods are used worldwide and have several commonalities: They focus on using what is provided by nature to prevent and heal illness, they believe in the interconnectedness of all living (and sometimes nonliving) things, and they believe that the balance of a person's energy flow with that of the rest of the universe is crucial to maintaining health.

The use of herbal medicines, music, special diet, meditative states, and healing touch are common to many of the traditional healing practices around the world. While some of these practices have been maintained only in small native communities within their countries of origin, other practices remain in use as complementary and alternative healing practices in Western countries.

SHAMANISM

Shamanism is considered by Westerners to be an alternative and nontraditional means of practicing medicine; however, it is actually the most traditional form of health care in existence today. Shamanism is a spiritual practice that has existed for tens of thousands of years. Many cultures have abandoned their ancient shamanic practices as the biomedical model has become the gold standard in several areas of the world. Recently, though, there has been a resurgence of interest in the traditional shamanic rituals, treatments, and herbal remedies.

Shamans practice an ancient way of healing that includes using objects from nature and songs, chants, dance, drums and other musical instruments, special items of clothing, spirit guides, and sacred rituals. In comparison with biomedical physicians who attempt to cure a disease, shamans strive to heal the condition. Also, this healing practice is typically more community-centered than personal. Shamans are traditionally highly regarded members of the tribe because of their ability to heal. The effectiveness of shamanic practices is difficult to study without impacting the cultures one is researching. The communities believe that their techniques are effective, and some researchers who have tried shamanic treatments personally have found them to be beneficial. Researchers have expressed concern over the potential loss of shamanic and herbalist knowledge from these cultures.

TRADITIONAL CHINESE MEDICINE

Aspects of traditional Chinese medicine (TCM) date back five thousand years. Variations are practiced in South Korea, Japan, and Vietnam. The first known medical text in the world was reportedly written in China by Emperor Huang-Ti in 2697 B.C.E. and focused on the interaction of the "tiny" human being with the immense universe.

TCM does not differentiate between the mind and the body, as does Western medicine, and it includes spiritual and religious elements. Huang-Ti wrote about the principles of yin and yang, which have separate meanings but also are ever-present together. The yin represents blood, spirit, and specific organs such as the heart, liver, and lungs, while the yang represents qi (pronounced "chee") and organs such as the stomach, intestines, and bladder. A major belief of TCM is that illness results from disruption or blockage of qi, or vital energy, which flows with blood through a network of twelve primary channels called meridians. Blockages are treated with acupuncture, acupressure, manipulative massage, or herbal medicines. Acupuncture has been demonstrated to decrease inflammation. Research to determine the mechanism of this effect is ongoing.

Huang-Ti also wrote about preventive medicine, stating that disease could be avoided by proper diet, regular habits, a proper amount of work and rest, and keeping the mind at peace. Qigong (breath exercise training) and Tai Chi (a focus on breath and specific postures) are practiced for health and for the prevention of disease and are used in hospitals to increase the stamina of patients. For example, people being treated with chemotherapy were found to have fared better when also participating in qigong therapy. They are able to eat more and to better tolerate the side effects of chemotherapy, and they have an increased rate of remission. Daoism, which believes that each person should follow the path intended for him or her by the universe, was promoted by Lao Tzu in the sixth century B.C.E. According to Daoism, one's youthfulness and longevity depend on one's behavior toward Dao ("the way").

AYURVEDIC MEDICINE

Ayurveda ("the science of life") is a traditional system of medicine practiced in India, Bangladesh, Sri Lanka, Nepal, and Pakistan. As with other traditional healing practices, Ayurveda focuses on the interconnectedness between humans and everything else in the universe. A major belief of Ayurveda is that one will find health if balance with the universe is maintained, while illness results from imbalance. The human constitution (*prakriti*), or one's stable state of physical and psychological characteristics, is another important concept in Ayurvedic medicine. *Prakriti* influences a person's likelihood of becoming ill as a result of imbalance. Another major Ayurvedic concept is the life forces (*doshas*): *vata*, *pitta*, and *kapha*. A person may have a dominant type of life force, and imbalances in the life forces are thought to cause illness. Prevention and treatment are tailored to the person's constitution and *dosha*. Treatment methods include meditation, stretching and breathing exercises, massage, purging toxins through enema, and tonics of herbs, vitamins, and protein.

HERBAL MEDICINE

Plants or portions of plants (roots, stems, leaves, flowers, seeds) that have been used traditionally for long periods of time for healing and are generally regarded as safe are known as traditional herbal medicines. Shamans often use herbs in their ceremonies or prescribe them after a healing session. For example, a researcher in 2003 found that plants used by *curanderos* (shamans) in the highlands of Mexico for the treatment of "sweet blood," or diabetes, could be shown to successfully treat rats and humans with type 2 diabetes. The researcher used a water decoction, the same way the *curandero* would use it, except that the dose was adjusted for a person's weight.

Traditional herbal medicine generally involves maintaining the combination of ingredients within a plant or mixture of herbs. Drug manufacturers, however, attempt to harvest the plants to isolate the one or few compounds they believe are "active" in affecting illness. TCM, conversely, usually involves a specific combination of herbs to heal an illness, as Chinese medicine has shown that a blend of herbs offers an enhanced therapeutic effect and a wider range of actions on the patient. Ayurvedic medicine uses more than 600 herbal formulas and about 250 single-plant

The Intersections of Traditional and Western Healing

Presented here is an excerpt from the online version of the exhibition "Native Voices: Native Peoples' Concepts of Health and Illness" at the National Library of Medicine. The exhibition, which "explores the interconnectedness of wellness, illness, and cultural life for Native Americans, Alaska Natives, and Native Hawaiians," highlights traditional healing practices among the indigenous peoples of North America.

Today, Native people of all groups are often faced with the question of whether to rely on traditional Native healing methods or to seek Western medical treatment. Until relatively recently, the two traditions operated in parallel, with little intersection between them. Today, however, Native Americans can access a continuum of health care. Many traditional healers still practice independently within tribal communities. Other healers may work with Western-trained primary care physicians to coordinate care for Native American patients. Some health care institutions offer both traditional and Western medicine, often at the same location.

In most areas, Native Americans get traditional healing from within the local tribal community, rather than through tribal health clinics or hospitals. In the Dakota and Lakota, and Mandan, Hidatsa, and Arikara, (MHA) Tribes of the Upper Plains, tribal members arrange for services by contacting local healers directly. Some Western-trained physicians also refer patients to traditional healers, and will sometimes help coordinate both Western and traditional medicine for a specific patient. . . .

The Dr. Agnes Kalaniho'okaha Cope Native Hawaiian Traditional Healing Center, Waianae Coast Comprehensive Health Center, in Oahu, Hawaii, provides a range of traditional healing practices offered by master practitioners. A Council of Elders oversees the practices, which are located onsite alongside Western primary medical care and comprehensive health and wellness services.

All practices start with Pule and Oli (prayer and chant). The Native practices at the Traditional Healing Center include:

- Lomilomi, or Hawaiian massage
- La'au Lapa'au, healing with herbal medicine
- La'au Kahea, spiritual healing
- Pale Keiki, art of midwifery
- Ho'oponopono, family conflict resolution and counseling
- Pule, healing through prayer
- Haha, healing through diagnostic observation
- He Ike Papalua, extrasensory perception or second sight

The Southcentral Foundation in Anchorage, Alaska, has become a leader in providing traditional healing services that complement services provided by the major Western medicine center, the Alaska Native Medical Center. The Traditional Healing Clinic offers traditional healing practices to patients upon request or referral, in coordination with Western-trained providers. The clinic also offers a range of wellness, lifestyle, and trauma recovery programs for Alaska Natives. The Native practices at the Southcentral Foundation Traditional Healing Clinic include healing hands and healing touch, prayer, cleansing, song and dance, counseling, talking circles, and a medicinal garden.

medicines. The naturally occurring variability in active ingredients in these mixtures makes standardization more difficult when one is attempting to study them scientifically.

Some traditional herbal treatments have been shown effective and safe through controlled clinical trials. For example, ginger root helps in the treatment of nausea. Cases of illness and poisoning have been reported, however, because the wrong plant was used, because of contamination with heavy metals, or because of interactions with other medications or herbs. Precautions to be taken when selecting herbal supplements include being certain that the bottle has a seal on it that states the herb has been tested for heavy metals and other toxic contaminants; using caution when taking herbs with prescription and over-the-counter medications, as some can have dangerous interactions; and notifying one's medical practitioner about the use of herbs in conjunction with prescription or over-the-counter medications.

REIKI

Reiki is an ancient form of energy healing from Japan, believed to have been "lost" for thousands of years and rediscovered in the nineteenth century by Mikao Usui. Practitioners train and receive "attunements" to reach certain levels of ability, including levels one through three, advanced, and master. There are many schools of Reiki that vary in the methods used. Typically, however, the hands of the practitioner are placed on twelve specific areas of the body (the seven chakras), or from head to toe, and energy is delivered from the source through the practitioner to the client. This method of healing is becoming mainstream, as it is increasingly being offered in many Western hospitals. It is believed to be relatively harmless, and some studies have demonstrated the potential benefits, including decreases in heart rate, blood pressure, levels of depression, and pain. Hematocrit, hemoglobin, and glucose levels in the blood have also been shown to be affected by Reiki treatment. Distance Reiki is also practiced by those with higher levels of training; however, there has been little clinical research regarding this type of treatment.

CONCLUSIONS

Scientific evidence for these traditional healing practices is considered lacking in most areas because of poorly designed studies with small sample sizes and because of the issues associated with creating a control condition (particularly a placebo control) that meets Western scientific standards. For example, a placebo for acupuncture is impossible; however, one can study the impact of treatment versus nontreatment. Certain types of traditional healing have been shown to be beneficial and to cause no harm, while others, such as herbal medicines, should be used with caution because of interactions with drugs and because of the possibility that the herbal is contaminated with high levels of heavy metals.

Dawn M. Bielawski, Ph.D.

FURTHER READING

Anhauser, Marcus. "Pharmacists Seek the Solution of a Shaman." *Drug Discovery Today* 8 (2003): 868-869. This article describes the scientific study of plant medicines to treat diabetes.

Hammerschlag, Carl Allen. "The Huichol Offering: A Shamanic Healing Journey." *Journal of Religion and Health* 48 (2009): 246-258. The author, a psychiatrist who practices shamanism, describes the intersection of science and medicine in the Huichol culture in Central Mexico.

Hou, Joseph P., and Jin Youyu. *The Healing Power of Chinese Herbs and Medicinal Recipes.* Binghamton, N.Y.: Haworth Press, 2005. An overview of the history of Chinese medicine in general and herbal medicine in particular. Includes chapters on specific herbal treatments and the treatment of specific issues, featuring herbal remedies for specific issues such as pain and fever.

Hyman, Mark. A. "Notes from Nepal: Reflections of a Medical Student on Shamans, Lamas, Serpents, and Fortunes." *Alternative Therapies* 12 (2006): 10-18. Journal entries written by the author during a public health project in the 1980s make up this article, which focuses mainly on the Tibetan shamans he encountered.

Ingerman, S. Interview by B. Horrigan. "Medicine for the Earth, Medicine for People." *Alternative Therapies* 9 (2003): 77-84. An interview with Ingerman about her expertise on the topic of shamanism.

Kavoussi, Ben, and Ross, B. Evan. "The Neuroimmune Basis of Anti-inflammatory Acupuncture." *Integrative Cancer Therapies* 6 (2007): 251-257. This review article describes the literature on basic research into the effects of acupuncture on inflammation.

Lenaerts, Mark. "Substances, Relationships, and the Omnipresence of the Body: An Overview of Asheninka Ethnomedicine (Western Amazonia)." *Journal of Ethnobiology and Ethnomedicine* 2 (2006): 49-68. This ethnographic report focuses on plant medicine used along the border of Peru and Brazil, using data collected between 1997 and 2000.

Rittner, Sabine. "Sound-Trance-Healing: The Sound Pattern Medicine of the Shipibo in the Amazon Lowlands of Peru." *Music Therapy Today* 8 (2007): 196-235. This article discusses field research with the Shipibo tribe about its use of Ayahuasca, songs, and visual structures in healing practices.

Villoldo, Alberto. "Jaguar Medicine." *Alternative Therapies* 13 (2007): 14-16. The author details his experiences studying with shamans in South America, using direct observation and quotations from the indigenous peoples.

Vitale, Ann. "An Integrative Review of Reiki Touch Therapy Research." *Holistic Nursing Practice* 21 (2007): 167-179. This review article focuses on research studies of the effectiveness and potential for improvement of research on Reiki.

Vuckovic, Nancy H., et al. "Feasibility and Short-Term Outcomes of a Shamanic Treatment for Temporomandibular Joint Disorders." *Alternative Therapies* 13 (2007): 18-29. This article describes a clinical trial of shamanic healing for temporomandibular joint disorders, or TMJ.

See also: Alternative versus traditional medicine; Ayurveda; Chinese medicine; Folk medicine; Herbal medicine; Home health; Naturopathy; Traditional Chinese herbal medicine; Whole medicine.

Tramadol

Category: Drug interactions

Definition: A non-narcotic and non-anti-inflammatory analgesic medication used for the treatment of moderate pain.

Interactions: 5-HTP (5-hydroxytryptophan), St. John's wort, SAMe (S-adenosylmethionine)

Trade name: Ultram

St. John's Wort, 5-HTP, SAMe

Effect: Possible Dangerous Interactions

There have been some case reports possibly implicating tramadol in serotonin syndrome. This syndrome is caused by excessive levels of serotonin, which bring about various dangerous side effects.

Because St. John's wort and 5-HTP might increase serotonin levels, and because SAMe has reportedly caused serotonin syndrome, combining any of these substances with tramadol could be risky.

EBSCO CAM Review Board

Further Reading

Hernandez, A. F., et al. "Fatal Moclobemide Overdose or Death Caused by Serotonin Syndrome?" *Journal of Forensic Sciences* 40 (1995): 128-130.

Mason, B. J., and K. H. Blackburn. "Possible Serotonin Syndrome Associated with Tramadol and Sertraline Coadministration." *Annals of Pharmacotherapy* 31 (1997): 175-177.

See also: 5-Hydroxytryptophan; Food and Drug Administration; Nonsteroidal anti-inflammatory drugs (NSAIDs); Pain management; St. John's wort; SAMe (S-adenosylmethionine); Supplements: Introduction.

Transcendental Meditation

Category: Therapies and techniques

Related term: Mantra meditation

Definition: A technique for relaxing the mind and body through the repetition of a mantra, or a sound without meaning.

Principal proposed uses: Blood pressure, mental functioning, pain, psychosocial stress

Other proposed uses: Cardiovascular disease, carotid artery thickness, high cholesterol, insulin resistance

Overview

Transcendental Meditation (TM) has its origins in ancient Vedic tradition in India. The TM technique was revived by the Indian guru Maharishi Mahesh Yogi and has been taught since 1958. It became widely popular in the 1960s and now claims to have millions of practitioners. The technique involves fifteen to twenty minutes of quiet meditation in the morning and evening. A mantra (a sound without meaning) is used as a form of thought during the sessions.

Mechanism of Action

During TM, the mind lets go of stimuli and concentration that otherwise keep it in an agitated state. The mind enters a state of restful awareness, and the body becomes completely relaxed. The mind is then considered to be in a transcendent state beyond the normal waking, dreaming, or sleep states. The transcendent state is believed to restore normal functioning of various systems in the body, particularly those systems involved in adapting to environmental stresses. All of the benefits deriving from TM can be attributed to the relaxed nonstressful state.

Uses and Applications

Proponents of TM claim that the program can benefit anyone who wants to achieve a better quality of life by reducing stress and increasing mental alertness and memory. All the secondary benefits from the use of TM can be attributed to a reduction in stress, including lowered blood pressure, reduced metabolic disease, and reduced cardiovascular disease.

SCIENTIFIC EVIDENCE

To perform a meta-analysis, data from many trials are combined for an overall statistical analysis. This procedure is thought to add strength to research findings. The value of a meta-analysis is only as strong as the quality of the component research trials.

A 2004 review article summarized controlled research studies on the effect of TM on risk factors related to cardiovascular disease. (It should be noted that most of the review articles consulted include a minimum of one author from the Institute for Natural Medicine and Prevention, Maharishi University of Management.) Several studies showed a reduction in blood pressure in both genders and in persons at high and low risk for hypertension. Two studies showed that TM reduced carotid artery thickness, a marker of atherosclerosis. Two other studies, involving elderly persons, showed a significant reduction in all-cause mortality in the groups practicing TM.

A 2002 review paper described studies on the effect of TM to change psychological or physiological indicators or consequences of stress. Several meta-analyses showed that TM significantly reduced anxiety or other negative psychological outcomes. Several studies showed TM decreased high blood pressure, compared with controls. Other studies showed TM reduced carotid artery thickness and exercise-induced ischemia, measures of cardiovascular disease.

An interesting study related TM to brain reactivity to pain. Practitioners of TM and healthy matched controls were subjected to thermally induced pain. The results indicated that TM practitioners experienced as much pain as the controls, but they were less affected by it. This was in spite of the fact that the TM mediators' brains showed a greater response to pain (reduced blood flow through certain regions).

Metabolic syndrome can be a condition of obese people, and it is thought to be a contributor to coronary heart disease. A sixteen-week study was conducted to evaluate the effect of TM on components of the syndrome. The results found that the group practicing TM, compared with the group receiving health education, showed significant reductions in blood pressure and insulin resistance and had a positive influence on cardiac autonomic tone as measured by heart rate variability.

Patient data were pooled from two studies originally designed to study the effects of TM on blood pressure. Statistical analysis of the combined data showed that the TM groups had a 23 percent decrease in all-cause mortality, compared with control groups receiving other meditation methods or no treatments. Furthermore, the TM groups showed a 30 percent decrease in cardiovascular mortality.

A 2007 review revisited previous studies and meta-analyses of the effect of relaxation techniques on reduction of high blood pressure. The authors identified 107 reports and applied rigorous criteria for selection of studies for reevaluation. Seventeen studies were selected and compiled into groups according to relaxation technique. These techniques included simple or relaxation-assisted biofeedback, progressive muscle relaxation, TM, and stress management with relaxation. Meta-analysis showed that only the TM group showed significant reductions in blood pressure.

CHOOSING A PRACTITIONER

Transcendental Meditation and TM are service marks registered in the U.S. Patent and Trademark Office, licensed to Maharishi Vedic Education Development Corporation. Only teachers certified by the foundation are permitted to teach the TM technique. The fee for the six-step process is high, but other techniques based on mantra meditation, such as primordial sound meditation and natural stress relief, are available at more accessible prices. The effectiveness of these other mantra meditation methods apparently has not been studied in randomized trials.

SAFETY ISSUES

There are no known safety risks with the use of TM, especially when taught by certified teachers.

David A. Olle, M.S.

FURTHER READING

Orme-Johnson, D., et al. "Neuroimaging of Meditation's Effect on Brain Reactivity." *NeuroReport* 17, no. 12 (2006): 1359-1363.

Paul-Labrador, M., et al. "Effects of a Randomized Controlled Trial of Transcendental Meditation on Components of the Metabolic Syndrome in Subjects with Coronary Artery Disease." *Archives of Internal Medicine* (2006): 1218-1224.

Rainforth, M., et al. "Stress Reduction Programs in

Patients with Elevated Blood Pressure." *Current Hypertension Report* 9, no. 6 (2007): 520-528.
Transcendental Meditation Program. http://www.tm.org.

See also: Atherosclerosis and heart disease prevention; Autogenic training; Cholesterol, high; Congestive heart failure; Diabetes; Hypnotherapy; Maharishi Mahesh Yogi; Meditation; Mind/body medicine; Pain management; Relaxation therapies; Stress.

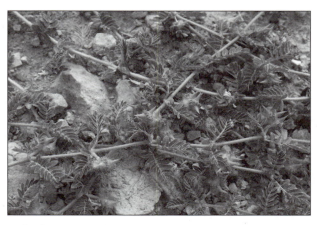

Tribulus terrestris has a long history of medicinal use in China, India, and Greece. (Nature's Images/Photo Researchers, Inc.)

Tribulus terrestris

CATEGORY: Herbs and supplements
RELATED TERM: Puncture vine
DEFINITION: Natural plant product used to treat specific health conditions.
PRINCIPAL PROPOSED USE: Sports performance enhancement
OTHER PROPOSED USES: Infertility in men and women, menopausal symptoms, sexual dysfunction in men and women

OVERVIEW

Tribulus terrestris (commonly known as puncture vine, the bane of bicycles in areas where it grows) has a long history of traditional medical use in China, India, and Greece. It was recommended as a treatment for female infertility, impotence, and low libido in both men and women, and to aid rejuvenation after long illness. The herb became widely known in the West when medal-winning Bulgarian Olympic athletes claimed that use of tribulus had contributed to their success. However, current evidence suggests that it does not enhance sports performance.

THERAPEUTIC DOSAGES

Tribulus terrestris is usually taken at a dose ranging from about 85 to 250 mg three times daily with meals. Some tribulus products are standardized to provide 40 percent furostanol saponins and taken at a dose providing 115 mg of saponins two to three times daily.

THERAPEUTIC USES

Studies performed in Bulgaria are the primary source of most current health claims regarding tribulus. According to this research, tribulus increases levels of various hormones in the steroid family, including testosterone, dehydroepiandrosterone (DHEA), and estrogen, and for this reason improves sports performance, fertility in men and women, sexual function in men and women, and symptoms of menopause, such as hot flashes. However, the design of these studies appears to fall far short of modern scientific standards, and there has not been any trustworthy scientific confirmation of these supposed benefits. One well-designed study failed to find that tribulus affects male sex hormone levels in young men.

Other studies that are far too preliminary to prove anything at all are quoted as proving that tribulus is helpful for the treatment of angina, high cholesterol, diabetes, and muscle spasms and for the prevention of kidney stones.

A properly designed, though small, human study compared the effects of tribulus (3.21 milligrams [mg] per kilogram of body weight–for example, 292 mg daily for a two-hundred-pound man) against placebo on body composition and endurance among fifteen men engaged in resistance training. At the end of the eight-week study, the only significant difference between the treatment and placebo groups was that the placebo group showed greater gains in endurance.

Another double-blind, placebo-controlled study enrolled twenty-two athletes and followed them for five weeks. The dose used in this trial was fixed at 450 mg daily for all participants. No benefits were seen.

SAFETY ISSUES

No significant adverse effects have been noted in any of the clinical trials or human research studies of tribulus. Animal studies performed in Bulgaria are said to have found the herb safe in both the short and the long terms. However, it is not clear whether these studies were performed in such a way that their conclusions can be trusted.

Women who are pregnant or nursing should not use any tribulus product. If the herb works as described, it might alter hormones in unsafe ways.

EBSCO CAM Review Board

FURTHER READING

Adimoelja, A. "Phytochemicals and the Breakthrough of Traditional Herbs in the Management of Sexual Dysfunctions." *International Journal of Andrology* 23 (2000): 82-84.

Antonio, J., et al. "The Effects of *Tribulus terrestris* on Body Composition and Exercise Performance in Resistance-Trained Males." *International Journal of Sport Nutrition and Exercise Metabolism* 10 (2000): 208-215.

Neychev, V. K., and V. I. Mitev. "The Aphrodisiac Herb *Tribulus terrestris* Does Not Influence the Androgen Production in Young Men." *Journal of Ethnopharmacology* 101, nos. 1-3 (2005): 319-323.

Rogerson, S., et al. "The Effect of Five Weeks of *Tribulus terrestris* Supplementation on Muscle Strength and Body Composition During Preseason Training in Elite Rugby League Players." *Journal of Strength and Conditioning Research* 21 (2007): 348-353.

See also: Infertility, men; Infertility, women; Sexual dysfunction in men; Sexual dysfunction in women; Sports and fitness support: Enhancing performance.

Tricyclic antidepressants

CATEGORY: Drug interactions
DEFINITION: Antidepressant medications mostly superseded by serotonin reuptake inhibitors.
INTERACTIONS: Coenzyme Q_{10}, 5-hydroxytryptophan (5-HTP), S-adenosylmethionine (SAMe), St. John's wort, yohimbe
DRUGS IN THIS FAMILY: Amitriptyline hydrochloride (Elavil), amoxapine (Asendin), clomipramine hydrochloride (Anafranil), desipramine hydrochloride (Norpramin), doxepin hydrochloride (Sinequan), imipramine (Tofranil), nortriptyline hydrochloride (Aventyl, Pamelor), protriptyline hydrochloride (Vivactil), trimipramine maleate (Surmontil)

COENZYME Q_{10} (CoQ_{10})

Effect: Supplementation Possibly Helpful

Preliminary evidence suggests that tricyclic antidepressants might deplete the body of CoQ_{10}, a substance that appears to be important for normal heart function. Based on this observation, it has been suggested (but not proved) that CoQ_{10} supplementation might help prevent the heart-related side effects that can occur with the use of tricyclic antidepressants.

ST. JOHN'S WORT, YOHIMBE, 5-HYDROXYTRYPTOPHAN (5-HTP), S-ADENOSYLMETHIONINE (SAMe)

Effect: Possible Dangerous Interactions

Based on one case report and general knowledge about the actions of these supplements, taking any of these in combination with some tricyclic antidepressants could present a risk of elevating serotonin levels too high.

ST. JOHN'S WORT

Effect: Possible Harmful Interaction

St. John's wort might decrease the effectiveness of tricyclic antidepressants by reducing blood levels of the drug. Conversely, if one is taking St. John's wort already and one's physician adjusts one's dose of medication, suddenly stopping the herb could cause blood levels of the drug to rise dangerously high.

EBSCO CAM Review Board

FURTHER READING

Iruela, L. M., et al. "Toxic Interaction of S-Adenosylmethionine and Clomipramine." *American Journal of Psychiatry* 150 (1993): 522.

Johne, A., et al. "Decreased Plasma Levels of Amitriptyline and Its Metabolites on Comedication with an Extract from St. John's Wort (Hypericum perforatum)." *Journal of Clinical Psychopharmacology* 22 (2002): 46-54.

Roots, J., et al. "Interaction of a Herbal Extract from St. John's Wort with Amitryptyline and Its Metabolites." *Clinical Pharmacology and Therapeutics* 67 (2000): 159.

See also: Food and Drug Administration; Supplements: Introduction.

Triglycerides, high

CATEGORY: Condition

RELATED TERMS: Hyperlipidemia, hypertriglyceridemia, pancreatitis, xanthomas

DEFINITION: Treatment for abnormally elevated levels of a fat-related substance that contributes to heart disease.

PRINCIPAL PROPOSED NATURAL TREATMENTS: Fish oil, niacin

OTHER PROPOSED NATURAL TREATMENTS: *Achillea wilhelmsii*, chromium, creatine, fenugreek, flax oil, pantethine, soy, vitamins C and E combined, walnut oil

INTRODUCTION

Triglycerides belong to a group of fat-related substances called lipids. An increase in levels of certain lipids (a condition called hyperlipidemia) contributes to heart disease.

To test for hyperlipidemia, physicians rely on blood tests called lipid profiles that measure triglycerides and two types of the lipid cholesterol: low-density lipoprotein (LDL) or bad cholesterol, and high-density lipoprotein (HDL) or good cholesterol. In many people with hyperlipidemia, elevation of LDL predominates. Drugs in the statin family work particularly well at treating this form of hyperlipidemia.

In some people with hyperlipidemia, however, high triglyceride levels are the primary problem. These persons are just as much at risk for heart disease as persons with elevated LDL cholesterol. Furthermore, if triglyceride levels get high enough, the pancreas may become inflamed, causing a dangerous condition called pancreatitis. Skin lesions called xanthomas also may occur.

Common causes of elevated triglyceride levels include genetic predisposition, diabetes, excessive alcohol intake, and various medications, including estrogen, tamoxifen, glucocorticoids, thiazide diuretics, and some beta-blockers. People with high triglycerides, or hypertriglyceridemia, do not respond well to statin drugs. Instead, they may need to use high-dose niacin or drugs in the fibrate family. Exercise (with or without weight loss) may also lower triglycerides. Diet, except when weight loss occurs, may not help, as a low-fat, high-carbohydrate diet can actually raise triglyceride levels.

PRINCIPAL PROPOSED NATURAL TREATMENTS

Fish oil. Fish oil has shown distinct promise for treating hypertriglyceridemia. More than two thousand people have participated in well-designed studies of fish oil for reducing triglyceride levels. Most studies ran from about seven to ten weeks.

It appears that fish oil supplements can reduce triglycerides by about 25 to 30 percent. Although not all studies have been positive, in a detailed review of forty-seven randomized trials, researchers concluded that fish oil is capable of significantly reducing triglyceride levels with no change in total cholesterol levels and only slight increases in HDL cholesterol

---

Dietary Fats, Omega-3, and Heart Disease

A 2004–2005 survey by the U.S. Food and Drug Administration found a wide range of consumer knowledge about the links between dietary fat intake and heart disease and between omega-3 supplements and heart disease. The survey results are excerpted here.

- More consumers know the linkage between saturated fat and heart disease than [know the linkage between] trans fat or omega-3 fatty acid and heart disease.
- Among the consumers who have heard of saturated fat, 78 percent say the fat raises the risk of heart disease, 1 percent say it lowers the risk, 1 percent say it has no effect on the risk, and 19 percent say they do not know.
- Among the consumers who have heard of trans fat or trans fatty acid, 48 percent say the fat raises the risk of heart disease, 5 percent say it lowers the risk, 4 percent say it has no effect on the risk, and 43 percent say they do not know.
- Regarding omega-3 fatty acid, 31 percent of consumers are correct about its relationship with the risk of heart disease, 6 percent have heard of it but are wrong about the relationship, 24 percent have heard of it but have no idea about the relationship, and 39 percent have never heard of the fat.

and LDL cholesterol. However, it should be noted that in some studies, the use of fish oil has markedly raised LDL cholesterol, which might offset some of the benefit.

Fish oil has been studied for reducing triglyceride levels specifically in people with diabetes, and it appears to do so safely and effectively. Furthermore, in people using statin drugs to control lipid levels, the addition of fish oil or its isolated component docosahexaenoic acid (DHA) appears to improve results.

Fish oil is a source of omega-3 fatty acids, healthy fats that the body needs as much as it needs vitamins. The most important omega-3 fatty acids found in fish oil are EPA (eicosapentaenoic acid) and DHA. According to some studies, EPA may be more important than DHA for reducing triglyceride levels.

In addition, a slightly modified form of fish oil (ethyl-omega-3 fatty acids) has been approved by the U.S. Food and Drug Administration (FDA) as a treatment for hypertriglyceridemia. This specially processed product, sold under the trade name Omacor, is widely advertised as more effective than ordinary fish oil. However, it should be noted that Omacor has undergone relatively little study itself; the prescribing information notes only two small trials to support its effectiveness for this use. This is far less evidence than is usually required for drug approval, and it is also substantially less than the body of evidence supporting standard fish oil as a treatment for hypertriglyceridemia.

OTHER PROPOSED NATURAL TREATMENTS

Numerous studies indicate that soy can reduce total and LDL cholesterol, especially when it replaces animal protein in the diet, and on this basis it has been approved for a "heart healthy" label by the FDA. Soy also appears to modestly improve triglyceride levels.

The supplement pantethine is widely promoted as a natural treatment for hypertriglyceridemia. However, the evidence that it works rests on small studies with somewhat inconsistent results.

In people with type 2 diabetes, the use of chromium may reduce triglyceride levels, according to some preliminary trials. However, chromium does not appear to be effective for reducing triglyceride levels in people without diabetes.

Other herbs and supplements that have shown promise for reducing triglyceride levels include fenugreek, creatine, and *Achillea wilhelmsii.*

The drug tamoxifen has a tendency to raise triglyceride levels. In an open study, the simultaneous use of vitamin C (500 milligrams [mg] daily) and vitamin E (400 mg daily) counteracted this side effect.

The supplement flax oil contains omega-3 fatty acids similar but not identical to those found in fish oil. It has been proposed as an alternative to fish oil because it does not cause fishy-smelling and fishy-tasting burps. However, evidence suggests that flax oil is not as effective as fish oil for reducing triglycerides.

Walnut oil has shown some promise for reducing triglycerides. Most natural treatments used to reduce cholesterol have the potential to also reduce triglyceride levels.

EBSCO CAM Review Board

FURTHER READING

Durrington, P. N., et al. "An Omega-3 Polyunsaturated Fatty Acid Concentrate Administered for One Year Decreased Triglycerides in Simvastatin Treated Patients with Coronary Heart Disease and Persisting Hypertriglyceridaemia." *Heart* 85 (2001): 544-548.

Eslick, G. D., et al. "Benefits of Fish Oil Supplementation in Hyperlipidemia." *International Journal of Cardiology* 136 (2009): 4-16.

Gupta, A., R. Gupta, and B. Lal. "Effect of *Trigonella foenum-graecum* (Fenugreek) Seeds on Glycaemic Control and Insulin Resistance in Type 2 Diabetes Mellitus." *Journal of the Association of Physicians of India* 49 (2001): 1057-1061.

McKenney, J. M., and D. Sica. "Prescription Omega-3 Fatty Acids for the Treatment of Hypertriglyceridemia." *American Journal of Health-System Pharmacy* 64 (2007): 595-605.

Meyer, B. J., et al. "Dose-Dependent Effects of Docosahexaenoic Acid Supplementation on Blood Lipids in Statin-Treated Hyperlipidaemic Subjects." *Lipids* 42 (2007): 109-115.

Schwellenbach, L. J., et al. "The Triglyceride-Lowering Effects of a Modest Dose of Docosahexaenoic Acid Alone Versus in Combination with Low-Dose Eicosapentaenoic Acid in Patients with Coronary Artery Disease and Elevated Triglycerides." *Journal of the American College of Nutrition* 25 (2006): 480-485.

Zibaeenezhad, M. J., et al. "Antihypertriglyceridemic Effect of Walnut Oil." *Angiology* 54 (2003): 411-414.

See also: Atherosclerosis and heart disease prevention; Cholesterol, high; Exercise; Fish oil; Flaxseed; Flaxseed oil; Gallstones; Heart attack; Hypertension; Pancreatitis.

Trimethoprim/sulfamethoxazole

RELATED NAME: TMP-SMZ
CATEGORY: Drug interactions
DEFINITION: An antibiotic combination that provides extra strength in fighting bacteria.
INTERACTIONS: Folate, PABA (para-aminobenzoic acid), potassium, St. John's wort and other herbs, white willow
TRADE NAMES: Bactrim, Cotrim, Septra, Sulfatrim

FOLATE
Effect: Supplementation Likely Helpful

Both trimethoprim and sulfamethoxazole interfere with folate: The sulfamethoxazole makes it hard for invading bacteria to manufacture folate, and the trimethoprim makes it hard for bacteria to use the folate. The net effect is to starve the bacteria of this necessary vitamin.

Humans and other mammals are much less affected by these antibiotics than are bacteria, because of the different way humans process folate. However, trimethoprim can still interfere to some extent with the body's ability to utilize this essential nutrient. Folate supplementation may be helpful if one takes this antibiotic for a long period of time (to prevent urinary tract infections, for example).

PABA (PARA-AMINOBENZOIC ACID)
Effect: Interference with Action of Drug

The supplement PABA may make trimethoprim/sulfamethoxazole less effective. Persons being treated with this drug should not take PABA except on medical advice.

POTASSIUM
Effect: Possible Harmful Interaction

Trimethoprim/sulfamethoxazole might increase levels of potassium in the body. Therefore, persons on long-term treatment with this antibiotic should not take potassium supplements except on the advice of a physician.

WHITE WILLOW
Effect: Possible Negative Interaction

The herb white willow contains substances very similar to aspirin. On this basis, one should not combine white willow with trimethoprim or sulfamethoxazole.

ST. JOHN'S WORT AND OTHER HERBS
Effect: Potential Increased Risk of Photosensitivity

Sulfa drugs can cause increased sensitivity to the sun. Various herbs, including St. John's wort and dong quai, can also cause this problem. Combined treatment with herb and drug might increase the risk further.

EBSCO CAM Review Board

FURTHER READING
Alappan, R., M. A. Perazella, and G. K. Buller. "Hyperkalemia in Hospitalized Patients Treated with Trimethoprim-Sulfamethoxazole." *Annals of Internal Medicine* 124 (1996): 316-320.
Vinnicombe, H. G., and J. P. Derrick. "Dihydropteroate Synthase from *Streptococcus pneumoniae*: Characterization of Substrate Binding Order and Sulfonamide Inhibition." *Biochemical and Biophysical Research Communications* 258 (1999): 752-757.

See also: Antibiotics, general; Folate; Food and Drug Administration; Herbal medicine; Potassium; St. John's wort; Supplements: Introduction; White willow.

Trimethylglycine

CATEGORY: Herbs and supplements
RELATED TERM: Betaine
DEFINITION: Natural substance of the human body used as a supplement to treat specific health conditions.
PRINCIPAL PROPOSED USE: High homocysteine levels
OTHER PROPOSED USES: Alcoholic liver disease, enhancing sports performance, nonalcoholic steatosis, substitute for S-adenosylmethionine (SAMe)

OVERVIEW

Trimethylglycine (TMG), also called betaine, is a substance manufactured by the body. It helps break down another naturally occurring substance called homocysteine.

In certain rare genetic conditions, the body cannot dispose of homocysteine, resulting in its accumulation to extremely high levels. This, in turn, leads to accelerated cardiovascular disease and other problems. Oral TMG is a treatment approved by the U.S. Food and Drug Administration (FDA) for this condition. It "methylates" homocysteine, removing it from circulation.

Meaningful, but not altogether consistent, evidence suggests that the relatively slight elevation of homocysteine that can occur in healthy people is also harmful. On this basis, it has been suggested that TMG might also reduce heart disease risk in healthy people. However, this has not been proven, and TMG has shown the potential for having adverse effects on cholesterol profile, which could counter any possible benefit from removing homocysteine. TMG is similar chemically to betaine hydrochloride, but it has entirely different actions.

REQUIREMENTS AND SOURCES

TMG is not required in the diet because the body can manufacture it from other nutrients. Grains, nuts, seeds, and meats contain small amounts of TMG. However, most TMG in food is destroyed during cooking or processing, so food is not a reliable way to get a therapeutic dosage.

After TMG has done its work on homocysteine, it is turned into another substance, dimethylglycine (DMG). Some manufacturers maintain that DMG is identical to TMG, but this is not true. DMG is not a methylating agent, so it cannot have any effect on homocysteine.

THERAPEUTIC DOSAGES

Optimal therapeutic dosages of TMG are not known. Common recommendations range from 375 to 3,000 milligrams daily.

THERAPEUTIC USES

There is no doubt that TMG greatly reduces homocysteine levels and improves health among people with the rare disease cystathionine beta-synthase deficiency, as well as related conditions. TMG also appears to reduce relatively mild homocysteine elevations in people without genetic defects. However, TMG also seems to worsen cholesterol profile, and this may counteract any possible benefits. For this reason, it may make more sense for people with elevated levels of homocysteine to reduce it by taking supplemental folate, vitamin B_6, and vitamin B_{12}; these supplements are known to reduce homocysteine levels, and unlike TMG, they also provide nutritional benefit.

TMG may help protect the liver against the effects of alcohol, perhaps by stimulating the formation of S-adenosylmethionine (SAMe). In addition, it may be helpful for nonalcoholic forms of fatty liver (nonalcoholic steatosis).

TMG has also been suggested as a less expensive substitute for SAMe in other conditions for which SAMe is used, such as osteoarthritis and depression. However, there is no evidence to show that it is effective.

A substance labeled pangamic acid or vitamin B_{15} has been extensively used as a performance enhancer by Russian athletes and has also become popular among American athletes. However, it is not clear that there really is any such substance; or, to state it another way, various substances have at various times been given that name. Most recently, the term has been associated with a mixture of calcium gluconate and DMG; one small study failed to find this form of pangamic acid effective for enhancing sports performance.

SAFETY ISSUES

The only known safety issue with TMG is regarding cholesterol profile. People with high or borderline-high cholesterol should use TMG only with caution. Maximum safe dosages for young children, pregnant or nursing mothers, and those with severe liver or kidney disease have not been established.

EBSCO CAM Review Board

FURTHER READING

Abdelmalek, M. F., et al. "Betaine, a Promising New Agent for Patients with Nonalcoholic Steatohepatitis." *American Journal of Gastroenterology* 96 (2001): 2711-2717.

Angulo, P., and K. D. Lindor. "Treatment of Nonalcoholic Fatty Liver: Present and Emerging Therapies." *Seminars in Liver Disease* 21 (2001): 81-188.

Kanbak, G., M. Inal, and C. Baycu. "Ethanol-Induced Hepatotoxicity and Protective Effect of Betaine." *Cell Biochemistry and Function* 19 (2001): 281-285.

Mangoni A. A., and S. H. Jackson. "Homocysteine and Cardiovascular Disease: Current Evidence and Future Prospects." *American Journal of Medicine* 112 (2002): 556-565.

Olthof, M. R., et al. "Effect of Homocysteine-Lowering Nutrients on Blood Lipids." *PLoS Medicine* 2, no. 5 (2005): e135.

_____. "Low Dose Betaine Supplementation Leads to Immediate and Long Term Lowering of Plasma Homocysteine in Healthy Men and Women." *Journal of Nutrition* 133 (2003): 4135-4138.

Schwab, U., et al. "Orally Administered Betaine Has an Acute and Dose-Dependent Effect on Serum Betaine and Plasma Homocysteine Concentrations in Healthy Humans." *Journal of Nutrition* 136 (2005): 34-38.

See also: Homocysteine, high; Liver disease; SAMe.

Tripterygium wilfordii

CATEGORY: Herbs and supplements
RELATED TERMS: Lei gong teng, thundergod vine
DEFINITION: Natural plant product used to treat specific health conditions.
PRINCIPAL PROPOSED USE: Rheumatoid arthritis
OTHER PROPOSED USES: Lupus, male contraceptive

OVERVIEW

Tripterygium wilfordii is a climbing vine with a long history of use in traditional Chinese herbal medicine. It is used in mixtures intended for the treatment of arthritis, muscle injury, skin diseases, and other problems. The roots, leaves, and flowers are the parts used medicinally.

Tripterygium is thought to be toxic or even fatal if taken to excess. Extracts made with ethyl acetate or chorloroform-methanol came into use in China in the 1970s and were said to be less toxic. However, the safety of these extracts has not been conclusively established, and experts recommend against using tripterygium except in the context of a scientific trial.

THERAPEUTIC DOSAGES

At present, experts recommend that tripterygium be used only in the context of a scientific trial.

THERAPEUTIC USES

In animal, test-tube, and preliminary human trials, tripterygium has shown immunosuppressive and anti-inflammatory affects. Because drugs with these properties are useful for conditions in which the immune system is overactive, such as rheumatoid arthritis and lupus, tripterygium has been proposed for similar use. However, there is only minimal evidence that it is effective.

One double-blind, placebo-controlled study performed in China in 1997 evaluated the topical use of a tripterygium extract in sixty-one people with rheumatoid arthritis The extract was applied five to six times daily to the affected joints. The results appeared to indicate that use of the herbal tincture over six weeks significantly reduced rheumatoid arthritis symptoms compared with placebo. However, due to problems in the study, researchers were compelled to use statistical methods that were somewhat questionable (technically, posthoc analysis). For this reason, the results are only somewhat meaningful.

Another study compared placebo to oral tripterygium extract, taken in a low or a high dose for twenty weeks. The results appeared to show benefit, but so many participants dropped out before the end of the study that the results are difficult to interpret.

At most, therefore, current evidence regarding tripterygium for rheumatoid arthritis remains preliminary. The National Institutes of Health (NIH) is currently conducting a much larger study on this herb that should provide more definitive information.

No other potential uses of tripterygium have undergone meaningful controlled clinical trials. Weak evidence hints that it might offer promise as a contraceptive for men.

SAFETY ISSUES

Tripterygium is a toxic herb: various components of tripterygium can cause liver injury, genetic damage, and birth defects. It is thought, but not proven, that certain chemical extracts of tripterygium are safe if used within proper dosage limits. All forms of the herb should be avoided by pregnant or nursing women, young children, and those with kidney or liver disease.

EBSCO CAM Review Board

FURTHER READING

Ho, L. J., and J. H. Lai. "Chinese Herbs as Immunomodulators and Potential Disease-Modifying Anti-rheumatic Drugs in Autoimmune Disorders." *Current Drug Metabolism* 5 (2004): 181-192.

Liu, Q., et al. "Triptolide." *Biochemical and Biophysical Research Communications* 319 (2004): 980-986.

Wan, Y., et al. "Multi-Glycoside of *Tripterygium wilfordii* Hook F. Ameliorates Proteinuria and Acute Mesangial Injury Induced by Anti-Thy1.1 Monoclonal Antibody." *Nephron Experimental Nephrology* 99 (February 17, 2005): e121-129.

Wang, X., et al. "Immunosuppressive Sesquiterpenes from *Tripterygium wilfordii*." *Chemical and Pharmacological Bulletin* 53 (2005): 607-610.

Wu, Y., et al. "The Suppressive Effect of Triptolide on Experimental Autoimmune Uveoretinitis by Down-Regulating Th1-Type Response." *International Immunopharmacology* 3 (2003): 1457-1465.

See also: Contraceptives, oral; Lupus; Rheumatoid arthritis.

Turmeric

CATEGORY: Herbs and supplements

RELATED TERMS: *Curcuma longa*, curcumin

DEFINITION: Herbal product used as a food spice and as a dietary supplement for specific health benefits.

PRINCIPAL PROPOSED USE: Dyspepsia

OTHER PROPOSED USES: Alzheimer's disease, cancer prevention, cataract prevention, chronic anterior uveitis, high cholesterol, lichen planus, liver protection, menstrual pain, multiple sclerosis, osteoarthritis, rheumatoid arthritis, ulcerative colitis

OVERVIEW

Turmeric is a widely used tropical herb in the ginger family. Its stalk is used both in food and in medicine, yielding the familiar yellow ingredient that colors and adds flavor to, or spices, curry. In the traditional Indian system of herbal medicine known as Ayurveda, turmeric is believed to strengthen the overall energy of the body and to relieve gas, dispel worms, improve digestion, regulate menstruation, dissolve gallstones, and relieve arthritis, among other uses.

Modern interest in turmeric began in 1971 when Indian researchers found evidence suggesting that turmeric may possess anti-inflammatory properties. Much of this observed activity appeared to be caused by the presence of a constituent called cur-cumin. Curcumin is also an antioxidant. Many of the studies mentioned here used curcumin rather than turmeric.

USES AND APPLICATIONS

Turmeric's antioxidant abilities make it a good food preservative, provided that the food is already yellow in color, and it is widely used for this purpose. Turmeric has been proposed as a treatment for dyspepsia. "Dyspepsia" is a catchall term that includes a variety of digestive problems, such as stomach discomfort, gas, bloating, belching, appetite loss, and nausea. Although many serious medical conditions can cause digestive distress, the term "dyspepsia" is most often used when no identifiable medical cause can be detected.

In Europe, dyspepsia is commonly attributed to inadequate bile flow from the gallbladder. While this has not been proven, turmeric does appear to stimulate the gallbladder. More important, one double-blind, placebo-controlled study suggests that turmeric does reduce dyspepsia symptoms. Another double-blind, placebo-controlled study suggests that, when taken with standard medications, curcumin can help maintain remission in people with ulcerative colitis.

Other proposed uses of turmeric or curcumin have little supporting evidence. Based on test-tube and animal studies, and on human trials too preliminary to provide any meaningful evidence, curcumin and turmeric are frequently described as anti-inflammatory substances and are recommended for the treatment of such conditions as osteoarthritis and menstrual pain. Some advocates state that curcumin is superior to standard medications in the ibuprofen family, because, at standard doses, it does not appear to harm the stomach. However, until turmeric is actually proven to meaningfully reduce pain and inflammation, such a comparison is premature. Also, high doses of curcumin might increase the risk of ulcers, and, contrary to some reports, turmeric does not appear to be effective for treating ulcers.

Animal and test-tube studies suggest (but do not prove) that turmeric might help prevent cancer. Weak evidence hints that curcumin might help prevent the heart and kidney injury potentially caused by the chemotherapy drug doxorubicin.

Some researchers have reported evidence that curcumin or turmeric might generally help protect the liver from damage. However, other researchers have failed to find any liver-protective effects, and there are

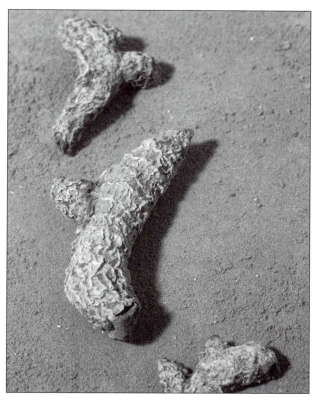

These turmeric roots are shown resting on pulverized turmeric. (Tom McHugh/Photo Researchers, Inc.)

even some indications that turmeric extracts can damage the liver when taken in high doses or for an extended period.

On the basis of even weaker evidence, curcumin or turmeric has also been recommended for preventing Alzheimer's disease, cataracts, chronic anterior uveitis (an inflammation of the iris of the eye), fungal infections, and multiple sclerosis, and for treating high cholesterol.

One preliminary study failed to find curcumin helpful for lichen planus, a disease of the skin and mucous membranes. A six-month, double-blind, placebo-controlled study of thirty-six elderly persons failed to find that the consumption of curcumin (at a dose of up to 4 grams [g] daily) led to improvements in cholesterol profile.

SCIENTIFIC EVIDENCE

Dyspepsia. A double-blind, placebo-controlled study performed in Thailand compared the effects of 500 milligrams (mg) curcumin four times daily with placebo and with a locally popular over-the-counter treatment. A total of 116 people were enrolled in the study. After seven days, 87 percent of the curcumin group experienced full or partial symptom relief from dyspepsia, compared with 53 percent of the placebo group; this difference was statistically significant.

Ulcerative colitis. Ulcerative colitis is a disease of the lower digestive tract marked by alternating periods of quiescence and flare-up. Curcumin has shown some promise for helping to maintain remission and prevent relapse. In a double-blind, placebo-controlled study, eighty-nine people with quiescent ulcerative colitis were given either placebo or curcumin (1 g twice daily) with standard treatment. In the six-month treatment period, the relapse rate was significantly lower in the treatment group than in the placebo group.

DOSAGE

For medicinal purposes, turmeric is frequently taken in a form standardized to curcumin content, at a dose that provides 400 to 600 mg of curcumin three times daily.

SAFETY ISSUES

Turmeric is on the GRAS (Generally Recognized As Safe) list of the U.S. Food and Drug Administration, and curcumin too is believed to be fairly nontoxic. Reported side effects are uncommon and are generally limited to mild stomach distress.

However, there is some evidence to suggest that turmeric extracts can be toxic to the liver when taken in high doses or for a prolonged time. For this reason, turmeric products should probably be avoided by persons with liver disease and by those who take medications that are hard on the liver.

In addition, because of curcumin's stimulating effects on the gallbladder, persons with gallbladder disease should use curcumin only on the advice of a physician. Safety in young children, pregnant or nursing women, and those with severe kidney disease also has not been established.

EBSCO CAM Review Board

FURTHER READING

Afaq, F., et al. "Botanical Antioxidants for Chemoprevention of Photocarcinogenesis." *Frontiers in Bioscience* 7 (2002): 784-792.

Baum, L., et al. "Curcumin Effects on Blood Lipid

Profile in a Six-Month Human Study." *Pharmacol Res.* 2007

Cheng, A. L., et al. "Phase I Clinical Trial of Curcumin, a Chemopreventive Agent, in Patients with High-Risk or Pre-malignant Lesions." *Anticancer Research* 21 (2001): 2895-2900.

Fowler, J. F., et al. "Innovations in Natural Ingredients and Their Use in Skin Care." *Journal of Drugs in Dermatology* 9, suppl. 6 (2010): S72-S81.

Hanai, H., et al. "Curcumin Maintenance Therapy for Ulcerative Colitis." *Clinical Gastroenterology and Hepatology* 4 (2006): 1502-1506.

See also: Dyspepsia; Functional foods: Introduction.

Tylophora

CATEGORY: Herbs and supplements
RELATED TERMS: *Tylophora asthmatica, T. indica*
DEFINITION: Natural plant product used to treat specific health conditions.
PRINCIPAL PROPOSED USE: Asthma
OTHER PROPOSED USES: Allergies (hay fever), bronchitis, colds

OVERVIEW

Tylophora indica is a climbing perennial plant indigenous to India, where it grows wild in the southern and eastern regions and has a long-standing reputation as a remedy for asthma (hence the name *T. asthmatica*). The leaves and roots of tylophora have been included in the *Bengal Pharmacopoeia* since 1884. It is said to have laxative, expectorant, diaphoretic (sweating), and purgative (vomiting) properties. Tylophora has been used for the treatment of various respiratory problems besides asthma, including allergies, bronchitis, and colds, as well as dysentery and osteoarthritis pain.

THERAPEUTIC DOSAGES

The typical dosage of tylophora leaf in dried or capsule form is 200 mg twice daily or 400 mg total in two doses.

THERAPEUTIC USES

Tylophora has become an increasingly popular treatment for asthma based on its traditional use for this purpose and several studies performed in the 1970s. However, the studies that found it effective were poorly designed, and a better-designed study found no benefits. Tylophora is also still recommended for some of its other traditional uses, including hay fever, bronchitis, and the common cold.

SCIENTIFIC EVIDENCE

Weak preliminary evidence hints that tylophora might have anti-inflammatory, antiallergic, and antispasmodic actions. All these effects could make it useful for the treatment of asthma. However, only double-blind, placebo-controlled studies can actually show a treatment effective. For tylophora and asthma, the evidence from this type of study is mixed at best.

In 1972, researchers reported the results of a double-blind, placebo-controlled crossover trial of 195 individuals with asthma who were given either placebo or 40 milligrams (mg) of a tylophora alcohol extract daily for six days. The results showed that people taking tylophora had fewer asthma symptoms, and the benefits endured for months after use of the herb was stopped. Similarly long-lasting results were seen in two double-blind, placebo-controlled studies involving more than two hundred individuals with asthma.

Even the researchers involved in these trials expressed surprise that short-term use of tylophora could produce long-lasting benefits; to outside observers, such findings make the results difficult to believe at all. Furthermore, most of these studies suffered from poor design and reporting. In 1979, researchers published the results of a double-blind study designed to remedy these problems. A total of 135 people with asthma were given either tylophora or placebo. No benefits were seen, and tylophora has not undergone much study since then. Better studies that show benefit will be necessary before tylophora can be considered a promising herb for asthma.

SAFETY ISSUES

In the second study mentioned above, tylophora caused nausea, vomiting, mouth soreness, and alterations in taste sensation in more than half of the participants. The other two studies found similar side effects, but far less frequently. The difference may have been because the second study had people chew the whole leaves from the plant, whereas other studies used dried leaves or powdered extract in capsule form.

Preliminary studies on animals have found ty-lophora extracts to be toxic only in extremely high doses; these extracts were apparently safe in the far smaller doses needed to produce a therapeutic effect. Due to the lack of comprehensive safety studies on tylophora, the herb should not be used by children, pregnant or nursing women, or individuals with severe kidney or liver disease. Whether tylophora interacts with any drugs is unknown.

EBSCO CAM Review Board

FURTHER READING

Bielory, L., and K. Lupoli. "Herbal Interventions in Asthma and Allergy." *Journal of Asthma* 36 (1999): 1-65.

Nandi, M. "Physical, Chemical, and Biological Assay of *Tylophora indica* Mother Tincture." *British Homeopathic Journal* 88 (1999): 161-165.

See also: Allergies; Asthma; Bronchitis; Colds and flu.

Tyrosine

CATEGORY: Herbs and supplements
RELATED TERM: L-tyrosine
DEFINITION: Natural substance of the human body used as a supplement to treat specific health conditions.
PRINCIPAL PROPOSED USES: None
OTHER PROPOSED USES: Attention deficit disorder, depression, enhancing mental function, fatigue, jet lag, enhancing sports performance

OVERVIEW

Tyrosine is an amino acid found in meat proteins. The body uses it as a starting material to make several neurotransmitters, chemicals that help the brain and nervous system function. Tyrosine has been proposed as a treatment for various conditions in which mental function is impaired or slowed down, such as fatigue and depression. It also has been tried for attention deficit disorder (ADD).

REQUIREMENTS AND SOURCES

The body makes tyrosine from another common amino acid, phenylalanine, so deficiencies are rare. However, they can occur in certain forms of severe kidney disease as well as in phenylketonuria (PKU), a metabolic disorder that requires complete avoidance of phenylalanine. Good sources of tyrosine include dairy products, meats, fish, and beans.

THERAPEUTIC DOSAGES

The typical therapeutic dosage of tyrosine used in studies ranges from 7 grams (g) to 30 g daily.

THERAPEUTIC USES

Preliminary evidence, including small double-blind trials, suggests that tyrosine supplements may help fight fatigue and improve memory and mental function in people who are deprived of sleep or exposed to other forms of stress. Based on these findings, it has been inferred that tyrosine might enhance alertness in people suffering from jet lag, but this has not been studied directly.

Tyrosine may also provide some temporary benefit for attention deficit disorder (ADD), but the benefits appear to wear off in about two weeks. Tyrosine is said to work better for this purpose when it is combined in an "amino acid cocktail" along with gamma-aminobutyric acid (GABA), phenylalanine, and glutamine; however, there is no scientific evidence to support this use.

Although one extremely tiny study found tyrosine helpful for depression, a larger study found no evidence of benefit. Tyrosine has also been suggested for enhancing sports performance. However, in a double-blind study of twenty men, one-time use of tyrosine at a dose 150 milligrams per kilogram body weight failed to improve any measurement of muscular performance.

SCIENTIFIC EVIDENCE

Sleep deprivation. A double-blind, placebo-controlled study that enrolled twenty U.S. Marines suggests that tyrosine can improve mental alertness during periods of sleep deprivation. In this study, the participants were deprived of sleep for a night and then tested frequently for their alertness throughout the day as they worked. Compared to placebo, 10 to 15 g of tyrosine given twice daily seemed to provide a "pick-up" for about two hours. Similar benefits were seen with 2 g of tyrosine daily in a double-blind, placebo-controlled trial of twenty-one military cadets exposed to physical and psychological stress.

Depression. A pilot study that enrolled nine individuals

is widely quoted as proving that tyrosine can help depression. However, this study was too small to provide reliable results. A subsequent double-blind, placebo-controlled study of sixty-five people with depression failed to find any benefit.

SAFETY ISSUES

Tyrosine seems to be generally safe, though at high dosages some people have reported nausea, diarrhea, vomiting, or nervousness. As with any other supplement taken in multigram doses, it is important to use a high-quality product; even a very small percentage of contaminant in the product might add up to a dangerous amount. Maximum safe dosages for young children, women who are pregnant or nursing, and those with severe liver or kidney disease have not been established.

EBSCO CAM Review Board

FURTHER READING

Deijen, J. B., et al. "Tyrosine Improves Cognitive Performance and Reduces Blood Pressure in Cadets After One Week of a Combat Training Course." *Brain Research Bulletin* 48 (1999): 203-209.

Mahoney, C. R., et al. "Tyrosine Supplementation Mitigates Working Memory Decrements During Cold Exposure." *Physiology and Behavior* 92, no. 4 (2007): 575-582.

Sutton, E. E., et al. Ingestion of Tyrosine: Effects on Endurance, Muscle Strength, and Anaerobic Performance." *International Journal of Sport Nutrition and Exercise Metabolism* 15 (2005): 173-185.

See also: Attention deficit disorder; Depression, mild to moderate; Fatigue; Jet lag.

U

Ulcerative colitis

CATEGORY: Condition

RELATED TERMS: Crohn's disease, inflammatory bowel disease

DEFINITION: Treatment of inflammation of the digestive tract.

PRINCIPAL PROPOSED NATURAL TREATMENTS: Aloe, fish oil, nutritional support, probiotics

OTHER PROPOSED NATURAL TREATMENTS: Acupuncture, blue-green algae, boswellia, bromelain, curcumin, evening primrose oil, food allergen avoidance, glutamine, mesoglycans, phosphatidylcholine, wheat grass juice

INTRODUCTION

Ulcerative colitis is a disease of the colon that is closely related to Crohn's disease. The two are grouped in a category called inflammatory bowel disease (IBD) because they both involve inflammation of the digestive tract.

The major symptoms of ulcerative colitis include abdominal pain and bloody diarrhea. When the disease becomes severe, those affected may develop fever, weight loss, dehydration, and anemia. Sometimes, constipation develops instead of diarrhea. Arthritis, skin sores, and liver inflammation also may occur.

One of the most feared consequences of ulcerative colitis is dramatic dilation of the colon, which can lead to fatal perforation of the colon. Ulcerative colitis also leads to a greatly increased risk of colon cancer.

Ulcerative colitis tends to wax and wane, with periods of remission punctuated by severe flare-ups. Medical treatment aims at reducing symptoms and inducing and maintaining remission.

Sulfasalazine is one of the most common medications for ulcerative colitis. Given either orally or as an enema, it can both decrease symptoms and prevent recurrences. Corticosteroids, such as prednisone, are used similarly in more severe cases, sometimes combined with other immunosuppressive drugs, such as azathioprine and cyclosporine. Partial removal of the colon may be necessary in severe cases.

PRINCIPAL PROPOSED NATURAL TREATMENTS

People with ulcerative colitis can easily develop deficiencies in numerous nutrients. Chronic bleeding leads to iron deficiency. Malabsorption, decreased appetite, drug side effects, and increased nutrient loss through the stool may lead to mild or profound deficiencies of protein, folate, calcium, copper, magnesium, selenium, zinc, and vitamins A, B_{12}, C, D, E, and K. For persons with ulcerative colitis, supplementation to restore adequate body stores of these nutrients is highly advisable and may improve specific symptoms and overall health. One should work closely with a physician to identify any nutrient deficiencies and to evaluate the success of supplementation in correcting them.

Essential fatty acids. Fish oil and evening primrose oil contain healthy fats called essential fatty acids. According to some of the small, double-blind, placebo-controlled trials reported, fish oil might be helpful for reducing symptoms of active ulcerative colitis. Evening primrose oil also has shown promise. However, larger studies will be necessary to discover for certain whether fish oil or evening primrose oil really help. Regular use of fish oil alone, or in combination with gamma-linolenic acid (found in evening primrose oil), has not been found effective for preventing disease flare-ups in people whose ulcerative colitis has gone into remission.

Probiotics. Friendly bacteria, or probiotics, might be helpful in ulcerative colitis. A double-blind trial of 116 people with ulcerative colitis compared probiotic treatment with a relatively low dose of the standard drug mesalazine. The results suggest that probiotic treatment might be just as effective as low-dose mesalazine for controlling symptoms and maintaining remission. Evidence of benefit was seen in other trials too. However, probiotics may be less useful for inducing remission; when they were added to standard medications used for induction of remission,

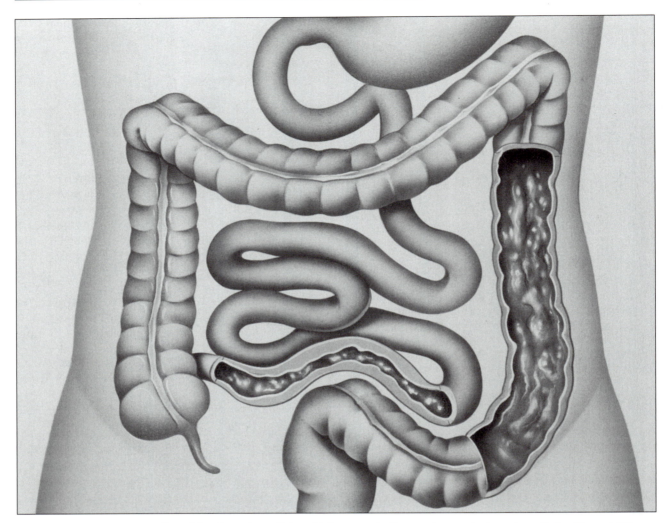

On the right, the colon is affected by ulcerative colitis, which causes inflammation and ulceration. (John Bavosi/Photo Researchers, Inc.)

no additional benefits were seen in a study of people with mild-to-moderate ulcerative colitis.

Probiotics might be useful for people with ulcerative colitis who have had part or all of the colon removed. Such persons frequently develop a complication called pouchitis, inflammation of part of the remaining intestine. Two double-blind, placebo-controlled studies found that probiotics can help prevent pouchitis and also reduce relapses in people who already have it. The probiotic mixture used in these trials contained four strains of *Lactobacillus*, three strains of *Bifidobacterium*, and one strain of *Streptococcus salivarius*. In addition, some evidence hints that probi-

otics might reduce the joint pain that commonly occurs in people with IBD.

Aloe. In a double-blind, placebo-controlled trial, forty-four people hospitalized with severe active ulcerative colitis were given oral aloe gel or placebo twice daily for four weeks. The results showed that aloe was more effective than placebo in inducing full or partial remission of symptoms.

OTHER PROPOSED NATURAL TREATMENTS

Researchers are now interested in the use of phosphadylcholine as a supportive treatment in severe ulcerative colitis. There may be an insufficient quantity

Aloe as a Possible Treatment for Ulcerative Colitis

The use of aloe, also called aloe vera, can be traced back six thousand years to early Egypt, where the plant was depicted on stone carvings. Known as the plant of immortality, aloe was presented as a burial gift to deceased pharaohs. Common names for the plant are burn plant, lily of the desert, and elephant's gall, and its Latin names are *Aloe vera* and *A. barbadensis*.

Traditionally, aloe was used topically to heal wounds and for various skin conditions. It also was used orally as a laxative. Aloe leaves contain a clear gel that is often used as a topical ointment. The gel has also been used orally to treat ulcerative colitis. The green part of the leaf that surrounds the gel can be used to produce a juice or a dried substance (called latex) that is taken by mouth.

According to the Natural Medicines Comprehensive Database, using aloe "with other stimulant laxative herbs may increase the risk of lowering potassium levels too much. Stimulant laxative herbs include blue flag rhizome, alder buckthorn, European buckthorn, butternut bark, cascara bark, castor oil, colocynth fruit pulp, gamboge bark exudate, jalap root, black root, manna bark exudate, podophyllum root, rhubarb root, senna leaves and pods, and yellow dock root."

of phosphatidylcholine in the mucus lining the colon in persons with ulcerative colitis. Taking phosphatidylcholine may correct this deficiency. A small, double-blind, placebo-controlled study of sixty persons whose ulcerative colitis was poorly responsive to corticosteroids were randomized to receive either phosphadylcholine (2 grams [g] per day) or placebo for twelve weeks. One-half of the participants taking phosphadylcholine showed a significant improvement in symptoms, compared to only 10 percent taking placebo. Moreover, 80 percent taking phosphadylcholine were able to completely discontinue their corticosteroids without disease flare-up, compared to 10 percent taking placebo.

A double-blind, placebo-controlled study of twenty-four people with ulcerative colitis examined the effects of wheat grass juice taken daily for one month. According to various measures of disease severity, participants given wheat grass juice improved to a greater ex-

tent than those given placebo. However, wheat grass juice is rather bitter, and it seems unlikely that the study could truly be blind, meaning that participants and doctors did not know who was getting the wheat grass juice and who was getting the placebo. Indeed, when researchers polled the participants, a majority of those given wheat grass juice correctly identified it. For this reason, as well as its small size, the results of the study are not convincing.

The substance curcumin (from the spice turmeric) has shown some promise for helping to maintain remission. In a double-blind, placebo-controlled study, eighty-nine people with quiescent ulcerative colitis were given either placebo or curcumin (1 g twice daily) with standard treatment. During the six-month treatment period, relapse rate was significantly lower in the treatment group than in the placebo group.

Glutamine, boswellia, bromelain, blue-green algae, colostrum, mesoglycan (glycosaminoglycans), and an extract of soy called Bowman-Birk inhibitor concentrate (BBI) have been suggested for the treatment of ulcerative colitis, but the evidence that they work remains preliminary at best. There are also weak indications that allergies to foods, such as milk, may play a role in ulcerative colitis. One study failed to find real acupuncture more effective than fake acupuncture for this condition.

HERBS AND SUPPLEMENTS TO USE ONLY WITH CAUTION

Various herbs and supplements may interact adversely with drugs used to treat ulcerative colitis.

EBSCO CAM Review Board

FURTHER READING

Ben-Arye, E., et al. "Wheat Grass Juice in the Treatment of Active Distal Ulcerative Colitis." *Scandinavian Journal of Gastroenterology* 37 (2002): 444-449.

Do, V. T., B. G. Baird, and D. R. Kockler. "Probiotics for Maintaining Remission of Ulcerative Colitis in Adults." *Annals of Pharmacotherapy* 44 (2010): 565-571.

Gionchetti, P., et al. "Prophylaxis of Pouchitis Onset with Probiotic Therapy." *Gastroenterology* 124 (2003): 1202-1209.

Joos, S., et al. "Acupuncture and Moxibustion in the Treatment of Ulcerative Colitis." *Scandinavian Journal of Gastroenterology* 41 (2006): 1056-1063.

Kato, K., et al. "Randomized Placebo-Controlled Trial

Assessing the Effect of Bifidobacteria-Fermented Milk on Active Ulcerative Colitis." *Alimentary Pharmacology and Therapeutics* 20 (2004): 1133-1141.

Langmead, L., et al. "Randomized, Double-Blind, Placebo-Controlled Trial of Oral Aloe Vera Gel for Active Ulcerative Colitis." *Alimentary Pharmacology and Therapeutics* 19 (2004): 739-748.

Lichtenstein, G. R., et al. "Bowman-Birk Inhibitor Concentrate: A Novel Therapeutic Agent for Patients with Active Ulcerative Colitis." *Digestive Diseases and Sciences* 53 (2008): 175-180.

Mallon, P., et al. "Probiotics for Induction of Remission in Ulcerative Colitis." *Cochrane Database of Systematic Reviews* (2007): CD005573. Available through *EBSCO DynaMed Systematic Literature Surveillance* at http://www.ebscohost.com/dynamed.

Stremmel, W., et al. "Phosphatidylcholine for Steroid-Refractory Chronic Ulcerative Colitis." *Annals of Internal Medicine* 147 (2007): 603-610.

See also: Aloe; Constipation; Crohn's disease; Diarrhea; Dyspepsia; Fish oil; Gastritis; Gastroesophageal reflux disease; Gastrointestinal health; Irritable bowel syndrome (IBS); Probiotics.

Ulcers

CATEGORY: Condition

DEFINITION: Treatment of a stomach-acid-burned hole in the tissue of the stomach and duodenum.

PRINCIPAL PROPOSED NATURAL TREATMENT: Probiotics (as an adjunct to standard therapy)

OTHER PROPOSED NATURAL TREATMENTS: Aloe, *Bacopa monniera*, beeswax extract (related to policosanol), butterbur, cayenne, colostrum, cranberry, deglycyrrhizinated licorice, fish oil, garlic, rhubarb, sea buckthorn oil, turmeric, vitamin B_{12}, vitamin C

INTRODUCTION

The highly concentrated acid produced by the stomach is quite capable of burning a hole through the tissue of the stomach and duodenum (part of the small intestine). That it usually does not do so is a tribute to the effectiveness of the methods that the body uses to protect itself. However, sometimes these protective mechanisms fail, and the ever-present acid begins to produce an ulcer.

Ulcer pain is caused by stomach acid coming into contact with unprotected tissue. Eating generally decreases ulcer pain temporarily, because food neutralizes the acid. As soon as the food begins to be digested, the pain returns.

Conventional medical treatment for ulcers has gone through a slow revolution. The prescribed response to ulcers used to be a bland diet, one low in spices and high in dairy products, which were believed to coat the stomach. However, eventually it was discovered that spicy foods are not the cause of ulcers and that milk itself is somewhat ulcer-forming. The only other option at that time was surgery.

Next in the line of treatment was antacids containing magnesium and aluminum. However, these were seldom strong enough to allow the ulcer to heal fully. Ulcer treatment took a big step forward with the development of Tagamet (cimetidine), followed by Zantac (ranitidine), Pepcid (famotidine), and others. These H_2-blocking drugs dramatically lower the stomach's production of acid. Later, a new class of even more potent acid suppressors appeared, the proton pump inhibitors, led by Prilosec (omeprazole).

When stomach acid is suppressed, ulcer pain rapidly diminishes and the ulcer heals. For a time, these drugs were regarded as the definitive answer to ulcers. This early enthusiasm began to fade when it became clear that ulcers frequently returned after the drugs were stopped. In the late 1980s, a new explanation for this problem began to surface. First regarded as an implausible theory, it has now become the accepted explanation.

It is now believed that ulcers are caused by the bacterium *Helicobacter pylori*. Apparently, this previously ignored organism has the capacity to infect the stomach and, by so doing, weaken the stomach lining. Only when antibiotics to kill *H. pylori* are combined with stomach acid suppressants do ulcers go away and stay away. However, it is not easy to kill *H. pylori*; antibiotic treatment is not always successful, and it has side effects. Friendly bacteria (probiotics) may help this treatment work better.

PRINCIPAL PROPOSED NATURAL TREATMENTS

Probiotics are healthful bacteria, the best known of which is *Lactobacillus acidophilus*, which is found in yogurt. There are many other probiotics too. Evidence suggests that various probiotics in the *Lactobacillus* family can inhibit the growth of *H. pylori*. While this

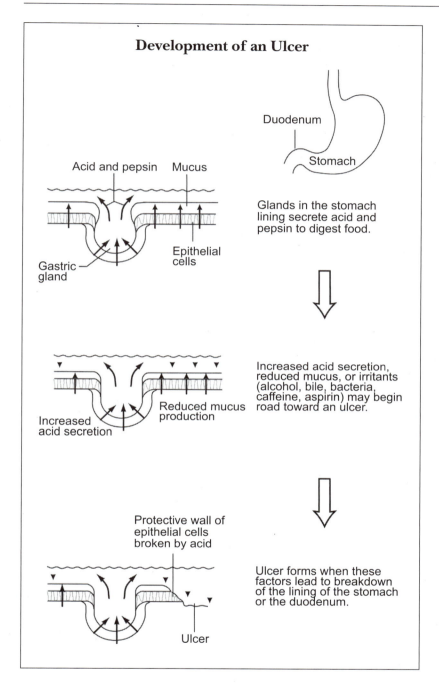

Development of an Ulcer

Duodenum

Stomach

Acid and pepsin   Mucus

Gastric gland

Epithelial cells

Glands in the stomach lining secrete acid and pepsin to digest food.

Increased acid secretion

Reduced mucus production

Increased acid secretion, reduced mucus, or irritants (alcohol, bile, bacteria, caffeine, aspirin) may begin road toward an ulcer.

Protective wall of epithelial cells broken by acid

Ulcer

Ulcer forms when these factors lead to breakdown of the lining of the stomach or the duodenum.

OTHER PROPOSED NATURAL TREATMENTS

Cranberry. The herb cranberry is thought to help prevent bladder infections by preventing adhesion of bacteria to the bladder. Preliminary evidence suggests that it might also help prevent the adhesion of *H. pylori* to the stomach wall.

A ninety-day, double-blind, placebo-controlled study performed in China tested the effects of daily consumption of cranberry juice in persons who were chronically infected with *Helicobacter* (but who did not necessarily have ulcers). The results indicated that the use of cranberry significantly decreased levels of *Helicobacter* in the stomach, presumably by causing some of the detached bacteria to be "washed away."

However, while this was a promising finding on a theoretical level, it did not directly address the treatment or prevention of ulcers. A more practical study evaluated the use of cranberry as a support to standard therapy. This double-blind trial enrolled 177 people with ulcers who were undergoing treatment with a common triple-drug therapy known as OAC (omeprazole, amoxicillin, and clarithromycin) used to eradicate *H. pylori*. All participants received standard therapy for one week. During this week and for two weeks after, they were additionally given either placebo or cranberry juice. Researchers also looked at a third group who were attending the same clinic and who received only OAC.

The results were somewhat promising. In the study group at large, OAC plus cranberry was no more effective than OAC plus placebo or OAC alone. However, among female participants in the study, the use of cranberry was associated with a significantly increased rate of *Helicobacter* eradication compared with placebo or no treatment.

Does this mean that women undergoing ulcer

effect does not appear to be strong enough for probiotic treatment to eradicate *H. pylori* on its own, preliminary studies, including several small double-blind trials, suggest that probiotics may help standard antibiotic therapy work better, reducing side effects, and improving the rate of eradication.

Vitamin B_{12} Absorption and Ulcer Treatments

Vitamin B_{12} is a water-soluble vitamin that is naturally present in some foods, is added to others, and is available as a dietary supplement and a prescription medication. The vitamin is required for proper red-blood-cell formation, neurological function, and deoxyribonucleic acid (DNA) synthesis.

Proton pump inhibitors, such as omeprazole (Prilosec) and lansoprazole (Prevacid), are used to treat peptic ulcer disease and gastroesophageal reflux disease, or GERD. These drugs can interfere with vitamin B_{12} absorption from food by slowing the release of gastric acid into the stomach. However, the evidence is conflicting on whether proton pump inhibitor use affects vitamin B_{12} status. As a precaution, health care providers should

monitor vitamin B_{12} status in patients taking proton pump inhibitors for prolonged periods.

Histamine H_2 receptor antagonists, also used to treat peptic ulcer disease, include cimetidine (Tagamet), famotidine (Pepcid), and ranitidine (Zantac). These medications can interfere with the absorption of vitamin B_{12} from food by slowing the release of hydrochloric acid into the stomach. Although H_2 receptor antagonists have the potential to cause vitamin B_{12} deficiency, no evidence indicates that they promote vitamin B_{12} deficiency, even after long-term use. Clinically significant effects may be more likely in patients with inadequate vitamin B_{12} stores, especially patients using H_2 receptor antagonists continuously for more than two years.

treatment may benefit from cranberry? Perhaps, but not necessarily. When a treatment fails to produce benefit in the entire group studied, researchers may, after the fact, look for a subgroup who did benefit. The laws of chance alone ensure that they can almost always find one. Therefore, it is not clear whether cranberry actually did provide benefit or whether this finding was merely a statistical fluke.

Other treatments. Persons who take H_2 blockers or proton pump inhibitors for ulcers may not be able to properly absorb vitamin B_{12} and might, therefore, benefit from vitamin B_{12} supplements. The best-known supplement used for ulcer disease is a special form of licorice known as deglycyrrhizinated licorice (DGL). However, the studies that supposedly showed it effective were not double-blind, and they involved a combination product that also contained antacids. Preliminary evidence does suggest that DGL might help protect the stomach from damage caused by nonsteroidal anti-inflammatory drugs.

One study found that the use of vitamin C supplements at a dose of 500 milligrams daily can improve the effectiveness of antibiotic therapy for *H. pylori*. Specifically, the use of vitamin C allowed a reduction in the dosage of clarithromycin, one of the most important antibiotics used to eradicate *H. pylori*. However, vitamin C did not help in cases where the species of *H. pylori* involved was resistant to clarithromycin.

Fish oil with antibiotic therapy has been tried as a treatment for eradicating *H. pylori*, but it did not prove

particularly effective. Preliminary studies suggest that various bioflavonoids, including citrus bioflavonoids, can inhibit the growth of *H. pylori*. All fruits and vegetables provide bioflavonoids, but these substances can also be taken as supplements. One study failed to find that the carotenoid astaxanthin is helpful for treating *H. pylori* infection.

Neither garlic nor cayenne appears to be helpful against *H. pylori*. However, some evidence suggests that cayenne can protect the stomach against damage caused by anti-inflammatory drugs.

Colostrum and butterbur might also help protect the stomach lining. *Bacopa monniera*, betaine hydrochloride, cat's claw, glutamine, marshmallow, methyl sulfonyl methane, reishi, sea buckthorn oil, selenium, suma, vitamin A, vitamin C, and zinc have also been suggested as aids to ulcer healing, but there is no meaningful scientific evidence that they are effective.

Contrary to some reports, the herb turmeric does not appear to be effective for treating ulcers, and it might increase the risk of developing ulcers if taken at excessive doses. Rhubarb and aloe have been suggested as treatments for bleeding ulcers. However, this condition is sufficiently dangerous that conventional medical treatment is far more appropriate.

HERBS AND SUPPLEMENTS TO USE ONLY WITH CAUTION

Various herbs and supplements may interact adversely with drugs used to treat ulcers.

EBSCO CAM Review Board

FURTHER READING

Al-Mofleh, I. A. "Spices, Herbal Xenobiotics, and the Stomach: Friends or Foes?" *World Journal of Gastroenterology* 16 (2010): 2710-2719.

Chuang, C. H., et al. "Adjuvant Effect of Vitamin C on Omeprazole-Amoxicillin-Clarithromycin Triple Therapy for *Helicobacter pylori* Eradication." *Hepatogastroenterology* 54 (2007): 320-324.

Gotteland, M., et al. "Modulation of *Helicobacter pylori* Colonization with Cranberry Juice and *Lactobacillus johnsonii* La1 in Children." *Nutrition* 24 (2008): 421-426.

Graham, D. Y, S. Y. Anderson, T. Lang. "Garlic or Jalapeno Peppers for Treatment of *Helicobacter pylori* Infection." *American Journal of Gastroenterology* 94 (1999): 1200-1202.

Kim, M. N., et al. "The Effects of Probiotics on PPI-triple Therapy for *Helicobacter pylori* Eradication." *Helicobacter* 13 (2008): 261-268.

Park, S. K., et al. "The Effect of Probiotics on *Helicobacter pylori* Eradication." *Hepatogastroenterology* 54 (2007): 2032-2036.

Shmuely, H., et al. "Effect of Cranberry Juice on Eradication of *Helicobacter pylori* in Patients Treated with Antibiotics and a Proton Pump Inhibitor." *Molecular Nutrition and Food Research* 51 (2007): 746-751.

See also: Constipation; Crohn's disease; Diarrhea; Dyspepsia; Gastritis; Gastroesophageal reflux disease; Gastrointestinal health; Irritable bowel syndrome (IBS); Peptic ulcer disease: Homeopathic remedies; Probiotics; Proton pump inhibitors.

Unani medicine

CATEGORY: Therapies and techniques

RELATED TERMS: Hikmat, homeopathy, Ionian medicine, Siddha medicine, Unani-Tibb

DEFINITION: The practice of balancing defined humours, or components, of the blood to sustain good health.

PRINCIPAL PROPOSED USES: Chronic diseases, mental illness

OTHER PROPOSED USES: Diabetes, hepatitis B, malaria, sexual dysfunction, skin problems

OVERVIEW

Unani is an Arabic spelling for the word "Ionian," which means "Greek." Unani medicine originated with the ancient philosopher-physician Hippocrates and his followers in Greece and was further developed in the Muslim world. The basic premise of Unani medicine is that disease is a natural process, with symptoms that are manifest by reactions of the body to disease. The function of a physician is to aid the natural forces and self-preservative powers of the body in combating a disease.

MECHANISM OF ACTION

Unani medicine concentrates on the presence of four humours (or components) in the body: blood, phlegm, yellow bile, and black bile. Each humour contributes its own characteristics and temperament to the body. Through proper care and treatment, the humours can be balanced to optimize the physical, emotional, and spiritual health of a person.

USES AND APPLICATIONS

The Central Council for Research in Unani Medicines claims that Unani medicine is highly effective in treating a variety of diseases, including hepatitis B,

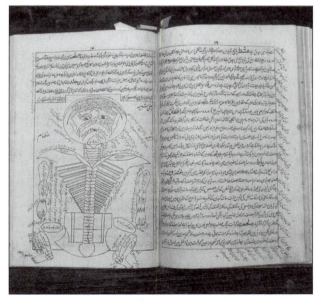

Unani medical textbook written in Arabic script. (Mark De Fraeye/Photo Researchers, Inc.)

malaria, and skin problems. It is further claimed to be unmatched for treating chronic diseases and other conditions, such as arthritis, asthma, cardiac disorders, urinary infections, and sexual disorders.

SCIENTIFIC EVIDENCE

In general, Unani medicine is relatively unknown, particularly in the Western world. It is actively practiced in Asia, particularly in India, Saudi Arabia, China, and Japan, where it is purported to be a sophisticated therapy that offers cures for a wide range of maladies. Depending on the disease involved, Unani medicine offers four levels of treatment: regimental therapy (exercise, massage, purging, cupping, spiritual awareness), dietotherapy (diet), pharmacotherapy (mild drugs, mostly herbal), and surgery. Prominent medical doctors, such as Stephen Barrett, question the validity of some aspects of the Unani regime and classify Unani medicine as a form of homeopathic medicine.

In practice, the scientific basis for Unani medicine involves a thorough examination of the tongue, pulse, urine, and stool of a patient to determine the balance of the four body humours. Once an imbalance is diagnosed, proper diet, mild drugs (ginkgo, ginseng, spices), and rest are prescribed to produce balance and improved health. If necessary, surgery is performed. During the 1990s, when a ten-year-old boy suffering from cerebral palsy was treated with the techniques of Unani medicine for an extended period of time by Hakim Jameel Ahmed, the boy's ability to think, talk, and walk improved significantly. Many other documented cases indicate that medical needs have been met using Unani medicine.

CHOOSING A PRACTITIONER

One should obtain a recommendation from a medical doctor for a person practicing Unani medicine. One should also ensure that the practitioner is licensed.

SAFETY ISSUES

Unani methods are generally safe. If used alone, there is the risk that a serious illness will remain undetected and untreated. Many Unani drugs are sugar-based and hence not suited for people suffering from diabetes.

Alvin K. Benson, Ph.D.

FURTHER READING

Alavi, Seema. *Islam and Healing: Loss and Recovery of an Indo-Muslim Medical Tradition, 1600–1900.* New York: Palgrave Macmillan, 2008.
Central Council for Research in Unani Medicine. http://unanimedicine.com/unanimed.
Chen, Nancy N. *Food, Medicine, and the Quest for Good Health.* New York: Columbia University Press, 2008.
Institute for Traditional Medicine. "Unani Medicine." Available at http://www.itmonline.org/arts/unani.htm.
Ministry of Health and Family Welfare, India. "Unani." Available at http://indianmedicine.nic.in.

See also: Cupping; Exercise; Faith healing; Herbal medicine; Homeopathy; Massage therapy; Meditation; Qigong; Spirituality; Traditional healing; Whole medicine.

Usui, Mikao

CATEGORY: Biography
IDENTIFICATION: Japanese Buddhist and teacher who developed the practice of Reiki
BORN: August 15, 1865; Taniani, Japan
DIED: March 9, 1929; Fukuyama, Japan

OVERVIEW

Mikao Usui, a Japanese Buddhist, developed Reiki, the spiritual and medicinal practice that involves using palm healing as a form of complementary and alternative medicine to treat physical and mental ailments. Practitioners claim that, using this technique, they can transfer healing energy to their patients.

The ultimate aim of many of Usui's teachings reportedly was to achieve enlightenment. However, no belief system or religion in particular was associated with his practices or teachings.

As a young child, Usui was sent to a monastery to receive his primary education. He went on to continue higher education and eventually received a doctorate in literature. Even late into life, he studied diverse subjects, including history, medicine, Buddhism, Christianity, and psychology.

Usui's teachings were influenced by Shintoism, the traditional faith of the Japanese people that is rooted in the presence of spirits that take the form of people, animals, mountains, and trees. During its early practice, Usui's method was known by another name (likely *Usui do*, or "the way of Usui"), and it was later changed to Reiki when it reached the Western world.

In 1922, Usui opened his first Reiki clinic in Harajuku, near Tokyo. Here, he began teaching classes about his system of healing. A couple of years later, in direct response to a devastating earthquake that hit parts of Japan, he opened a new clinic in Nakano, also near Tokyo. By this time, Usui had acquired some fame for his efforts throughout Japan, and he was even given an award by the Japanese emperor. Because of his distinction and reported successes in practice, many physicians and other healers sought Usui out for teaching sessions. As a result, Usui began teaching a simplified version of his principles to the public to meet the growing demand.

After developing and refining Reiki for many years, he founded a society of Japanese Reiki masters, which included a group of his many disciples. Many of Usui's disciples made significant contributions to the field and continued to practice this system. According to the inscription on his memorial stone, Usui taught Reiki to more than two thousand people during his lifetime.

Usui's popularity led him to travel extensively, which reportedly took a toll on his health. He is said to have fallen ill late in his life, possibly as a consequence of the stress of his position. Mikao Usui died of a stroke in 1929.

Brandy Weidow, M.S.

FURTHER READING

Beckett, Don. *Reiki, the True Story: An Exploration of Usui Reiki*. Berkeley, Calif.: Frog, 2009.

Petter, Frank Arjava. *Reiki: The Legacy of Dr. Usui (Shangri-La)*. Twin Lakes, Wis.: Lotus Press, 1998.

Stiene, Bronwen, and Frans Stiene. *The Japanese Art of Reiki: A Practical Guide to Self-Healing*. Hampshire, England: O Books, 2005.

Usui, Mikao, and Christine M. Grimm. *The Original Reiki Handbook of Dr. Mikao Usui*. Twin Lakes, Wis.: Lotus Press, 1999.

See also: Energy medicine; Massage therapy; Reiki; Traditional healing.

Uva ursi

CATEGORY: Herbs and supplements
RELATED TERMS: Arctostaphylos uva-ursi, bearberry
DEFINITION: Natural plant product used as a dietary supplement for specific health benefits.
PRINCIPAL PROPOSED USE: Bladder infection treatment

OVERVIEW

The uva ursi plant is a low-lying evergreen bush whose berries are a favorite of bears, hence the related name "bearberry." However, the leaves of the plant are used medicinally.

Uva ursi has a long history of use for treating urinary conditions both in the Americas and in Europe. Until the development of sulfa antibiotics, its principal active component, arbutin, was frequently prescribed as a urinary antiseptic.

THERAPEUTIC DOSAGES

European recommendations indicate that the dosage of uva ursi should be adjusted to provide 400 to 800 milligrams of arbutin daily. Because of fears of toxicity, this dosage should not be exceeded; furthermore, the herb should not be used for more than two weeks and no more than five times a year.

Uva ursi should be taken with meals to minimize gastrointestinal upset. Uva ursi (based on its arbutin content) is thought to be most effective in alkaline urine and for this reason, it should not be combined with vitamin C or cranberry juice. Some herbal experts recommend taking it with calcium citrate to alkalinize the urine.

Uva ursi is also frequently sold in combination with other herbs traditionally thought to be helpful for bladder infections, including dandelion, cleavers, juniper berry, buchu, and parsley.

THERAPEUTIC USES

Uva ursa is widely marketed today for the treatment of bladder infections. However, it has not been proven effective, and safety concerns exist.

SCIENTIFIC EVIDENCE

Despite uva ursi's popularity for treating bladder infections, there is no meaningful evidence that it works.

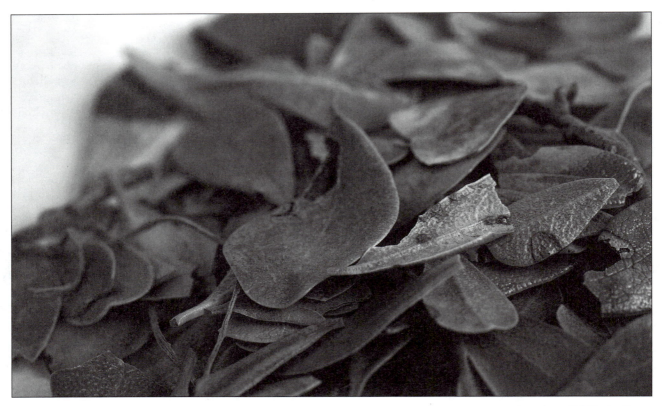

The leaves of the uva ursi plant have a long medicinal history in the treatment of urinary tract disorders. (UIG via Getty Images)

Two studies evaluated the antibacterial power of the urine of people who were taking uva ursi and found activity against most major bacteria that infect the urinary tract. However, while such findings are interesting, what is really needed is a double-blind, placebo-controlled trial to discover whether using uva ursi actually helps people with established urinary tract infections. No study of this type has been reported.

One study evaluated the continuous use of uva ursi for prevention of bladder infections. This double-blind, placebo-controlled trial followed fifty-seven women for one year. One-half were given a standardized dose of uva ursi (in combination with dandelion leaf, intended to promote urine flow), while the others received placebo. Over the course of the study, none of the women on uva ursi developed a bladder infection, whereas five of the untreated women did. However, this study is little more than a curiosity because most experts do not believe that continuous treatment with uva ursi is safe.

SAFETY ISSUES

There are significant safety concerns with uva ursi. The arbutin contained in uva ursi leaves is broken down in the intestine to another chemical, hydroquinone. This chemical is altered a bit by the liver and then sent to the kidneys for excretion. Hydroquinone then acts as an antiseptic in the bladder. However, hydroquinone is also a liver toxin, carcinogen, and irritant. For this reason, uva ursi is not recommended for long-term use. In addition, it should not be taken by young children, pregnant or nursing women, or those with severe liver or kidney disease.

EBSCO CAM Review Board

FURTHER READING

Cybulska, P., et al. "Extracts of Canadian First Nations Medicinal Plants, Used as Natural Products, Inhibit *Neisseria gonorrhoeae* Isolates with Different Antibiotic Resistance Profiles." *Sexually Transmitted*

Diseases (February 4, 2011): DOI: 10.1097/OLQ. 0b013e31820cb166.

Head, K. A. "Natural Approaches to Prevention and Treatment of Infections of the Lower Urinary Tract." *Alternative Medicine Review* 13, no. 3 (2008): 227-244.

See also: Antibiotics, general; Bladder infection; Cranberry; Herbal medicine.

Uveitis

CATEGORY: Condition
RELATED TERMS: Acute anterior uveitis, anterior uveitis, irido-cyclitis, iritis
DEFINITION: Treatment of the inflammation of the uvea, the middle layer of the tissues surrounding the eyeball.
PRINCIPAL PROPOSED NATURAL TREATMENTS: None
OTHER PROPOSED NATURAL TREATMENTS: Turmeric, vitamin E with vitamin C

INTRODUCTION

Uveitis is a condition marked by inflammation of the uvea. The uvea is the middle layer of the tissues surrounding the eyeball, stretching from the iris at the front of the eye to a lining beneath the retina at the back of the eye. The three main types of uveitis are named based on where the inflammation occurs: iritis (or "anterior uveitis"), which affects the front of the eye; cyclitis (or "intermediate uveitis"), for inflammation along the body of the eye; and choroiditis (or "posterior uveitis"), which affects the rear of the eye. Uveitis can also be called acute or chronic, depending on whether it is short or long in duration.

Uveitis usually occurs in only one eye. In the most common forms of uveitis, the eye is reddened, and the redness reaches into the area just next to the iris. The affected pupil may be smaller than the other and its shape may be irregular. Vision is often blurred or misty, and blinking will not clear it. Deep, aching pain generally accompanies uveitis.

Uveitis can begin after injury to the eye or after eye surgery, but it can also start with no obvious trigger. While the underlying cause of uveitis is unknown, autoimmune processes are thought to play a role.

Antioxidants for Treating Uveitis

Antioxidants are substances that may prevent potentially disease-producing cell damage that can result from natural bodily processes or from exposure to certain chemicals. There are a number of different antioxidants found in foods and available as dietary supplements, including vitamins C and E.

Oxidation—one of the body's natural chemical processes—can produce free radicals, which are highly unstable molecules that can damage cells. For example, free radicals are produced when the body breaks down foods for use or storage. They are also produced when the body is exposed to tobacco smoke, radiation, and environmental contaminants. Free radicals can cause damage, known as oxidative stress, which is thought to play a role in the development of many diseases, including eye disease, Alzheimer's disease, cancer, heart disease, Parkinson's disease, and rheumatoid arthritis. In laboratory experiments, antioxidant molecules counter oxidative stress and its associated damage.

If left untreated, uveitis can cause permanent damage to vision, including blindness. For this reason, one should seek medical examination and treatment. The diagnosis of uveitis is made by means of a special medical tool called a slit lamp. Treatment involves medications to reduce inflammation and to control pressure in the eye.

PROPOSED NATURAL TREATMENTS

No natural treatment can substitute for standard medical care for uveitis. However, two natural substances taken together, vitamin C and vitamin E, have shown promise when used in addition to standard treatment.

In a double-blind trial of 145 people undergoing treatment for acute anterior uveitis, participants were additionally given either placebo or combined treatment with vitamin C (500 milligrams [mg] twice daily) and vitamin E (100 mg twice daily). People receiving the real treatment had better visual acuity at the end of the eight-week study period. Researchers hypothesized that free radicals (a class of dangerous, naturally occurring chemicals) play a role in the eye injury caused by uveitis. Vitamin C and vitamin E are antioxidants, and they tend to neutralize free radicals.

While further study is necessary to corroborate these results, it appears plausible that the use of these antioxidants may help keep the eye healthy while it recovers from the condition.

Other antioxidants have also been recommended for acute uveitis, but there is no real evidence that they are helpful. These include beta-carotene, bilberry, citrus bioflavonoids, lipoic acid, lutein, oligomeric proanthocyanidins, selenium, and vitamin A.

Antioxidants are also often recommended for chronic uveitis (combined with conventional care). One study examined the potential benefits of an antioxidant extract made from the herb turmeric and appeared to find benefit. However, this study lacked a placebo group and, therefore, cannot be taken as reliable.

Manufacturers of natural treatments for uveitis make numerous other recommendations, based on speculation only. These treatments include fish oil, flax oil, manganese, vitamin B complex (a mixture of vitamins B_1, B_2, B_3, B_6, and B_{12}; pantothenic acid; biotin; and folate), olive leaf extract, red clover, and zinc.

EBSCO CAM Review Board

FURTHER READING

Gaby, A. R. "Nutritional Therapies for Ocular Disorders." *Alternative Medicine Review* 13 (2008): 191-204.

Lal, B., et al. "Efficacy of Curcumin in the Management of Chronic Anterior Uveitis." *Phytotherapy Research* 13 (1999): 318-322.

Van Rooij, J., et al. "Oral Vitamins C and E as Additional Treatment in Patients with Acute Anterior Uveitis." *British Journal of Ophthalmology* 83 (1999): 1277-1282.

See also: Blepharitis; Cataracts; Conjunctivitis; Glaucoma; Turmeric; Vitamin C; Vitamin E.

V

Vaginal infection

CATEGORY: Condition

RELATED TERMS: Bacterial vaginosis, *Candida*, candidal yeast infection, *Gardnerella*, trichomonas, vaginal yeast infection, vaginitis, yeast infection

DEFINITION: Treatment of bacterial, fungal, and parasitic infections of the vagina.

PRINCIPAL PROPOSED NATURAL TREATMENTS: None

OTHER PROPOSED NATURAL TREATMENTS: Boric acid, essential oils, garlic, goldenseal, probiotics, *Solanum nigrescens*, *Tabebuia avellanedae*, tea tree oil, vitamin C

INTRODUCTION

There are three main causes of vaginal infections: the fungus (yeast) *Candida albicans*, the parasite *Trichomonas vaginalis*, and the bacterial organism *Gardnerella vaginalis*. Factors that can contribute to vaginal infections include antibiotics (which kill friendly bacteria, allowing yeast to grow), corticosteroids and human immunodeficiency virus infection (which suppress the immune system), oral contraceptives and pregnancy (which alter the vaginal environment by changing hormone levels), and diabetes (increased sugar levels provide a friendly environment for yeast).

Conventional medical treatment for vaginal infections caused by *Candida* includes vaginal suppositories containing antifungal medications or, in some cases, oral antifungal medications. Women with diabetes often find that yeast infections are less common when their blood sugar levels are well controlled.

Trichomonas infections are treated with oral metronidazole, and *Gardnerella* infections are treated with oral or vaginal metronidazole or vaginal clindamycin. Nonspecific vaginitis is usually caused by *Gardnerella*, but there are other causes.

PROPOSED NATURAL TREATMENTS

There are some promising natural treatments for vaginal infections caused by *Candida* and other organisms, but the scientific evidence for them is not strong.

Probiotics (friendly bacteria) such as *Lactobacillus acidophilus* are normally found in the vagina. When colonies of these organisms are present, it is difficult for unfriendly organisms, such as *Candida*, to become established. Probiotic supplements can help restore a normal balance of vaginal organisms, which could, in theory, reduce the chance of developing a vaginal yeast infection. For this reason, women who frequently experience yeast infections or who are taking antibiotics are often advised to consume probiotics. However, evidence that probiotics really help prevent vaginal yeast infections remains incomplete and inconsistent. A fairly large study (278 participants) failed to find *Lactobacillus* helpful for preventing yeast infections caused by antibiotics.

Another kind of vaginal infection, called bacterial vaginosis, is most often caused by *G. vaginalis*. In a study of women with a history of bacterial vaginosis, researchers found that vaginally inserting a daily capsule containing the probiotics *L. rhamnosus*, *L. acidophilus*, and *Streptococcus thermophilus* did reduce recurrence. Although this study found benefit, other studies have produced mixed results regarding the benefits of probiotics in the treatment and prevention of bacterial vaginosis.

Tea tree oil, an essential oil from the plant *Melaleuca alternifolia*, possesses antibacterial and antifungal properties and appears to spare friendly bacteria in the *Lactobacillus* family. Tea tree oil has been tried for various forms of vaginal infection, but there is little scientific evidence that it works. In an open trial, ninety-six women with trichomonal vaginitis were treated with tampons saturated in tea tree oil, which were left in the vagina for twenty-four hours, and then followed by daily vaginal douches with a tea tree oil solution. The researcher reported good results with this regimen in three to four weeks. However, because this was not a double-blind trial, the results mean little.

A double-blind study of one hundred women found vitamin C vaginal tablets (250 milligrams) at most marginally helpful for nonspecific vaginitis. Boric acid, a chemical substance with antiseptic properties, was part of a double-blind comparison study of 108 women with yeast infections. The study found that 92 percent of those who used boric acid suppositories nightly for two weeks experienced full recovery, compared to 64 percent of those given suppositories of the "outdated" antifungal drug nystatin. However, there are safety concerns with boric acid. If taken internally, it is quite toxic. For this reason, it should not be applied to open wounds. In addition, it should not be used by pregnant women or be applied to the skin of infants.

A single-blind trial, involving one hundred women with *Candida* vaginitis, compared nystatin suppositories with suppositories made from the plant *Solanum nigrescens* and found equivalent benefits. However, this plant can be toxic and should not be used except under physician supervision.

Test-tube studies have found antifungal properties in numerous herbs, including the tropical tree *Tabebuia avellanedae*, garlic extracts, the plant alkaloid berberine sulfate (found in goldenseal), and essential oils of various plants, including cinnamon, eucalyptus, lemongrass, oregano, palmarosa, and peppermint.

EBSCO CAM Review Board

FURTHER READING

Barrons, R., and D. Tassone. "Use of *Lactobacillus* Probiotics for Bacterial Genitourinary Infections in Women." *Clinical Therapeutics* 30 (2008): 453-468.

Falagas, M.E., G. I. Betsi, and S. Athanasiou. "Probiotics for the Treatment of Women with Bacterial Vaginosis." *Clinical Microbiology and Infection* 13 (2007): 657-664.

Jeavons, H. S. "Prevention and Treatment of Vulvovaginal Candidiasis Using Exogenous *Lactobacillus*." *Journal of Obstetric, Gynecologic, and Neonatal Nursing* 32 (2003): 287-296.

Larsson, P. G., et al. "Human Lactobacilli as Supplementation of Clindamycin to Patients with Bacterial Vaginosis Reduce the Recurrence Rate." *BMC Women's Health* 8 (2008): 3.

Petersen, E. E., and P. Magnani. Efficacy and Safety of Vitamin C Vaginal Tablets in the Treatment of Non-specific Vaginitis." *European Journal of Obstetrics, Gynecology, and Reproductive Biology* 117 (2004): 70-75.

Petricevic, L., and A. Witt. "The Role of *L Actobacillus casei rhamnosus* Lcr35 in Restoring the Normal Vaginal Flora After Antibiotic Treatment of Bacterial Vaginosis." *BJOG: An International Journal of Obstetrics and Gynaecology* 115 (2008): 1369-1374.

Pirotta, M., et al. "Effect of *Lactobacillus* in Preventing Post-Antibiotic Vulvovaginal Candidiasis." *British Medical Journal* 329 (2004): 548.

Ya, W., C. Reifer, and L. E. Miller. "Efficacy of Vaginal Probiotic Capsules for Recurrent Bacterial Vaginosis." *American Journal of Obstetrics and Gynecology* 203 (2010): e1-6.

See also: Bladder infection; Candida/yeast hypersensitivity syndrome; Endometriosis; Polycystic ovary syndrome; Pregnancy support; Probiotics; Women's health.

Valerian

CATEGORY: Herbs and supplements
RELATED TERM: *Valeriana officinalis*
DEFINITION: Natural plant product used to treat specific health conditions.
PRINCIPAL PROPOSED USE: Insomnia
OTHER PROPOSED USES: Anxiety, nervous stomach, stress

OVERVIEW

More than two hundred plant species belong to the genus *Valeriana*, but the one most commonly used as an herb is *V. officinalis*. The root is used for medicinal purposes.

Galen recommended valerian for insomnia in the second century. Beginning in the sixteenth century, this herb became popular as a sedative in Europe, and it later became popular in the United States. Scientific studies on valerian in humans began in the 1970s, leading to its approval as a sleep aid by Germany's Commission E in 1985. However, the scientific evidence showing that valerian really works remains incomplete.

As with most herbs, experts are not exactly sure which ingredients in valerian are most important. Early research focused on a group of chemicals known as valepotriates, but they are no longer considered candidates. A constituent called valerenic acid has also undergone study, but its role is far from clear. Another substance in valerian, called linarin, has also attracted research interest.

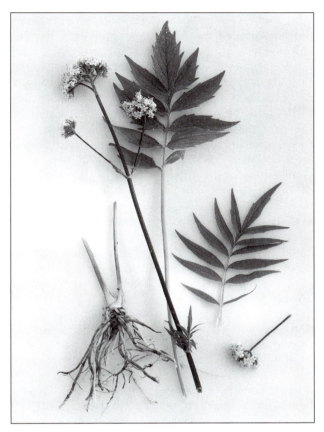

Valerian plant with flowers and root. (Michael Rosenfeld/ Getty Images)

The understanding of how valerian might function remains similarly incomplete. Several studies suggest that valerian affects GABA, a naturally occurring amino acid that appears to be related to the experience of anxiety. Conventional tranquilizers in the valium family are known to bind to GABA receptors in the brain, and valerian may work similarly. However, there are some significant flaws in these hypotheses, and the reality is that experts do not really know how valerian works, or, indeed, whether it does work.

THERAPEUTIC DOSAGES

For insomnia, the standard adult dosage of valerian is 2 grams (g) to 3 g of dried herb, 270 to 450 mg of an aqueous valerian extract, or 600 mg of an ethanol extract, taken thirty to sixty minutes before bedtime. The same amount, or a reduced dose, can be taken twice daily for anxiety.

Because of valerian's unpleasant odor, European manufacturers have created odorless valerian products. However, these are not widely available in the United States. Valerian is not recommended for children under three years old.

THERAPEUTIC USES

Valerian is commonly recommended as a mild treatment for occasional insomnia. However, evidence from the best positive study on valerian suggests that it is useful only when taken over an extended period of time for chronic sleep disorders. Overall, it is not clear whether valerian is effective for sleep at all.

Like other treatments used for insomnia, valerian has also been proposed as a treatment for anxiety, but there is no reliable evidence that it is effective. Finally, valerian is sometimes suggested as a treatment for a nervous stomach; however, there is no supporting scientific evidence for this use.

SCIENTIFIC EVIDENCE

Insomnia. Overall, the evidence supporting valerian as a sleep aid remains substantially incomplete and contradictory. A systematic review published in 2007 concluded that valerian is probably not effective for treating insomnia. In a subsequent review of eighteen randomized trials, researchers found that people who took valerian did report an improvement in their sleep, but this finding was not supported by more objective measures of sleep quality.

However, there have been some positive results, both with valerian alone and with valerian combined with other herbs. The best positive study of valerian for insomnia followed 121 people for twenty-eight days. In this double-blind, placebo-controlled trial, half of the participants took 600 milligrams (mg) of an alcohol-based valerian extract one hour before bedtime, while the other half took placebo. Valerian did not work right away. For the first couple of weeks, valerian and placebo were running neck and neck. However, by day twenty-eight, valerian pulled far ahead. Effectiveness was rated as good or very good by participant evaluation in 66 percent of the valerian group and in 61 percent by doctor evaluation, whereas in the placebo group, effectiveness was so rated by only 29 percent of participants and doctors.

Although positive, these results are a bit confusing. In another large study, valerian was immediately more effective than placebo, which is more in keeping with how the herb is typically used. This trial followed 128 subjects who had no sleeping problems. On nine nonconsecutive nights, each participant took one of three treatments: valerian, a combination of valerian and the herb hops, or placebo. The results showed that on the nights they took valerian alone, participants fell asleep faster than when they were taking placebo or the combination. In contradiction to this, other studies have failed to find any immediate mental-depressant effects with valerian; most substances that rapidly induce sleep also sedate the mind.

Furthermore, the more recent and best-designed studies have generally failed to find valerian more helpful at all. One of these was a four-week study in which 135 people were given valerian and 135 were given placebo. Another was a two-week study of 405 people that found "modest benefits at most."

A six-week, double-blind study of 202 people with insomnia compared valerian extract (600 mg at bedtime) with the standard drug oxazepam (10 mg at bedtime) and found equal efficacy. Equivalent benefits were also seen in a similar study of 75 people. However, the absence of a placebo group in these two studies decreases the reliability of the results.

A study of 184 people tested a standardized combination of valerian and hops, with mixed results. Researchers tested quite a few aspects of sleep, such as time to fall asleep, length of sleep, and number of awakenings, and found evidence of benefit in only a few. This use of "multiple outcome measures" makes the results somewhat unreliable.

A much smaller study also found evidence that a combination of hops and valerian extract is more effective as a sleep aid than placebo. The results of this trial also hint that hops plus valerian is more effective than valerian alone, but this possible finding did not reach statistical significance.

A double-blind comparative study that enrolled forty-six patients compared the effects of the standard drug bromazepam to a mixture of valerian and hops with either treatment taken half an hour before bedtime. The results suggest that the two treatments were equally effective. One study found that this valerian-hops combination can antagonize the arousal produced by caffeine.

A combination of valerian and lemon balm has also been tried for insomnia. A rather poorly designed thirty-day, double-blind, placebo-controlled study of ninety-eight individuals without insomnia found mar-

ginal evidence that a valerian-lemon balm combination improved sleep quality compared with placebo. However, a double-blind crossover study of twenty people with insomnia compared the benefits of the sleeping drug Halcion (0.125 mg) against placebo and a combination of valerian and lemon balm and failed to find the herb effective. The drug, however, did prove effective. In addition, valerian has shown some promise for helping people sleep better after discontinuing conventional sleeping pills in the benzodiazepine family.

Anxiety and stress. In a double-blind, placebo-controlled study, thirty-six people with generalized anxiety disorder were given either valerian extract, Valium, or placebo for a period of four weeks. The study failed to find statistically significant differences between the groups, presumably due to its small size.

Valerian has also been tested for possible benefits during stressful circumstances. Two preliminary double-blind studies found weak evidence that valerian may produce calming effects in induced stressful situations. Another study evaluated the effects of a combination containing valerian and lemon balm taken in various doses. Some benefits were seen with doses of 600 mg or 1200 mg three times daily, but the highest dose, 1,800 mg three times daily, actually appeared to increase anxiety symptoms during a stressful situation. Furthermore, people taking the herbal treatment at any dose showed slightly decreased cognitive function compared with those given placebo.

SAFETY ISSUES

Valerian is on the U.S. Food and Drug Administration's (FDA) Generally Recognized As Safe (GRAS) list and is approved for use as a food. In animals, it takes enormous doses of valerian to produce any serious adverse effects. Valerian has shown an excellent safety profile in clinical trials.

In a suicide attempt, one young woman took approximately 20 g of valerian, twenty to forty times the recommended dose. Only mild symptoms developed, including stomach cramps, fatigue, chest tightness, tremors, and light-headedness. All of these symptoms were resolved within twenty-four hours after two treatments with activated charcoal. The woman's laboratory tests, including tests of her liver function, remained normal. However, this does not mean that people can safely exceed the recommended dose.

One report did find toxic results from herbal remedies containing valerian mixed with several other herbal ingredients, including skullcap. Four individuals who took these remedies later developed liver problems. However, skullcap products are sometimes contaminated with the liver-toxic herb germander, and this could have been the explanation.

There have also been about fifty reported cases of overdose with a combination preparation called Sleep-Qik, which contains valerian, as well as conventional medications. Researchers specifically looked for liver injury, but they found no evidence that it occurred.

There are some safety concerns about valepotriates, constituents of valerian, because in test-tube studies they have been found to affect deoxyribonucleic acid (DNA) and cause other toxic effects. However, valepotriates are not present to a significant extent in any commercial preparations.

Although no animal studies or controlled human trials have found evidence that valerian causes withdrawal symptoms when stopped, one case report is sometimes cited in support of the possibility that this might occur. It concerns a fifty-eight-year-old man who developed delirium and rapid heartbeat after surgery. According to the patient's family, he had been taking high doses of valerian root extract, about 2.5 to 10 g per day, for many years. His physicians decided that he was suffering from valerian withdrawal. However, considering the many other factors involved, such as multiple medications and general anesthesia, it is not really possible to conclude that valerian caused his symptoms.

In clinical trials, use of valerian has not been associated with any significant side effects. A few people experience mild gastrointestinal distress, and there have been rare reports of people developing a paradoxical mild stimulant effect from valerian.

Valerian does not appear to impair driving ability or produce morning drowsiness when taken at night. As noted above, most studies have failed to find any immediate sedative effect with valerian. However, one study reported finding mild impairment of attention for a couple of hours after taking valerian. For this reason, it is not a good idea to drive immediately after taking it.

There have been no reported drug interactions with valerian, and two studies found reasons to believe that valerian should not raise or lower the blood levels of too many medications. Nonetheless, there are at least theoretical concerns that valerian might amplify the effects of sedative drugs. A 1995 study was somewhat reassuring on this score because it found no interaction between alcohol and valerian. However, animal studies have found that valerian extracts may prolong the effects of some sedatives, and there have been some worrisome case reports suggesting that the combination of valerian and alcohol can lead to excessive sedation in some people. For this reason, experts recommend that people not combine valerian with central nervous system depressants, except under a doctor's supervision.

Safety in young children, pregnant or nursing women, and those with severe liver or kidney disease has not been established. People who are taking sedative drugs, such as benzodiazepines, should not take valerian in addition to them, except under physician supervision.

EBSCO CAM Review Board

FURTHER READING

Bent, S., et al. "Valerian for Sleep." *American Journal of Medicine* 119 (2006): 1005-1012.

Donovan, J. L., et al. "Multiple Night-Time Doses of Valerian (*Valeriana officinalis*) Had Minimal Effects on CYP3A4 Activity and No Effect on CYP2D6 Activity in Healthy Volunteers." *Drug Metabolism and Disposition: The Biological Fate of Chemicals* 32 (2004): 1333-1336.

Fernández-San-Martín, M. I., et al. "Effectiveness of Valerian on Insomnia." *Sleep Medicine* 11, no. 6 (2010): 505-511.

Gurley, B. J., et al. "In Vivo Effects of Goldenseal, Kava Kava, Black Cohosh, and Valerian on Human Cytochrome P450 1A2, 2D6, 2E1, and 3A4/5 Phenotypes." *Clinical Pharmacology and Therapeutics* 77 (2005): 415-426.

Jacobs, B. P., et al. "An Internet-Based Randomized, Placebo-Controlled Trial of Kava and Valerian for Anxiety and Insomnia." *Medicine* 84, no. 4 (2005): 197-207.

Kennedy, D. O., et al. "Anxiolytic Effects of a Combination of *Melissa officinalis* and *Valeriana officinalis* During Laboratory Induced Stress." *Phytotherapy Research* 20 (2006): 96-102.

Koetter, U., et al. "A randomized, Double Blind, Placebo-Controlled, Prospective Clinical Study to Demonstrate Clinical Efficacy of a Fixed Valerian Hops Extract Combination (Ze 91019) in Patients

Suffering from Non-organic Sleep Disorder." *Phytotherapy Research* 21, no. 9 (2007): 847-851.

Morin, C. M., et al. "Valerian-Hops Combination and Diphenhydramine for Treating Insomnia." *Sleep* 28 (2005): 1465-1471.

Oxman, A. D., et al. "A Televised, Web-Based Randomised Trial of an Herbal Remedy (Valerian) for Insomnia." *PLoS One* 2, no. 10 (2007): e1040.

Taibi, D. M., et al. "A Randomized Clinical Trial of Valerian Fails to Improve Self-Reported, Polysomnographic, and Actigraphic Sleep in Older Women with Insomnia." *Sleep Medicine* 10, no. 3 (2009): 319-328.

_____. "A Systematic Review of Valerian as a Sleep Aid: Safe but Not Effective." *Sleep Medicine Reviews* 11 (2007): 209-230.

See also: Anxiety and panic attacks; Insomnia; Stress.

Valproic acid

CATEGORY: Drug interactions

DEFINITION: A commonly used anticonvulsant treatment.

INTERACTIONS: Biotin, carnitine, dong quai, folate, ginkgo, glutamine, melatonin, St. John's wort, vitamin A, vitamin D, white willow

TRADE NAMES: Depakene

DRUGS IN THIS FAMILY: Depakene syrup, depakote, depakote sprinkle, divalproex sodium, sodium valproate

CARNITINE

Effect: Supplementation Possibly Helpful

Carnitine is an amino acid that has been used for heart conditions, Alzheimer's disease, and intermittent claudication. Intermittent claudication is a possible complication of atherosclerosis in which impaired blood circulation causes severe pain in calf muscles during walking or exercising.

Long-term therapy with anticonvulsant agents, particularly valproic acid, is associated with low levels of carnitine. However, it is not clear whether the anticonvulsants cause the carnitine deficiency or whether it occurs for other reasons. It has been hypothesized that low carnitine levels may contribute to valproic acid's damaging effects on the liver. The risk of this liver damage increases in children younger than twenty-four months, and carnitine supplementation does seem to be protective. However, in one double-blind crossover study, carnitine supplementation produced no real improvement in "well-being" as assessed by parents of children receiving either valproic acid or carbamazepine. L-carnitine supplementation may be advisable in certain cases, such as in infants and young children (especially those younger than two years) who have neurologic disorders and are receiving valproic acid and multiple anticonvulsants.

VITAMIN D

Effect: Supplementation Possibly Helpful

Valproic acid slows down the liver's conversion of vitamin D into the active form of the vitamin that can be used by the body. This effect might lead to reduced calcium absorption, since the body needs active vitamin D to absorb calcium properly. Therefore, it might be advisable to take vitamin D supplements at the U.S. Adequate Intake (AI) dosage.

FOLATE

Effect: Supplementation Possibly Helpful

Folate (also known as folic acid) is a B vitamin that plays an important role in many vital aspects of health, including preventing neural tube birth defects and possibly reducing the risk of heart disease. Because inadequate intake of folate is widespread, if one is taking any medication that depletes or impairs folate even slightly, one may need supplementation. Valproic acid appears to decrease the body's absorption of folate, and other antiseizure drugs can also reduce levels of folate in the body. The low serum folate caused by anticonvulsants can raise homocysteine levels, a condition believed to increase the risk of heart disease.

Adequate folate intake is also necessary to prevent neural tube birth defects, such as spina bifida and anencephaly. Because anticonvulsant drugs deplete folate, babies born to women taking anticonvulsants are at increased risk for such birth defects. Anticonvulsants may also play a more direct role in the development of birth defects.

However, the case for taking extra folate during anticonvulsant therapy is not as simple as it might seem. It is possible that folate supplementation might itself impair the effectiveness of anticonvulsant drugs, and physician supervision is necessary.

MELATONIN

Effect: Supplementation Possibly Helpful

One double-blind study in children found that use of melatonin improved general quality of life in children on valproic acid. The most obvious way melatonin might help would involve improvements in sleep, as melatonin is a widely used treatment for insomnia. Another rather theoretical study by the same author suggests it might help in other more subtle ways that involve the body's biochemistry.

BIOTIN

Effect: Supplementation Possibly Helpful, but Take at a Different Time of Day

Many antiseizure medications, including valproic acid, are believed to interfere with the absorption of biotin. For this reason, persons taking valproic acid may benefit from extra biotin. Biotin should be taken two to three hours apart from antiseizure medication. One should not exceed the recommended daily intake, because it is possible that too much biotin might interfere with the effectiveness of the medication.

VITAMIN A

Effect: Possible Increased Risk of Birth Defects

Both valproic acid and vitamin A can increase the risk of birth defects. The effect might be additive, indicating that pregnant women should avoid such combination treatment.

GLUTAMINE

Effect: Theoretical Harmful Interaction

Because valproic acid works (at least in part) by blocking glutamate pathways in the brain, high dosages of glutamine might possibly overwhelm the drug and increase the risk of seizures.

WHITE WILLOW

Effect: Possible Negative Interaction

The herb white willow contains substances very similar to aspirin. On this basis, it might not be advisable to combine white willow with valproic acid.

GINKGO

Effect: Possible Harmful Interaction

The herb ginkgo is widely used for improving memory and mental function. Seizures also have been reported with the use of ginkgo leaf extract in people with previously well-controlled epilepsy; in one case, the seizures were fatal. One possible explanation is contamination of ginkgo leaf products with ginkgo seeds. It has also been suggested that ginkgo might interfere with the effectiveness of some antiseizure medications, including phenytoin. Finally, it has been noted that the drug tacrine (also used to improve memory) has been associated with seizures, and ginkgo may affect the brain in ways similar to tacrine.

DONG QUAI, ST. JOHN'S WORT

Effect: Possible Harmful Interaction

Valproic acid has been reported to cause increased sensitivity to the sun, amplifying the risk of sunburn or skin rash. Because St. John's wort and dong quai may also cause this problem, taking them during treatment with this drug might add to this risk.

EBSCO CAM Review Board

FURTHER READING

De Vivo, D. C., et al. "L-carnitine Supplementation in Childhood Epilepsy: Current Perspectives." *Epilepsia* 39 (1998): 1216-1225.

Granger, A. S. "*Ginkgo biloba* Precipitating Epileptic Seizures." *Age and Ageing* 30 (2001): 523-525.

Gupta, M., S. Aneja, and K. Kohli. "Add-on Melatonin Improves Quality of Life in Epileptic Children on Valproate Monotherapy." *Epilepsy and Behavior* 5 (2004): 316-321.

Kupiec, T., and V. Raj. "Fatal Seizures Due to Potential Herb-Drug Interactions with *Ginkgo biloba*." *Journal of Analytical Toxicology* 29 (2006): 755-758.

Lewis, D. P., et al. "Drug and Environmental Factors Associated with Adverse Pregnancy Outcomes: Part 1–Antiepileptic Drugs, Contraceptives, Smoking, and Folate." *Annals of Pharmacotherapy* 32 (1998): 802-817.

See also: Biotin; Carnitine; Dong quai; Folate; Food and Drug Administration; Ginkgo; Glutamine; Melatonin; St. John's wort; Supplements: Introduction; Vitamin A, Vitamin D; White willow.

Varicose veins

CATEGORY: Condition

RELATED TERM: Venous insufficiency

DEFINITION: Treatment of the condition that causes damage to veins that are near the surface of the skin.

PRINCIPAL PROPOSED NATURAL TREATMENTS: Butcher's broom, gotu kola, horse chestnut, oligomeric proanthocyanidins, oxerutins and other bioflavonoids, red vine leaf (grape leaf)

OTHER PROPOSED NATURAL TREATMENTS: Balneotherapy, bromelain, calendula, *Collinsonia*, comfrey, mesoglycan, *Mimosa tenuiflora*, witch hazel

INTRODUCTION

Walking upright places a burden on the veins of the leg. Although they lack the strong muscular lining of arteries, the leg veins must constantly return a large volume of blood to the heart. The movements of the legs act as a pump to push the blood upward, while flimsy valves stop gravity from pulling the blood back down.

However, over time these valves often begin to fail. The blood then begins to pool in the deep veins of the leg, stretching the vein wall and injuring its lining. This leads to venous insufficiency. Typically, the legs begin to feel heavy, swollen, achy, and tired. Varicose veins, a condition closely related to venous insufficiency, occur when veins near the surface of the skin are damaged. They visibly dilate and become distorted, resulting in a cosmetically unpleasant appearance.

Varicose veins affect women about two to three times as often as men. Occupations involving prolonged standing also increase the incidence of venous insufficiency. Pregnancy and obesity do so as well, because the increase of pressure in the abdomen makes it more difficult for the blood to flow upward.

Conventional medical treatment of venous insufficiency consists mainly of reducing weight, elevating the legs, and wearing elastic support hose. Unsightly damaged veins can be destroyed by injection therapy or be surgically removed.

PRINCIPAL PROPOSED NATURAL TREATMENTS

When it comes to natural products, some illnesses are far more responsive than others. While there are no well-documented natural therapies for asthma (as an example), more than half a dozen natural therapies have meaningful supporting evidence as treatments for varicose veins or venous insufficiency.

These treatments have much in common. All of them appear to work by strengthening the walls of veins and other vessels, with the net effect of reducing fluid leakage. Studies indicate that the use of such products reduces leg swelling and pain. However,

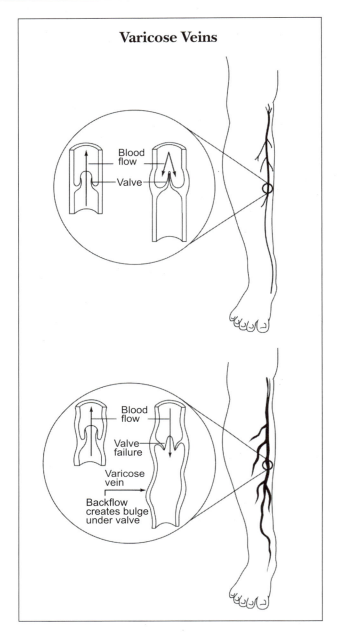

Varicose Veins

there is no meaningful evidence that any natural product can cure unsightly varicose veins that already exist or prevent new ones from developing.

Symptoms similar to those caused by varicose veins can actually be caused by dangerous conditions such as phlebitis or thrombosis. One should consult a doctor before self-treating with the natural supplements described here.

Horse chestnut. The most popular herbal treatment

for venous insufficiency and varicose veins is horse chestnut. More than eight hundred people have been involved in double-blind, placebo-controlled studies of horse chestnut for treating venous insufficiency. One of the largest of these trials followed 212 people for forty days using a crossover design. Participants initially received either horse chestnut or placebo and were then crossed over to the other treatment (without their knowledge) after twenty days. Horse chestnut treatment significantly reduced leg edema, pain, and the sensation of heaviness when compared with placebo. However, the design of this study was not quite up to modern standards. A better-designed double-blind study of seventy-four people also found benefit.

Good results were also seen in a partially double-blind, placebo-controlled study that compared the effectiveness of horse chestnut to that of compression stockings in 240 people for twelve weeks (horse chestnut and placebo were blinded, but the compression stockings were not). Compression stockings worked faster to lessen swelling, but by twelve weeks, the results were equivalent between the two treatments, and both were better than placebo.

Unlike many herbs, the active ingredients in horse chestnut have been identified to a reasonable degree of certainty. The ingredients appear to be a complex of related chemicals known as aescin. Aescin reduces the rate of fluid leakage from stressed and irritated vessel walls. It is not known how this works, but the most prominent theory proposes that aescin plugs leaking capillaries, prevents the release of enzymes that break down collagen and open holes in capillary walls, and forestalls other forms of vein damage.

Oxerutins and other bioflavonoids. Oxerutins have been widely used in Europe since the mid-1960s but remain hard to find in North America. Derived from a naturally occurring bioflavonoid called rutin, oxerutins were specifically developed to treat varicose veins and related venous problems. It is not clear whether this particular derivative of rutin is more effective than other bioflavonoids used for these conditions, but oxerutins are by far the best studied.

About twenty double-blind, placebo-controlled studies, enrolling a total of more than two thousand persons, have examined the effectiveness of oxerutins for treating varicose veins and venous insufficiency. Virtually all have found oxerutins significantly more effective than placebo, giving substantial relief from swelling, aching, leg pains, and other uncomfortable symptoms, while causing no significant side effects. Together, these studies make a strong case for the use of oxerutins in these conditions.

For example, a twelve-week, double-blind, placebo-controlled study enrolled 133 women with moderate, chronic venous insufficiency. One-half received 1,000 milligrams (mg) of oxerutins daily, and the rest of the participants took placebo. All participants were also fitted with standard compression stockings and wore them for the duration of the trial. The researchers measured subjective symptoms, such as aches and pains, and objective measures of edema in the leg.

Those who took oxerutins experienced significantly less lower-leg edema than the placebo group. Furthermore, these better results lasted through a six-week follow-up period, even though participants were no longer taking oxerutins. The stockings produced no lasting benefit after participants stopped wearing them. They gave symptomatic relief while they were worn, but they did not improve capillary circulation in a lasting way, as oxerutins apparently did.

Several other double-blind, placebo-controlled studies have also found benefits with oxerutins. Additionally, there is some evidence that troxerutin, one of the compounds in the standardized mixture sold as oxerutins, may be effective when taken alone, though perhaps not as effective as the standard mixture of oxerutins.

Oxerutins are closely related to the natural flavonoid rutin, which is found primarily in citrus fruits and buckwheat. Two double-blind, placebo-controlled studies suggest that buckwheat tea might also be effective against varicose veins, presumably because of its rutin content. Other citrus-derived bioflavonoids, such as diosmin, hesperidin, and hidrosmin, may also be effective.

Oligomeric proanthocyanidins. Grape seed and pine bark contain high levels of special bioflavonoids called oligomeric proanthocyanidin complexes (OPCs). Similar substances are found in cranberry, bilberry, blueberry, hawthorn, and other plants.

OPCs are antioxidant chemicals that appear to have the ability to improve collagen (a type of strengthening tissue found in many parts of the body), reduce capillary leakage, and control inflammation.

Placebo-controlled studies (most of them double-blind) involving about four hundred participants, suggest that OPCs provide significant benefit for varicose veins. For example, a double-blind study

Treating Varicose Veins with Horse Chestnut

The horse chestnut tree (*Aesculus hippocastanum*) is native to the Balkan Peninsula but grows throughout the Northern Hemisphere. Although horse chestnut is sometimes called buckeye, it should not be confused with the Ohio or California buckeye trees, which are related but not the same species.

For centuries, horse chestnut seeds, leaves, bark, and flowers have been used for a variety of conditions and diseases. Horse chestnut seed extract has been used to treat chronic venous insufficiency (a condition in which the veins do not efficiently return blood from the legs to the heart). This condition is associated with varicose veins, pain, ankle swelling, feelings of heaviness, itching, and nighttime leg cramping.

Studies have found that horse chestnut seed extract is indeed beneficial in treating chronic venous insufficiency. There is also preliminary evidence that horse chestnut seed extract may be as effective as wearing compression stockings. There is not enough scientific evidence to support the use of horse chestnut seed, leaf, or bark for any other conditions.

When properly processed, horse chestnut seed extract contains little or no aesculin (or esculin), a poison, and is considered generally safe when used for short periods of time. However, the extract can cause some side effects, including itching, nausea, or gastrointestinal upset.

---

comparing grape seed OPCs with placebo in seventy-one persons showed improvement in 75 percent of the treated group, compared to 41 percent in the control group. Similarly, a two-month, double-blind, placebo-controlled trial of forty persons with chronic venous insufficiency found that 100 mg three times daily of OPCs from pine bark significantly reduced edema, pain, and the sensation of leg heaviness. Another double-blind, placebo-controlled study of twenty persons also found OPCs from pine bark effective. In addition, evidence from small double-blind trials suggests that OPCs might be more effective for venous insufficiency than either diosmin or horse chestnut.

Gotu kola. There is significant scientific evidence for the effectiveness of the herb gotu kola in varicose veins and venous insufficiency. A vacuum suction chamber has been used in some gotu kola studies to evaluate the rate of fluid leakage in venous insufficiency. The vacuum produces swelling when applied to the skin of the ankle. When leg veins are leaking a lot of fluid, this swelling takes longer to disappear.

In one study of people with venous insufficiency, two weeks of treatment with gotu kola extracts was shown to reduce the time necessary for the swelling to disappear. A placebo-controlled study (whether it was double-blind was not stated) of fifty-two persons with venous insufficiency compared the effects of gotu kola extract at 180 and 90 mg daily with placebo. After four weeks of treatment, researchers observed improvement in various measurements of vein function in all treated persons, but not in the placebo group. They also found that the higher dose was more effective than the lower dose. This kind of dose responsiveness is generally taken as good evidence that a treatment is actually effective.

Another study of double-blind design followed eighty-seven people with varicose veins and compared the benefits of gotu kola at 60 and 30 mg daily with placebo. Again, the results showed improvements in both of the treated groups, but greater improvement at the higher dose.

A double-blind study of ninety-four people with venous insufficiency of the lower limb compared the benefits of gotu kola extract at 120 and 60 mg daily with placebo. The results also showed a significant dose-related improvement in the treated groups in symptoms such as subjective heaviness, discomfort, and edema.

A 1992 review of all the gotu kola studies available concluded that gotu kola extract provides a dose-related improvement in venous insufficiency symptoms, reducing foot swelling, ankle edema, and fluid leakage from the veins.

Red vine leaf. Extracts of red vine leaf (*Folia vitis viniferae*, or grape leaf) have also been tried as a treatment for chronic venous insufficiency. One twelve-week, double-blind, placebo-controlled study followed 219 people with chronic venous insufficiency. In this study, daily doses of 360 and 720 mg of red vine leaf extract both proved significantly more effective than placebo in reducing edema and in improving pain and other symptoms. The researchers concluded that the higher dosage resulted in a slightly greater, more sustained improvement. Benefits were also seen in a much smaller study. (The usual dose of red vine leaf is 360 or 720 mg taken once daily.)

In the foregoing double-blind study, side effects were largely limited to mild gastrointestinal distress and occasional reports of headaches. Blood tests and physical examination did not reveal any harmful effects. However, comprehensive safety studies have not been performed, and red vine leaf is not recommended for pregnant or nursing women or for persons with severe liver or kidney disease.

Butcher's broom. Butcher's broom (*Ruscus aculeatus*) is so named because its branches were a traditional source of broom straw used by butchers. This Mediterranean evergreen bush has a long history of traditional use in the treatment of urinary conditions. More recent European interest has focused on the possible value of butcher's broom in the treatment of hemorrhoids and varicose veins.

A well-designed and well-reported double-blind trial evaluated the effectiveness of a standardized butcher's broom extract in 166 women with chronic venous insufficiency. For twelve weeks, participants received either placebo or butcher's broom (one tablet twice daily containing 36 to 37.5 mg of a methanol dry extract concentrated at 15-20:1). The results showed that leg swelling (the primary measurement used) decreased significantly in the butcher's broom group compared with the placebo group. Similar results were seen in a twelve-week, double-blind, placebo-controlled trial with 148 participants.

Other Proposed Natural Treatments

A minimum of twenty double-blind, placebo-controlled studies have evaluated the efficacy of a popular European treatment containing butcher's broom extract combined with the bioflavonoid hesperidin methyl chalcone as well as vitamin C. Although not all studies were positive, and many had design flaws, in general it appears that this combination treatment is more effective than placebo.

A substance extracted from pig intestines known as mesoglycan has been investigated in Italy as a remedy for varicose veins and related conditions. In the best of the reported trials, 183 persons with leg ulcers caused by poor vein function were treated with either placebo or mesoglycan (first by injection and then orally) for twenty-four weeks. The results of this double-blind study suggest that mesoglycan significantly improved the rate at which the leg ulcers healed.

The bark of the tree *Mimosa tenuiflora* is used in Mexico to treat skin problems. One small, double-blind, placebo-controlled study hints that the use of a gel containing *M. tenuiflora* extract might also help heal such vein-related leg ulcerations.

Bromelain is not actually a single substance but, rather, a collection of protein-digesting enzymes found in pineapple juice and in the stems of pineapple plants. Although there is no direct evidence on its use for varicose veins, bromelain has antiedema effects similar to those of treatments used for varicose veins, suggesting that it might be helpful.

The herb *Collinsonia*, or stone root, has a long history of use as an oral treatment for varicose veins and hemorrhoids, but it has not been scientifically evaluated to any meaningful extent. The same is true of topical witch hazel, comfrey, and calendula.

Balneotherapy, which involves the use of aqueous spa treatments such as warm and cold baths, mud packs, saunas, and steam baths, has been promoted for the treatment of varicose veins. A small randomized trial in France found that four daily balneotherapy sessions for three weeks significantly improved skin changes and quality of life in subjects with moderate to severe varicose veins, compared to a group waiting to undergo the therapy.

EBSCO CAM Review Board

Further Reading

Boyle, P., C. Diehm, and C. Robertson. "Meta-analysis of Clinical Trials of Cyclo 3 Fort in the Treatment of Chronic Venous Insufficiency." *International Angiology* 22 (2003): 250-262.

Carpentier, P. H., and B. Satger. "Evaluation of Balneotherapy Associated with Patient Education in Patients with Advanced Chronic Venous Insufficiency." *Journal of Vascular Surgery* 49 (2009): 163-170.

Petruzzellis, V., et al. "Oxerutins (Venoruton): Efficacy in Chronic Venous Insufficiency." *Angiology* 53 (2002): 257-263.

Rivera-Arce, E., et al. "Therapeutic Effectiveness of a *Mimosa tenuiflora* Cortex Extract in Venous Leg Ulceration Treatment." *Journal of Ethnopharmacology* 109 (2007): 523-528.

See also: Aging; Butcher's broom; Citrus bioflavonoids; Horse chestnut; Gotu kola; Oligomeric proanthocyanidin; Oxerutins; Venous insufficiency: Homeopathic remedies; Women's health.

Vega test

CATEGORY: Therapies and techniques

RELATED TERMS: Electroacupuncture according to Voll, electrodermal testing, honeycomb device, Vega-test machine

DEFINITION: A technique that measures the body's electrical resistance at acupuncture points.

OVERVIEW

An unconventional device called the Vega-test machine is promoted by some alternative medicine practitioners for diagnosing illnesses and determining appropriate treatments. Other names for this approach include electrodermal testing (EDT) and electroacupuncture according to Voll (EAV). The method, which has many variations, generally involves measuring the body's electrical resistance at acupuncture points. Possible allergens or toxins, or prospective treatments, are placed within a device called a honeycomb that is said to test the effects of that substance on the body. More recent devices use a computer that reportedly simulates the presence of test substances.

There is no commonly accepted scientific basis for the use of this method. To the limited extent that it has been tested, it has not proven itself a valid diagnostic technique.

SCIENTIFIC EVIDENCE

Four Vega-test practitioners, each with a minimum of ten years experience, agreed to participate in a study conducted by a proponent of EDT testing. Thirty people volunteered to participate as subjects in the study. One-half of the volunteers had known allergies to house dust mites or cat dander (as determined by skin testing), while the others were not allergic to these allergens. Each participant was tested with six items in three separate sessions by each of three different operators of the Vega machine, resulting in more than fifteen hundred separate allergy tests over the course of the study. The results showed that the Vega-test practitioners were unable to distinguish between allergic and nonallergic participants. In addition, no individual operator of the machine was more accurate than any other.

In another study, the Vega test failed to distinguish between people with respiratory allergies to a defined set of substances and those without them. One smaller double-blind study did find the Vega test capable of distinguishing between allergens and nonallergens. However, one of the authors of this study felt that it suffered from significant flaws, and he went on to conduct the foregoing first trial.

On the basis of this information, the only fair assessment is that the Vega test has not been shown to be a meaningful method of identifying allergies to dust mites or cat dander. Proponents of the Vega device and other EDT techniques object that the device's primary use is not to identify respiratory allergens. However, there is no reliable evidence that the method has validity for any use.

EBSCO CAM Review Board

FURTHER READING

González-Correa, C. A. "Toward a Binary Interpretation of Acupuncture Theory: Principles and Practical Consequences." *Journal of Alternative and Complementary Medicine* 10 (2004): 573-579.

Krop, J., G. T. Lewith, and W. Gziut. "A Double Blind, Randomized, Controlled Investigation of Electrodermal Testing in the Diagnosis of Allergies." *Journal of Alternative and Complementary Medicine* 3 (1997): 241-248.

Lewith, G. T. "Can We Evaluate Electrodermal Testing?" *Complementary Therapies in Medicine* 11 (2003): 115-117.

Lewith, G. T., et al. "Is Electrodermal Testing as Effective as Skin Prick Tests for Diagnosing Allergies?" *British Medical Journal* 322 (2001): 131-134.

Semizzi, M., et al. "A Double-Blind, Placebo-Controlled Study on the Diagnostic Accuracy of an Electrodermal Test in Allergic Subjects." *Clinical and Experimental Allergy* 32 (2002): 928-932.

See also: Acupressure; Acupuncture; Hara diagnosis; Meridians; Pulse diagnosis; Tongue diagnosis.

Vegan diet

RELATED TERMS: Strict vegetarianism, veganism

CATEGORY: Therapies and techniques

DEFINITION: Alternative diet that excludes meat, fish, eggs, honey, and dairy products.

PRINCIPAL PROPOSED USE: Rheumatoid arthritis

OTHER PROPOSED USES: Cancer prevention, fibromyalgia, heart disease prevention

OVERVIEW

The vegan diet can also be called strict vegetarianism because it excludes not only meat and fish but also eggs, honey, and milk (dairy) products. Many practitioners of the vegan diet additionally avoid the use of animal products in other forms, such as clothing (wool, leather, silk), jewelry (pearls) and cosmetics (lanolin). People who adopt veganism may do so for health reasons, ethical considerations, or both.

There are several forms of veganism, and these may disagree on various major and minor points. For example, the raw-food diet and the macrobiotics diet are both vegan, but while macrobiotic practitioners believe that raw food is unhealthy, raw-foodists believe that cooked food is the source of many health problems.

The word "vegan" was created in 1944 by Elsie Shrigley and Donald Watson, "pure" vegetarians who were annoyed that many people who called themselves vegetarian ate dairy products and even fish. They combined the first three and last two letters of the word "vegetarian" to form "vegan," thereby intending to indicate that veganism was "the beginning and end of vegetarian."

SCIENTIFIC EVIDENCE

Some proponents of veganism claim that a vegan diet can cure many health conditions. However, in attempting to scientifically verify such claims, one runs into a significant problem: It is difficult, if not impossible, to design a scientifically reliable study of diet. For the results of a study to be trustworthy, participants and researchers must not know (be "blinded") who received the treatment under study (the active group) and who received a placebo treatment (the control group). If practitioners and researchers know who is in which group, numerous confounding factors will take over and produce misleading results. These factors include observer bias, reporting bias, and the placebo effect. To briefly summarize this complex issue, unblinded studies usually mean little to nothing. It is difficult to keep knowledge of the vegan diet from study participants.

USES AND APPLICATIONS

Rheumatoid arthritis is the prime condition for which veganism has been advocated. In several studies, people put on a vegan diet showed improvement in symptoms compared with those who were allowed to eat in an ordinary fashion. However, the absence of blinding makes these results unreliable. These studies would have been more meaningful if, for example, all participants ate a vegan diet and in addition consumed cookies that, without participants' knowing, contained either animal or vegetable fats. No studies using this or any other properly blinded control treatment have been reported.

A small study of similarly inadequate design weakly hints that a vegan diet might be helpful for fibromyalgia. Another small study compared a vegan diet to an antidepressant for treatment for fibromyalgia, and the antidepressant appeared to be more effective. Here, however, unconscious bias may have been working in the opposite direction: This study was conducted in Bangladesh, where a vegan diet is not exceptional, whereas the Western drug used could have had something of an aura. Even weaker evidence hints that vegan diets might be helpful for treating hypertension and for preventing heart disease and cancer.

SAFETY ISSUES

A vegan diet can in principle provide all necessary nutrients, with the exception of vitamin B_{12}. However, in practice, vegans are frequently deficient in calcium, iron, vitamin D, selenium, phosphorous, and zinc.

Vitamin B_{12} presents a special issue. This vitamin is not provided to any meaningful extent by nonplant foods. (The alga spirulina contains B_{12}, but in a nonabsorbable form.) Deficiency in B_{12} is therefore inevitable among those who follow a strict vegan diet and who do not take supplements. Such deficiency has led to serious health consequences among vegans and among breast-fed infants of vegan mothers. When severe, B_{12} deficiency can cause irreversible nerve damage. Mild deficiency leads to anemia and, in association with other common deficiencies, increased risk of bone thinning and fracture.

There is an additional potential issue for athletes to consider: A vegan diet is very low in the nonessential nutrient creatine. It is possible that creatine supplements may be particularly helpful for vegan athletes.

EBSCO CAM Review Board

FURTHER READING

Berkow, S. E., and N. D. Barnard. "Blood Pressure Regulation and Vegetarian Diets." *Nutrition Reviews* 63 (2005): 1-8.

Davis, B. C., and P. M. Kris-Etherton. "Achieving Optimal Essential Fatty Acid Status in Vegetarians: Current Knowledge and Practical Implications." *American Journal of Clinical Nutrition* 78 (2003): 640S-646S.

Fuhrman, J., and D. M. Ferreri. "Fueling the Vegetarian (Vegan) Athlete." *Current Sports Medicine Reports* 9 (2010): 233-241.

Kaartinen, K., et al. "Vegan Diet Alleviates Fibromyalgia Symptoms." *Scandinavian Journal of Rheumatology* 29 (2000): 308-313.

Trapp, C. B., and N. D. Barnard. "Usefulness of Vegetarian and Vegan Diets for Treating Type 2 Diabetes." *Current Diabetes Reports* 10 (2010): 152-158.

Turner-McGrievy, G. M., et al. "Effects of a Low-Fat Vegan Diet and a Step II Diet on Macro- and Micronutrient Intakes in Overweight Postmenopausal Women." *Nutrition* 20 (2004): 738-746.

Venderley, A. M., and W. W. Campbell. "Vegetarian Diets: Nutritional Considerations for Athletes." *Sports Medicine* 36 (2006): 293-305.

See also: Rheumatoid arthritis; Cancer risk reduction; Fibromyalgia: Homeopathic remedies.

Vegetarian diet

CATEGORY: Therapies and techniques

RELATED TERMS: Lacto-ovo vegetarian diet, vegan diet

DEFINITION: A diet that avoids the consumption of meats.

PRINCIPAL PROPOSED USES: Blood pressure, heart disease prevention, high cholesterol, weight loss

OTHER PROPOSED USES: Anxiety, allergies, arthritis, asthma, cancer, dementia, depression, diabetes, gout, hemorrhoids, kidney stones, osteoporosis, premenstrual syndrome

OVERVIEW

A vegetarian diet has many health benefits and may actually reduce the incidence of some diseases. The American Dietetic Association (ADA) states that properly managed vegetarian diets "are healthful, nutritionally adequate, and provide health benefits in the prevention and treatment of certain diseases."

The defining characteristic of a vegetarian diet is abstention from meat consumption. There are, however, a number of different types of vegetarian diets, ranging from the lacto-ovo vegetarian diet, which includes dairy products and eggs, to the vegan diet, which excludes all meats and animal products. The focus here is the lacto-ovo vegetarian diet.

MECHANISM OF ACTION

A vegetarian diet works through eliminating the consumption of meat products that are high in saturated fat and cholesterol, while increasing the intake of high-fiber, cholesterol-free, plant-based foods.

USES AND APPLICATIONS

The transition to a healthy vegetarian diet can be simple with some education and planning. A healthy vegetarian diet centers on decreasing fat intake and increasing fiber intake. This can be accomplished through emphasizing fresh fruits and vegetables, beans and other legumes, and whole-grain foods that are high in fiber and low in cholesterol and saturated fat. The diet avoids processed foods and refined sugar. A healthy vegetarian diet fulfills all these criteria.

Many nutritionists, however, recommend that a person transition to a vegetarian diet in stages, allowing the body to adjust by substituting a few meat meals each week with vegetarian food. One should start by reducing and eliminating red meat, then gradually eliminating pork, poultry, and fish. A simple way to make the transition is to use readily available soy-based meat substitutes such as tofu, tempeh, and textured vegetable protein, which are high in protein and can have a meat-like texture and taste.

In 2003, the ADA published a set of guidelines for North American vegetarian diets, recommending the following elements:

Whole grains. Six servings per day, including wheat, oatmeal, quinoa, couscous, and rice. Grains provide fiber, iron, and B vitamins. If possible, one should soak grains overnight to increase their digestibility.

Vegetables and fruits. Six servings per day, including carrots, leafy greens, collards, brassicas (broccoli, cabbage, brussels sprouts), apples, oranges, and bananas. Brassicas are rich in vitamin C, fiber, and carotenoids. Leafy greens and collards are sources of calcium, protein, and many vitamins, including C and A. Fruits are rich in vitamins B and C and calcium. Fresh vegetables and fruits have the highest vitamin content. One should steam or lightly cook vegetables to maintain higher nutrient value.

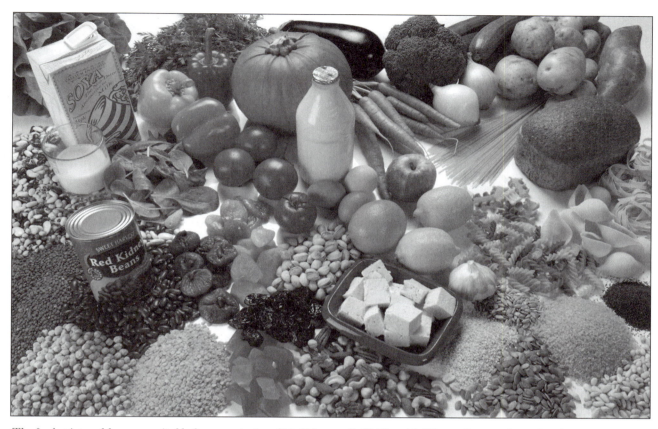

The foods pictured here are suitable for a vegetarian diet. (Martyn F. Chillmaid/Photo Researchers, Inc.)

Legumes, nuts, and other protein-rich foods. Five servings per day, including beans, peas, soy, nuts, dairy foods, and eggs.

Fats. Two servings per day, including vegetable oils, walnuts, mayonnaise, butter, and margarine.

Calcium-rich foods. Eight servings per day, including milk, cheese, fortified soy and fruit juices, and leafy greens.

SCIENTIFIC EVIDENCE

Research has shown that people who eat a healthy vegetarian diet weigh less and have lower cholesterol levels, lower blood pressure, and lower rates of many diseases. Research also has shown that this diet can reverse the effects of atherosclerosis. The risk of men contracting prostate cancer and women getting breast cancer are almost four times as high for meat eaters, compared with those on a largely vegetarian diet. In addition, a vegetarian diet has been used successfully to treat osteoporosis, arthritis, allergies, asthma, gout, hemorrhoids, kidney stones, premenstrual syndrome, anxiety, and depression. A 2000 study of members of the Seventh-day Adventist Church (who practice a lacto-ovo vegetarian diet) indicated that these members live, on average, two years longer than persons on a meat-based diet.

SAFETY ISSUES

A well-planned vegetarian diet is a healthy and safe diet; however, vegetarians need to be aware of particular nutrients that may be lacking in diets without meat. These nutrients include protein, vitamin B_{12}, vitamin A, vitamin D, calcium, iron, zinc, and N-3 fatty acids. It is possible to get these nutrients from plant-based foods, but they are not as abundant as in animal-based foods. To reap the benefits of a vegetarian diet, it is important to eat a diverse mix of whole grains, fresh vegetables, fruits, leafy greens, legumes, and nuts and to consciously reduce cholesterol and saturated fat intake by limiting dairy, eggs, and high-fat foods.

Animal-based proteins are complete proteins but are high in cholesterol. Research has shown that plant sources can meet the body's need for protein as long as a variety of plant foods are consumed. Most plant proteins are incomplete, lacking one or more of the essential amino acids. However, vegetarians can easily overcome this lack by combining a variety of complementary plant sources. In general, combining legumes such as beans, soy, and peas with grains such as rice, wheat, and couscous (for example, in beans and rice, hummus and crackers, or peanut butter and bread) forms a complete protein.

Those vegetarians who regularly eat eggs and dairy foods get adequate amounts of vitamin B_{12}, yet the ADA recommends regular B_{12} supplements or foods fortified with B_{12}. Vitamin A requirements can be met through eating carrots, leafy greens, or fruits (such as apricots, mangos, and pumpkins) that are rich in beta-carotene or by taking supplements. Vegetarians can get adequate amounts of vitamin D through regular exposure to the sun, by eating fortified foods, and by taking supplements.

Calcium is readily obtained by eating enriched soy products, nuts, legumes, dairy, and dark green vegetables such as broccoli and kale. Iron is available in raisins, legumes, tofu, potatoes, and leafy greens. Iron is absorbed more efficiently in the body if iron-rich foods are combined with those containing vitamin C, such as oranges, apples, and tomatoes. Zinc is abundant in pumpkin seeds, legumes, peas, lentils, whole grains, and soy products.

Vegetarians need to get adequate amounts of N-3 or omega-3 fatty acids. Vegetarian diets tend to be high in N-6 fatty acids but low in N-3 fatty acids (found in abundance in seafood and in some plants and nut oils). The body needs a balance of both. Vegetarian sources of N-3 fats include soy, walnuts, pumpkin seeds, and hemp seeds. Flaxseed oil is particularly rich in these fats.

Robert Flatley, M.L.S.

FURTHER READING

Hagler, Louise, and Dorothy R. Bates, eds. *The New Farm Vegetarian Cookbook.* 2d ed. Summertown, Tenn.: Book Publishing, 1989. A classic book of simple soy-based vegetarian recipes.
International Vegetarians Union. http://www.ivu.org.
"A New Food Guide for North American Vegetarians." Available at http://www.metabolicdiet.com/pdfs/ veg_food_guide.pdf. Outlines the basics of a balanced and healthy vegetarian diet.
Vegetarian Resource Group. http://www.vrg.org.

See also: Anti-inflammatory diet; Calcium; Diet-based therapies; Low-carbohydrate diet; Low glycemic-index diet; Macrobiotic diet; Nondairy milk; Raw foods diet; Soy; Vegan diet; Vitamins and minerals.

Venous insufficiency: Homeopathic remedies

CATEGORY: Homeopathy
DEFINITION: The use of highly diluted remedies to treat damage to veins near the surface of the skin.
STUDIED HOMEOPATHIC REMEDIES: *Arnica; Calcarea carbonica; Hamamelis;* combination homeopathic remedy containing *Meliotus offic, Aesculus, Hamamelis, Carduus marianus, Lycopodium, Lachesis, Arnica,* and *Rutin*

SCIENTIFIC EVALUATIONS OF HOMEOPATHIC REMEDIES

No homeopathic remedies have been shown to be effective for the treatment of venous insufficiency. In one study, a partly homeopathic remedy for venous insufficiency failed to prove conclusively effective. This twenty-four-day, double-blind, placebo-controlled study of sixty-one people with varicose veins evaluated the effect of a remedy containing *Meliotus offic, Aesculus, Hamamelis, Carduus marianus, Lycopodium, Lachesis, Arnica,* and *Rutin.* (While some of these ingredients were included at homeopathic potencies, others were taken at small dilutions, making them herbal therapies rather than true homeopathic remedies.) For twenty-four days, the participants took twenty drops of the remedy or placebo. The tested treatment failed to achieve significant effects on most standard measures of disease severity.

In another double-blind trial, 130 people undergoing surgery for varicose veins were given homeopathic *Arnica* 5x (decimal scale) or placebo. No comparative benefits were seen.

TRADITIONAL HOMEOPATHIC TREATMENTS

Homeopathic *Calcarea carbonica* may be used for

people with painful varicose veins who also have the following symptom picture: easily fatigued, cold hands and feet, generally flabby musculature, a tendency toward being overweight, and a taste for sweet foods. Anxiety and a propensity to become overwhelmed by life are also part of the symptom picture.

Homeopathic *Hamamelis* is sometimes used when varicose veins are relatively large, easily damaged or torn (leading to bleeding), and tender to the touch. The legs have a purple or mottled appearance. Bleeding hemorrhoids may accompany the vein problems in the legs.

EBSCO CAM Review Board

FURTHER READING

Allen, L. "Assessment and Management of Patients with Varicose Veins." *Nursing Standard* 23 (2009): 49-57.

Ernst, E., T. Saradeth, and K. L. Resch. "Complementary Therapy of Varicose Veins." *Phlebologie* 5 (1990): 157-163.

Ramelet, A. A., et al. "Homoeopathic *Arnica* in Postoperative Haematomas." *Dermatology* 201 (2000): 347-348.

See also: Homeopathy; Obesity and excess weight; Restless legs syndrome; Varicose veins.

Vertigo

CATEGORY: Condition
RELATED TERMS: Benign paroxysmal positional vertigo, benign positional vertigo, dizziness, Meniere's disease, vertiginous syndrome
DEFINITION: Treatment of dizziness accompanied by the sense of movement.
PRINCIPAL PROPOSED NATURAL TREATMENTS: None
OTHER PROPOSED NATURAL TREATMENTS: Ginger, ginkgo, hypnosis, oxerutins, vitamin B_6

INTRODUCTION

Vertigo is closely related to dizziness but involves the perception of seeing a room spin. The experience is similar to what happens when one spins around rapidly and then stops. Often, vertigo is accompanied by nausea and a loss of balance. Vertigo may pass quickly, or it may last for hours or even days.

There are many possible causes of vertigo, including motion sickness, infection in the inner ear, vision problems, head injury, insufficient blood supply to the brain, and brain tumors. A condition called benign paroxysmal positional vertigo leads to attacks of vertigo triggered by certain head positions; its cause is believed to be deposits of calcium in the inner ear. Another condition, Meniere's disease, is characterized by sudden, intense attacks of vertigo often accompanied by nausea and vomiting, ringing in the ears, and progressive deafness. Its cause is unknown.

Conventional treatments for vertigo depend upon the cause and severity of the condition. Drugs for motion sickness and mild vertigo of any cause include meclizine, dimenhydrinate, and perphenazine. Scopolamine is prescribed for severe motion sickness. Benign paroxysmal positional vertigo is often treated through a series of exercises that help to alleviate symptoms. For Meniere's disease, changes in diet are often recommended (including limiting sodium, sugar, and alcohol intake), sometimes with diuretic drugs.

PROPOSED NATURAL TREATMENTS

Several natural treatments have been tried for vertigo; however, the scientific evidence for these treatments is preliminary. A double-blind, placebo-controlled study of sixty-seven people with vertigo found that 160 milligrams (mg) of *Ginkgo biloba* extract per day significantly reduced symptoms compared with placebo. At the end of the three-month study, 47 percent of the ginkgo group had completely recovered, compared to only 18 percent of the placebo group.

The supplements oxerutins and vitamin B_6 are sometimes recommended for vertigo; however, the evidence supporting these treatments is extremely preliminary. Hypnosis has been tried for vertigo resulting from head trauma, with some apparent success.

EBSCO CAM Review Board

FURTHER READING

Grontved, A., et al. "Ginger Root Against Seasickness: A Controlled Trial on the Open Sea." *Acta Oto-Laryngologica* 105 (1988): 45-49.

Haguenauer, J. P., et al. "Treatment of Balance Disorders Using *Ginkgo biloba* Extract." *Presse médicale* 15 (1986): 1569-1572.

Schneider, B., P. Klein, and M. Weiser. "Treatment of

Vertigo with a Homeopathic Complex Remedy Compared with Usual Treatments." *Arzneimittel-Forschung* 55 (2005): 23-29.

Stewart, J. J., et al. "Effects of Ginger on Motion Sickness Susceptibility and Gastric Function." *Pharmacology* 42 (1991): 111-120.

See also: Altitude sickness; Ginger; Ginkgo; Hypnotherapy; Morning sickness; Nausea; Oxerutins; Vitamin B$_6$.

Vertigo: Homeopathic remedies

CATEGORY: Homeopathy

DEFINITION: The use of highly diluted remedies to treat dizziness accompanied by the sense of movement.

STUDIED HOMEOPATHIC REMEDIES: *Cocculus*; *Conium*; homeopathic remedy containing *Ambra grisea*, *Conium*, *Petroleumm*, and *Cocculus*

SCIENTIFIC EVALUATIONS OF HOMEOPATHIC REMEDIES

One double-blind study found that a particular combination homeopathic remedy sold as Vertigoheel was just as effective as standard treatment for vertigo. This study followed 105 people with acute or chronic vertigo of various causes, including Meniere's disease and positional vertigo. The homeopathic treatment used contained *Ambra grisea*, *Conium*, *Petroleumm*, and *Cocculus*. The treatment was compared with betahistine hydrochloride, an antihistamine widely used in Europe for vertigo symptoms.

To evaluate the success of the treatment, researchers recorded the frequency, duration, and self-reported intensity of participants' vertigo attacks. The results showed that the homeopathic mixture was as effective as the antihistamine during the six weeks of the treatment period. However, these results are not as meaningful as they appear; betahistine is at most modestly effective for vertigo, and because there was no placebo group in the study, it is quite possible that the benefits seen in the Vertigoheel group were no different than what would have been seen with placebo treatment.

Another study found this same remedy just as effective as the herb *Ginkgo biloba* for vertigo. However, because ginkgo itself has not been proven effective for this purpose, these results mean little.

TRADITIONAL HOMEOPATHIC TREATMENTS

Classical homeopathy offers possible homeopathic treatments for vertigo. These therapies are chosen based on various specific details of the person seeking treatment.

The homeopathic remedy *Cocculus* is often recommended for the treatment of vertigo, especially when the vertigo is a result of motion sickness. The symptom picture of this remedy includes a pattern of symptoms being made worse by eating or drinking, rising up from bed, or exposure to bright light, along with a sense of confusion and possibly a sick headache. Lying down usually relieves the symptoms. In contrast, the homeopathic remedy *Conium* is associated with a symptom picture in which vertigo is made worse by lying down, turning over, or moving the head.

EBSCO CAM Review Board

FURTHER READING

Issing, W., P. Klein, and M. Weiser. "The Homeopathic Preparation Vertigoheel Versus *Ginkgo biloba* in the Treatment of Vertigo in an Elderly Population." *Journal of Alternative and Complementary Medicine* 11 (2005): 155-160.

Karkos, P. D., et al. "'Complementary ENT': A Systematic Review of Commonly Used Supplements." *Journal of Laryngology and Otology* 121 (2007): 779-782.

Weiser, M., W. Strosser, and P. Klein. "Homeopathic vs. Conventional Treatment of Vertigo." *Archives of Otolaryngology: Head Neck Surgery* 124 (1998): 879-885.

See also: Homeopathy; Nausea.

Vervain

CATEGORY: Herbs and supplements

RELATED TERM: *Verbena officinalis*

DEFINITION: Natural plant product used to treat specific health conditions.

PRINCIPAL PROPOSED USE: Stimulating flow of breast milk

OTHER PROPOSED USES: Insomnia, menstrual pain

OVERVIEW

The herb vervain is a common perennial wildflower in England, found growing at the edge of roads and in meadows. It has a long history of use in Celtic religious tradition and has been used as medicine by many cultures. The leaf and flower are the parts used medicinally.

Like other bitter plants, vervain has been used to stimulate appetite and digestion. Other traditional uses include treating abdominal spasms, fevers, depression (especially following illness or childbirth), and inadequate flow of breast milk.

THERAPEUTIC DOSAGES

A typical dosage of vervain is 2 to 3 grams three times daily, taken as dry herb or made into tea. Equivalent dosages are also available in tincture form and may be more palatable.

THERAPEUTIC USES

Vervain is commonly recommended today to increase flow of breast milk, as well as to treat insomnia and menstrual pain. However, there is no meaningful evidence to support any of these uses.

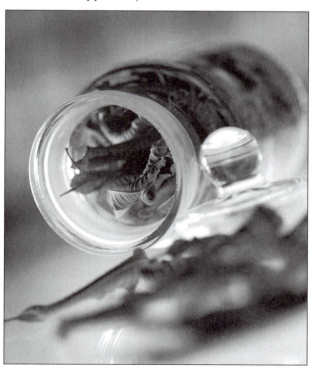

Jar containing dried leaves of vervain. (Philippe Garo/ Photo Researchers, Inc.)

One study in rats found possible sedative effects with a vervain extract. A test-tube study found hints of potential anticancer effects. However, evidence like this is far, far too preliminary to show efficacy. Only double-blind, placebo-controlled studies can prove that a treatment really works, and no studies of this type have been performed on vervain.

SAFETY ISSUES

Although vervain is thought to be a relatively safe herb, it has not undergone any meaningful safety testing at a modern scientific level. There is some reason to believe it may not be safe for use in pregnancy. Despite its reputation for enhancing flow of breast milk, safety in nursing women has also not been established. Additionally, safety in young children and people with severe liver or kidney disease remains unknown.

EBSCO CAM Review Board

FURTHER READING

Dudai, N., et al. "Citral Is a New Inducer of Caspase-3 in Tumor Cell Lines." *Planta Medica* 71 (2005): 484-488.

See also: Breast-feeding support; Insomnia; Women's health.

Vinpocetine

CATEGORY: Herbs and supplements
RELATED TERM: Periwinkle
DEFINITION: Natural plant product used to treat specific health conditions.
PRINCIPAL PROPOSED USE: Alzheimer's disease and other forms of dementia
OTHER PROPOSED USES: Enhancing mental function in healthy people, strokes

OVERVIEW

Vinpocetine is a chemical derived from vincamine, a constituent found in the leaves of common periwinkle (*Vinca minor* L.), as well as the seeds of various African plants. It is used as a treatment for memory loss and mental impairment.

Developed in Hungary more than twenty years ago, vinpocetine is sold in Europe as the drug Cavinton. In the United States it is available as a dietary supplement, although the substance probably does not fit that category by any rational definition. Vinpocetine does not exist to any significant extent in nature. Producing it requires significant chemical work performed in the laboratory.

THERAPEUTIC DOSAGES

The usual dose of vinpocetine is a 10-milligram capsules three times per day, although dosages ranging from half to twice that amount have been used in studies. Vinpocetine reportedly is better absorbed when taken with a meal.

THERAPEUTIC USES

Some evidence supports the idea that vinpocetine can enhance memory and mental function, especially in those with Alzheimer's disease and related conditions. It is also widely marketed for enhancing memory in healthy people, but there is no real evidence that it is helpful for this purpose.

It has been hypothesized that vinpocetine helps people with Alzheimer's disease by enhancing blood flow in the brain, safeguarding brain cells against damage, and inhibiting a substance known as phosphodiesterase. Based on these proposed actions, vinpocetine has also been tried as a treatment for reducing brain damage following strokes.

SCIENTIFIC EVIDENCE

Alzheimer's disease and related conditions (dementia). A sixteen-week, double-blind, placebo-controlled trial of 203 individuals with mild to moderate dementia found significant benefit in the treated group. Benefits have also been seen in other studies. However, a major review found that overall, the evidence that vinpocetine works remains too weak to rely upon, due to limitations in study quality.

Strokes. In a single-blind, placebo-controlled trial, thirty individuals who had just experienced a stroke received either placebo or vinpocetine along with conventional treatment for thirty days. The results showed that participants in the vinpocetine group experienced a significantly reduced level of residual disability as measured at three months.

A few other studies, some of poor design, also provide suggestive evidence that vinpocetine may be helpful for strokes. However, much of the existing evidence is too preliminary to rely on, and a recent review combining two relatively high-quality studies in-

volving sixty-three subjects was unable to determine whether or not vinpocetine provided any benefit for stroke patients.

People who have had strokes are sometimes advised to take blood-thinning drugs. There are concerns that vinpocetine may interact adversely with some medications of this type.

SAFETY ISSUES

No serious side effects have been reported in any of the clinical trials. However, there is one case report of vinpocetine apparently causing agranulocytosis (loss of certain white blood cells).

Vinpocetine inhibits blood platelets from forming clots, and for this reason it could cause problems if it is taken by individuals with bleeding problems, during the period immediately before or after surgery or labor and delivery, or in combination with medications or natural substances that also affect platelet activity. These substances include aspirin, clopidogrel (Plavix), ticlopidine (Ticlid), pentoxifylline (Trental), garlic, ginkgo, policosanol, and high-dosage vitamin E

The drug warfarin (Coumadin) affects blood clotting, but not through actions on platelets. One study found only a minimal interaction between warfarin and vinpocetine. Interestingly, it was in the direction of decreased clotting. Nonetheless, combination therapy with vinpocetine and warfarin should not be attempted except under the supervision of a physician. In addition, safety in pregnant or nursing women, young children, and those with severe liver or kidney disease has not been established.

IMPORTANT INTERACTIONS

People who are taking blood-thinning drugs, such as aspirin, clopidogrel (Plavix), ticlopidine (Ticlid), or pentoxifylline (Trental), might have bleeding problems if they are simultaneously using vinpocetine. Taking vinpocetine with natural substances that have blood-thinning properties, such as garlic, ginkgo, policosanol, or high-dose vitamin E, might in theory also cause bleeding problems. Taking warfarin (Coumadin) with vinpocetine might impair warfurin's blood-thinning actions.

EBSCO CAM Review Board

FURTHER READING

Bereczki, D., and I. Fekete. "Vinpocetine for Acute Ischaemic Stroke." *Cochrane Database of Systematic Reviews* 1 (2008): CD000480.

Bonoczk, P., G. Panczel, and Z. Nagy. "Vinpocetine Increases Cerebral Blood Flow and Oxygenation in Stroke Patients: A Near Infrared Spectroscopy and Transcranial Doppler Study." *European Journal of Ultrasound* 15 (2002): 85-91.

Feigin, V. L., et al. "Vinpocetine Treatment in Acute Ischaemic Stroke." *European Journal of Neurology* 8 (2001): 81-85.

Szilagyi, G., et al. "Effects of Vinpocetine on the Redistribution of Cerebral Blood Flow and Glucose Metabolism in Chronic Ischemic Stroke Patients: A PET Study." *Journal of Neurological Science* (March 15, 2005): 229-230, 275-284.

See also: Alzheimer's disease; Strokes.

Vitamin A

CATEGORY: Herbs and supplements

RELATED TERM: Retinol

DEFINITION: Organic compound used to treat specific health conditions.

PRINCIPAL PROPOSED USE: Viral infections in children

OTHER PROPOSED USES: Acne, aging skin, Crohn's disease, diabetes, eczema, human immunodeficiency virus infection support, menorrhagia, psoriasis, retinitis pigmentosa, rosacea, seborrhea

OVERVIEW

Vitamin A is a fat-soluble antioxidant that protects the body's cells against damaging free radicals and plays other vital roles in the body. However, it is potentially more dangerous than most other vitamins because it can build up to toxic levels. For this reason, it should be used with caution.

It has long been assumed that beta-carotene supplements taken at nutritional doses are a safer way for people to get their needed vitamin A. However, while this may be true in general, beta-carotene also appears to present some risks.

REQUIREMENTS AND SOURCES

Vitamin A is an essential nutrient, meaning one must obtain it from the diet. The official U.S. recommendations for daily intake of vitamin A are expressed in international units (IUs) or retinol activity equiva-lents (RAE), which are measured in micrograms (mcg), as follows:

Infants, 0 to 6 months of age (400 mcg RAE or 1,330 IU) and 7 to 12 months of age (500 mcg RAE or 1,665 IU); children aged 1 to 3 years (300 mcg RAE or 1,000 IU) and 4 to 8 years (400 mcg RAE or 1,330 IU); boys 9 to 13 years (600 mcg RAE or 2,000 IU); boys 14 to 18 years and adult men (900 mcg RAE or 3,000 IU); girls 9 to 13 years of age (600 mcg RAE or 2,000 IU); girls 14 to 18 years and adult women (700 mcg RAE or 2,330 IU); pregnant girls (750 mcg RAE or 2,500 IUs); pregnant women (770 mcg RAE or 2,560 IU); nursing girls (1,200 mcg RAE or 4,000 IUs); and nursing women (1,300 mcg RAE or 4,300 IU).

Pregnant women should not take vitamin A supplements. They should instead take beta-carotene.

Vitamin A is obtained from many food, in the form of either vitamin A or beta-carotene. Liver and dairy products are excellent sources of vitamin A. Carrots, apricots, collard greens, kale, sweet potatoes, parsley, and spinach are also good sources.

Deficiency in vitamin A is common in developing countries. In the developed world, deficiency is relatively rare. However, certain diseases can cause vitamin A deficiency by impairing the ability of the digestive tract to absorb nutrients. These include Crohn's disease, ulcerative colitis, and cystic fibrosis.

THERAPEUTIC DOSAGES

Although some studies have used high doses of vitamin A, intake above the safe upper limit level is not recommended except on the advice of a physician.

THERAPEUTIC USES

There is some evidence that vitamin A supplements reduce deaths from measles and other infectious illnesses among children in developing countries, presumably because they correct a deficiency in the children's diets. However, this does not mean that vitamin A supplements above and beyond the basic nutritional requirement are a useful treatment for measles or any other childhood disease.

Vitamin A might improve blood sugar control in people with diabetes. However, people with diabetes may also be especially vulnerable to liver damage from excessive amounts of vitamin A. Therefore, people with diabetes should take vitamin A only on the advice of a physician.

Vitamin A has shown some potential for preventing

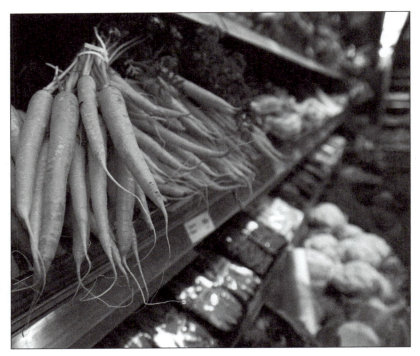
Carrots are a good source of vitamin A. (AP Photo)

one type of skin cancer: squamous cell cancer. However, in these studies, doses above the standard safe upper limits have been used. With proper monitoring this may be safe, but experts do not recommend trying it without physician supervision. High-dose vitamin A has been tried for a variety of other skin diseases, including acne, psoriasis, rosacea, seborrhea, and eczema, as well as menorrhagia (heavy menstruation) and retinitis pigmentosa (a chronic disease of the eyes). However, the benefits seen have been modest at best, and again the recommended dosages of vitamin A are so high as to raise concerns about toxic risk.

Vitamin A might be beneficial for people with human immunodeficiency virus (HIV). However, results of studies have been contradictory, and some evidence even suggests that vitamin A supplements might increase transmission of the disease from a pregnant mother to her newborn.

Topical vitamin A may be helpful for treatment of aging skin. One double-blind, placebo-controlled study found that a 0.4 percent vitamin A lotion applied three times a week significantly reduced the number of "fine" wrinkles in seniors. Benefits were

also seen in terms of some biochemical measures of skin health.

On the basis of very weak evidence, too weak to be relied upon at all, vitamin A has been proposed as a treatment for a wide variety of other conditions, including Down syndrome, ear infections, eating disorders, glaucoma, gout, impaired night vision, kidney stones, lupus, multiple sclerosis, ulcerative colitis, and ulcers. One study suggests that vitamin A is not effective for Crohn's disease.

SCIENTIFIC EVIDENCE

Diabetes. According to many but not all studies, people with diabetes tend to be deficient in vitamin A. An observational study suggests that vitamin A supplements may improve blood sugar control in people with diabetes. However, due to safety concerns, people should not supplement with vitamin A except under medical supervision.

Menorrhagia (heavy menstruation). One study suggests that women with heavy menstrual bleeding can benefit from taking 25,000 IU daily of vitamin A. However, vitamin A cannot be recommended as an ongoing treatment for menorrhagia, since women who menstruate can become pregnant, and even fairly low doses of supplemental vitamin A may cause birth defects.

HIV support. One small double-blind study suggested that taking beta-carotene might raise white blood cell count in people with HIV. However, two subsequent, larger controlled trials found no significant differences between those taking beta-carotene and those taking placebo in white blood cell count, CD4+ count, or other measures of immune function.

Two observational studies lasting six to eight years suggest that higher intakes of vitamin A or beta-carotene may be helpful, but they also found that caution is in order with regard to dosage. This group of researchers generally linked higher intake of vitamin A or beta-carotene to lower risk of acquired immunodeficiency syndrome (AIDS) and lower death rates, with an important exception: People with the highest intake of either nutrient (more than 11,179 IU per day of beta-carotene, more than 20,268 IU per day of vitamin A) did worse than those who took somewhat less.

Despite hope that vitamin A given to pregnant, HIV-positive women might decrease the infection rate of their babies, two double-blind studies found no significant differences between those babies whose mothers took vitamin A and those babies whose mothers took placebo. In any case, vitamin A is not considered safe for use during pregnancy; beta-carotene is preferred.

Crohn's disease. According to a double-blind study of eighty-six people with Crohn's disease, vitamin A does not help prevent flare-ups.

Lower respiratory tract infections. Lower respiratory tract infections include conditions like pneumonia and bronchiolitis. Young children are especially susceptible to these infections. A review of ten trials involving more than thirty-three hundred children under age seven years of age found that, in the majority of cases, vitamin A did not reduce the incidence of infection or severity of symptoms. In two of the studies, vitamin A was beneficial for undernourished children. However, children with adequate nutrition actually faired worse.

SAFETY ISSUES

The safe upper intake levels of vitamin A have been set as follows:

Infants aged 0 to 12 months (600 mcg RAE or 2,000 IU); children aged 1 to 3 years (600 mcg RAE or 2,000 IU) and 4 to 8 years (900 mcg RAE or 3,000 IU); boys and girls aged 9 to 13 years (1,700 mcg RAE or 5,660 IU); boys and girls aged 14 to 18 years (2,800 mcg RAE or 9,320 IU); adults (3,000 mcg RAE or 10,000 IU); pregnant girls (2,800 mcg RAE or 9,320 IUs); pregnant women (3,000 mcg RAE or 10,000 IU); nursing girls (2,800 mcg RAE or 9,320 IUs); and nursing women (3,000 mcg RAE or 10,000 IU).

It is thought that dosages of vitamin A above 50,000 IU per day taken for several years can cause liver injury, bone problems, fatigue, hair loss, headaches, and dry skin. However, one recent study found no harm with dosages as high as 75,000 IU taken for one year. Nonetheless, experts do not recommend using vitamin A at doses above the upper limits, except under close physician supervision. Some people may be more likely to develop toxic symptoms than others.

People who already have liver disease should check with their doctors before taking vitamin A supple-ments because even small doses may be harmful. It is thought that people with diabetes may have trouble releasing vitamin A stored in the liver. This may mean that they are at greater risk for vitamin A toxicity.

Excessive intake of vitamin A, or beta-carotene, appears to accelerate liver injury in people with alcoholism. In addition, relatively high intake of vitamin A (but not beta-carotene) has been associated with increased risk of osteoporosis.

Women should avoid taking vitamin A supplements during pregnancy, because at toxic levels it might increase the risk of birth defects. Pregnant women taking valproic acid medications (Depakote, Depacon, or Depakene) may be even more at risk of vitamin A toxicity.

Vitamin A may increase the anticoagulant effects of warfarin (Coumadin). In addition, because vitamin A chemically resembles the drug isotretinoin (Accutane), it may amplify that drug's toxic effects.

IMPORTANT INTERACTIONS

People who are taking isotretinoin (Accutane) should not take vitamin A, as the two might enhance each other's toxicity. Pregnant women taking valproic acid (Depakote, Depacon, or Depakene) should not take vitamin A supplements unless advised to do so by a physician. People taking warfarin (Coumadin) should not take vitamin A supplements unless advised to do so by a physician.

EBSCO CAM Review Board

FURTHER READING

Berson, E. L., et al. "Clinical Trial of Docosahexaenoic Acid in Patients with Retinitis Pigmentosa Receiving Vitamin A Treatment." *Archives of Ophthalmology* 122 (2004): 1297-1305.

Chen, H., et al. "Vitamin A for Preventing Acute Lower Respiratory Tract Infections in Children up to Seven Years of Age." *Cochrane Database of Systematic Reviews* 1 (2011): CD006090.

Kafi, R., et al. "Improvement of Naturally Aged Skin with Vitamin A (Retinol)." *Archives of Dermatology* 143 (2007): 606-612.

Mehta, S., and W. Fawzi. "Effects of Vitamins, Including Vitamin A, on HIV/AIDS Patients." *Vitamins and Hormones* 75 (2007): 355-383.

Michaelsson, K., et al. "Serum Retinol Levels and the Risk of Fracture." *New England Journal of Medicine* 348 (2003): 287-294.

See also: Acne; Aging; Children's health; Diabetes; Eczema; HIV support; Psoriasis; Retinitis pigmentosa; Rosacea; Seborrheic dermatitis.

Vitamin B$_1$

CATEGORY: Herbs and supplements

RELATED TERM: Thiamin

DEFINITION: Organic compound used to treat specific health conditions.

PRINCIPAL PROPOSED USE: Congestive heart failure

OTHER PROPOSED USES: Alzheimer's disease, canker sores, enhancing mental function, epilepsy, fibromyalgia, human immunodeficiency virus support

OVERVIEW

Vitamin B$_1$, also called thiamin, was the first B vitamin discovered. Every cell in the body needs thiamin to make adenosine triphosphate, or ATP, the body's main energy-carrying molecule. The heart, in particular, has considerable need for thiamin to keep up its constant work. Severe deficiency of thiamin results in beriberi, a disease common in the nineteenth century but rare today. Many of the principal symptoms of beriberi involve impaired heart function.

REQUIREMENTS AND SOURCES

The need for vitamin B$_1$ varies with age and gender. The official U.S. and Canadian recommendations for daily intake are as follows:

Infants aged 0 to 6 months (0.2 mg) and 7 to 12 months (0.3 mg); children aged 1 to 3 years (0.5 mg), 4 to 8 years (0.6 mg), and 9 to 13 years (0.9 mg); males aged 14 years and older (1.2 mg); females aged 14 to 18 years (1.0 mg); women (1.1 mg); and pregnant or nursing women (1.4 mg).

Although vitamin B$_1$ deficiency is rare in the developed world, it may occur in certain medical conditions, such as alcoholism, anorexia, Crohn's disease, and folate deficiency. People undergoing kidney dialysis or taking loop diuretics may also become deficient in vitamin B$_1$. Certain foods may impair the body's absorption of B$_1$ including fish, shrimp, clams, mussels, and the herb horsetail.

Brewer's and nutritional yeast are the richest sources of B$_1$. Peas, beans, nuts, seeds, and whole grains also provide fairly good amounts.

THERAPEUTIC DOSAGES

A typical dose of vitamin B$_1$ for therapeutic purposes is 200 milligrams (mg) daily, although much higher dosages have also been tried. Some nutritional experts recommend taking B$_1$ with other B vitamins in the form of a B-complex supplement. However, there is no meaningful evidence that this offers any advantage.

THERAPEUTIC USES

Congestive heart failure (CHF) is a condition in which the pumping ability of the heart declines, and fluid begins to accumulate in the lungs and legs. Standard treatment for CHF includes strong "water pills" called loop diuretics. These drugs, however, deplete the body of B$_1$. Since the heart depends on vitamin B$_1$ for its proper function, this is potentially quite worrisome. Preliminary evidence, including a small double-blind, placebo-controlled trial, hints that supplementation with B$_1$ can improve symptoms.

One double-blind study suggests that thiamin taken at a dose of 50 mg daily might enhance mental function. Other potential uses of thiamin have even less scientific support. Observational studies of people with human immunodeficiency virus (HIV) infection suggest–but definitely do not prove–that increased intake of vitamin B$_1$ might slow progression to acquired immunodeficiency syndrome (AIDS) and enhance overall survival rate. Weak and contradictory evidence hints that vitamin B$_1$ may be helpful for Alzheimer's disease. Vitamin B$_1$ has also been proposed as a treatment for epilepsy, canker sores, and fibromyalgia, but the evidence for these uses is too preliminary to cite.

SAFETY ISSUES

Vitamin B$_1$ appears to be quite safe, even when taken in very high doses. People who are taking loop diuretics, such as furosemide or Lasix, may need extra vitamin B$_1$.

EBSCO CAM Review Board

FURTHER READING

Benton, D., et al. "Thiamine Supplementation, Mood and Cognitive Functioning." *Psychopharmacology (Berl)* 129 (1997): 66-71.

Bettendorff, L., et al. "Low Thiamine Diphosphate

Levels in Brains of Patients with Frontal Lobe Degeneration of the Non-Alzheimer's Type." *Journal of Neurochemistry* 69 (1997): 2005-2010.

Brady, J. A., C. L. Rock, and M. R. Horneffer. "Thiamin Status, Diuretic Medications, and the Management of Congestive Heart Failure." *Journal of the American Dietetic Association* 95 (1995): 541-544.

Gold, M., R. A. Hauser, and M. F. Chen. "Plasma Thiamine Deficiency Associated with Alzheimer's Disease but Not Parkinson's Disease." *Metabolic Brain Disease* 13 (1998): 43-53.

Mimori Y., H. Katsuoka, and S. Nakamura. "Thiamine Therapy in Alzheimer's Disease." *Metabolic Brain Disease* 11 (1996): 89-94.

Shimon, I., et al. "Improved Left Ventricular Function After Thiamine Supplementation in Patients with Congestive Heart Failure Receiving Long-Term Furosemide Therapy." *American Journal of Medicine* 98 (1995): 485-490.

See also: Alzheimer's disease; Canker sores; Epilepsy; Fibromyalgia: Homeopathic remedies; HIV support.

Vitamin B$_2$

CATEGORY: Herbs and supplements
RELATED TERMS: Riboflavin, riboflavin-5-phosphate
DEFINITION: Organic compound used to treat specific health conditions.
PRINCIPAL PROPOSED USE: Migraine headaches
OTHER PROPOSED USES: Cataracts, human immunodeficiency virus support, sickle cell anemia, sports performance enhancement

OVERVIEW

Riboflavin, also known as vitamin B$_2$, is an essential nutrient required for life. This vitamin works with two enzymes critical to the body's production of adenosine triphosphate (ATP), its main energy source. Vitamin B$_2$ is also used to process amino acids and fats and to activate vitamin B$_6$ and folate. Preliminary evidence suggests that riboflavin supplements may offer benefits for two illnesses: migraine headaches and cataracts.

REQUIREMENTS AND SOURCES

The official U.S. and Canadian recommendations for daily intake of riboflavin are as follows:

Infants aged 0 to 6 months (0.3 mg) and 7 to 12 months (0.4 mg); children aged 1 to 3 years (0.5 mg), 4 to 8 years (0.6 mg), and 9 to 13 years (0.9 mg); males aged 14 years and older (1.3 mg); females aged 14 to 18 years (1.0 mg); women (1.1 mg); pregnant women (1.4 mg); and nursing women (1.6 mg).

Riboflavin is found in organ meats, such as liver, kidney, and heart, and in many vegetables, nuts, legumes, and leafy greens. The richest sources are torula (nutritional) yeast, brewer's yeast, and calf liver. Almonds, wheat germ, wild rice, and mushrooms are also good sources.

Although serious riboflavin deficiencies are rare, slightly low levels can occur in children, the elderly, and those in poverty. Oral contraceptives used in the 1970s and 1980s appeared to reduce levels of riboflavin. However, it is not clear whether more recent versions of these medications, which contain much lower levels of estrogen, would have the same effect.

THERAPEUTIC DOSAGES

For migraine headaches, the typical recommended dosage of riboflavin is much higher than nutritional needs: 400 milligrams (mg) daily. For cataract prevention, riboflavin may be taken at the nutritional dosages described. Since the B vitamins tend to work together, many nutritional experts recommend taking B$_2$ with other B vitamins, perhaps in the form of a B-complex supplement.

THERAPEUTIC USES

Preliminary evidence suggests that riboflavin supplements taken at high dosages may reduce the frequency of migraine headaches. One very large study suggests that riboflavin at nutritional doses may be helpful for cataracts, but in this study it was combined with another B vitamin—niacin (vitamin B$_3$)—so it is hard to say which vitamin was responsible for the effect. Riboflavin has also been proposed as a treatment for sickle cell anemia, for human immunodeficiency virus (HIV) infection, and as a performance enhancer for athletes, but there is no real evidence that it is effective for these uses.

SCIENTIFIC EVIDENCE

Migraine headaches. According to a three-month, double-blind, placebo-controlled study of fifty-five people with migraines, riboflavin can significantly reduce the frequency and duration of migraine attacks. This study found that, when given a minimum of two months to work, a daily dose of riboflavin (400 mg) can produce dramatic migraine relief. The majority of the participants experienced a more than 50 percent decrease in the number of migraine attacks, as well as in the total days with headache pain. However, a larger and longer study is needed to follow up on these results.

Cataracts. Riboflavin supplements may help prevent cataracts, but the evidence remains unclear. In a large double-blind, placebo-controlled study, 3,249 people were given either placebo or one of four nutrient combinations (vitamin A/zinc, riboflavin/niacin, vitamin C/molybdenum, or selenium with beta-carotene and vitamin E) for six years. Those receiving the riboflavin/niacin supplement showed a significant (44 percent) reduction in the incidence of cataracts. However, it is unclear whether the benefits seen in this group came from the niacin, the riboflavin, or the combination of the two. There was a small but statistically significantly higher incidence of a special type of cataract, called a subcapsular cataract, in the niacin/riboflavin group.

SAFETY ISSUES

Riboflavin seems to be an extremely safe supplement.

EBSCO CAM Review Board

FURTHER READING

Schoenen J., J. Jacquy, and M. Lenaerts. "Effectiveness of High-Dose Riboflavin in Migraine Prophylaxis." *Neurology* 50 (1998): 466-470.

Tang, A. M, N. M. Graham, and A. J. Saah. "Effects of Micronutrient Intake on Survival in Human Immunodeficiency Virus Type 1 Infection." *American Journal of Epidemiology* 143 (1996): 1244-1256.

See also: Cataracts; HIV support; Migraines; Sickle cell disease; Sports and fitness support: enhancing recovery.

Vitamin B$_3$

CATEGORY: Herbs and supplements
RELATED TERMS: Niacin, niacinamide, nicotinamide, inositol hexaniacinate

DEFINITION: Organic compound used to treat specific health conditions.

PRINCIPAL PROPOSED USES: Niacin: High cholesterol/triglycerides; niacinamide: diabetes treatment, osteoarthritis, photosensitivity; inositol hexaniacinate: intermittent claudication, Raynaud's phenomenon

OTHER PROPOSED USES: Aging skin, cataracts, human immunodeficiency virus support, pregnancy support, rosacea, schizophrenia, tardive dyskinesia

PROBABLY NOT EFFECTIVE USES: Diabetes prevention in children at high risk, passing a urine drug screen

OVERVIEW

Vitamin B$_3$ is required for the proper function of more than fifty enzymes. Without it, the body would not be able to release energy or make fats from carbohydrates. Vitamin B$_3$ is also used to make sex hormones and other important chemical signal molecules.

Vitamin B$_3$ comes in two principal forms: niacin (nicotinic acid) and niacinamide (nicotinamide). When taken in low doses for nutritional purposes, these two forms of the vitamin are essentially identical. However, each has its own particular effects when taken in high doses. Additionally, a special form of niacin called inositol hexaniacinate has shown some promise as a treatment with special properties of its own.

REQUIREMENTS AND SOURCES

The official U.S. and Canadian recommendations for daily intake of niacin are as follows:

Infants aged 0 to 6 months (2 mg) and 7 to 12 months (4 mg); children aged 1 to 3 years (6 mg), 4 to 8 years (8 mg), and 9 to 13 years (12 mg); males aged 14 years and older (14 mg); females aged 14 and older (14 mg); pregnant women (18 mg); and nursing women (17 mg).

Because the body can make niacin from the common amino acid tryptophan, niacin deficiencies are rare in developed countries. However, the antituberculosis drug isoniazid (INH) impairs the body's ability to produce niacin from tryptophan and may create symptoms of niacin deficiency.

Good food sources of niacin are seeds, yeast, bran, peanuts (especially with skins), wild rice, brown rice, whole wheat, barley, almonds, and peas. Tryptophan is found in protein foods, such as meat, poultry, dairy products, and fish. Turkey and milk are particularly excellent sources of tryptophan.

THERAPEUTIC DOSAGES

When used as therapy for a specific disease, niacin, niacinamide, and inositol hexaniacinate are taken in dosages much higher than nutritional needs, about 1 to 4 grams (g) daily. Because of the risk of liver inflammation at these doses, medical supervision is essential.

Many people experience an unpleasant flushing sensation and headache when they take niacin. These symptoms can usually be reduced by gradually increasing the dosage over several weeks or by using slow-release niacin. However, slow-release niacin appears to be more likely to cause liver inflammation than other forms of niacin. Inositol hexaniacinate may also cause less flushing than plain niacin, and if aspirin is taken along with niacin, the flushing reaction will usually decrease.

THERAPEUTIC USES

There is no question that niacin (but not niacinamide) can significantly improve cholesterol profile, reducing levels of total and low-density lipoprotien (LDL, or bad) cholesterol and raising high-density lipoprotein (HDL, or good) cholesterol. However, unpleasant flushing reactions, as well as a risk of liver inflammation and dangerous interactions with other cholesterol-lowering drugs, have kept niacin from being widely used.

Niacinamide may improve blood sugar control in both children and adults who already have diabetes. In addition, some evidence has suggested that regular use of niacinamide (but not niacin) might help prevent diabetes in children at special risk of developing it; however, subsequent studies indicate that it probably does not work.

Preliminary evidence suggests that niacinamide may be able to decrease symptoms of osteoarthritis and help control polymorphous light eruption, a type of photosensitivity. Somewhat surprisingly, topical niacinamide has shown some promise for skin conditions. In a double-blind study of fifty women with signs of aging skin, use of a niacinamide cream significantly improved skin appearance and elasticity compared with placebo cream. Niacinamide cream has also shown promise for rosacea.

The inositol hexaniacinate form of niacin (taken orally) may be helpful for intermittent claudication14 and Raynaud's phenomenon. In addition, weak and in some cases contradictory evidence suggests one of the several forms of niacin might be helpful for people with bursitis, cataracts, human immunodeficiency virus (HIV) infection, pregnancy, schizophrenia, and tardive dyskinesia.

A new use of niacin was reported in 2007: It appears that some people take very high doses of niacin (about 2.5 to 5 grams at a time) in the belief that it will mask drugs in the urine. However, not only does niacin fail to conceal the presence of drugs on a urine drug screen, but also, when taken suddenly at doses this high, niacin can cause life-threatening problems involving the liver and heart. In addition, it can dangerously disturb blood sugar regulation and blood coagulation.

SCIENTIFIC EVIDENCE

Niacin is one of the best-researched of all the vitamins, and the evidence for using it to treat at least one condition–high cholesterol–is strong enough that it has become an accepted mainstream treatment.

High cholesterol/triglycerides. Niacin has been used since the 1950s to improve cholesterol profile. Several well-designed double-blind, placebo-controlled studies have found that niacin can reduce LDL (bad) cholesterol by approximately 10 percent and triglycerides by 25 percent, while raising HDL (good) cholesterol by 20 to 30 percent. Niacin also lowers levels of lipoprotein (a)–another risk factor for atherosclerosis–by about 35 percent. Long-term studies have shown that use of niacin can significantly reduce death rates from cardiovascular disease. Niacin also appears to be a safe and effective treatment for high cholesterol in people with diabetes and, contrary to previous reports, does not seem to raise blood sugar levels.

Treating diabetes. When a child develops diabetes, there is an interval called the honeymoon period in which the pancreas can still make some insulin and there is little to no need for injected insulin. Weak evidence suggests that niacinamide might slightly delay the onset of more severe symptoms. A cocktail of niacinamide plus antioxidant vitamins and minerals has also been tried, but the results were disappointing in one study. However, in another study, use of intensive insulin therapy along with niacinamide and vitamin E

Niacin Deficiency

Between 1907 and 1940, approximately three million Americans contracted pellagra, a disfiguring skin disease caused by niacin deficiency. An online exhibition of the National Institutes of Health's Office of NIH History highlights the role of U.S. Public Health Service surgeon Joseph Goldberger in helping to determine the cause of the disease. Scientists who followed in the footsteps of Goldberger would determine that pellagra was caused by a diet deficient in niacin. Part of the story is recounted here.

In 1914, a worried Congress asked the surgeon general to investigate pellagra, and Goldberger was assigned to the case. His theory on pellagra, often mistaken for leprosy, contradicted commonly held medical opinions. The work of Italian investigators and Goldberger's own observations in mental hospitals, orphanages, and cotton mill towns convinced him that germs did not cause the disease. In such institutions, inmates contracted the disease, but staff never did. Goldberger knew from his years of experience working on infectious diseases that germs did not distinguish between, for example, inmates and employees. Italian criminologist Cesare Lombroso had speculated that spoiled maize caused pellagra.

Goldberger found no evidence for Lombroso's hypothesis, but diet certainly seemed the crucial factor. Shipments of food that Goldberger had requested from Washington were provided to children in two Mississippi orphanages and to inmates at the Georgia State Asylum. Results were dramatic: Those who were fed a diet of fresh meat, milk, and vegetables instead of a corn-based diet recovered from pellagra. Those without the disease who ate the new diet did not contract pellagra.

Critics, many unable to part from the germ theory of pellagra, raised doubts. Goldberger hoped to squelch those reservations by demonstrating the existence of a particular substance that, when removed from the diet of healthy individuals, resulted in pellagra. With the cooperation of Mississippi's progressive governor, Earl Brewer, Goldberger experimented on eleven healthy volunteer prisoners at the Rankin State Prison Farm in 1915. Offered pardons in return for their participation, the volunteers ate a corn-based diet. Six of the eleven showed pellagra rashes after five months.

was more effective than insulin plus niacinamide alone in prolonging the honeymoon period.

A recent study suggests that niacinamide may also improve blood sugar control in type 2 diabetes, but it did not use a double-blind design.

Intermittent claudication. Double-blind studies involving a total of about four hundred individuals have found that inositol hexaniacinate can improve walking distance for people with intermittent claudication. For example, in one study, one hundred individuals were given either placebo or 4 g of inositol hexaniacinate daily. Over a period of three months, participants improved significantly in the number of steps they could take on a special device before experiencing excessive pain.

Osteoarthritis. There is some evidence that niacinamide may provide some benefits for those with osteoarthritis. In a double-blind study, seventy-two people with arthritis were given either 3,000 milligrams (mg) daily of niacinamide in six equal doses or placebo for twelve weeks. The results showed that treated participants experienced a 29 percent improvement in symptoms, whereas those given placebo worsened by 10 percent. However, at this dose, liver inflammation is a concern that must be taken seriously.

Raynaud's phenomenon. According to one small double-blind study, the inositol hexaniacinate form of niacin may be helpful for Raynaud's phenomenon. The dosage used was 4 g daily—once again, a dosage high enough for liver inflammation to be a real possibility.

SAFETY ISSUES

When taken at a dosage of more than 100 mg daily, niacin frequently causes annoying skin flushing, especially in the face, as well as stomach distress, itching, and headache. In studies, as many as 43 percent of individuals taking niacin quit because of unpleasant side effects.

A more dangerous effect of niacin is liver inflammation. Although some reports suggest that it occurs most commonly with slow-release niacin, it can occur with any type of niacin when taken at a daily dose of more than 500 mg (usually 3 g or more). Regular blood tests to evaluate liver function are therefore mandatory when using high-dose niacin (or niacinamide or inositol hexaniacinate). This reaction almost always goes away when niacin is stopped. Contrary to claims on some manufacturers' Web sites, there is no reliable evidence that inositol hexaniacinate is safer than ordinary niacin.

As noted above, a single dose of 2.5 to 5 g of niacin, used in the vain hope of passing a urine drug test despite the presence of drugs in the system, can cause life-threatening disturbances in body function. Since this range includes the high-end of the dosage used for treating cholesterol, presumably people who gradually work up to taking several grams of niacin daily can accommodate it in a way that those who take it suddenly cannot.

People who have liver disease, ulcers (presently or in the past), or gout, or drink too much alcohol should not take high-dose niacin except on medical advice. While there has been some concern that niacin may raise blood sugar levels in diabetics, the effect appears to be slight, and it carries little, if any, clinical significance.

Combining high-dose niacin with statin drugs, the most effective medications for high cholesterol, further improves cholesterol profile by raising HDL (good) cholesterol. However, there are real concerns that this combination therapy could cause a potentially fatal condition called rhabdomyolysis.

A growing body of evidence, however, suggests that the risk is relatively slight in individuals with healthy kidneys. Furthermore, even much lower doses of niacin than the usual dose given to improve cholesterol levels (100 mg versus 1,000 mg or more) may provide a similar benefit. At this dose, the risk of rhabdomyolysis should be decreased. Nonetheless, it is not safe to try this combination except under close physician supervision. Rhabdomyolysis can be fatal.

Another potential drug interaction involves the anticonvulsant drugs carbamazepine and primidone. Niacinamide might increase blood levels of these drugs, possibly requiring reduction in drug dosage. People should not use this combination except under physician supervision. The maximum safe dosage of niacin for pregnant or nursing women has been set at 35 mg daily (30 mg if eighteen years old or younger).

IMPORTANT INTERACTIONS

For people who are taking cholesterol-lowering drugs in the statin family, niacin might offer potential benefits; however, there are real dangers to this combination. People should not try it except under physician supervision.

People taking the antituberculosis drug isoniazid (INH) may need extra niacin. People who take anticonvulsant drugs, such as carbamazepine or primidone, should not take niacinamide except under physician supervision. Similarly, people who drink alcohol excessively should not take niacin except under physician supervision.

EBSCO CAM Review Board

FURTHER READING

Bissett, D. L., et al. "Niacinamide: A B Vitamin That Improves Aging Facial Skin Appearance." *Dermatological Surgery* 31 (2005): 860-865.

Cabrera-Rode, E., et al. "Effect of Standard Nicotinamide in the Prevention of Type 1 Diabetes in First Degree Relatives of Persons with Type 1 Diabetes." *Autoimmunity* 39 (2006): 333-340.

Crino, A., et al. "A Randomized Trial of Nicotinamide and Vitamin E in Children with Recent Onset Type 1 Diabetes (IMDIAB IX)." *European Journal of Endocrinology* 150 (2004): 719-724.

Draelos, Z. D., et al. "Niacinamide-Containing Facial Moisturizer Improves Skin Barrier and Benefits Subjects with Rosacea." *Cutis: Cutaneous Medicine for the Practitioner* 76 (2005): 135-141.

Gale, E. A., et al. "European Nicotinamide Diabetes Intervention Trial (ENDIT): A Randomised Controlled Trial of Intervention Before the Onset of Type 1 Diabetes." *The Lancet* 363 (2004): 925-931.

Goldberg, R. B., and T. A. Jacobson. "Effects of Niacin on Glucose Control in Patients with Dyslipidemia." *Mayo Clinic Proceedings* 83 (2008): 470-478.

Grundy, S. M., et al. "Efficacy, Safety, and Tolerability of Once-Daily Niacin for the Treatment of Dyslipidemia Associated with Type 2 Diabetes: Results of the Assessment of Diabetes Control and Evaluation of the Efficacy of Niaspan Trial." *Archives of Internal Medicine* 162 (2002): 1568-1576.

Mittal, M. K., et al. "Toxicity from the Use of Niacin to Beat Urine Drug Screening." *Annals of Emergency Medicine* 50, no. 5 (2007): 587-590.

Wink, J., G. Giacoppe, and J. King. "Effect of Very-Low-Dose Niacin on High-Density Lipoprotein in Patients Undergoing Long-Term Statin Therapy." *American Heart Journal* 143 (2002): 514-518.

Wolfe, M. L., et al. "Safety and Effectiveness of Niaspan When Added Sequentially to a Statin for

Treatment of Dyslipidemia." *American Journal of Cardiology* 87 (2001): 476-479.

See also: Aging; Cataracts; Cholesterol, high; Diabetes; HIV support; Inositol; Osteoarthritis; Photosensitivity; Pregnancy support; Raynaud's phenomenon; Rosacea; Schizophrenia; Tardive dyskinesia; Triglycerides, high.

Vitamin B$_6$

CATEGORY: Herbs and supplements
RELATED TERMS: Pyridoxine, pyridoxine hydrochloride, pyridoxal-5-phosphate
DEFINITION: Organic compound used to treat specific health conditions.
PRINCIPAL PROPOSED USES: Nausea of pregnancy (morning sickness)
OTHER PROPOSED USES: Asthma, depression, heart disease prevention, human immunodeficiency virus support, kidney stones, monosodium glutamate sensitivity, photosensitivity, reducing homocysteine levels, rheumatoid arthritis, schizophrenia, seborrheic dermatitis, tardive dyskinesia, vertigo
PROBABLY NOT EFFECTIVE USES: Alzheimer's disease, autism (combined with magnesium), carpal tunnel syndrome, diabetic neuropathy, eczema, premenstrual syndrome, side effects of oral contraceptives

OVERVIEW

Vitamin B$_6$ plays a major role in making proteins, hormones, and neurotransmitters—chemicals that carry signals between nerve cells. Because mild deficiency of vitamin B$_6$ is common, this is one vitamin that is probably worth taking as insurance. However, there is little evidence that taking vitamin B$_6$ above nutritional needs offers benefits in the treatment of any particular illnesses, except, possibly, nausea of pregnancy (morning sickness).

REQUIREMENTS AND SOURCES

Vitamin B$_6$ requirements increase with age. The official U.S. and Canadian recommendations for daily intake are as follows:

Infants aged 0 to 6 months (0.1 mg) and 7 to 12 months (0.3 mg); children aged 1 to 3 years (0.5 mg),
4 to 8 years (0.6 mg), and 9 to 13 years (1.0 mg); males aged 14 years to fifty years (1.3 mg); females aged 14 to 18 years (1.2 mg); women aged 19 to fifty years (1.3 mg); pregnant women (1.9 mg); and nursing women (2.0 mg).

Severe deficiencies of vitamin B$_6$ are rare, but mild deficiencies are extremely common. In a survey of 11,658 adults, 71 percent of men and 90 percent of women were found to have diets deficient in B$_6$. Vitamin B$_6$ is the most commonly deficient water-soluble vitamin in the elderly, and children often do not get enough B$_6$. In addition, evidence has been presented that current recommended daily intakes should be increased.

Vitamin B$_6$ deficiency might be worsened by use of hydralazine (for high blood pressure), penicillamine (used for rheumatoid arthritis and certain rare diseases), theophylline (an older drug for asthma), monoamine oxidase (MAO) inhibitors, and the antituberculosis drug isoniazid (INH), all of which are thought to interfere with B$_6$ to some degree. Good sources of B$_6$ include nutritional (torula) yeast, brewer's yeast, sunflower seeds, wheat germ, soybeans, walnuts, lentils, lima beans, buckwheat flour, bananas, and avocados.

THERAPEUTIC DOSAGES

One study found that 30 milligrams (mg) of vitamin B$_6$ daily was effective for symptoms of morning sickness. While far above nutritional needs, this dosage should be safe. However, for the treatment of other conditions, B$_6$ has been recommended at doses as high as 300 mg daily. There are potential risks at this level of vitamin B$_6$ intake.

THERAPEUTIC USES

The results of a large double-blind, placebo-controlled study suggest that vitamin B$_6$ at a dose of 30 mg daily may be helpful for treating nausea in pregnancy (morning sickness). Vitamin B$_6$ has been proposed for numerous other uses, but without much, if any, scientific substantiation. For example, the two most famous uses of vitamin B$_6$, carpal tunnel syndrome and premenstrual syndrome (PMS), have no reliable supporting evidence, and the best-designed studies found this vitamin ineffective for either of these purposes.

Higher intake of vitamin B$_6$ reduces the level in the blood of homocysteine, a substance that might accelerate cardiovascular diseases, such as heart disease, strokes, and related conditions. However, there is no meaningful evidence that reducing homocysteine is beneficial, and considerable evidence that it is not.

A series of studies suggests that vitamin B$_6$ may be helpful for the treatment of tardive dyskinesia (TD). In the first study, a four-week, double-blind crossover trial of fifteen people, treatment with vitamin B$_6$ significantly improved TD symptoms compared with placebo. Benefits were seen beginning at one week of treatment. The subsequent follow-up study tested the benefits of vitamin B$_6$ used over a period of twenty-six weeks in fifty people with tardive dyskinesia, and once again the supplement proved more effective than placebo.

For the following other conditions, current evidence for benefit with vitamin B$_6$ remains incomplete or contradictory: allergy to monosodium glutamate (MSG), asthma, depression, diabetes of pregnancy, human immunodeficiency virus (HIV) infection, photosensitivity, preventing kidney stones, schizophrenia, seborrheic dermatitis, tardive dyskinesia and other side effects of antipsychotic drugs, and vertigo.

Despite some claims in the media, vitamin B$_6$ has not shown benefit for enhancing mental function. Research investigating the benefits of B$_6$ in combination with folate and vitamin B$_{12}$ as a potential treatment for cognitive decline due to Alzheimer's disease has also shown disappointing results.

One study failed to find B$_6$ at a dose of 50 mg daily helpful for rheumatoid arthritis, despite a general B$_6$ deficiency seen in people with this condition. Vitamin B$_6$, alone or in combination with magnesium, showed some early promise for the treatment of autism, but the best-designed studies failed to find it effective.

Additionally, current evidence suggests that vitamin B$_6$ is not effective for treating diabetic neuropathy or eczema, or for helping control the side effects of oral contraceptives.

SCIENTIFIC EVIDENCE

Nausea and vomiting: Morning sickness. Vitamin B$_6$ supplements have been used for years by conventional physicians as a treatment for morning sickness. In 1995, a large double-blind study validated this use. A total of 342 pregnant women were given placebo or 30 mg of vitamin B$_6$ daily. Subjects then graded their symptoms by noting the severity of their nausea and recording the number of vomiting episodes. The women in the B$_6$ group experienced significantly less nausea than those in the placebo group, suggesting that regular use of B$_6$ can be helpful for morning sickness. However, vomiting episodes were not significantly reduced.

At least three studies have compared vitamin B$_6$ to ginger for the treatment of morning sickness. Two studies found them to be equally beneficial, while the other found ginger to be somewhat better. However, because ginger is not an established treatment for this condition, these studies alone do not provide any additional evidence in favor of B$_6$.

Chemotherapy-induced nausea and vomiting. Researchers also investigated whether vitamin B$_6$ can reduce the nausea and vomiting that often accompanies chemotherapy. A total of 142 women with ovarian cancer who were undergoing chemotherapy were randomized into three groups: acupuncture plus B$_6$ injection into the P6 acupuncture point (located on the inside of the forearm, about two inches above the wrist crease), acupuncture alone, or B$_6$ alone. Those that received both acupuncture and B$_6$ experienced less nausea and vomiting compared with the other two groups.

Premenstrual syndrome. A properly designed double-blind study of 120 women found no benefit of vitamin B$_6$ for premenstrual syndrome (PMS). In this study, three prescription drugs were compared against vitamin B$_6$ (pyridoxine, at 300 mg daily) and placebo. All study participants received three months of treatment and three months of placebo. Vitamin B$_6$ proved to be no better than placebo.

Approximately a dozen other double-blind studies have investigated the effectiveness of vitamin B$_6$ for PMS, but none were well designed; overall, the evidence for any benefit is weak at best. Some books on natural medicine report that the negative results in some of these studies were due to insufficient B$_6$ dosage, but in reality there was no clear link between dosage and effectiveness.

However, preliminary evidence suggests that the combination of B$_6$ and magnesium might be more effective than either treatment alone.

Autism. One double-blind, placebo-controlled crossover study found indications that very high doses of vitamin B$_6$ may produce beneficial effects in the treatment of autism. However, this study was small and poorly designed; furthermore, it used a dose of vitamin B$_6$ so high that it could cause toxicity.

It has been suggested that combining magnesium with vitamin B$_6$ could offer additional benefits, such as reducing side effects or allowing a reduced dose of the vitamin. However, the two reasonably well-designed studies using combined vitamin B$_6$ and magnesium have failed to find benefits. Therefore, it is not possible at present to recommend vitamin B$_6$ with or without magnesium as a treatment for autism.

Asthma. A double-blind study of seventy-six children with asthma found significant benefit from vitamin B$_6$ after the second month of usage. Children in the vitamin B$_6$ group were able to reduce their doses of asthma medication (bronchodilators and steroids). However, a recent double-blind study of thirty-one adults who used either inhaled or oral steroids did not show any benefit. The dosages of B$_6$ used in these studies were quite high, in the range of 200 to 300 mg daily. Because of the risk of nerve injury, it is not advisable to take this much B$_6$ without medical supervision.

SAFETY ISSUES

The safe upper levels for daily intake of vitamin B$_6$ are as follows:

Children aged 1 to 3 years (30 mg), 4 to 8 years (40 mg), 9 to 13 years (60 mg), and 14 to 18 years (18 mg); adults (100 mg); pregnant girls (80 mg); and pregnant women (100 mg).

At higher dosages, especially above 2 g daily, there is a very real risk of nerve damage. Nerve-related symptoms have even been reported at doses as low as 200 mg. (This is a bit ironic, given that B$_6$ deficiency also causes nerve problems.) In some cases, very high doses of vitamin B$_6$ can cause or worsen acne symptoms.

In addition, doses of vitamin B$_6$ over 5 mg may interfere with the effects of the drug levodopa when it is taken alone. However, vitamin B$_6$ does not impair the effectiveness of drugs containing levodopa and carbidopa. Maximum safe dosages for individuals with severe liver or kidney disease have not been established.

IMPORTANT INTERACTIONS

People who are taking isoniazid (INH), penicillamine, hydralazine, theophylline, or MAO inhibitors may need extra vitamin B$_6$, but they should take only nutritional doses. Higher doses of B$_6$ might interfere with the action of the drug. People who are taking levodopa without carbidopa for Parkinson's disease should not take more than 5 mg of vitamin B$_6$ daily,

except on medical advice. In addition, B$_6$ might reduce the side effects for people taking antipsychotic medications.

EBSCO CAM Review Board

FURTHER READING

Aisen, P. S., et al. "High-Dose B Vitamin Supplementation and Cognitive Decline in Alzheimer Disease." *JAMA: The Journal of the American Medical Association* 300, no. 15 (2008): 1774-1783.

Chiang, E. P., et al. "Pyridoxine Supplementation Corrects Vitamin B$_6$ Deficiency but Does Not Improve Inflammation in Patients with Rheumatoid Arthritis." *Arthritis Research and Therapy* 7 (2005): R1404-1411.

Ensiyeh, J., and M. A. Sakineh. "Comparing Ginger and Vitamin B$_6$ for the Treatment of Nausea and Vomiting in Pregnancy." *Midwifery* 25, no. 6 (2009): 649-653.

Huang, S. C., et al. "Vitamin B$_6$ Supplementation Improves Pro-Inflammatory Responses in Patients with Rheumatoid Arthritis." *European Journal of Clinical Nutrition* 64, no. 9 (2010): 1007-1013.

Lerner, V., et al. "Vitamin B$_6$ Treatment for Tardive Dyskinesia." *Journal of Clinical Psychiatry* 68 (2007): 1648-1654.

_____. "Vitamin B$_6$ Treatment in Acute Neuroleptic-Induced Akathisia." *Journal of Clinical Psychiatry* 65 (2004): 550-1554.

Malouf, R., and E. J. Grimley. "The Effect of Vitamin B$_6$ on Cognition." *Cochrane Database of Systematic Reviews* 4 (2003): CD004393.

Miodownik, C., et al. "Vitamin B$_6$ Add-on Therapy in Treatment of Schizophrenic Patients with Psychotic Symptoms and Movement Disorders." *Harefuah* 142 (2003): 592-566, 647.

Schwammenthal, Y., and D. Tanne. "Homocysteine, B-Vitamin Supplementation, and Stroke Prevention: From Observational to Interventional Trials." *Lancet Neurology* 3 (2004): 493-495.

Smith, C., et al. "A Randomized Controlled Trial of Ginger to Treat Nausea and Vomiting in Pregnancy." *Obstetrics and Gynecology* 103 (2004): 639-645.

Sripramote, M., and N. Lekhyananda. "A Randomized Comparison of Ginger and Vitamin B$_6$ in the Treatment of Nausea and Vomiting of Pregnancy." *Journal of the Medical Association of Thailand* 86 (2003): 846-853.

You, Q., et al. "Vitamin B$_6$ Points PC6 Injection During

Acupuncture Can Relieve Nausea and Vomiting in Patients with Ovarian Cancer." *International Journal of Gynecological Cancer* 19 (2009): 567-771.

See also: Asthma, Depression, mild to moderate; HIV support; Kidney stones; Morning sickness; Photosensitivity; Rheumatoid arthritis; Schizophrenia; Seborrheic dermatitis; Tardive dyskinesia; Vertigo.

Vitamin B_{12}

CATEGORY: Herbs and supplements
RELATED TERMS: Cobalamin, cyanocobalamin, hydrocobalamin, methylcobalamin
DEFINITION: Organic compound used to treat specific health conditions.
PRINCIPAL PROPOSED USE: Correcting deficiency
OTHER PROPOSED USES: Alzheimer's disease, amyotrophic lateral sclerosis (Lou Gehrig's disease), asthma, Bell's palsy, depression, diabetic neuropathy, eczema, human immunodeficiency virus support, male infertility, multiple sclerosis, osteoporosis, periodontal disease, recurrent miscarriage, restless legs syndrome, tinnitus, vitiligo

OVERVIEW

Vitamin B_{12}, an essential nutrient, is also known as cobalamin. The "cobal" in the name refers to the metal cobalt contained in B_{12}. Vitamin B_{12} is required for the normal activity of nerve cells and works with folate and vitamin B_6 to lower blood levels of homocysteine, a chemical in the blood that might contribute to heart disease. B_{12} also plays a role in the body's manufacture of S-adenosylmethionine (SAMe).

Anemia is usually (but not always) the first sign of B_{12} deficiency. Early in the twentieth century, doctors coined the name "pernicious anemia" for a stubborn form of anemia that did not improve even when the patient was given iron supplements. Experts now know that pernicious anemia comes about when the stomach fails to excrete a special substance called intrinsic factor. The body needs the intrinsic factor for efficient absorption of vitamin B_{12}. In 1948, vitamin B_{12} was identified as the cure for pernicious anemia. B_{12} deficiency also causes nerve damage, and this may, in some cases, occur without anemia first developing.

Vitamin B_{12} has also been proposed as a treatment for numerous other conditions, but there is no definitive evidence that it is effective for any purpose other than correcting deficiency.

REQUIREMENTS AND SOURCES

Extraordinarily small amounts of vitamin B_{12} suffice for daily nutritional needs. The official U.S. and Canadian recommendations for daily intake (in micrograms, or mcg) are as follows:

Infants aged 0 to 6 months (0.4 mcg) and 7 to 12 months (0.5 mcg); children aged 1 to 3 years (0.9 mcg), 4 to 8 years (1.2 mcg), and 9 to 13 years (1.8 mcg); males and females aged 14 years and older (2.4 mcg); pregnant women (2.6 mcg); and nursing women (2.8 mcg).

Vitamin B_{12} deficiency is rare in the young, but it is not unusual in older people: Probably 10 to 20 percent of the elderly are deficient in B_{12}. This may be because older people have lower levels of stomach acid. The vitamin B_{12} in food comes attached to proteins and must be released by acid in the stomach in order to be absorbed. When stomach acid levels are low, people do not absorb as much vitamin B_{12} from their food. Vitamin B_{12} supplements do not need acid for absorption and should therefore get around this problem. However, for reasons that are unclear, one study found that B_{12}-deficient seniors need very high dosages of the supplements to normalize their levels, as high as 600 to 1,000 mcg daily. Similarly, people who take medications that greatly reduce stomach acid, such as omeprazole (Prilosec) or ranitidine (Zantac), also may have trouble absorbing B_{12} from food and could benefit from supplementation.

Stomach surgery and other conditions affecting the digestive tract can also lead to B_{12} deficiency. Vitamin B_{12} absorption or levels in the blood may also be impaired by colchicine (for gout), metformin and phenformin (for diabetes), and azidothymidine ([AZT] for acquired immunodeficiency syndrome [AIDS]). Exposure to nitrous oxide, such as may be experienced by dentists and dental hygienists, might cause B_{12} deficiency, but studies disagree. Slow-release potassium supplements might also impair B_{12} absorption.

Vitamin B_{12} is found in most animal foods; it is also found only in animal food. Beef, liver, clams, and lamb provide a whopping 80 to 100 mcg of B_{12} per 3.5-ounce serving, at least forty times the dietary requirement. Sardines, chicken liver, beef kidney, and calf

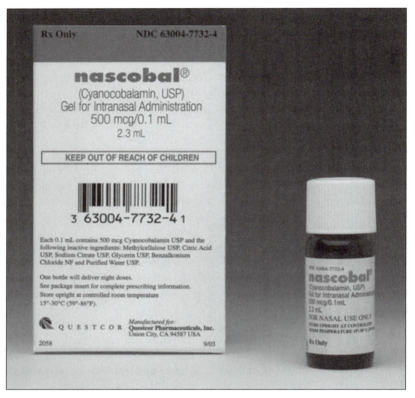

A prescription nasal vitamin B$_{12}$ supplement can be used by people who have difficulty absorbing B$_{12}$ through the digestive tract. (PR Newswire)

liver are also good sources, providing between 25 and 60 mcg per serving. Trout, salmon, tuna, eggs, whey, and many cheeses provide at least the recommended daily intake.

Total vegetarians (vegans) must take vitamin B$_{12}$ supplements or consume B$_{12}$-fortified foods, or they will eventually become deficient. Contrary to some reports, seaweed and tempeh do not provide B$_{12}$. Some forms of blue-green algae, such as spirulina, contain B$_{12}$, but it is not in an absorbable state.

Vitamin B$_{12}$ is available in three forms: cyanocobalamin, hydrocobalamin, and methylcobalamin. The first is the most widely available and least expensive, but some experts think that the other two forms are preferable.

Severe B$_{12}$ deficiency can cause anemia and, potentially, nerve damage. The latter may become permanent if the deficiency is not corrected in time. Anemia most often develops first, leading to treatment before permanent nerve damage develops. However, folate supplements can get in the way of this "early warning system." This is why people are cautioned against taking high doses of folate without medical supervision. When taken at a dosage higher than 400 mcg daily, folate can prevent anemia caused by B$_{12}$ deficiency, thereby allowing permanent nerve damage to develop without any warning. More mild deficiencies of vitamin B$_{12}$ may cause elevated levels of homocysteine in the blood, potentially increasing risk of heart disease. Mild B$_{12}$ deficiency, too slight to cause anemia, may also impair brain function.

THERAPEUTIC DOSAGES

For correcting absorption problems caused by medications, taking vitamin B$_{12}$ at the level of dietary requirements should suffice. For other purposes, enormously higher daily doses—ranging from 100 to 2,000 mcg—are sometimes recommended.

THERAPEUTIC USES

It appears that individuals who take medications that dramatically lower stomach acid, such as H$_2$ blockers or proton pump inhibitors, would benefit by taking B$_{12}$ supplements. Other individuals likely to be deficient in B$_{12}$, such as the elderly and those taking the medications listed above in Requirements and Sources, might well benefit from a daily B$_{12}$ supplement to prevent B$_{12}$ deficiency.

For pernicious anemia, B$_{12}$ injections are traditionally used. However, research has shown that oral B$_{12}$ works just as well, provided people take enough of it: between 300 and 1,000 mcg daily.

Weak evidence suggests that B$_{12}$ supplements may improve sperm activity and sperm count; on this basis, they could be useful for male infertility. Some cases of recurrent miscarriage might be due to vitamin B$_{12}$ deficiency.

One placebo-controlled, double-blind study, enrolling forty-nine people with eczema, found benefit with a cream containing vitamin B$_{12}$ at a concentration of 0.07 percent. Topical B$_{12}$ is hypothesized to work for eczema by reducing local levels of the substance nitric oxide (not related to nitrous oxide).

On the basis of weak and sometimes contradictory evidence, vitamin B$_{12}$ has been suggested for human immunodeficiency virus (HIV), amyotrophic lateral sclerosis, carpal tunnel syndrome, diabetic neuropathy, multiple sclerosis, restless legs syndrome, and tinnitus. Some evidence suggests that people with vitiligo (splotchy loss of skin pigmentation) might be deficient in vitamin B$_{12}$, and supplementation along with folate may be helpful. However, the evidence is very weak and not all studies agree.

Some alternative practitioners recommend the use of injected vitamin B$_{12}$ for Bell's palsy. However, the only scientific support for this approach comes from one study that was not double-blind.

Vitamin B$_{12}$ is also sometimes recommended for numerous other problems, including asthma, osteoporosis, periodontal disease, and depression. However, there is not much evidence that it really works.

A double-blind trial of vitamin B$_{12}$ for seasonal affective disorder, a type of depression related to lack of light during the winter, failed to find evidence of benefit. In addition, a randomized trial involving older adults with mild depression found that taking folate (400 mcg) and vitamin B$_{12}$ (100 mcg) daily for two years was no better than a placebo for reducing depressive symptoms.

One double-blind, placebo-controlled study of 140 people with mildly low B$_{12}$ levels failed to find the supplement helpful for improving mental function and mood. Another study failed to find evidence that vitamin B$_{12}$ improved general sense of well-being among seniors with signs of mild B$_{12}$ deficiency.

Although vitamin B$_{12}$ has been proposed as a treatment for Alzheimer's disease, this recommendation is based solely on the results of one small, poorly designed study. More recent and better-designed studies found little to no benefit.

SCIENTIFIC EVIDENCE

Vitamin B$_{12}$ deficiencies in men can lead to reduced sperm counts and lowered sperm mobility. For this reason, B$_{12}$ supplements have been tried for improving fertility in men with abnormal sperm production. In one double-blind study of 375 infertile men, supplementation with vitamin B$_{12}$ produced no benefits on average in the group as a whole. However, in a particular subgroup of men with sufficiently low

sperm count and sperm motility, B$_{12}$ appeared to be helpful. Such "dredging" of the data is suspect from a scientific point of view, however, and this study cannot be taken as proof of effectiveness.

SAFETY ISSUES

Vitamin B$_{12}$ appears to be extremely safe. However, in some cases, very high doses of the vitamin can cause or worsen acne symptoms.

IMPORTANT INTERACTIONS

People who are taking colchicine; AZT; medications that reduce stomach acid, such as the H$_2$ blocker ranitidine (Zantac) or the proton pump inhibitor omeprazole (Prilosec); oral hypoglycemics, such as metformin or phenformin; and slow-release potassium supplements; and people who are exposed to nitrous oxide anesthesia may need extra B$_{12}$. Another option is to take extra calcium, which may, in turn, improve B$_{12}$ absorption.

EBSCO CAM Review Board

FURTHER READING

Hvas, A. M., et al. "No Effect of Vitamin B$_{12}$ Treatment on Cognitive Function and Depression." *Journal of Affective Disorders* 81 (2004): 269-273.

_____. "Vitamin B$_{12}$ Treatment Has Limited Effect on Health-Related Quality of Life Among Individuals with Elevated Plasma Methylmalonic Acid." *Journal of Internal Medicine* 253 (2003): 146-152.

Malouf, R., and J. Grimley Evans. "Folic Acid with or Without Vitamin B$_{12}$ for the Prevention and Treatment of Healthy Elderly and Demented People." *Cochrane Database of Systematic Reviews* 4 (2008): CD004514.

Reznikoff-Etievant, M. F., et al. "Low Vitamin B$_{12}$ Level as a Risk Factor for Very Early Recurrent Abortion." *European Journal of Obstetrics, Gynecology, and Reproductive Biology* 104 (2002): 156-159.

Sato, Y., et al. "Amelioration by Mecobalamin of Subclinical Carpal Tunnel Syndrome Involving Unaffected Limbs in Stroke Patients." *Journal of Neurological Sciences* 231 (2005): 13-18.

Seussen, S. J., et al. "Oral Cyanocobalamin Supplementation in Older People with Vitamin B$_{12}$ Deficiency." *Archives of Internal Medicine* 165 (2005): 1167-1172.

Stucker, M., et al. "Topical Vitamin B, a New Therapeutic Approach in Atopic Dermatitis: Evaluation of Efficacy and Tolerability in a Randomized Placebo-Controlled Multicentre Clinical Trial." *British Journal of Dermatology* 150 (2004): 977-983.

Ting, R. Z., et al. "Risk Factors of Vitamin B_{12} Deficiency in Patients Receiving Metformin." *Archives of Internal Medicine* 166 (2006): 1975-1999.

Walker, J. G., et al. "Mental Health Literacy, Folic Acid and Vitamin B_{12}, and Physical Activity for the Prevention of Depression in Older Adults." *British Journal of Psychiatry* 197, no. 1 (2010): 45-54.

See also: Alzheimer's disease; Amyotrophic lateral sclerosis; Asthma; Bell's palsy; Depression, mild to moderate; Diabetes, complications of; Eczema; HIV support; Infertility, male; Multiple sclerosis; Osteoporosis; Periodontal disease; Restless legs syndrome; Tinnitus; Vitiligo.

Vitamin C

CATEGORY: Herbs and supplements

RELATED TERMS: Ascorbate, ascorbic acid

DEFINITION: Natural substance essential for health and promoted as a dietary supplement for specific health benefits.

PRINCIPAL PROPOSED USES: None

OTHER PROPOSED USES: Acute anterior uveitis, aging skin, allergies, asthma, autism, bedsores, bladder infections in pregnancy, cancer prevention, cancer treatment, cataracts, common cold treatment, easy bruising, gallbladder disease prevention, glaucoma, heart disease prevention, human immunodeficiency virus infection, hypertension, insomnia, low sperm count, macular degeneration, maintaining effectiveness of nitrate drugs, menopausal symptoms, minor injuries, muscle soreness after exercise, osteoarthritis, photosensitivity, preeclampsia prevention, reflex sympathetic dystrophy prevention, sunburn prevention, vascular dementia prevention, ulcers, weight loss

PROBABLY NOT EFFECTIVE USES: Cervical dysplasia, common cold prevention

OVERVIEW

Although most animals can make vitamin C, humans have lost the ability to do so through evolution. Because of this, humans must get the vitamin from food, chiefly fresh fruits and vegetables. One of this vitamin's main functions is helping the body manufacture collagen, a key protein in connective tissues, cartilage, and tendons.

From ancient times through the early nineteenth century, sailors and others deprived of fresh fruits and vegetables developed a disease called scurvy. Scurvy involves scorbutic symptoms, which include nonhealing wounds, bleeding gums, bruising, and overall weakness. It is now known that scurvy is nothing more than vitamin C deficiency. Scurvy was successfully treated with citrus fruit during the mid-eighteenth century. In 1931–1932, Hungarian physiologist Albert Szent-Györgyi isolated the active ingredient of citrus fruits, calling it the antiscorbutic principle, or ascorbic acid (vitamin C).

Vitamin C is a powerful antioxidant that neutralizes damaging natural substances called free radicals. It works in water, both inside and outside cells. Vitamin C complements another antioxidant vitamin, vitamin E, which works in lipid (fatty) parts of the body.

Vitamin C is the single most popular vitamin supplement in the United States and perhaps the most controversial too. In the 1960s, two-time Nobel Prize winner Linus Pauling claimed that vitamin C could effectively treat both cancer and the common cold. Subsequent research has mostly discounted these claims but has not dampened enthusiasm for this essential nutrient. The vitamin C "movement" has led to hundreds of clinical studies testing the vitamin on dozens of illnesses; at present, however, no dramatic benefits have been discerned.

REQUIREMENTS AND SOURCES

Vitamin C is an essential nutrient that must be obtained from food or supplements; the body cannot manufacture it. The official U.S. and Canadian recommendations for daily intake (in milligrams) are as follows:

Infants to six months of age (40) and seven to twelve months of age (50); children one to three years of age (15), four to eight years of age (25), and nine to thirteen years of age (45); boys aged fourteen to eighteen years (75) and girls aged fourteen to eighteen years (65); men (90) and women (75); pregnant girls (80) and pregnant women (85); nursing girls (115) and nursing women (120).

Smoking cigarettes significantly reduces levels of

vitamin C in the body. The recommended daily intake for smokers is 35 mg higher across all age groups.

Scurvy, the classic vitamin C deficiency disease, is now a rarity in the developed world, although a more subtle deficiency of vitamin C is fairly common. According to one study, 40 percent of Americans do not get enough vitamin C. Also, vitamin C deficiency great enough to cause bleeding problems during surgery turns out to be more common than previously thought.

Aspirin and other anti-inflammatory drugs might lower body levels of vitamin C, as might oral contraceptives. Supplementation may be helpful if one is taking any of these medications.

Most people think of orange juice as the quintessential source of vitamin C, but many vegetables are actually even richer sources. Red chili peppers, sweet peppers, kale, parsley, collard, and turnip greens are full of vitamin C, as are broccoli, Brussels sprouts, watercress, cauliflower, cabbage, and strawberries. (Oranges and other citrus fruits are good sources too.)

One great advantage of getting vitamin C from foods rather than from supplements is that many other potentially healthful nutrients are obtained at the same time, nutrients such as bioflavonoids and carotenes. However, vitamin C in food is partially destroyed by cooking and exposure to air, so for maximum nutritional benefit, one could try eating freshly made salads rather than dishes that require a lot of cooking.

Vitamin C supplements are available in two forms: ascorbic acid and ascorbate. The latter is less intensely sour.

THERAPEUTIC DOSAGES

Since the time of Pauling, proponents have recommended taking vitamin C in enormous doses, as high as 20,000 to 30,000 mg daily. However, some evidence suggests that there might not be any reason to take more than 200 mg of vitamin C daily (ten to one hundred times less than the amount recommended by vitamin C proponents). The reason is that if a person consumes more than 200 mg daily (researchers have tested up to 2,500 mg), the kidneys begin to excrete the excess at a steadily increasing rate, matching the increased dose. The digestive tract also stops absorbing it well. The net effect is that no matter how much is taken, the blood levels of vitamin C do not increase very much.

However, there are some flaws in this research. It is possible that vitamin C levels might rise in other tissues even if they remain constant in the blood. Furthermore, this study did not evaluate the possible effects of taking vitamin C several times daily rather than once daily.

Many nutritional experts recommend 500 mg of vitamin C daily. This dose is almost undoubtedly safe. Others recommend taking as much vitamin C as possible, up to 30,000 mg daily, cutting back only when one starts to develop stomach cramps and diarrhea. This recommendation seems based more on a semireligious enthusiasm for vitamin C than on any evidence that such huge doses of the vitamin are beneficial.

Intravenous vitamin C can easily raise vitamin C levels to a level 140 times higher than the maximum achievable with oral vitamin C. However, there is no meaningful evidence that intravenous vitamin C provides any medical benefits.

THERAPEUTIC USES

According to numerous double-blind, placebo-controlled studies, the regular use of vitamin C supplements can slightly reduce symptoms of colds and modestly shorten the length of the illness. However, taking vitamin C at the onset of a cold probably will not work.

Regular use of vitamin C does not seem to help prevent colds. One exception is the "postmarathon sniffle," colds that develop after heavy exercise. Vitamin C may be helpful for preventing this condition, although not all studies agree.

Two double-blind studies suggest that the use of vitamin C with vitamin E might slightly reduce the risk of developing preeclampsia, a complication of pregnancy. However, a much larger follow-up study failed to find benefits. Two studies conducted by a single research group have found that vitamin C at a dose of 500 mg daily might help prevent reflex sympathetic dystrophy, a poorly understood condition that can follow injuries such as fractures.

Over time, the body develops tolerance to drugs in the nitrate family (such as nitroglycerin). Some evidence suggests that the use of vitamin C can help maintain the effectiveness of these medications.

Other small double-blind trials suggest that vitamin C might be helpful for anterior uveitis (when taken with vitamin E), autism, easy bruising, minor injuries, protecting the liver in nonalcoholic steatohepatitis, speeding recovery from bedsores, treating female

Vitamin C for Preventing Reflex Sympathetic Dystrophy

Reflex sympathetic dystrophy (RSD) is a set of symptoms that can develop in the legs, arms, feet, and hands after fractures and other injuries. Also called complex regional pain syndrome, its symptoms include changes in skin temperature and color over the affected area, accompanied by burning pain, sensitivity to touch, sweating, and limitation of range of motion. The cause of RSD is unknown, and it is very difficult to treat.

Two studies performed by a single research group suggest that RSD might be preventable by timely use of vitamin C following a fracture. The most recent of these studies compared placebo with three different dosages of vitamin C in 416 people with wrist fractures.

For fifty days, participants received either placebo or vitamin C at a dose of 200 milligrams (mg), 500 mg, or 1,500 mg daily. They were then followed to see how many developed RSD. The results indicated that approximately 10 percent of those given placebo developed RSD, while less than 2 percent of those given vitamin C in the 500 mg or the 1,500 mg daily dose did so. (This difference was statistically significant.) The 200-mg dose of vitamin C did appear to offer some protection too, but not as much.

Based on these findings, the researchers concluded that people who have been injured, placing them at risk for RSD, should take vitamin C at a dose of 500 mg daily. However, it should be noted that confirmation by an independent research group is still lacking.

Steven Bratman, M.D.

infertility (specifically, a condition called luteal phase defect), and preventing early rupture of the chorio-amniotic membranes in pregnancy. Vitamin C might also improve the effectiveness of antibiotic treatment for *Helicobacter pylori*, the cause of most peptic ulcers.

Preliminary evidence suggests that cream containing vitamin C may improve the appearance of aging or sun-damaged skin. Inconsistent evidence suggests that oral or topical vitamin C, taken by itself or with vitamin E, may also help protect the skin from sun damage.

Double-blind studies of vitamin C for the following conditions have yielded mixed results: asthma, male infertility, reducing the muscle soreness that typically develops after exercise, and hypertension. Unexpectedly, one study found that a combination of vitamin C (500 mg daily) and grape seed oligomeric proanthocyanidins (1,000 mg daily) slightly increased blood pressure. Whether this was a fluke of statistics or a real combined effect remains unclear.

Limited and in some cases contradictory evidence suggests possible benefit in the prevention or treatment of allergies, atrial fibrillation following coronary artery bypass grafting, bladder infections during pregnancy, gallbladder disease (in women), glaucoma, gout, obesity, and vascular dementia. Also, the intravaginal use of vitamin C tablets might be helpful for nonspecific vaginitis.

Observational studies indicate that people with a higher intake of vitamin C have a lower incidence of cataracts, macular degeneration, heart disease, cancer, and osteoarthritis. However, these findings do not indicate that vitamin C supplements will help prevent or treat these conditions. Observational studies are notoriously unreliable for showing the efficacy of treatments; only double-blind studies can do that, and only one has been performed that directly examined vitamin C's potential benefits for preventing these conditions. Two large double-blind trials exploring the effectiveness of vitamin C for heart disease prevention, one in women at high risk and the other in men at low risk, failed to find any benefit. Vitamin C has been proposed as a treatment for cancer, but this claim is very controversial, and there is no scientifically meaningful evidence that it works.

Massive doses of vitamin C have at times been popular among people with human immunodeficiency virus (HIV) infection, based on preliminary evidence. An observational study linked high doses of vitamin C with slower progression to acquired immunodeficiency syndrome (AIDS). However, a double-blind study of forty-nine people with HIV who took combined vitamins C and E or placebo for three months did not show any significant effects on the amount of HIV detected or the number of opportunistic infections. Furthermore, one study found that vitamin C at a dose of 1 g daily substantially reduced blood levels of the drug indinavir, a protease inhibitor used for the treatment of HIV infection. This could potentially cause the drug to fail.

In a study of eighty women with *Chlamydia tracho-matis* infection, adding vitamin C to doxycycline and triple sulfa vaginal cream reduced discharge and pain associated with intercourse. According to a double-blind, placebo-controlled study of 141 women with cervical dysplasia (early cervical cancer), vitamin C, taken at a dosage of 500 mg daily, does not help to reverse the dysplasia.

One substantial study failed to find vitamin C useful for improving high cholesterol. Vitamin C also does not appear to be helpful for treating Raynaud's phenomenon caused by scleroderma.

SCIENTIFIC EVIDENCE

Colds. As the best known of all natural treatments for the common cold, vitamin C has been subjected to irresponsible hype from both proponents and opponents. Enthusiasts claim that if one takes vitamin C daily, one will never get sick, while critics of the treatment insist that vitamin C has no benefit.

However, a reasoned evaluation of the research indicates something in between. Numerous studies have found that vitamin C supplements taken at a dose of 1,000 mg daily or more throughout the cold season can modestly reduce symptoms of colds and help a person get over a cold faster, but they do not generally help prevent colds.

Reducing cold symptoms. Most studies on vitamin C have evaluated the potential benefits of taking vitamin C throughout the cold season. A review of twenty-nine placebo-controlled trials involving more than eleven thousand people found that the use of vitamin C in this way can reduce symptoms and decrease the duration of colds. Other studies have found similar results.

Many people begin taking vitamin C only when cold symptoms start. Vitamin C is probably not effective when used in this way. One double-blind trial enrolled four hundred persons with new-onset cold symptoms and divided them into four different daily vitamin-C-dosage groups: 30 mg daily (a dose lower than the minimum daily requirement and used by the researchers as a placebo), 1,000 mg, 3,000 mg, or 3,000 mg with bioflavonoids. Participants were instructed to take the vitamin at the onset of symptoms and for the following two days. The results showed no difference in the duration or severity of cold symptoms among the groups. High-dose vitamin C taken at the onset of a cold, in other words, did not help. A review of seven randomized and nonrandomized trials

also found that taking vitamin C at the start of a cold did not offer any benefits. Indeed, there are numerous other natural treatments for the common cold, some of which may be more helpful than vitamin C.

Preventing colds. Although two relatively late studies suggest that regular use of vitamin C throughout the cold season can help prevent colds, these studies had a variety of flaws, and most other studies have found little to no benefit along these lines. However, people who are truly deficient in vitamin C, such as elderly people in nursing homes, may show increased resistance to infection if they take vitamin C (or other nutrients).

In addition, vitamin C might be helpful for preventing the respiratory infections that can follow heavy endurance exercise. Marathon running and similar forms of exertion can temporarily weaken the immune system, leading to infections. Vitamin C may be helpful. According to a double-blind, placebo-controlled study involving ninety-two runners, taking 600 mg of vitamin C for twenty-one days before a race made a significant difference in the incidence of sickness afterward. Within two weeks of the race, 68 percent of the runners taking placebo developed cold symptoms, versus only 33 percent of those taking the vitamin C supplement. As part of the same study, nonrunners of similar age and gender to those running were also given vitamin C or placebo. The supplement had no apparent effect on the incidence of upper respiratory infections in this group. Vitamin C seemed to be effective in this capacity only for those who exercised intensively.

Two other studies found that vitamin C could reduce the number of colds experienced by groups of people involved in rigorous exercise in extremely cold environments. One study involved 139 children attending a skiing camp in the Swiss Alps, while the other enrolled 56 military men engaged in a training exercise in northern Canada during the winter months. In both cases, the participants took either 1 g of vitamin C or placebo daily at the time their training program began. Cold symptoms were monitored for one to two weeks following training, and significant differences in favor of vitamin C were found.

However, one large study of 674 U.S. Marine Corps recruits in basic training found no such benefit. The results showed no difference in the number of colds between the treatment and placebo groups.

There are many possibilities for this discrepancy.

Perhaps basic training in the Marine Corps is significantly different from the other forms of exercise studied. Another point to consider is that the Marine recruits did not start taking vitamin C right at the beginning of training, but waited three weeks. The study also lasted a bit longer than the positive studies mentioned above, continuing for two months; maybe vitamin C is more effective at preventing colds in the short term. Another possibility is that vitamin C does not work. More research is needed to know for sure.

Preeclampsia prevention. Preeclampsia is a dangerous complication of pregnancy that involves high blood pressure, swelling of the whole body, and improper kidney function. A double-blind, placebo-controlled study of 283 women at increased risk for preeclampsia found that supplementation with vitamin C (1,000 mg daily) and vitamin E (400 international units daily) significantly reduced the chances of developing this disease.

While this research is promising, larger studies are necessary to confirm whether vitamins C and E will actually work. The authors of this study point out that similarly sized studies found benefits with other treatments, such as aspirin, that later proved to be ineffective when large-scale studies were performed. Furthermore, it is not known whether such high dosages of these vitamins are absolutely safe for pregnant women.

Cancer treatment. Cancer treatment is one of the more controversial proposed uses of vitamin C. An early study tested vitamin C in eleven hundred terminally ill people with cancer. One hundred participants received 10,000 mg daily of vitamin C, while one thousand other participants (the control group) received no treatment. Those taking the vitamin survived more than four times longer on average (210 days) than those in the control group (50 days). A large (1,826-participant) follow-up study by the same researchers found a nearly doubled survival rate (343 days versus 180 days) in vitamin-C-treated participants whose cancers were deemed incurable compared with untreated controls. However, these studies were poorly designed, and other generally better-constructed studies have found no benefit of vitamin C in cancer. Vitamin C cannot be regarded as a proven treatment for cancer.

Reflex sympathetic dystrophy. Reflex sympathetic dystrophy (RSD) is a set of symptoms that can develop in the legs, arms, feet, and hands after fractures and other injuries. It is also called complex regional pain syndrome. Symptoms include changes in skin temperature and color over the affected area, accompanied by burning pain, sensitivity to touch, sweating, and limited of range of motion. The cause of RSD is unknown, and the condition is very difficult to treat.

Two studies performed by a single research group reported evidence that vitamin C can help prevent RSD after wrist fractures. In one of these studies, 123 adults with wrist fractures were enrolled and followed for one year. All were given 500 mg of vitamin C or placebo daily for fifty days. The results showed significantly fewer cases of RSD in the treated group.

A subsequent study conducted by the same research group compared placebo with three dosages of vitamin C in 416 people who had a wrist fracture. Again, treatment continued for fifty days. The results indicated that approximately 10 percent of those given placebo developed RSD, while less than 2 percent of those given either 500 or 1,500 mg of vitamin C daily did so. According to the statistical analysis used by the authors, this relative benefit was statistically significant. The 200-mg dose of vitamin C did appear to offer some protection too, but not as much.

Easy bruising. A two-month, double-blind study of ninety-four elderly people with marginal vitamin C deficiency found that vitamin C supplements decreased their tendency to bruise.

Hypertension. According to a thirty-day, double-blind study of thirty-nine persons taking medications for hypertension (high blood pressure), treatment with 500 mg of vitamin C daily can reduce blood pressure by about 10 percent. Smaller benefits were seen in studies of persons with normal blood pressure or borderline hypertension. However, other studies have failed to find any significant blood-pressure-lowering effect. This mixed evidence suggests, on balance, that if vitamin C does have any blood-pressure-lowering effect, it is at most quite small.

Maintaining the effectiveness of nitrate drugs. Nitroglycerin and related nitrate medications are used for the treatment of angina. However, the effectiveness of these medications tends to diminish over time. According to a double-blind study of forty-eight people, the use of vitamin C at a dose of 2,000 mg three times daily helped maintain the effectiveness of nitroglycerin. These findings are supported by other studies too.

Angina is too serious a disease for self-treatment. Persons with angina should not take vitamin C (or any other supplement) except on a physician's advice.

SAFETY ISSUES

The U.S. government has issued recommendations regarding tolerable upper intake levels (ULs) for vitamin C. The UL can be thought of as the highest daily intake over a prolonged time known to pose no risks to most members of a healthy population. The ULs for vitamin C are as follows: children one to three years of age (400), four to eight years of age (650), and nine to thirteen years of age (1,200); boys and girls aged fourteen to eighteen years (1,800); men and women (2,000); pregnant girls (1,800) and pregnant women (2,000); nursing girls (1,800) and nursing women (2,000).

Even within the safe intake range for vitamin C, some persons may develop diarrhea. This side effect will likely go away with continued use of vitamin C, but one might have to cut down the dosage for a while and then gradually build up again.

Concerns have been raised that long-term vitamin C treatment can cause kidney stones. However, in large-scale observational studies, persons who consume large amounts of vitamin C have shown either no change or a decreased risk of kidney stone formation. Still, there may be certain persons who are particularly at risk for vitamin-C-induced kidney stones. People with a history of kidney stones and those with kidney failure who have a defect in vitamin-C or oxalate metabolism should probably restrict vitamin C intake to approximately 100 mg daily. Persons with glucose-6-phosphate dehydrogenase deficiency, iron overload, or a history of intestinal surgery should also avoid high-dose vitamin C.

Vitamin C supplements increase absorption of iron. Because it is not good to get more iron than needed, persons using iron supplements should not take vitamin C at the same time as the iron supplements except under a physician's supervision.

One study from the 1970s suggests that high doses of vitamin C (3 g daily) might increase the levels of acetaminophen (such as Tylenol) in the body. This could potentially put a person at higher risk for acetaminophen toxicity. This interaction is probably relatively unimportant when acetaminophen is taken in single doses for pain and fever, or for a few days during a cold. However, if one uses acetaminophen daily or has kidney or liver problems, simultaneous use of high-dose vitamin C is probably not advisable.

Weak evidence suggests that vitamin C, when taken in high doses, might reduce the blood-thinning effects of warfarin (Coumadin) and heparin. One study found that vitamin C at a dose of 1 g daily substantially reduced blood levels of the drug indinavir, a protease inhibitor used for the treatment of HIV infection.

Heated disagreement exists regarding whether it is safe or appropriate to combine antioxidants such as vitamin C with standard chemotherapy drugs. The reasoning behind the concern is that some chemotherapy drugs may work in part by creating free radicals that destroy cancer cells, and antioxidants might interfere with this beneficial effect. However, there is no good evidence that antioxidants actually interfere with chemotherapy drugs; in fact, there is growing evidence that they do not. Finally, the maximum safe dosages of vitamin C for people with severe liver or kidney disease have not been determined.

IMPORTANT INTERACTIONS

Persons taking aspirin, other anti-inflammatory drugs, or oral contraceptives may need more vitamin C. The risk of liver damage from high doses of acetaminophen may be increased if one also takes large doses of vitamin C. High-dose vitamin C might reduce the effectiveness of warfarin and heparin.

High-dose vitamin C can cause a person to absorb too much iron. This is especially a problem for people with diseases that cause them to store too much iron. Vitamin C may help maintain the effectiveness of medications in the nitrate family.

Persons who have angina should not take vitamin C (or any other supplement) except on a physician's advice. High-dose vitamin C may reduce the effectiveness of protease inhibitors for HIV infection. Finally, persons undergoing cancer chemotherapy should not use vitamin C except on a physician's advice.

EBSCO CAM Review Board

FURTHER READING

Bryer, S. C., and A. H. Goldfarb. "Effect of High Dose Vitamin C Supplementation on Muscle Soreness, Damage, Function, and Oxidative Stress to Eccentric Exercise." *International Journal of Sport Nutrition and Exercise Metabolism* 16 (2006): 270-280.

Chuang, C. H., et al. "Adjuvant Effect of Vitamin C on Omeprazole-Amoxicillin-Clarithromycin Triple Therapy for *Helicobacter pylori* Eradication." *Hepatogastroenterology* 54 (2007): 320-324.

Connolly, D. A., et al. "The Effects of Vitamin C Supplementation on Symptoms of Delayed Onset

Muscle Soreness." *Journal of Sports Medicine and Physical Fitness* 46 (2006): 462-467.

Cook, N. R., et al. "A Randomized Factorial Trial of Vitamins C and E and Beta Carotene in the Secondary Prevention of Cardiovascular Events in Women: Results from the Women's Antioxidant Cardiovascular Study." *Archives of Internal Medicine* 167 (2007): 1610-1618.

Hemila, H., E. Chalker, and B. Douglas. "Vitamin C for Preventing and Treating the Common Cold." *Cochrane Database of Systematic Reviews* (2010): CD000980. Available online through *EBSCO DynaMed Systematic Literature Surveillance* at http:// www.ebscohost.com/dynamed.

Rumbold, A. R., et al. "Vitamins C and E and the Risks of Preeclampsia and Perinatal Complications." *New England Journal of Medicine* 354 (2006): 1796-1806.

Sesso, H. D., et al. "Vitamins E and C in the Prevention of Cardiovascular Disease in Men." *Journal of the American Medical Association* 300 (2008): 2123-2133.

Tecklenburg, S. L., et al. "Ascorbic Acid Supplementation Attenuates Exercise-Induced Bronchoconstriction in Patients with Asthma." *Respiratory Medicine* 101 (2007): 1770-1778.

Zollinger, P. E., et al. "Can Vitamin C Prevent Complex Regional Pain Syndrome in Patients with Wrist Fractures?" *Journal of Bone and Joint Surgery: American Volume* 89 (2007): 1424-1431.

See also: Colds and flu; Supplements: Introduction; Vitamins and minerals.

Vitamin D

CATEGORY: Herbs and supplements

RELATED TERMS: Cholecalciferol (vitamin D_3), ergocalciferol (vitamin D_2)

DEFINITION: Natural substance promoted as a dietary supplement for specific health benefits.

PRINCIPAL PROPOSED USE: Osteoporosis prevention and treatment

OTHER PROPOSED USES: Cancer prevention, diabetes prevention, hypertension prevention, polycystic ovary syndrome, psoriasis, seasonal affective disorder

OVERVIEW

Vitamin D is both a vitamin and a hormone. It is a vitamin because the body cannot absorb calcium without it, and it is a hormone because the body manufactures it in response to the skin's exposure to sunlight.

There are two major forms of vitamin D, and both have the word "calciferol" in their names. In Latin, calciferol means "calcium carrier." Vitamin D_3 (cholecalciferol) is made by the body and is found in some foods. Vitamin D_2 (ergocalciferol) is the form most often added to milk and other foods, and the form that one is most likely to use as a supplement.

Strong evidence suggests that using both vitamin D and calcium supplements can be helpful for preventing and treating osteoporosis. Other potential uses of vitamin D have little supporting evidence.

REQUIREMENTS AND SOURCES

As with vitamin A, dosages of vitamin D are often expressed in terms of international units (IU) rather than milligrams. The official U.S. and Canadian recommendations for daily (IU) intake of vitamin D are as follows:

Infants to twelve months of age (200); children one year to eighteen years of age (200); adults to fifty years of age (200), adults to seventy years of age (400); adults aged seventy-one years and older (600); pregnant females (200); and nursing females (200).

However, growing evidence suggests that these recommendations may be too low.

In a study of military personnel in submarines, the use of 400 IU of vitamin D daily was inadequate to maintain bone health, while six days of sun exposure proved capable of supplying enough vitamin D for forty-nine sunless days. In addition, a study of veiled Islamic women living in Denmark found that 600 IU of vitamin D daily was insufficient to raise vitamin D levels in the blood to normal levels. The authors of this study recommend that sun-deprived persons should receive 1,000 IU of vitamin D daily.

There is very little vitamin D found naturally in the foods that humans eat (the best source is cold-water fish). In many countries, vitamin D is added to milk and other foods like breakfast cereals and margarine, contributing to daily intake.

As indicated by the study of submarine personnel, by far the best source of vitamin D is sunlight. However, current recommendations that stress sun avoidance and the use of sunblock may have the unintended effect of increasing the prevalence of vitamin D deficiency. Severe vitamin D deficiency was common in England in the nineteenth century because coal smoke often obscured the sun. During that time, cod liver oil, which is high in vitamin D, became popular as a supplement for children to help prevent rickets, a disease caused by vitamin D deficiency in which developing bones soften and curve because they are not receiving enough calcium.

Vitamin D deficiency is known to occur today in the elderly (who often receive less sun exposure) and in people who live in northern latitudes and do not drink vitamin-D-enriched milk. The consequences of this deficiency may be increased risk of hypertension, osteoporosis, and several forms of cancer.

Additionally, phenytoin (Dilantin), primidone (Mysoline), and phenobarbital for seizures; corticosteroids; cimetidine (Tagamet) for ulcers; the blood-thinning drug heparin; and the antituberculosis drugs isoniazid (INH) and rifampin may interfere with vitamin D absorption or activity.

THERAPEUTIC DOSAGES

For therapeutic purposes, vitamin D is taken at the nutritional doses described in the foregoing Requirements and Sources section (and sometimes in even higher amounts). Persons who wish to exceed nutritional levels of vitamin D intake should consult a physician.

THERAPEUTIC USES

Persons concerned about osteoporosis should take calcium and vitamin D. The combination appears to help prevent bone loss. This is true even if one is taking other treatments for osteoporosis; after all, one cannot build bone without calcium, and one cannot properly absorb and utilize calcium without adequate intake of vitamin D. Vitamin D may also help prevent the falls that lead to osteoporotic fractures.

Some evidence suggests that getting adequate vitamin D may help prevent cancer of the breast, colon, pancreas, prostate, and skin, but the research on this question has yielded mixed results. One study suggests that the combined use of calcium plus vitamin D, but not either supplement separately, can help reduce the risk of colon cancer. However, an extremely large study involving more than thirty-six thousand postmenopausal women found that supplementing

the diet with 1,000 milligrams (mg) of calcium plus 400 IU of vitamin D daily did not lower the risk of breast cancer in seven years. Based on the results of this placebo-controlled study, there does not appear to be a connection between vitamin D and breast cancer risk.

Weak evidence hints that adequate vitamin D intake might reduce the risk of hypertension and diabetes. A large, randomized, placebo-controlled trial of more than thirty-six thousand postmenopausal women found daily supplementation with 1,000 mg of calcium plus 400 IU of vitamin D did not reduce or prevent hypertension during seven years of follow-up. These results are possibly limited by nonstudy calcium use.

One preliminary study suggests that supplementation with vitamin D and calcium may be helpful for women with polycystic ovary syndrome. A meta-analysis (formal statistical review) of published studies found some evidence that the use of vitamin D at recommended levels may reduce overall mortality. This article suggested, but did not attempt to establish, just how vitamin D might accomplish this.

Vitamin D is sometimes mentioned as a treatment for psoriasis. However, this recommendation is based on Danish studies using calcipotriol, a variation of vitamin D_3 that is used externally (applied to the skin). Calcipotriol does not affect the body's absorption of calcium, so it is a very different substance from the vitamin D one can purchase at a store.

It has been suggested that because vitamin D levels in the body drop in the wintertime, vitamin D supplements might be helpful for seasonal affective disorder. A small, double-blind, placebo-controlled trial conducted in winter with forty-four people found that vitamin D supplements produced improvements in various measures of mood. However, a double-blind, placebo-controlled study of 2,217 women older than age seventy years failed to find benefit. It has been hypothesized that light therapy (used successfully for seasonal affective disorder) works by raising vitamin D levels, but there is some evidence that this is not the case. Finally, vitamin D supplements also do not appear to help enhance growth in healthy children.

SCIENTIFIC EVIDENCE

Osteoporosis. Persons with severe osteoporosis often have low levels of vitamin D. Supplementing with vitamin D alone is probably no more than minimally

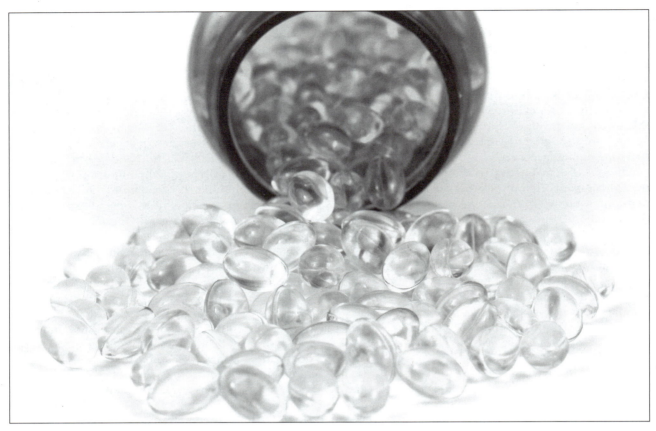

Strong evidence suggests that the combination of vitamin D and calcium supplements can be quite helpful for preventing and treating osteoporosis. (© Dreamstime.com)

helpful, at best, but the combination of calcium and vitamin D is probably more effective.

Vitamin D may offer another benefit for osteoporosis in the elderly: Most studies have found that vitamin D supplementation improves balance in the elderly (especially in women) and reduces risk of falling. Because the most common adverse consequence of osteoporosis is a fracture caused by a fall, this could be a meaningful benefit. Why vitamin D should offer this benefit, however, remains a mystery. Supplementation with vitamin D plus calcium may also aid healing after a fracture has occurred.

SAFETY ISSUES

When taken at recommended dosages, vitamin D appears to be safe. However, when used at considerable excess, vitamin D can build up in the body and cause toxic symptoms. At an intake level of about 40,000 IU daily (about one hundred times the recommended daily intake), vitamin D can cause dangerous elevations in blood calcium levels. Doses five times higher than this were consumed by a few persons because of a manufacturing error; the resulting toxicity was severe and may have caused one death.

However, short of these vastly excessive dosages, it is not clear at what level vitamin D becomes toxic. The official safe upper limits for vitamin D daily intake are as follows: infants to twelve months of age (1,000), children one year to eighteen years of age (2,000); adults (2,000); pregnant and nursing females (2,000). Some experts believe these upper limits have been set a bit too low.

There is no disagreement that people with sarcoidosis or hyperparathyroidism should never take vitamin D without first consulting a physician. Also, taking vitamin D and calcium supplements might interfere with some of the effects of drugs in the calcium-channel blocker family. It is very important that one consult a physician before trying this combination.

The combination of calcium, vitamin D, and thiazide diuretics could potentially lead to excessive calcium levels in the body. Persons taking thiazide diuretics should consult with a physician about the right doses of vitamin D and calcium.

IMPORTANT INTERACTIONS

Persons who may need extra vitamin D include those who are taking antiseizure drugs, such as phenobarbital, primidone (Mysoline), valproic acid (Depakene), phenytoin (Dilantin), corticosteroids, cimetidine (Tagamet), heparin, isoniazid, (INH), and rifampin. Persons taking calcium-channel blockers should not take high-dose vitamin D (with calcium) except under physician supervision. Finally, persons taking thiazide diuretics should not take calcium and vitamin D supplements unless under a doctor's supervision.

EBSCO CAM Review Board

FURTHER READING

Autier, P., and S. Gandini. "Vitamin D Supplementation and Total Mortality." *Archives of Internal Medicine* 167 (2007): 1730-1737.

Bischoff-Ferrari, H. A., and B. Dawson-Hughes. "Where Do We Stand on Vitamin D?" *Bone* 41, suppl. 1 (2007): S13-S19.

Bischoff-Ferrari, H. A., et al. "Is Fall Prevention by Vitamin D Mediated by a Change in Postural or Dynamic Balance?" *Osteoporosis International* 17 (2006): 656-663.

Chlebowski, R. T., et al. "Calcium plus Vitamin D Supplementation and the Risk of Breast Cancer." *Journal of the National Cancer Institute* 100 (2008): 1581-1591.

Dumville, J. C., et al. "Can Vitamin D Supplementation Prevent Winter-time Blues?" *Journal of Nutrition, Health, and Aging* 10 (2006): 151-153.

Fosnight, S. M., W. J. Zafirau, and S. E. Hazelett. "Vitamin D Supplementation to Prevent Falls in the Elderly: Evidence and Practical Considerations." *Pharmacotherapy* 28 (2008): 225-234.

Hypponen, E., and C. Power. "Vitamin D Status and Glucose Homeostasis in the 1958 British Birth Cohort: The Role of Obesity." *Diabetes Care* 29 (2006): 2244-2246.

Margolis, K. L., et al. "Effect of Calcium and Vitamin D Supplementation on Blood Pressure: The Women's Health Initiative Randomized Trial." *Hypertension* 52 (2008): 847-855.

See also: Calcium; Osteoporosis; Vitamins and minerals.

Vitamin E

CATEGORY: Herbs and supplements

RELATED TERMS: Alpha tocopherol, d-alpha-tocopherol, d-beta-tocopherol, d-delta-tocopherol, d-gamma-tocopherol, d-tocopherol, dl-alpha-tocopherol, dl-tocopherol, mixed tocopherols, tocopheryl acetate, tocopheryl succinate

DEFINITION: Natural substance essential for health and promoted as a dietary supplement for specific health benefits.

PRINCIPAL PROPOSED USE: Prostate cancer prevention

OTHER PROPOSED USES: Acute anterior uveitis (with vitamin C), Alzheimer's disease, cancer treatment support, cataracts, cyclical mastalgia, deep venous thrombosis prevention, diabetic neuropathy, epilepsy, immune support, macular degeneration, male infertility, menopausal symptoms, menstrual pain, premenstrual syndrome, preeclampsia prevention, restless leg syndrome, rheumatoid arthritis, sports performance, tardive dyskinesia, vascular dementia

PROBABLY NOT EFFECTIVE USES: Amyotrophic lateral sclerosis, cancer prevention, cataract prevention, congestive heart failure, diabetes prevention, fibrocystic breast disease, heart disease prevention, human immunodeficiency virus infection, kidney damage in diabetes, macular degeneration, osteoarthritis, Parkinson's disease

OVERVIEW

Vitamin E is an antioxidant that fights damaging natural substances known as free radicals. It works in lipids (fats and oils), which makes it complementary to vitamin C, which fights free radicals dissolved in water. As an antioxidant, vitamin E has been widely advocated for preventing heart disease and cancer. However, the results of large, well-designed trials have generally not been encouraging. Many other proposed benefits of vitamin E have also failed to prove useful in studies. There are no medicinal uses for vitamin E with solid scientific support.

REQUIREMENTS AND SOURCES

Vitamin E dosage recommendations are a bit complex because the vitamin exists in many forms. New vitamin E recommendations are in milligrams (mg) of alpha-tocopherol. Alpha-tocopherol can come from either natural vitamin E (called, somewhat incorrectly, d-alpha-tocopherol) or synthetic vitamin E (called, also somewhat incorrectly, dl-alpha-tocopherol). However, much of the alpha-tocopherol in synthetic vitamin E is inactive. For this reason, one has to take about twice as much of it to get the same effect.

There are other forms of vitamin E too, such as beta-, delta-, and gamma-tocopherols, all of which occur in food. These other forms may be important; for example, preliminary evidence hints that gamma-tocopherol may be the most important (or, perhaps, the only) form of vitamin E for preventing prostate cancer. On this basis, it has been suggested that the best vitamin E supplement would be a mixture of all these.

Vitamin E dosages are commonly listed on labels as international units (IU). One IU natural vitamin E equals 0.67 mg alpha-tocopherol; one IU synthetic vitamin E equals 0.45 mg alpha-tocopherol. Therefore, to meet the new dietary recommendations for vitamin E (15 mg per day), one needs to get either 22 IU natural vitamin E (22 IU x 0.67 = 15 mg) or 33 IU synthetic vitamin E (33 IU x 0.45 = 15 mg). The official U.S. and Canadian recommendations for daily intake (in milligrams) of vitamin E are as follows:

Infants to six months of age (4) and seven to twelve months of age (5); children one to three years of age (6), four to eight years of age (7), and nine to thirteen years of age (11); males and females aged fourteen years and older (15); pregnant females (15); and nursing females (19).

In developed countries, mild dietary deficiency of vitamin E is relatively common. The best food sources of vitamin E are polyunsaturated vegetable oils, seeds, nuts, and whole grains. To get a therapeutic dosage, though, one needs to take a supplement.

THERAPEUTIC DOSAGES

The optimal therapeutic dosage of vitamin E has not been established. Most studies have used between 50 and 800 IU daily, and some have used even higher doses. This would correspond to about 50 to 800 mg of synthetic vitamin E (dl-alpha-tocopherol) or 25 to 400 mg of natural vitamin E (d-alpha-tocopherol or mixed tocopherols).

In purchasing natural vitamin E, one should look for a label that reads "mixed tocopherols." However, some manufacturers use this term to mean the synthetic dl-alpha-tocopherol, so the contents need to be read closely. Natural tocopherols come as d-alpha-, d-gamma-, d-delta-, and d-beta-tocopherol.

THERAPEUTIC USES

Observational studies raised hopes that vitamin E supplements could help prevent various forms of cancer and also heart disease. However, observational studies are notoriously unreliable for determining the effectiveness of treatments. Only double-blind trials can do that, and such studies have, on balance, found vitamin E ineffective for preventing heart disease or any common form of cancer other than, possibly, prostate cancer. The use of high-dose vitamin E for a long time might slightly increase the death rate. Other potential uses of vitamin E have limited supporting evidence.

Intriguing but far from definitive studies suggest that vitamin E might improve immune response to vaccinations, control symptoms of restless leg syndrome, help prevent deep venous thrombosis, reduce symptoms of premenstrual syndrome, and decrease symptoms of menstrual pain. Vitamin E, combined with evening primrose, has also been studied as a way to alleviate premenstrual breast pain (mastalgia).

While there is weak evidence that vitamin E supplements can reduce discomfort in rheumatoid arthritis, there is strong evidence that it does not prevent it. Although preliminary studies hinted that the use of vitamin E might prevent or slow the progression of cataracts, in a ten-year study of almost forty thousand female healthcare professionals, the use of natural vitamin E at a dose of 600 mg every other day failed to have any effect on cataract development.

Evidence regarding whether vitamin E can slow the progression of Alzheimer's disease is inconsistent. A large study failed to find vitamin E helpful for preventing mental decline (resulting from any cause) in women older than sixty-five years of age. Studies of vitamin E in combination with vitamin C for the prevention of preeclampsia have yielded inconsistent results.

Vitamin E has also shown equivocal promise in

Selected Food Sources of Vitamin E (Alpha-Tocopherol)

Food	Milligrams (mg) per Serving	Percent Daily Value
Wheat germ oil (1 tablespoon)	20.3	100
Sunflower seeds, dry roasted (1 ounce)	7.4	37
Almonds, dry roasted (1 ounce)	6.8	34
Sunflower oil (1 tablespoon)	5.6	28
Safflower oil (1 tablespoon)	4.6	23
Hazelnuts, dry roasted (1 ounce)	4.3	22
Peanut butter (2 tablespoons)	2.9	15
Peanuts, dry roasted (1 ounce)	2.2	11
Corn oil (1 tablespoon)	1.9	10
Spinach, boiled (1/2 cup)	1.9	10
Broccoli, chopped, boiled (1/2 cup)	1.2	6
Soybean oil (1 tablespoon)	1.1	6
Kiwifruit (1 medium)	1.1	6
Mango, sliced (1/2 cup)	0.7	4
Tomato, raw (1 medium)	0.7	4
Spinach, raw (1 cup)	0.6	3

diabetes. One double-blind trial found benefits for cardiac autonomic neuropathy, a complication of diabetes. Weaker evidence hints at possible benefits for diabetic peripheral neuropathy. However, the best-designed study of all, a long-term trial involving 3,654 people with diabetes, found that the use of vitamin E did not protect against diabetes-induced kidney or heart damage. Similarly, while a few studies performed by one research group suggested that vitamin E might be helpful for improving glucose control in people with diabetes, subsequent evidence showed that the benefits are limited to the short term. In addition, in an extremely large double-blind study, the use of vitamin E at a dose of 600 IU every other day failed to reduce the risk of participants developing type 2 diabetes. Finally, a study unexpectedly found that when people with diabetes took 500 mg of vitamin E daily (either as natural alpha tocopherol or as a mixture of alpha and gamma tocopherol), their blood pressure increased. Similarly, studies on whether vitamin E is helpful for allergic rhinitis (hay fever) have produced conflicting results.

A small double-blind study conducted in Iran reported that vitamin E (400 IU daily) was more effective than placebo for treating menopausal hot flashes. However, a larger study in the United States failed to find vitamin E significantly helpful for hot flashes associated with breast cancer treatment.

Vitamin E might help reduce the lung-related side effects caused by the drug amiodarone, which is used to prevent abnormal heart rhythms. A trial of 108 persons undergoing chemotherapy with cisplatin found that vitamin E supplementation (extended three months past chemotherapy) reduced cisplatin-related neurotoxicity (damage to nerves common during treatment with cisplatin). Studies have yielded mixed results on whether vitamin E is helpful for controlling seizures in people with epilepsy, reducing symptoms of tardive dyskinesia, aiding recovery during heavy exercise, and treating male infertility.

When combined with vitamin C, vitamin E may protect against sunburn to a small extent. The same combination has also shown promise for acute anterior uveitis. A separate study failed to find vitamin E alone (at the high dose of 1,600 mg daily) helpful for macular edema (swelling of the center of the retina) associated with uveitis.

Vitamin E has been tried for amyotrophic lateral sclerosis (Lou Gehrig's disease), but the results in the first reported double-blind study showed questionable benefits, if any. Some vitamin E proponents felt that the dose of vitamin E used in this study might have been too low. Accordingly, they conducted another study using ten times the dose, this one lasting eighteen months and enrolling 160 people. Once again, vitamin E failed to prove significantly more effective than placebo.

In one observational study, the high intake of vitamin E was linked to decreased risk of progression to acquired immunodeficiency syndrome in people with human immunodeficiency virus (HIV) infection. However, a double-blind study of forty-nine people with HIV who took combined vitamins C and E or placebo for three months did not show any significant effects on the amount of HIV detected or the number of opportunistic infections. It has been suggested that vitamin E may enhance the antiviral effects of the drug AZT, but evidence for this is minimal.

Vitamin E has been suggested for preventing the cardiac toxicity caused by the drug doxorubicin. However, while it has shown promise in animal studies, when studied in people, vitamin E has persistently failed to prove effective for this purpose.

Vitamin E is sometimes recommended for osteoarthritis. However, a two-year, double-blind, placebo-controlled study of 136 people with osteoarthritis of the knee failed to find any benefit in terms of symptom control or slowing disease progression. An earlier six-month, double-blind, placebo-controlled trial of seventy-seven people with osteoarthritis also failed to find benefit.

A four-year, double-blind, placebo-controlled trial of 1,193 people with macular degeneration failed to find vitamin E alone helpful for preventing or treating macular degeneration. Vitamin E has also so far failed to prove helpful for preventing or treating alcoholic hepatitis, asthma, congestive heart failure, fibrocystic breast disease, or Parkinson's disease.

In a very large study involving more than 29,000 male smokers, researchers failed to find benefit of alpha-tocopherol (50 IU per day), beta-carotene (20 mg per day), or the two taken together for the prevention of type 2 diabetes in a five-to-eight-year period.

Scientific Evidence

Cancer prevention. The results of observational trials have been mixed, but on balance, they suggest that high intake of vitamin E and other antioxidants is associated with reduced risk of lung cancer and many other forms of cancer, including bladder, stomach, mouth, throat, laryngeal, liver, and prostate. Based on these and other results, researchers developed the hypothesis that antioxidants can help prevent cancer and set in motion large, long-term, double-blind, placebo-controlled studies to verify it. However, these studies generally failed to find vitamin E helpful for the prevention of cancer in people at high risk for it.

The one positive note came in a double-blind trial of 29,133 smokers. In this study, 50 mg of synthetic vitamin E (dl-alpha-tocopherol) daily for five to eight years led to a 32 percent reduction in the incidence of prostate cancer and a 41 percent drop in prostate cancer deaths.

Results were seen soon after the beginning of supplementation. This was unexpected because prostate cancer grows very slowly. The fact that vitamin E almost immediately lowered the incidence of prostate cancer suggests that it somehow blocks the step at which a hidden prostate cancer makes the leap to being detectable.

Nonetheless, the negative results regarding most other types of cancer have made scientists hesitant to place too much hope in these findings. It has been suggested that alpha-tocopherol alone is less effective than the multiple forms of tocopherol that occur in nature; in particular, it has been suggested that gamma-tocopherol rather than alpha-tocopherol might be the most relevant form of vitamin E for cancer prevention. The use of alpha-tocopherol supplements may deplete both gamma- and delta-tocopherol levels, potentially producing a negative effect. However, gamma-tocopherol has not been tested in meaningful controlled trials, and it is quite possible that were one to be performed, the results would prove as disappointing as those for other forms of vitamin E. In addition, under certain circumstances, vitamin E may have a pro-oxidant effect (the reverse of what is desired).

Cardiovascular disease. Most observational studies have found associations between high intake of vitamin E and reduced risk of cardiovascular disease (heart disease and strokes). However, observational studies by themselves cannot be relied upon to identify useful treatments. Double-blind studies, which provide much more convincing evidence of effectiveness, have generally failed to find vitamin E supplements effective.

The Heart Outcomes Prevention Evaluation trial found that natural vitamin E (d-alpha-tocopherol) at a dose of 400 IU daily did not reduce the number of heart attacks, strokes, or deaths from heart disease any more than placebo. The trial followed more than nine thousand men and women who had existing heart disease or who were at high risk for it.

Negative results were seen in numerous other large trials too. When the results of these studies began to come in, some antioxidant proponents suggested that the people enrolled in these trials already had disease too advanced for vitamin E to help. However, a subsequent large trial found vitamin E ineffective for slowing the progression of heart disease also in healthy people. Moreover, in an extremely large placebo-controlled trial involving more than fourteen thousand male physicians in the United States at low risk for heart disease, 400 IU of vitamin E every other day failed to lower the risk of major cardiovascular events or mortality in a period of eight years. On the contrary, vitamin E was associated with a slightly increased risk of stroke.

As with preventing cancer, critics have suggested that the form of vitamin E used in these studies (alpha-tocopherol) was not the best choice, and that gamma-tocopherol might be more helpful. Gamma-tocopherol is present in the diet much more abundantly than alpha-tocopherol, and it could be that the studies showing benefits with dietary vitamin E actually tracked the influence of gamma-tocopherol. However, an observational study specifically examining if gamma-tocopherol levels were associated with the risk of heart attack found no relationship between the two.

In addition, under certain circumstances, vitamin E may have a pro-oxidant effect, and this could explain the negative outcomes. One study found that vitamin E might help prevent serious cardiovascular events in persons with diabetes who also have the particular genetic marker Hp 2. It has been hypothesized that people with the Hp 2 gene have an inadequate endogenous (built-in) antioxidant defense system, and for this reason they might be particularly benefited by taking antioxidant supplements such as vitamin E. However, this concept remains highly preliminary.

Preeclampsia prevention. Preeclampsia is a dangerous complication of pregnancy that involves high blood pressure, swelling of the whole body, and improper kidney function. A double-blind, placebo-controlled study of 283 women at increased risk for preeclampsia found that supplementation with vitamin E (400 IU daily of natural vitamin E) and vitamin C (1,000 mg daily) significantly reduced the chances of developing this disease.

While this research is promising, larger studies are necessary to confirm whether vitamins E and C will actually work. The authors of this study point out that studies of similar size found benefits with other treatments, such as aspirin, that later proved to be ineffective when large-scale studies were performed. Furthermore, it is not known if such high dosages of these vitamins are absolutely safe for pregnant women.

Tardive dyskinesia. Between 1987 and 1998, several double-blind studies were published that indicated vitamin E was beneficial in treating tardive dyskinesia (TD). Although most of these studies were small and lasted only four to twelve weeks, one thirty-six-week study enrolled forty people. Three small double-blind studies reported that vitamin E was not helpful. Nonetheless, a statistical analysis of the double-blind studies done before 1999 found good evidence that vitamin E was more effective than placebo. Most studies found that vitamin E worked best for TD of more recent onset.

However, in 1999, the picture on vitamin E changed with the publication of one more study, the largest and longest to date. This double-blind study included 107 participants from nine different research sites who took 1,600 IU of vitamin E or placebo daily for a minimum of one year. In contrast to most of the previous studies, this trial did not find vitamin E effective in decreasing TD symptoms.

Researchers proposed a number of possible explanations for the discrepancy. One explanation was that the earlier studies were too small or too short to be accurate, and that vitamin E really did not help. Another was the most complicated: that vitamin E might help only a subgroup of people who have TD (those with milder TD symptoms of more recent onset) and that fewer of these people had participated in the latest study. They also pointed to changes in schizophrenia treatment since the last study was done, including the growing use of antipsychotic medications that do not cause TD.

The effectiveness of vitamin E for an individual person is simply not known. Given the lack of other good treatments for TD and the general safety of the vitamin, it may be worth discussing with one's physician.

Immune support. The elderly often do not respond adequately to vaccinations. One double-blind study suggests that vitamin E may be able to strengthen the immune response to vaccines. In this trial, eighty-eight people older than age sixty-five years were given either placebo or vitamin E at 60, 200, or 800 IU dl-alpha-tocopherol daily. The researchers then gave all participants immunizations against hepatitis B, tetanus, diphtheria, and pneumonia and looked at participants' immune response to these vaccinations. The researchers also used a skin test that evaluates the overall strength of the immune response.

The results were promising. Vitamin E at 200 mg per day and, to a lesser extent, at 800 mg per day significantly increased the strength of the immune response. However, it is not clear whether vitamin E has a general "immune support" effect.

One study in the elderly found that the use of vitamin E did not help prevent colds and other respiratory infections, and even seemed to slightly increase the severity of infections that did occur. In a similar-sized double-blind study of long-term-care residents, the use of vitamin E at 200 IU daily failed to reduce incidence or number of days of respiratory infection or antibiotic use. The researchers found some evidence of benefit by breaking down the respiratory infections by type, but such after-the-fact analysis is questionable from a statistical perspective. The same researchers repeated the study with a larger group and did find a reduction in frequency of colds. Another researcher found evidence that vitamin E can have either a harmful or a helpful effect, depending on who takes it (the exact differences remaining undefined).

Alzheimer's disease. Evidence is conflicting regarding whether high-dose vitamin E can slow the progression of Alzheimer's disease. In a double-blind, placebo-controlled study, 341 people with Alzheimer's disease received either 2,000 IU daily of vitamin E (dl-alpha-tocopherol), the antioxidant drug selegiline, or placebo. Those given vitamin E took nearly two hundred days longer to reach a severe state of the disease than the placebo group. (Selegiline was even more effective.)

However, negative results were seen in a study of 769 people at high risk of developing Alzheimer's disease (judging on the basis of early symptoms). Partici-

pants were given either 2,000 IU of vitamin E, the drug donepezil, or placebo for three years. Neither treatment reduced the percentage of people who went on to develop Alzheimer's disease. Such high dosages of vitamin E should not be taken except under a doctor's supervision.

Dysmenorrhea. In a double-blind, placebo-controlled trial, one hundred young women with significant dysmenorrhea (menstrual pain) were given either 500 IU of vitamin E or placebo for five days. Treatment began two days before, and continued for three days after, the expected onset of menstruation. While both groups showed significant improvement in pain in the two months of the study (presumably because of the power of placebo), pain reduction was greater in the treatment group than in the placebo group.

Benefits were also seen in a four-month, double-blind, placebo-controlled study of 278 adolescent girls in Iran. The dose used in this study was 200 IU twice daily.

Mastalgia. Eight-five women with premenstrual mastalgia (breast pain) were randomized to receive one of four treatments for six months: vitamin E (1,200 IU) and placebo, evening primrose (3,000 mg) and placebo, vitamin E and evening primrose, or placebo alone. In this small study, none of the treatment groups experienced better results than the placebo group.

Male infertility. In a double-blind, placebo-controlled study of 110 men whose sperm showed subnormal activity, treatment with 100 IU of vitamin E daily resulted in improved sperm activity and higher actual fertility (measured in pregnancies). However, a smaller double-blind trial found no benefit.

Cardiac autonomic neuropathy. People with diabetes sometimes develop cardiac autonomic neuropathy, irregular heart beats. A four-month, double-blind, placebo-controlled trial found that vitamin E at a dose of 600 mg daily might improve these symptoms.

SAFETY ISSUES

The safe upper intake level (UL) for vitamin E for adults is set at 1,000 mg daily. The equivalent amounts are 1,500 IU of natural vitamin E and 1,100 IU of synthetic vitamin E. For pregnant girls (females eighteen years old and younger), the upper limit is 800 mg.

Vitamin E has a blood-thinning effect that could lead to problems in certain situations. In one study of 28,519 men, vitamin E supplementation at the low dose of about 50 IU synthetic vitamin E per day caused an increase in fatal hemorrhagic strokes, the kind of stroke caused by bleeding. (However, it reduced the risk of a more common type of stroke, and the two effects essentially canceled out.) Based on its blood-thinning effects, there are concerns that vitamin E could cause problems if it is combined with medications that also thin the blood, such as warfarin (Coumadin), heparin, clopidogrel (Plavix), ticlopidine (Ticlid), pentoxifylline (Trental), and aspirin. Theoretically, the net result could be to thin the blood too much, causing bleeding problems. A study that evaluated vitamin E plus aspirin did find an additive effect. In contrast, the results of a study on vitamin E and Coumadin found no evidence of interaction, but it would still not be advisable to combine these treatments except under a physician's supervision.

There is also a remote possibility that vitamin E could also interact with supplements that possess a mild blood-thinning effect, such as garlic, policosanol, and ginkgo. Persons with bleeding disorders, such as hemophilia, and those about to undergo surgery or labor and delivery should also approach vitamin E with caution.

In addition, vitamin E might temporarily enhance the body's sensitivity to its own insulin in persons with type 2 diabetes. This could lead to a risk of blood sugar levels falling too low. In addition, one study found that the use of vitamin E can raise blood pressure in people with diabetes. Persons with diabetes should not take high-dose vitamin E without first consulting a physician.

When all major vitamin E studies are statistically combined through meta-analysis, some evidence appears to suggest that the long-term usage of vitamin E at high doses might increase the overall death rate, for reasons that are unclear. The results of one large study involving 29,000 males indicate that vitamin E supplementation may increase the risk of tuberculosis in heavy smokers. Curiously, however, this was true only in those participants who also consumed high levels of vitamin C (a minimum of 90 mg daily) in their diet. Consuming high levels of vitamin C without supplemental vitamin E actually led to a reduction in tuberculosis risk.

Finally, considerable controversy exists regarding whether it is safe or appropriate to combine vitamin E with standard chemotherapy drugs. The reasoning behind this concern is that some chemotherapy drugs may work in part by creating free radicals that destroy cancer cells. Antioxidants like vitamin E might interfere with this beneficial effect. However, there is no good evidence that antioxidants actually interfere with chemotherapy drugs, growing evidence that they do not, and some evidence of potential benefit under certain circumstances. Nonetheless, in view of the high stakes involved, it is strongly recommend that persons should not take any supplements while undergoing cancer chemotherapy, except on the advice of a physician.

Important Interactions

One should seek medical advice before taking vitamin E if also taking blood-thinning drugs, such as Coumadin, heparin, Plavix, Ticlid, Trental, and aspirin. Vitamin E may help protect from lung-related side effects if one is taking amiodarone. Vitamin E may help reduce side effects if one is taking phenothiazine drugs. One should seek medical advice before taking vitamin E if also taking chemotherapy drugs. High-dose vitamin E might cause blood sugar levels to fall too low, requiring an adjustment in medication dosage, if one is taking oral hypoglycemic medications.

EBSCO CAM Review Board

Further Reading

Christen, W. G., et al. "Vitamin E and Age-Related Cataract in a Randomized Trial of Women." *Ophthalmology* 115 (2008): 822-829.

Kang, J. H., et al. "A Randomized Trial of Vitamin E Supplementation and Cognitive Function in Women." *Archives of Internal Medicine* 166 (2006): 2462-2468.

Karlson, E. W., et al. "Vitamin E in the Primary Prevention of Rheumatoid Arthritis." *Arthritis and Rheumatism* 59 (2008): 1589-1595.

Kataja-Tuomola, M., et al. "Effect of Alpha-tocopherol and Beta-carotene Supplementation on Macrovascular Complications and Total Mortality from Diabetes." *Annals of Medicine* 42 (2010): 178-186.

Keith, M. E., et al. "A Controlled Clinical Trial of Vitamin E Supplementation in Patients with Congestive Heart Failure." *American Journal of Clinical Nutrition* 73 (2001): 219-224.

Manning, P. J., et al. "Effect of High-Dose Vitamin E on Insulin Resistance and Associated Parameters in Overweight Subjects." *Diabetes Care* 27 (2004): 2166-2171.

Meydani, S. N., et al. "Vitamin E and Respiratory

Infection in the Elderly." *Annals of the New York Academy of Sciences* 1031 (2005): 214-222.

Pace, A., et al. "Vitamin E Neuroprotection for Cisplatin Neuropathy." *Neurology* 74 (2010): 762-766.

Peters, U., et al. "Vitamin E and Selenium Supplementation and Risk of Prostate Cancer in the Vitamins and Lifestyle (VITAL) Study Cohort." *Cancer Causes and Control* 19 (2008): 75-87.

Pruthi, S., et al. "Vitamin E and Evening Primrose Oil for Management of Cyclical Mastalgia." *Alternative Medicine Review* 15 (2010): 59-67.

Sesso, H. D., et al. "Vitamins E and C in the Prevention of Cardiovascular Disease in Men." *Journal of the American Medical Association* 300 (2008): 2123-2133.

Shahar, E., G. Hassoun, and S. Pollack. "Effect of Vitamin E Supplementation on the Regular Treatment of Seasonal Allergic Rhinitis." *Annals of Allergy, Asthma, and Immunology* 92 (2004): 654-658.

Ziaei, S., A. Kazemnejad, and M. Zareai. "The Effect of Vitamin E on Hot Flashes in Menopausal Women." *Gynecologic and Obstetric Investigation* 64 (2007): 204-207.

Ziaei, S., et al. "A Randomised Controlled Trial of Vitamin E in the Treatment of Primary Dysmenorrhoea." *BJOG: An International Journal of Obstetrics and Gynaecology* 112 (2005): 466-469.

See also: Antioxidants; Cancer prevention; Prostatitis; Supplements: Introduction; Vitamins and minerals.

Vitamin K

CATEGORY: Herbs and supplements

RELATED TERMS: Vitamin K_1 (phylloquinone), vitamin K_2 (menaquinone), vitamin K_3 (menadione)

DEFINITION: Organic compound used to treat specific health conditions.

PRINCIPAL PROPOSED USES: Osteoporosis, treating medication-induced vitamin K deficiency

OTHER PROPOSED USES: Menorrhagia (heavy menstruation), nausea

OVERVIEW

Vitamin K plays a major role in the body's blood-clotting system. There are three forms of vitamin K: K_1 (phylloquinone), found in plants; K_2 (menaquinone), produced by bacteria in the intestines; and K_3 (menadione), a synthetic form.

Vitamin K is used medically to reverse the effects of "blood-thinning" drugs, such as warfarin (Coumadin). Growing evidence suggests that it may also be helpful for osteoporosis.

REQUIREMENTS AND SOURCES

Vitamin K is an essential nutrient, but a person needs only a tiny amount of it. The official U.S. recommendations for daily intake (in micrograms, or mcg) have been set as follows:

Infants aged 0 to 6 months (2 mcg) and 7 to 12 months (2.5 mcg); children aged 1 to 3 years (30 mcg) and 4 to 8 years (55 mcg); boys aged 9 to 13 years (60 mcg) and aged 14 to 18 years (75 mcg); men (120 mcg); girls aged 9 to 13 years (60 mcg) and aged 14 to 18 years (75 mcg); women (90 mcg); pregnant girls (75 mcg); pregnant women (90 mcg, preferably the K_1 variety [phylloquinone]); and nursing girls (75 mcg) and women (90 mcg, preferably phylloquinone).

Vitamin K (in the form of K_1) is found in green leafy vegetables. Kale and turnip greens are the best food sources, providing about ten times the daily adult requirement in a single serving. Spinach, broccoli, lettuce, and cabbage are also very rich sources, and people can get perfectly respectable amounts of vitamin K in such common foods as oats, green peas, whole wheat, and green beans, as well as watercress and asparagus.

Vitamin K (in the form of K_2) is also manufactured by bacteria in the intestines. This is a major source of vitamin K. Long-term use of antibiotics can cause a vitamin K deficiency by killing these bacteria. However, this effect seems to be significant only in people who are deficient in vitamin K to begin with. Pregnant and postmenopausal women are also sometimes deficient in this vitamin. In addition, children born to women taking anticonvulsants while pregnant may be significantly deficient in vitamin K, causing them to have bleeding problems and facial bone abnormalities. Vitamin K supplementation during pregnancy may be helpful for preventing this.

The blood-thinning drug warfarin (Coumadin) works by antagonizing the effects of vitamin K. Conversely, vitamin K supplements, or intake of foods containing high levels of vitamin K, block the action of this medication and can be used as an antidote.

What Is the Best Source of Vitamin K?

Researchers with the U.S. Department of Agriculture (USDA) studied vitamin K to see the effects of the supplement on volunteers who consumed a vegetable or fortified oil, both rich in vitamin K. A discussion of the study was presented in the USDA magazine Agricultural Research *in January 2000. The discussion is excerpted here.*

Worldwide, only a handful of researchers study vitamin K—long known for its critical role in blood clotting. But with the aging of the U.S. population, this vitamin may command a bigger following as its importance to the integrity of bones becomes increasingly clear. It activates at least three proteins involved in bone health, says Sarah Booth. She is in the Vitamin K Laboratory at the Jean Mayer USDA Human Nutrition Research Center on Aging at Tufts University in Boston.

Vegetables provide the lion's share of this vitamin [K] in the diet, but nutritionists have assumed that people absorb more from oil or oil-based supplements than from vegetables. To find out, Booth led a study with colleagues at Yale University School of Medicine to compare the absorption and use—known as bioavailability—of vitamin K from broccoli and from oil fortified with the vitamin. For five days each, volunteers consumed a helping of broccoli or fortified oil along with a base diet. This increased their phylloquinone [vitamin K_1] intake to around 400 micrograms per day—five to six times the recommended dietary allowance.

"What's really exciting," Booth says, "is to look at the functional markers for vitamin K status. There were no differences between vitamin K from broccoli and vitamin K from oil overall. That's good because green leafy vegetables contain so many other nutrients." For instance, when the volunteers ate broccoli, blood levels of an important carotenoid—lutein—increased compared to when they ate the base diet only.

Cephalosporins and possibly other antibiotics may also interfere with vitamin-K-dependent blood clotting. However, this interaction seems to be significant only in people who have diets poor in vitamin K..

People with disorders of the digestive tract, such as chronic diarrhea, celiac sprue, ulcerative colitis, or Crohn's disease, may become deficient in vitamin K. Alcoholism can also lead to vitamin K deficiency.

THERAPEUTIC DOSAGES

In one study of osteoporosis, vitamin K was taken at the high dose of 1 milligram (mg) daily, more than ten times the necessary nutritional intake.

THERAPEUTIC USES

Growing, but not definitive, evidence suggests that vitamin K should be added to the list of nutrients helpful for preventing osteoporosis. Based on its ability to help blood clot normally, vitamin K has also been proposed as a treatment for excessive menstrual bleeding. However, the last actual study testing this idea was carried out more than fifty-five years ago. Vitamin K has also been recommended for nausea, although there is no meaningful evidence that it really works.

Preliminary evidence suggests that vitamin K supplementation may help prevent liver cancer. Very high doses of intravenous vitamin K have also been used to treat advanced liver cancer, with, perhaps, marginal benefits.

SCIENTIFIC EVIDENCE

Vitamin K plays a known biochemical role in the formation of bone. This has led researchers to look for relationships between vitamin K intake and osteoporosis.

Observational studies have found that people with osteoporosis often have low levels of vitamin K and that people with higher intake of vitamin K have a lower incidence of osteoporosis. Research also suggests that supplemental vitamin K can reduce the amount of calcium lost in the urine. This is indirect evidence of a beneficial effect on bone.

However, while these studies are interesting, only double-blind, placebo-controlled trials can actually prove a treatment effective. Several such studies have been performed on vitamin K for osteoporosis, with generally positive results.

One of these was a three-year, double-blind, placebo-controlled trial of 181 women; it found that vitamin K significantly enhanced the effectiveness of supplementation with calcium, vitamin D, and magnesium. Participants, postmenopausal women between the ages of fifty and sixty, were divided into three groups: receiving either placebo, calcium plus vitamin D plus magnesium, or calcium plus vitamin D plus magnesium plus vitamin K_1 (at the high dose of 1 mg daily). Researchers monitored bone loss by using a standard DEXA bone density scan. The results showed that the study participants using vitamin K along with the other nutrients lost less bone than those in the other two groups.

Benefits were also seen in other studies. However, another placebo-controlled trial involving 452 older men and woman with normal levels of calcium and vitamin D failed to demonstrate any beneficial effects of 500 micrograms (mcg) per day of vitamin K supplementation on bone density and other measures of bone health over a three-year period.

If there is a favorable effect, it is appears to be quite modest. Vitamin K may show its influence most strongly when, instead of a DEXA scan alone, more complex tests of bone strength are used. Some evidence hints that vitamin K works by reducing bone breakdown, rather than by enhancing bone formation.

SAFETY ISSUES

Vitamin K is quite safe at the recommended therapeutic dosages. The vitamin directly counters the effects of the anticoagulant warfarin (Coumadin). Persons who are taking warfarin should not take vitamin K supplements or alter their dietary intake of vitamin K without doctor supervision.

One study suggests a novel way of using this effect deliberately. Researchers gave people on warfarin a fixed daily dose of vitamin K to override the changes in warfarin action caused by the natural variation in day-to-day dietary vitamin K consumption. The results were positive: INR values (the standard measurement of warfarin's blood thinning effect) became more stable. However, this method should not be used except under close physician supervision.

Newborns are commonly given vitamin K_1 injections to prevent bleeding problems. Although some have suggested that this practice may increase the risk of cancer, enormous observational studies have found no such connection (one such trial involved more than one million participants).

IMPORTANT INTERACTIONS

People who are taking warfarin (Coumadin) should not take vitamin K supplements or eat foods high in vitamin K except under the supervision of a physician. (They will need to have their medication dosages adjusted.) People taking cephalosporins or other antibiotics may need more vitamin K if they are already deficient in this nutrient. People taking anticonvulsants, such as phenytoin (Dilantin), carbamazepine, phenobarbital, and primidone (Mysoline), and are pregnant may also need more vitamin K.

EBSCO CAM Review Board

FURTHER READING

Bolton-Smith, C., et al. "A Two-Year Randomized Controlled Trial of Vitamin K1 (Phylloquinone) and Vitamin D3 Plus Calcium on the Bone Health of Older Women." *Journal of Bone and Mineral Research* 22, no. 4 (2007): 509-519.

Booth, S. L., et al. "Dietary Vitamin K Intakes Are Associated with Hip Fracture but Not with Bone Mineral Density in Elderly Men and Women." *American Journal of Clinical Nutrition* 71 (2000): 1201-1208.

_____. "Effect of Vitamin K Supplementation on Bone Loss in Elderly Men and Women." *Journal of Clinical Endocrinology and Metabolism* 93, no. 4 (2008): 1217-1223.

Braam, L. A., et al. "Vitamin K_1 Supplementation Retards Bone Loss in Postmenopausal Women Between Fifty and Sixty Years of Age." *Calcified Tissue International* 73 (2003): 21-26.

Cockayne, S., et al. "Vitamin K and the Prevention of Fractures." *Archives of Internal Medicine* 166 (2006): 1256-1261.

Habu, D., et al. "Role of Vitamin K2 in the Development of Hepatocellular Carcinoma in Women with Viral Cirrhosis of the Liver." *JAMA: The Journal of the American Medical Association* 292 (2004): 358-361.

Knapen, M. H., L. J. Schurgers, and C. Vermeer. "Vitamin K2 Supplementation Improves Hip Bone Geometry and Bone Strength Indices in Postmenopausal Women." *Osteoporosis International* 18, no. 7 (2007): 963-972.

Martini, L. A., et al. "Dietary Phylloquinone Depletion and Repletion in Postmenopausal Women: Effects on Bone and Mineral Metabolism." *Osteoporosis International* 17, no. 6 (2006): 929-935.

Purwosunu, Y., et al. "Vitamin K Treatment for Postmenopausal Osteoporosis in Indonesia." *Journal of Obstetrics and Gynaecology Research* 32 (2006): 230-234.

Rombouts, E. K., F. R. Rosendaal, and F. J. van der

Meer. "Daily Vitamin K Supplementation Improves Anticoagulant Stability." *Journal of Thrombosis and Haemostasis* 5, no. 10 (2007): 2043-2048.

Sarin, S. K., et al. "High Dose Vitamin K3 Infusion in Advanced Hepatocellular Carcinoma." *Journal of Gastroenterology and Hepatology* 21 (2006): 1478-1482.

See also: Nausea; Osteoporosis; Vitamin K.

Vitamins and minerals

CATEGORY: Herbs and supplements

DEFINITION: Organic compounds used to treat specific health conditions.

PRINCIPAL PROPOSED USE: Correct nutrient deficiencies

OTHER PROPOSED USES: Cancer treatment support (radiation therapy), cataract prevention, depression, enhancing mental function, enhancing sports performance, female infertility, immune support, morning sickness, premenstrual syndrome, pregnancy support, stress

OVERVIEW

There are two main ways to use vitamins and mineral supplements: megadose and nutritional therapy. The megadose approach involves taking supplements at doses far above nutritional needs in the hope of producing a specific medical benefit. This technique essentially uses nutrients as natural drugs.

The second approach, taking nutrients at the level of nutritional needs, is addressed here. Also covered are "nutritional insurance" and the nutrients one should consider taking on a daily basis.

REQUIREMENTS AND SOURCES

There is no doubt that it is important to get enough of all necessary nutrients. However, the process of determining proper daily intake levels for vitamins and minerals is far from an exact science, and the recommendations issued by experts in various countries often disagree to a certain extent.

THERAPEUTIC DOSAGES

In general, while it is fairly easy to determine the minimum nutrient intakes that are necessary to avoid frank malnutrition, there is no straightforward way to determine optimum intake levels. Furthermore, individual needs undoubtedly vary based on numerous factors, including age, genetics, lifestyle, other foods in the diet, and many additional environmental influences. No schedule of official recommendations could possibly take all these factors into account, even if all the necessary data existed (which they do not). Thus, all recommendations for daily nutrient intake must be regarded as approximate.

Common nutritional deficiencies. Severe deficiencies of vitamins or minerals are rare in the developed world. However, evidence suggests that slight deficiencies in certain nutrients may be relatively common. These include calcium, chromium, folate, magnesium, vitamin B_6, vitamin C, vitamin B_{12} (primarily in the elderly), vitamin D, vitamin E, and zinc.

While few people are so deficient in these nutrients as to show symptoms of outright malnutrition, subtle deficiencies may increase the risk of a number of diseases. For example, insufficient intake of calcium and vitamin D may increase the chances of developing osteoporosis, and inadequate folate and vitamin B_6 may speed the development of heart disease.

Thus, taking supplements to supply these important vitamins and minerals as a form of insurance may be a

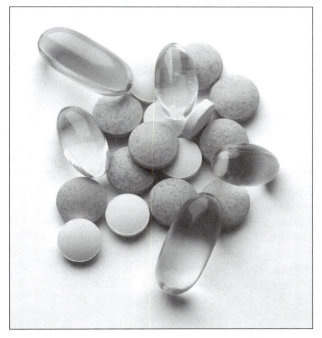

Dietary supplements. (Jon Stokes/Photo Researchers, Inc.)

good idea. Besides vitamins and minerals, intake of essential fatty acids may commonly be inadequate.

Women may develop iron deficiency, but men hardly ever do. Even in women, iron supplements are not beneficial in the absence of true deficiency. Experts recommend avoiding iron supplements unless tests show they are really needed.

Multivitamin/mineral supplements. The simplest way for individuals to support their nutrition is to take a general multivitamin and mineral supplement providing a broad range of nutrients at standard nutritional levels. However, there are a few caveats to keep in mind.

Some supplements include very high doses of certain nutrients, such as antioxidants. When nutrients are taken in this fashion, individuals are using them as drugs rather than as nutrients; these persons are no longer in the world of nutritional supplementation and have passed into the riskier world of megadose treatment. Experts recommend the use of an iron-free multivitamin and mineral supplement, unless a person has been tested and found to be deficient in iron.

The minerals calcium and magnesium are very bulky, and few multivitamin/mineral supplements provide the daily requirement. These minerals generally must be taken in the form of additional pills. It is not possible for the body to absorb a day's worth of calcium in a single dose. A minimum of two doses are necessary.

Finally, note that food may contain many nonessential substances, such as carotenoids and bioflavonoids, that nonetheless enhance health. For this reason, no nutrient supplement should be regarded as a substitute for a healthy and varied diet.

Individual supplements. One problem with multivitamin/mineral supplements is that some nutrients may interfere with the absorption of others. For this reason, there may be advantages to taking supplements separately. (The hassle factor is a strong disadvantage.) In addition, this method allows one to avoid taking vitamins and minerals one does not need.

Individuals who use this approach should keep in mind the following: Minerals come in many different chemical forms, technically called salts. For example, calcium can be purchased as calcium carbonate, calcium citrate, calcium orotate, and in half a dozen or more other forms. In some cases, certain salts of minerals are known to be better absorbed than others. This is particularly the case with calcium. In addi-

tion, individuals who take zinc should balance it with copper.

There may be advantages to taking certain nutrients at levels a bit higher than the standard recommendations, but each nutrient presents its own issues. More is not necessarily better.

Natural versus synthetic vitamins. Many people wonder whether "natural" vitamins are better than "synthetic" ones. Ultimately, no vitamin or mineral supplement is natural. Purified vitamins and minerals are refined, processed products analogous to white sugar or artificial fertilizer. It does not much matter whether they are extracted from foods or manufactured in a laboratory: The result is the same. For example, vitamin C made from rose hips is chemically identical to vitamin C synthesized from scratch. Both are ascorbic acid.

Rose hips themselves, however, supply many nutrients along with vitamin C. Individuals who truly wish to get their vitamins naturally might consider taking them as freeze-dried or condensed whole-food supplements rather than as purified vitamins. This might offer a specific advantage over purified vitamins. In addition, fruits and vegetables may provide substances that are not actually essential but that promote better health.

THERAPEUTIC USES

Under certain conditions, the need for many nutrients may increase. These include illnesses such as diabetes, Crohn's disease, human immunodeficiency virus (HIV), and ulcerative colitis. Furthermore, individuals who smoke cigarettes or overuse alcohol may need additional nutrients.

Also, medications may increase the need for certain nutrients. Other potential uses of multivitamins generally lack strong support.

SCIENTIFIC EVIDENCE

Some but not all evidence hints that multivitamin/multimineral supplements may help prevent infections in seniors or otherwise enhance immunity. However, there are strong suspicions that scientific fraud may have tainted this research, and when the potentially fraudulent studies are disregarded, the evidence looks more negative than positive.

Similarly, some but not all studies suggest that multivitamin/multimineral supplements can enhance mental function, and here, too, there are concerns about potential fraud. In general, the best-designed

Recommended Intake Levels of Selected Supplements and the Known Risks Associated with Excessive Amounts (Adults to Age Fifty Years)

Vitamin or Mineral	Why You Need It	Recommended Daily Dose	Tolerable Upper Intake Level (UL)	Overuse	Good Food Sources
Vitamin A	Vision, growth, and immune function	900 micrograms (mcg) for men (equivalent to 2,997 International Units [IU]), 700 mcg for women (2,333 IU)	3,000 mcg (10,000 IU)	Too much may cause hair loss, nausea, and vomiting and may increase the risk of bone fracture. Very high intakes can cause liver disease and fetal malformations.	Preformed vitamin A sources include fortified cereal, eggs, and dairy products; provitamin A carotenoids (like beta-carotene) are found in deep orange and dark green fruits and vegetables.
Vitamin B$_6$	Protein metabolism, neurotransmitter formation, red blood cell function, hormone function	1.3 milligrams (mg) per day	100 mg	If taken at very high doses, may result in painful neurologic symptoms and difficulty walking.	Fortified cereals, beans, meat, poultry, fish, some fruits and vegetables
Folic acid (folate)	DNA metabolism and the metabolism of several important amino acids	0.4 mg	1,000 mcg	High doses, while safe in themselves, may mask symptoms of pernicious anemia, allowing it to progress unchecked.	Fruits and vegetables, fortified grain foods
Niacin	Necessary for energy metabolism	16 mg for men, 14 mg for women	35 mg	In doses fifty times higher than the tolerable UL, can damage the liver and cause severe gastrointestinal problems.	Meat, poultry, fish, fortified cereals, legumes, milk, seeds
Vitamin C	Required for the synthesis of collagen and the neurotransmitter norepinephrine	90 mg for men, 75 mg for women	2,000 mg	Generally safe, but at high doses can cause diarrhea and might increase risk of urinary tract stones.	Citrus fruits
Vitamin D	Helps to form and maintain strong bones and is needed to maintain blood levels of calcium and phosphorus	5 mcg (200 IU)	50 mcg (2,000 IU)	Continuous high intakes might lead to liver and kidney failure.	Fatty fish (herring, salmon, sardines), eggs from hens that have been fed vitamin D, and fortified milk; exposure to sunlight
Iron	An essential component of hundreds of proteins involved in the transport and storage of oxygen	8 mg for men, 18 mg for women age 19–50 years, 8 mg for women older than age 50 years	45 mg	Can poison a child, causing nausea, vomiting, lethargy, fever, difficulty breathing, coma, and even death; in adults, excess iron is theorized to increase risk of heart disease.	Lean red meats, shellfish, legumes, dried fruit, and green leafy vegetables. (Iron from nonmeat sources is best absorbed when vitamin C also is present.)
Selenium	Necessary for the function of numerous enzymes	55 mcg	400 mcg	Toxic effects of overdose include hair and nail brittleness and loss, gastrointestinal disturbances, skin rashes, fatigue, irritability, and nervous system abnormalities.	Organ meats, seafood, grains

studies have failed to find benefit. However, it is quite possible that multivitamin/multimineral supplements are helpful for people with marked vitamin or mineral malnutrition.

One study found that the use of a multivitamin tablet improved mood, but not cognitive function, in hospitalized acutely ill seniors. Another study failed to find that a mix of multivitamins (either general, or consisting of B-complex vitamins) was more effective than placebo for treating depression in healthy young adults.

Incomplete, and in some cases contradictory, evidence suggests that use of multivitamin or multimineral supplements might reduce antisocial behavior in children and young adults (especially those who are malnourished), prevent bedsores, lower blood pressure, improve fertility in women, improve general well-being, enhance sports performance, enhance growth in children, speed healing of minor wounds, reduce the pain of osteoarthritis, reduce pregnancy-related nausea ("morning sickness"), decrease risk of numerous birth defects, help control menopausal hot flashes, decrease symptoms of premenstrual stress syndrome (PMS) and ordinary stress, reduce risk of prostate cancer, and help prevent cataracts.

In a double-blind study of forty people undergoing radiation therapy for breast cancer, use of a standard multivitamin preparation failed to reduce fatigue compared with placebo. In fact, people in the placebo group may have done somewhat better than those given the vitamin.

SAFETY ISSUES

Standard multivitamin/multimineral tablets contain nutrients at levels believed to be safe for the majority of healthy people, as indicated by amounts at or below the recommended daily allowance. However, even these supplements could be harmful for people with certain diseases, such as kidney or liver disease, or for people taking certain medications, such as warfarin (Coumadin).

There are other multivitamin/multimineral tablets that contain high levels of certain nutrients far above nutritional needs. These could conceivably present risks for healthy people, particularly if they are taken in combination with additional specific supplements. Almost any mineral can be toxic if taken to excess, and there are also risks with excessive intake of vitamins A, B_6, and D.

One study found that use of multivitamin/mineral supplements may actually increase the infectivity of women with HIV. The reasons for this are unclear.

EBSCO CAM Review Board

FURTHER READING

de Souza Fede, A. B., et al. "Multivitamins Do Not Improve Radiation Therapy-Related Fatigue." *American Journal of Clinical Oncology* 30 (2007): 432-436.

Fry, A. C., et al. "Effect of a Liquid Multivitamin/Mineral Supplement on Anaerobic Exercise Performance." *Research in Sports Medicine* 14 (2006): 53-64.

Gariballa, S., and S. Forster. "Effects of Dietary Supplements on Depressive Symptoms in Older Patients." *Clinical Nutrition* 26, no. 5 (2007): 545-551.

Goh, Y. I., et al. "Prenatal Multivitamin Supplementation and Rates of Congenital Anomalies." *Journal of Obstetrics and Gynaecology Canada* 28 (2006): 680-689.

Kirby, R. S. "Menopacenutrient Therapy: An Alternative Approach to Pharmaceutical Treatments for Menopause." *International Journal of Fertility and Women's Medicine* 51 (2006): 125-129.

McNeill, G., et al. "Effect of Multivitamin and Multimineral Supplementation on Cognitive Function in Men and Women Aged Sixty-five Years and Over." *Nutrition Journal* 6 (May 2, 2007): 10.

Meyer, F., et al. "Antioxidant Vitamin and Mineral Supplementation and Prostate Cancer Prevention in the SU.VI.MAX Trial." *International Journal of Cancer* 116, no. 2 (2005): 182-186.

Sternberg, S., and S. Roberts. "Nutritional Supplements and Infection in the Elderly: Why Do the Findings Conflict?" *Nutrition Journal* 5 (November 23, 2006): 30.

See also: Cancer treatment support; Cataracts; Depression, mild to moderate; Sports and fitness support: Enhancing sports performance; Infertility, female; Morning sickness; Premenstrual syndrome (PMS); Pregnancy support; Stress.

Vitiligo

CATEGORY: Condition
RELATED TERM: Depigmentation
DEFINITION: Treatment of the skin disease in which pigment-making cells are destroyed.

PRINCIPAL PROPOSED NATURAL TREATMENTS: Khellin, L-phenylalanine

OTHER PROPOSED NATURAL TREATMENTS: Folate, *Ginkgo biloba*, para-aminobenzoic acid, *Picrorhiza kurroa*, ultraviolet light, vitamin B_{12}

INTRODUCTION

Vitiligo is a skin disease in which pigment-making cells, called melanocytes, are destroyed, leaving white irregular patches of skin where pigment used to be. The patches usually appear on the hands, feet, arms, face, and lips but can also occur on the skin around the mouth, nose, eyes, and genitals. Hair growing from areas affected by vitiligo may also turn white. Although vitiligo in itself is not painful, it can cause emotional distress.

Science has not identified the cause of vitiligo, but some researchers theorize that an autoimmune process plays a role. In an autoimmune disease, the body's immune system starts attacking innocent tissues. In vitiligo, antibodies may develop against melanocytes, ultimately destroying some of them. Vitiligo seems to be more common in people who have other autoimmune diseases; however, most people with vitiligo have no other autoimmune disease.

Most conventional vitiligo treatments combine ultraviolet light (UVA) exposure with oral or topical drugs that selectively sensitize the skin to UVA; such drugs are called psoralens because they are most commonly used to treat psoriasis. The results of this treatment are generally reasonably good. Another option is topical corticosteroids, which may be best for localized vitiligo. In severe cases, surgical procedures including skin grafting and melanocyte transplantation, may be considered, although these approaches are still experimental.

PRINCIPAL PROPOSED NATURAL TREATMENTS

Most natural therapies for vitiligo also employ exposure to UVA or natural sunlight in conjunction with an oral or topical treatment.

Khellin. Khellin, an extract of the fruit of the Mediterranean plant khella (*Ammi visnaga*), is closely related to the standard psoralen drug methoxsalen. Both are used with UVA to repigment vitiligo patches. A double-blind, placebo-controlled study of sixty people indicated that the combination of oral khellin and natural sun exposure caused repigmentation in 76.6 percent of the treatment group; in comparison,

no improvement was seen in the control group receiving sunlight plus placebo. A subsequent placebo-controlled study of thirty-six people found that a topical khellin gel plus UVA caused repigmentation in 86.1 percent of the treated cases, as opposed to 66.6 percent in the placebo group. A typical oral dosage of khellin is 100 milligrams (mg) daily. Khellin has no reported side effects when used topically. Oral doses, however, have caused various side effects ranging from nausea and vomiting to liver inflammation.

L-phenylalanine. A small number of preliminary studies suggest that oral L-phenylalanine, a natural amino acid, might also be helpful for vitiligo. It too is combined with either sunlight or controlled ultraviolet light.

Of four studies, only one was double-blind. It found positive results; however, because only twenty-four people were enrolled, further research will be necessary to confirm its conclusions. The other studies were open, uncontrolled trials, so they prove little.

OTHER PROPOSED NATURAL TREATMENTS FOR VITILIGO

A double-blind study of fifty-two people found that the use of *Ginkgo biloba* extract (40 mg three times daily) helped slow the spread of vitiligo in people with limited, slowly spreading symptoms. There is some evidence that people with vitiligo have lower than average levels of both vitamin B_{12} and folate. In addition, there is a particularly high incidence of vitiligo among persons with pernicious anemia, a condition in which vitamin B_{12} is poorly absorbed. However, this information does not prove that taking extra vitamin B_{12} and folate will help. Furthermore, a much larger study of one hundred people found no significant association between vitiligo and low levels of either vitamin. One uncontrolled study does suggest that vitamin B_{12} and folate supplements might improve pigmentation in vitiligo, but because of the study's poor design, the results prove little. Also, one poorly designed single-blind study suggests that the herb *Picrorhiza kurroa* might increase effectiveness of the standard drug methoxsalen.

Para-aminobenzoic acid (PABA) is best known as an active ingredient in sunscreen. Based on a 1942 study, oral PABA has been suggested as a vitiligo treatment. The study, however, lacked a control group, so the results are not meaningful. Another study suggests that high oral doses of PABA can actually cause vitiligo.

Vitiligo is sometimes associated with pernicious anemia. Pernicious anemia in turn is often linked to low levels of stomach gastric acid, a condition called achlorhydria. For this reason, some physicians specializing in natural medicine recommend supplemental hydrochloric acid (often in the form of betaine hydrochloride) to augment low gastric acid, but there is no evidence that it helps.

EBSCO CAM Review Board

FURTHER READING

Camacho, F., and J. Mazuecos. "Treatment of Vitiligo with Oral and Topical Phenylalanine." *Archives of Dermatology* 135 (1999): 216-217.

Kim, S. M., Y. K. Kim, and S-K Hann. "Serum Levels of Folic Acid and Vitamin B12 in Korean Patients with Vitiligo." *Yonsei Medical Journal* 40 (1999): 195-198.

Njoo, M. D., et al. "Nonsurgical Repigmentation Therapies in Vitiligo." *Archives of Dermatology* 134 (1998): 1532-1540.

Parsad, D., R. Pandhi, and A. Juneja. "Effectiveness of Oral *Ginkgo biloba* in Treating Limited, Slowly Spreading Vitiligo." *Clinical and Experimental Dermatology* 28 (2003): 285-287.

See also: Acne; Eczema; Phenylalanine; Photosensitivity; Rosacea; Scar tissue; Seborrheic dermatitis; Skin, aging; Sunburn.

Walking, mind/body

CATEGORY: Therapies and techniques
RELATED TERMS: Mindful walking, spiritual walking
DEFINITION: An aerobic activity to rest the mind, body, and soul.

OVERVIEW

Mind/body walking has been practiced for hundreds, possibly thousands, of years. In the mid-1890s, naturalist Henry David Thoreau cautioned about the need for the spirit to be present when walking in the woods. He was practicing mind/body walking before the modern term was officially coined.

In the busy modern world, in which instant communication and overstimulation are the norm, mindful walking may be difficult to understand. However, mind/body walking requires that a person leave all interference and thoughts behind. Instead, the walker focuses on becoming connected mentally and physically.

MECHANISM OF ACTION

Mindful walking does not look any different from regular walking. The legs move forward, one at a time, and the arms swing with each step. The movement exercises the entire body. Walking and allowing the mind to relax dissipate all physical and mental tension.

USES AND APPLICATIONS

Walking is one of the best weight-bearing exercises. It stimulates bone growth, thereby strengthening bones. At the same time, walking tones muscles and enhances circulation, so all organs benefit.

Mindful walking allows a person to slow a hectic lifestyle and improve well-being. This simple exercise helps people maintain a healthy weight; lowers blood pressure; decreases low-density lipoprotein (LDL), or bad cholesterol, in the body; and increases high-density lipoprotein (HDL), or good cholesterol. Mindful walking also improves circulation and reduces stress and stress-related illnesses such as heart disease, stroke, and diabetes.

Walkers are calmer and sleep better at night. An added benefit is that mind/body walking enhances self-esteem and stimulates creativity.

CHOOSING A PRACTITIONER

Fitness professionals can teach methods to enhance mind/body walking and calm the mind. However, mind/body walking is most often self-taught. Like everything else, it takes practice to learn how to relax the mind and pay attention to the world. The only equipment needed is a good pair of supportive walking shoes and loose, comfortable clothing.

SAFETY ISSUES

People new to walking should slowly build up their stamina. One should start with shorter walks, maybe ten to fifteen minutes, and walk on flat surfaces, then slowly build up to longer walks in hilly areas. Before taking a walk, it is important to first warm up the muscles by walking in place or in small circles. A warmup helps improve circulation and muscle elasticity; it also prevents injury. After a short warmup, it is important to stretch leg and arm muscles for a few minutes. After a brisk walk, a cool-down (walking in place) and a short stretch also will help prevent injuries and muscle cramping. When walking at night or early in the morning, one should wear light colors or reflective tape as a precautionary measure.

Renée Euchner, R.N., B.S.N.

FURTHER READING

Baker, P. R., et al. "Community Wide Interventions for Increasing Physical Activity." *Cochrane Database of Systematic Reviews* (2011): CD008366.

Harp, David. *Mindfulness to Go: How to Meditate While You're on the Move.* Oakland, Calif.: Harbinger, 2011.

Hölzel, B. K., et al. "Mindfulness Practice Leads to Increases in Regional Brain Gray Matter Density." *Psychiatry Research: Neuroimaging* 191, no. 1 (2011): 36-43.

See also: Alexander technique; Dance movement therapy; Exercise; Exercise-based therapies; Feldenkrais method; Hellerwork; Mind/body medicine; Progressive muscle relaxation; Relaxation therapies; Restless legs syndrome; Sciatica; Varicose veins; Wellness therapies.

Warfarin

CATEGORY: Drug interactions

DEFINITION: An anticoagulant used to thin the blood and prevent it from clotting.

INTERACTIONS: Alfalfa, bromelain, chamomile, chondroitin, coenzyme Q_{10}, cranberry, danshen, devil's claw, dong quai, feverfew, garlic, ginger, ginkgo, ginseng, green tea, ipriflavone, papain, PC-SPES, policosanol, Reishi, royal jelly, St. John's wort, soy, vinpocetine, vitamin A, vitamin C, vitamin E, vitamin K, white willow

TRADE NAME: Coumadin

RELATED DRUGS: Anisindione (Miradon), dicumarol

ALFALFA

Effect: Possible Harmful Interaction

The herb alfalfa (*Medicago sativa*) is promoted for a variety of conditions. The relatively high vitamin K content in alfalfa could reduce the effectiveness of warfarin. Vitamin K directly counteracts warfarin's blood-thinning effects. Since the amount of vitamin K in alfalfa varies widely, it is difficult to give an exact safe upper dose. As a precaution, avoid alfalfa supplements during warfarin therapy except under medical supervision.

CHAMOMILE

Effect: Possible Harmful Interaction

The herb chamomile contains substances in the coumarin family. Some coumarins have blood-thinning actions that could interact with warfarin. One case report exists of a person in whom it appears that combined use of chamomile and warfarin led to internal bleeding.

CHONDROITIN

Effect: Possible Harmful Interaction

Based on chondroitin's chemical similarity to the anticoagulant drug heparin, it has been suggested that chondroitin might have anticoagulant effects as well. There are no case reports of any problems relating to this, and studies suggest that chondroitin has at most a mild anticoagulant effect. Nonetheless, chondroitin should not be combined with warfarin except under physician supervision.

COENZYME Q_{10} (CoQ_{10})

Effect: Possible Harmful Interaction

CoQ_{10} is a vitamin-like substance that plays a fundamental role in the body's energy production. This substance is somewhat similar in structure to vitamin K, and reportedly, it too can reduce the therapeutic effects of warfarin. In three case reports, CoQ_{10} was found to interfere with warfarin's blood-thinning effects. A double-blind study found no interaction between CoQ_{10} and warfarin. However, in view of warfarin's low margin of safety, one should consult a physician before combining CoQ_{10} with warfarin.

CRANBERRY

Effect: Possible Harmful Interaction

Several case reports suggest that cranberry juice can increase warfarin's action, causing dangerous and potentially fatal bleeding problems. However, formal studies have failed to find evidence of such an interaction. Nonetheless, one should be cautious, especially when taking cranberry juice in dosages higher than eight ounces daily.

DANSHEN

Effect: Possible Harmful Interaction

The herb danshen, the root of *Salvia miltiorrhiza,* is used in traditional Chinese medicine for treating heart disease. Preliminary evidence, including several case reports, suggests that danshen can dangerously increase the effects of warfarin and cause significant bleeding problems. Persons taking warfarin should avoid danshen except under a physician's supervision.

DEVIL'S CLAW

Effect: Possible Harmful Interaction

The herb devil's claw (*Harpogophytum procumbens*) is used for various types of arthritis and digestive problems. According to one case report, devil's claw might increase the risk of abnormal bleeding when taken with warfarin. As a precaution, one should not combine devil's claw and warfarin except under a physician's supervision.

DONG QUAI

Effect: Possible Harmful Interaction

The herb dong quai (*Angelica sinensis*) is used for menstrual disorders. According to one case report, dong quai may add to the blood-thinning effects of warfarin, thus increasing the risk of abnormal bleeding. One should probably avoid combining dong quai and warfarin without medical supervision.

FEVERFEW

Effect: Possible Harmful Interaction

The herb feverfew (*Tanacetum parthenium*) is primarily used for the prevention and treatment of migraine headaches. In vitro studies suggest that feverfew thins the blood by interfering with the ability of blood platelets to clump together. This raises the concern that feverfew might increase the risk of abnormal bleeding when combined with warfarin. However, there is as yet no evidence that the blood-thinning effect of feverfew is significant in humans. Though an additive effect of feverfew and warfarin appears to be theoretical at this time, it may be best to avoid this combination except under medical supervision.

GARLIC

Effect: Possible Harmful Interaction

The herb garlic (*Allium sativum*) is taken to lower cholesterol, among many other proposed uses. One of the possible side effects of garlic is an increased tendency to bleed. This blood-thinning effect has been demonstrated in a double-blind trial of garlic in sixty volunteers, as well as in other studies and one case report.

According to two other case reports, the blood-thinning effects of warfarin were greatly enhanced in persons taking garlic. This could amplify the risk of bleeding problems. Based on these findings, one should avoid combining garlic and warfarin except under a physician's supervision.

GINGER

Effect: Possible Harmful Interaction

The herb ginger (*Zingiber officinale*) is used for nausea associated with motion sickness, morning sickness in pregnancy, and the postsurgical period. Ginger appears to thin the blood by interfering with the ability of blood platelets to clump together. As with feverfew, this raises the concern that ginger might increase the risk of abnormal bleeding when taken with warfarin. However, there is no evidence at present that the blood-thinning effect of ginger is significant in humans.

Though an additive effect of ginger and warfarin appears to be theoretical based on current evidence, it may be best to avoid this combination except under medical supervision. Ginger-flavored drinks should not present a problem, but candies containing whole dried ginger are potentially of concern.

GINKGO

Effect: Possible Harmful Interaction

The herb ginkgo (*Ginkgo biloba*) has been used to treat Alzheimer's disease and ordinary age-related memory loss, among many other uses. Inconsistent evidence suggests that ginkgo might reduce the ability of platelets (blood-clotting cells) to stick together. In addition, several case reports suggest that use of ginkgo may be associated with an increased risk of serious abnormal bleeding episodes in persons taking the herb. These findings raise concern that ginkgo might add to the blood-thinning effects of warfarin, and there is one report of abnormal bleeding in an individual who had been taking the herb and drug together. However, two double-blind studies found no interaction between ginkgo and warfarin. These findings are reassuring. Nonetheless, in view of warfarin's low margin of safety, one should consult a physician before combining ginkgo with warfarin.

GINSENG

Effect: Possible Harmful Interaction

The herb ginseng (*Panax ginseng*) is promoted as an adaptogen, a treatment that is said to help the body adapt to stress of all types. A case report suggests that *P. ginseng* can reduce the anticoagulant effects of warfarin; however, three double-blind studies failed to find any interaction. In general, double-blind studies are far more reliable than case reports, and therefore, it would appear that there is not too much reason for concern regarding this potential interaction. However, another double-blind trial that evaluated the closely related American ginseng species (*P. quinquefolius*) found that use of the herb reduced the anticoagulant effects of warfarin, similar to what was seen in the case report. At this point, therefore, it is reasonable to suggest that caution should be exercised when combining ginseng and warfarin.

LOW-CARBOHYDRATE, HIGH-PROTEIN DIET

Effect: Possible Harmful Interaction

Low-carbohydrate, high-protein diets have been advocated for weight loss. According to two case reports, adoption of such diets may decrease the effectiveness of warfarin, possibly by increasing blood levels of a substance called albumin that might tend to bind and inactivate warfarin in the body.

GREEN TEA

Effect: Possible Harmful Interaction in Very High Doses

Dried green tea leaf contains significant levels of vitamin K on a per-weight basis. On this basis, it has been stated that people using blood thinners in the warfarin family should avoid green tea. However, green tea taken as a beverage provides such small amounts of the vitamin that the risk seems minimal for normal consumption. There is one case report of problems that developed in a person on warfarin who consumed as much as a gallon of green tea daily.

IPRIFLAVONE

Effect: Possible Harmful Interaction

Ipriflavone, a synthetic isoflavone that slows bone breakdown, is used to treat osteoporosis. Warfarin use increases the risk of osteoporosis. Because ipriflavone has been found to help prevent osteoporosis in certain circumstances, one might be tempted to consider taking this supplement while also using warfarin. However, some evidence indicates that ipriflavone might interfere with the body's normal breakdown of warfarin. This could raise the levels of warfarin in the body and could increase the risk of abnormal bleeding.

PAPAIN, BROMELAIN

Effect: Possible Harmful Interaction

One case report suggests that papain, a digestive enzyme found in papaya extract (*Carica papaya*), might add to warfarin's blood-thinning effect.

VINPOCETINE

Effect: Possible Harmful Interaction

The substance vinpocetine is sold as a dietary supplement for the treatment of age-related memory loss and impaired mental function. Vinpocetine is thought to inhibit blood platelets from forming clots. For this reason, it should not be combined with medications or natural substances that impair the blood's ability to clot normally, as this may lead to excessive bleeding. One study found only a minimal interaction between the blood-thinning drug warfarin and vinpocetine (and it actually involved an increased tendency for blood clotting), so one should use caution.

PC-SPES

Effect: Possible Harmful Interaction

PC-SPES is an herbal combination that has shown promise for the treatment of prostate cancer. One case report suggests that PC-SPES might increase risk of bleeding complications if combined with blood-thinning medications. Subsequent evidence has indicated that PC-SPES actually contains warfarin, making this interaction inevitable.

POLICOSANOL

Effect: Possible Harmful Interaction

Policosanol, derived from sugarcane, is used to reduce cholesterol levels. It also interferes with platelet clumping, creating a risk of interactions with blood-thinning drugs.

For example, a thirty-day, double-blind, placebo-controlled trial of twenty-seven persons with high cholesterol levels found that policosanol at 10 milligrams (mg) a day markedly reduced the ability of blood platelets to clump together. Another double-blind, placebo-controlled study of thirty-seven healthy volunteers found evidence that the blood-thinning effect of policosanol increased as the dose was increased: the larger the policosanol dose, the greater the effect. Another double-blind, placebo-controlled study of forty-three healthy volunteers compared the effects of policosanol (20 mg daily), the blood-thinner aspirin (100 mg daily), and policosanol and aspirin combined at these same doses. The results again showed that policosanol substantially reduced the ability of blood platelets to stick together, and that the combined therapy exhibited additive effects. Based on these findings, persons should not combine warfarin and policosanol except under medical supervision.

REISHI

Effect: Possible Harmful Interaction

One study suggests that reishi impairs platelet clumping. This creates the potential for an interaction with any blood-thinning medication.

ROYAL JELLY

Effect: Possible Harmful Interaction

One case report indicates that use of royal jelly can increase the effectiveness of warfarin, creating risk of bleeding.

SOY

Effect: Possible Harmful Interaction

One case report indicates that soy milk might decrease warfarin's effectiveness.

ST. JOHN'S WORT

Effect: Possible Harmful Interaction

The herb St. John's wort (*Hypericum perforatum*) is primarily used to treat mild to moderate depression. Evidence suggests that St. John's wort may interfere with warfarin, possibly requiring an increased dosage of the drug to maintain the proper therapeutic effect. Seven cases have been reported in which the blood-thinning effects of warfarin have been impaired in persons taking St. John's wort. A hidden risk lies in this type of interaction. If taking warfarin, one should avoid St. John's wort except under a physician's supervision.

VITAMIN A

Effect: Possible Harmful Interaction

Supplemental vitamin A might increase the blood-thinning effects of warfarin, and this could potentially lead to an increased risk of abnormal bleeding. For this reason, it may be best to avoid combining vitamin A with warfarin unless supervised by a physician.

VITAMIN C

Effect: Possible Harmful Interaction

Vitamin C taken in high dosages (more than 1,000 mg daily) has been reported to reduce the blood-thinning effect of warfarin. In one case, the person was taking 1,000 mg of vitamin C daily; another involved megadoses (about 16,000 mg daily). As a precaution, if taking warfarin, one should consult with a physician before taking high-dose vitamin C supplements.

VITAMIN E

Effect: Possible Harmful Interaction

On the basis that vitamin E thins the blood, it has been suggested not to combine vitamin E with warfarin. However, a four-week, double-blind study of twenty-five persons taking warfarin found no additive effect. None of the participants taking vitamin E at a daily dose of 800 or 1,200 IU showed an increased risk for abnormal bleeding.

In contrast, a case report indicated that vitamin E (800 IU daily) added to the effects of warfarin and resulted in abnormal bleeding. Because this effect did not become apparent until the fourth week, it is possible that problems might take longer to develop than the four-week period covered by the double-blind study, or that certain persons might be more prone to an interaction. An unpublished, thirty-day study of three volunteers taking a warfarin-like drug also found an additive effect with only 42 IU of vitamin E daily.

Though the evidence supporting a possible interaction is scanty, it is best not to risk serious bleeding problems. One should avoid combining vitamin E with warfarin except under the supervision of a physician.

VITAMIN K

Effect: Possible Harmful Interaction

Vitamin K is an antidote to warfarin; it directly counteracts warfarin's blood-thinning effects. This is true for both supplemental vitamin K and foods high in vitamin K. For this reason, eating more vitamin K-rich vegetables can decrease warfarin's therapeutic effect, and eating less of these foods can increase the drug's effect. Either situation can lead to potential life-threatening complications.

Therefore, once established on a certain dose of warfarin, one should not change one's usual intake of vitamin K without consulting a physician.

One study suggests a novel way of using this effect deliberately. Researchers gave people on warfarin a fixed daily dose of vitamin K to override the changes in warfarin action caused by the natural variation in day-to-day dietary vitamin K consumption. The results were positive: INR values (the standard measurement of warfarin's blood-thinning effect) became more stable. However, this method should not be used except under close physician supervision.

WHITE WILLOW

Effect: Possible Harmful Interaction

The herb white willow (*Salix alba*), also known as willow bark, is used to treat pain and fever. White willow contains a substance that is converted by the body into a salicylate similar to the blood-thinner aspirin.

Because white willow, like aspirin, may enhance the blood-thinning effects of warfarin, this combination should be avoided unless medically supervised.

OTHER HERBS AND SUPPLEMENTS

Effect: Possible Harmful Interaction

One case report suggests that a combination of the herbs boldo and fenugreek increased the effects of warfarin. Another isolated case report suggests that the same can happen when fish oil is combined with warfarin.

Based on their known effects or the effects of their constituents, the following herbs and supplements might not be safe to combine with warfarin, though this has not been proven: chamomile (*Matricaria recutita*), *Coleus forskohlii*, ginger (*Zingiber officinale*), horse chestnut (*Aesculus hippocastanum*), papaya (*Carica papaya*), red clover (*Trifolium pratense*), reishi (*Ganoderma lucidum*), mesoglycan, fish oil, oligomeric proanthocyanidins (OPC's), and phosphatidylserine.

EBSCO CAM Review Board

FURTHER READING

Beatty S. J., B. H. Mehta, and J. L. Rodis. "Decreased Warfarin Effect After Initiation of High-Protein, Low-Carbohydrate Diets." *Annals of Pharmacotherapy* 39 (2005): 744-747.

Buckley, M. S., et al. "Fish Oil Interaction with Warfarin." *Annals of Pharmacotherapy* 38 (2004): 50-52.

Greenblatt, D. J., et al. "Interaction of Flurbiprofen with Cranberry Juice, Grape Juice, Tea, and Fluconazole." *Clinical Pharmacology and Therapeutics* 79 (2006): 125-133.

Jiang, X., et al. "Effect of Ginkgo and Ginger on the Pharmacokinetics and Pharmacodynamics of Warfarin in Healthy Subjects." *British Journal of Clinical Pharmacology* 59 (2005): 425-432.

Lee, N. J., and J. D. Fermo. "Warfarin and Royal Jelly Interaction." *Pharmacotherapy* 26 (2006): 583-586.

Lee, S. H., et al. "Interaction Between Warfarin and *Panax ginseng* in Ischemic Stroke Patients." *Journal of Alternative and Complementary Medicine* 14, no. 6 (2008): 715-721.

Pham, D. Q., and A. Q. Pham. "Interaction Potential Between Cranberry Juice and Warfarin." *American Journal of Health-System Pharmacy* 64 (2007): 490-494.

Welch, J. M., and K. Forster. "Probable Elevation in International Normalized Ratio from Cranberry Juice." *Journal of Pharmacy Technology* 23 (2007): 104-107.

Yuan, C. S., et al. "American Ginseng Reduces Warfarin's Effect in Healthy Patients." *Annals of Internal Medicine* 141 (2004): 23-27.

See also: Alfalfa; Bromelain; Chamomile; Chondroitin; Coenzyme Q_{10}; Cranberry; Danshen; Devil's claw; Dong quai; Feverfew; Food and Drug Administration; Garlic; Ginger; Ginkgo; Ginseng; Green Tea; Ipriflavone; Papain; PC-SPES; Policosanol; Reishi; Royal jelly; St. John's wort; Soy; Supplements: Introduction; Vinpocetine; Vitamin A; Vitamin C; Vitamin E; Vitamin K; White Willow.

Warts

CATEGORY: Condition

RELATED TERMS: Common warts, condyloma acuminata, flat warts, plantar warts, verruca vulgaris

DEFINITION: Treatment of a common, benign skin growth caused by a viral infection.

PRINCIPAL PROPOSED NATURAL TREATMENT: Hypnosis

OTHER PROPOSED NATURAL TREATMENTS: Aloe, bloodroot, colloidal silver, echinacea, essential oils, greater celandine, neem, tea tree oil, zinc

INTRODUCTION

A wart is a noncancerous skin growth that occurs when a virus called human papillomavirus infects the surface layer of the skin. In most cases, warts have a roughened surface and a clearly defined boundary. They most commonly occur on the fingers, hands, and arms but can occur almost anywhere. Warts on the bottom of the feet are called plantar warts, and those that occur in the genital area are called genital warts.

Warts are usually painless. However, when they occur in an area that causes them to be subjected to pressure or rubbing, such as the bottom of the foot (plantar warts), they can become extremely tender. Genital warts that occur on the cervix are associated with a significantly increased risk of cervical dysplasia.

Conventional treatment for warts primarily involves a variety of methods to directly remove them. Over-the-counter topical treatments containing salicylic acid gradually dissolve the wart but may take

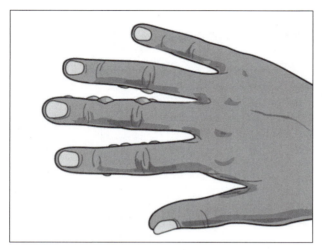

Warts come in more than fifty varieties; a common site is on the fingers of the hand.

many weeks to work. (One should not use this method on genital warts.) Podophyllin, trichloroacetic acid, and cantharidin are other substances that may be applied to a wart to remove it and may be more effective, but they are generally applied only by a physician in an office setting. Other methods of wart removal include freezing the wart with liquid nitrogen (cryotherapy), burning the wart, removing it with a laser, or cutting it out.

A completely different approach involves stimulating the immune system to destroy the wart. The drug Aldara (imiquimod) is the most common approach of this type, although injections of the immune-stimulating substance interferon are also sometimes tried.

PRINCIPAL PROPOSED NATURAL TREATMENTS

Warts often disappear on their own, as if the body "decided" to mount an immune response to remove them. Some evidence indicates that the body can be encouraged to do so through the use of the power of suggestion.

Hypnotherapy may be regarded as the deliberate use of the power of suggestion for therapeutic benefit. In three controlled studies enrolling 180 people with warts, the use of hypnosis caused warts to regress to a significantly greater extent than no treatment, placebo treatment, or (in one of the studies) salicyclic acid treatment. Another study found that fake treatment with a fake X-ray machine can cause children's warts to disappear.

OTHER PROPOSED NATURAL TREATMENTS

Numerous herbs and supplements are marketed as part of topical products said to help remove warts. However, there is no meaningful scientific evidence to indicate that any of them are effective. The herb bloodroot (*Sanguinaria canadensis*) is traditionally made into a paste and applied directly to the surface of a wart to dissolve it. Other proposed topical treatments include aloe, colloidal silver, greater celandine, neem, tea tree oil, and other essential oils. These herbs are said to kill viruses. The herb echinacea is also sometimes recommended because it is thought to have immune-stimulating effects. However, there is no meaningful evidence that any of these approaches has any greater wart-removal powers than placebo therapy. One somewhat poorly conducted double-blind study hints that high (and potentially toxic) doses of the mineral zinc, taken orally, may be helpful for warts.

EBSCO CAM Review Board

FURTHER READING

Meineke, V., et al. "Verrucae Vulgares in Children: Successful Simulated X-Ray Treatment (A Suggestion-Based Therapy)." *Dermatology* 204 (2002): 287-289.

Spanos, N. P., R. J. Stenstrom, and J. C. Johnston. "Hypnosis, Placebo, and Suggestion in the Treatment of Warts." *Psychosomatic Medicine* 50 (1988): 245-260.

Spanos, N. P., V. Williams, and M. I. Gwynn. "Effects of Hypnotic, Placebo, and Salicylic Acid Treatments on Wart Regression." *Psychosomatic Medicine* 52 (1990): 109-114.

See also: Acne; Eczema; Hypnotherapy; Peyronie's disease; Rosacea; Warts: Homeopathic remedies.

Warts: Homeopathic remedies

CATEGORY: Homeopathy

DEFINITION: The use of highly diluted remedies to treat a common, benign skin growth caused by a viral infection.

STUDIED HOMEOPATHIC REMEDIES: *Antimonium crudum*; *Calcarea carbonica*; *Causticum*; combination treatment of oral *A. crudum* plus topical *Thuja* and *Nitric acidum*; *Natrum muriaticum*; *Nitric acidum*; *Sepia*; staphysagria; sulphur; *Thuja occidentalis*

SCIENTIFIC EVALUATIONS OF HOMEOPATHIC REMEDIES

While the list of classical homeopathic treatments for warts is rather long, there is no real evidence that any of them are effective. One large, randomized, double-blind, placebo-controlled trial with 174 participants tested a fixed homeopathic treatment plan for plantar warts (warts on the soles of the feet). The trial involved a six-week course of treatment consisting of one tube of *Thuja* 30c (centesimal) weekly, five pellets of *Antimonium crudum* 7c daily, and one tube of *Nitric acidum* 7c daily. The results of this complex protocol were not encouraging: At the end of the treatment period and the post-treatment follow-up, homeopathic treatment of plantar warts had not proved itself any more effective than placebo.

Another double-blind, placebo-controlled trial with a negative outcome enrolled seventy children with warts on the backs of their hands. These children were assessed according to classical homeopathy for assignment to one of ten preselected remedies. Each participant was then randomly treated either with the remedy indicated by the assessment or with placebo. Once more, the results were disappointing.

TRADITIONAL HOMEOPATHIC TREATMENTS

Classical homeopathy offers possible homeopathic treatments for warts. These therapies are chosen based on various specific details of the person seeking treatment.

People who can be described as romantic, gluttonous, sleepy, weary, peevish, and sulky and who have horny warts on the hands and feet or flat warts fit the symptom picture for *A. crudum*. Those who have cold hands, feet, knees, and head; whose hands are clammy; and who sweat on the top of the head at night fit the picture for *Calcarea carbonica*. This treatment is often used for babies and children. Homeopathic practitioners use *N. acidum* to treat large jagged warts that bleed when washed and *Thuja occidentalis* to treat warts that are large, seedy, and pedunculated (meaning they have a stalk at the base).

Natrum muriaticum might be the right classical remedy for responsible, reserved people who have hot, moist palms but skin that is drying and cracking around the nail beds; who do not like direct prolonged exposure to the sun; who have headaches; and who have skin conditions such as warts, fever blisters, or eczema.

Sepia (the ink from a cuttlefish) is a remedy used for many skin conditions. The skin of a patient needing sepia is described as blotchy, dry, rough, and cracked or crusty, and pigmented with freckles, moles, sun spots, and age spots. The warts of a person who could use sepia may, over time, have also developed pigmentation.

The warts of a person who may fit the picture for staphysagria are said to look like figs or cauliflowers on stalks. Itching is another characteristic of the skin symptoms indicating this remedy.

The homeopathic indications for sulphur are numerous. Among its many other uses, sulphur is traditionally used to treat skin symptoms, including warts. The skin of a person who might respond well to sulphur is typically dry, warm, and red. However, this remedy has a reputation for aggravating the skin symptoms of some people.

Finally, persons who have warts located on the tips of their fingers or nose might benefit from *Causticum*. The warts described for this remedy are large and jagged and bleed easily.

EBSCO CAM Review Board

FURTHER READING

Kainz, J. T., et al. "Homeopathic Versus Placebo Therapy of Children with Warts on the Hands." *Dermatology* 193 (1996): 318-320.

Labrecque, M., et al. "Homeopathic Treatment of Warts." *CMAJ: Canadian Medical Association Journal* 146 (1992): 1749-1753.

Simonart, T., and V. D. Maertelaer. "Systemic Treatments for Cutaneous Warts." *Journal of Dermatological Treatment* (November 6, 2010): DOI:10.3109/09546634.2010.500324.

See also: Homeopathy; Warts.

Weight loss, undesired

CATEGORY: Condition

RELATED TERMS: Cachexia, enhancing appetite, excessive weight loss, tumor-induced weight loss, weight loss caused by illness

DEFINITION: Treatment for undesired or unintentional weight loss.

PRINCIPAL PROPOSED NATURAL TREATMENT: Fish oil

OTHER PROPOSED NATURAL TREATMENTS: Arginine, beta-hydroxy beta-methylbutyrate, branched-chain amino acids, creatine, conjugated linoleic acid, fish oil, glutamine, lipoic acid, medium-chain triglycerides, melatonin, N-acetylcysteine, ornithine alpha-ketoglutarate

INTRODUCTION

While many more people experience excessive appetite and would rather decrease that appetite so they can lose weight, some people find that they have insufficient desire to eat food and, thus, lose weight unintentionally. Mild weight loss can occur in relatively healthy people with stomach problems such as dyspepsia or gastric atonia (sluggish action of the stomach). More severe loss of weight can occur among people who are receiving cancer chemotherapy or who have serious diseases such as human immunodeficiency virus infection, emphysema, Crohn's disease, or congestive heart failure. In extreme cases, inadequate caloric and fat intake leads to a form of starvation (cachexia) that can hamper recovery and increase the risk of death.

Conventional treatment of undesired weight loss primarily involves concentrated protein-calorie supplements, often taken in liquid form. However, among people who have cancer, simply increasing nutritional intake may not help. Cancer can cause a condition called tumor-induced weight loss (TIWL), in which symptoms of starvation occur despite apparently adequate nutrition. The cause is thought to be a particular form of inflammation caused by the cancer. For this reason, nonsteroidal anti-inflammatory drugs have been tried for the treatment of TIWL, with some positive results. Progesterone-related drugs also may be helpful for TIWL, for reasons that are not clear.

PRINCIPAL PROPOSED NATURAL TREATMENTS

Fish oil contains omega-3 fatty acids, "good fats" that have many potential health-promoting properties. Cancer-induced weight loss involves inflammation and responds to treatment with anti-inflammatory drugs. Fish oil also has anti-inflammatory effects. According to some, though not all, studies, fish oil supplements can help people with cancer gain weight. A typical dosage of fish oil used for cancer-induced weight loss is about 12 grams (g) daily.

OTHER PROPOSED NATURAL TREATMENTS

Fats are a concentrated form of energy. For this reason, people with undesired weight loss are often encouraged to increase fat intake. People with cancer have an additional reason to consume more fat: Cancer interferes with the normal process of fat storage, making it less efficient. Certain special fats may be particularly helpful for correcting this fat deficiency. These include conjugated linoleic acid and medium-chain triglycerides (MCTs), along with fish oil.

People with human immunodeficiency virus (HIV) infection or acquired immunodeficiency syndrome may have trouble absorbing fats. Two small double-blind studies have found that MCTs are more easily absorbed than ordinary fats in people with these conditions. However, there is no direct evidence that MCTs actually help people with HIV infection gain weight. In both of the studies noted here, participants consumed nothing but a special nutritional formula containing MCTs. Taking MCTs in this way requires medical supervision to determine the dose.

People with excessive weight loss caused by serious illness may also need extra protein. Amino acids are the basic building blocks of proteins, and they may be easier to digest than whole proteins. Certain amino acid supplements have shown particular usefulness in treating cancer cachexia. One such supplement is branched-chain amino acids (BCAAs), a collection of the amino acids leucine, isoleucine, and valine. A double-blind study tested BCAAs on twenty-eight people with cancer who had lost their appetites because of the disease itself or because of its treatment. Appetite improved in 55 percent of those taking BCAAs (4.8 g daily) compared to only 16 percent of those who took placebo.

Promising results for both cancer-induced and HIV-induced weight loss have also been seen with the amino acids arginine, glutamine, and ornithine alpha-ketoglutarate.

Other treatments found useful for cancer- or HIV-induced weight loss include the antioxidants lipoic acid and N-acetylcysteine, a cocktail containing the sports supplement beta-hydroxy-beta-methylbutyrate and the amino acids arginine and glutamine, and the hormone melatonin.

Traditional remedies for mild, occasional loss of appetite involve the use of bitter-tasting herbs, such as gentian (sold as "bitters" in liquor stores), devil's claw, goldenseal, hops, and horehound. In one study, use of creatine failed to help maintain muscle mass in people undergoing chemotherapy for colon cancer.

HERBS AND SUPPLEMENTS TO USE ONLY WITH CAUTION

Various herbs and supplements may interact adversely with drugs used to treat the underlying condition or conditions causing weight loss, so persons should be cautious when considering the use of herbs and supplements.

HOMEOPATHIC REMEDIES

A double-blind, placebo-controlled study evaluated the potential benefits of homeopathic thyroid hormone for weight loss. A total of 208 people were enrolled in the study. All study participants were undergoing a fast and had reached a plateau where they were no longer rapidly losing weight. The use of homeopathic thyroid significantly enhanced the rate of weight loss.

EBSCO CAM Review Board

FURTHER READING

Barber, M. D. "Cancer Cachexia and Its Treatment with Fish-Oil-Enriched Nutritional Supplementation." *Nutrition* 17 (2001): 751-755.

Bruera, E., et al. "Effect of Fish Oil on Appetite and Other Symptoms in Patients with Advanced Cancer and Anorexia/Cachexia." *Journal of Clinical Oncology* 21 (2003): 129-134.

Inui, A. "Cancer Anorexia-Cachexia Syndrome: Current Issues in Research and Management." *CA: A Cancer Journal for Clinicians* 52 (2002): 72-91.

Mantovani, G., et al. "Managing Cancer-Related Anorexia/Cachexia." *Drugs* 61 (2001): 499-514.

Norman, K., et al. "Effects of Creatine Supplementation on Nutritional Status, Muscle Function, and Quality of Life in Patients with Colorectal Cancer." *Clinical Nutrition* 25 (2006): 596-605.

Schmidt, J. M., and B. Ostermayr. "Does a Homeopathic Ultramolecular Dilution of Thyroidinum 30cH Affect the Rate of Body Weight Reduction in Fasting Patients?" *Homeopathy* 91 (2002): 197-206.

Yoshida, S., et al. "Glutamine Supplementation in Cancer Patients." *Nutrition* 17 (2001): 766-768.

See also: Adolescent and teenage health; Cancer treatment support; Eating disorders; Fish oil; Obesity and excess weight.

Weil, Andrew T.

CATEGORY: Biography

IDENTIFICATION: American physician and a foremost practitioner of integrative medicine in the United States

BORN: June 8, 1942; Philadelphia, Pennsylvania

OVERVIEW

Andrew Weil, an American physician and writer, is perhaps best known for popularizing and practicing what is called integrative medicine (a term he coined). In general, Weil believes that mainstream and complementary and alternative medical practices should be combined for treatment. He also advocates regular exercise, nutrition, and stress control for promoting health.

Weil completed both his undergraduate and medical training at Harvard University, but he chose to skip a traditional residency program and instead obtained a medical internship at Mt. Zion Hospital in San Francisco. He also worked for the National Institute of Mental Health and served as a fellow for the Institute of Current World Affairs.

Weil has written several best-selling books and has founded a company that promotes the use of integrative medicine to ensure general health. He also is a noted opponent of the U.S. government's so-called war on drugs, arguing that many banned plants (such as medicinal mushrooms) have useful medicinal purposes. He was reportedly a proponent of mind-altering drugs as early as his undergraduate years, when he and other students obtained mescaline and used themselves as test subjects. He has been open about his own use of numerous drugs for both experimental and recreational purposes. Critics of Weil have said that he promotes unverified belief systems that may have detrimental effects on others who believe in these systems.

Weil founded the Arizona Center for Integrative Medicine in 1994 and has since acted as its program director. A number of respected medical institutions have since introduced integrative medicine programs and centers for training and treatment.

Weil also focuses on the health concerns of the elderly, and he has expanded his teachings to include healthy lifestyle and health care practices in general, building on his original investigations of consciousness and mental health. In particular, he has articulated the importance of including fish and organic fruits and vegetables in one's diet.

Brandy Weidow, M.S.

Further Reading

Weil, Andrew. *Health and Healing: The Philosophy of Integrative Medicine and Optimum Health.* Rev. ed. Orlando, Fla.: Mariner Books, 2004.

_____. *Healthy Aging: A Lifelong Guide to Your Physical and Spiritual Well-Being.* New York: Knopf, 2005.

_____. *Spontaneous Healing: How to Discover and Enhance Your Body's Natural Ability to Maintain and Heal Itself.* New York: Knopf, 1995.

_____. *Why Our Health Matters: A Vision of Medicine That Can Transform Our Future.* New York: Hudson Street Press, 2009.

See also: Chopra, Deepak; Integrative medicine; Popular practitioners.

Well-being

Category: Issues an overviews
Related term: Wellness
Definition: Treatment that improves a person's overall sense of wellness through resolving specific medical conditions.
Principal proposed natural treatments: Ginseng, multivitamin-multimineral supplements
Other proposed natural treatments: Ashwagandha, astragalus, dehydroepiandrosterone, *Eleutherococcus*, garlic, maitake, "natural" thyroid hormone, reishi, *Rhodiola rosacea*, schisandra, selenium, shiitake, spirulina, suma, various alternative therapies, vitamin B_{12}, yoga

Introduction

It is one of the cardinal principles of natural medicine that treatment should aim not only to treat illness but also to enhance well-being, or wellness. According to this ideal, a proper course of treatment should improve the sense of general well-being, enhance immunity to illness, raise physical stamina, and increase mental alertness; it should also resolve specific medical conditions.

While there can be little doubt that this is a laudable goal, it is easier to laud it than to achieve it. Conventional medicine tends to focus on treating diseases rather than on increasing wellness, not as a matter of philosophical principle, but because it is easier to accomplish.

One strong force affecting wellness is genetics. Beyond this, commonsense steps endorsed by all physicians include increasing exercise, reducing stress, improving diet, getting enough sleep, and living a life of moderation without bad habits, such as smoking or overeating. However, it is difficult to make strong affirmations, and the optimum forms of diet and exercise and other aspects of lifestyle remain unclear. They may always remain unclear, as it is impossible to perform double-blind, placebo-controlled studies on most lifestyle habits.

Principal Proposed Natural Treatments

Although no natural treatments have been proven effective for enhancing overall wellness, two have shown promise: multivitamin-multimineral tablets and the herb *Panax ginseng*.

Multivitamin-multimineral supplements. To function at their best, humans need good nutrition. However, the modern diet often fails to provide people with sufficient amounts of all the necessary nutrients. For this reason, the use of a multivitamin-multimineral supplement might be expected to enhance overall health and well-being, and preliminary double-blind trials generally support this view.

For example, in one double-blind study, eighty healthy men between the ages of eighteen and forty-two were given either a multivitamin-multimineral supplement or placebo and followed for twenty-eight days. The results showed that the use of the nutritional supplement improved several measures of well-being. Similarly, an eight-week, double-blind, placebo-controlled study of ninety-five people with careers in middle management also found improvements in well-being. Furthermore, several studies have found that multivitamin-multimineral supplements can improve immunity in older people. General nutritional supplements may also help improve response to stress.

Panax ginseng. The herb *Panax ginseng* has an ancient reputation as a healthful tonic. According to a more modern concept developed in the former Soviet Union, ginseng functions as an adaptogen. An adaptogen helps the body adapt to stresses of various kinds, whether heat, cold, exertion, trauma, sleep deprivation, toxic exposure, radiation, infection, or psychologic stress. In addition, an adaptogen causes no side effects, is effective in treating many illnesses, and helps return an organism toward balance no matter what may have gone wrong.

From a modern scientific perspective, it is not truly clear that such things as adaptogens actually exist. However, there is some evidence that ginseng may satisfy some of the definition's requirements.

Several studies have found that ginseng can improve the overall sense of well-being. For example, such benefits were seen in a twelve-week double-blind trial that evaluated the effects of *P. ginseng* extract in 625 people. The average age of the participants was just under forty years old. Each participant received a multivitamin supplement daily, but for one set of participants, the multivitamin also contained ginseng. Level of well-being was measured by a set of eleven questions. The results showed that people taking the ginseng-containing supplement reported significant improvement compared to those taking the supplement without ginseng.

Similarly positive findings were reported in a double-blind, placebo-controlled study of thirty-six people newly diagnosed with diabetes. After eight weeks, participants who had been taking 200 milligrams of ginseng daily reported improvements in mood, well-being, vigor, and psychophysical performance that were significant compared to the reports of control participants.

A twelve-week, double-blind, placebo-controlled study of 120 people found that ginseng improved general well-being among women aged thirty to sixty years and men aged forty to sixty years, but not among men aged thirty to thirty-nine years. This finding is possibly consistent with the traditional theory that ginseng is more effective for older people. Other results suggest this as well. A double-blind, placebo-controlled trial of thirty young people found marginal benefits at most, and a sixty-day, double-blind, placebo-controlled trial of eighty-three adults in their mid-twenties found no effect.

In addition, ginseng has shown some potential for enhancing immunity, mental function, and sports performance. These are all effects consistent with the adaptogen concept.

OTHER PROPOSED NATURAL TREATMENTS

Besides *P. ginseng*, certain other herbs are regarded as adaptogens, including *Eleutherococcus senticosus* (Si-berian ginseng), *Rhodiola rosacea*, ashwagandha, astragalus, suma, schisandra, and the Asian mushrooms maitake, shiitake, and reishi. Meaningful supporting evidence for their benefits, however, is scant. In one of the better studies, a small, double-blind, placebo-controlled trial of *R. rosacea*, the herb seemed to improve physical and mental performance and sense of well-being in students under stress.

Although garlic is not generally regarded as an adaptogen, one study found that garlic powder (but not garlic oil) enhanced well-being. However, another study failed to find such benefits with garlic powder.

So-called green juices made from such substances as spirulina and wheat grass are widely marketed for enhancing well-being. A double-blind study found that the use of one such product improved general vitality, but so did placebo, and the differences between the outcomes in the two groups were marginal.

Levels of the hormone dehydroepiandrosterone (DHEA) naturally decrease with age, and for this reason DHEA supplements have been widely hyped as a kind of fountain of youth. However, several studies have found that DHEA supplementation does not improve mood or increase the general sense of well-being in older people. A relatively large (about five hundred participants) double-blind study also failed to find selenium helpful in the elderly. Also, a smaller study failed to find evidence that vitamin B_{12} improved the general sense of well-being among elderly people with signs of mild B_{12} deficiency.

In some branches of alternative medicine, low levels of thyroid hormone are believed to be a common cause of impaired well-being. As part of this theory, it is said that the most commonly used medical form of thyroid replacement therapy (thyroxine, also called T4) is inadequate. Supposedly, better results are obtained when T4 is taken with the thyroid hormone known as T3, often in the form of "natural thyroid" extracted from animal thyroid glands. However, a double-blind study of 110 people designed to test this theory failed to find combined T3-T4 more effective than T4 alone.

Practitioners and other proponents of yoga have long claimed that its gentle stretching exercises, special breathing techniques, and deep meditative states enhance overall health. However, there is only limited evidence that yoga improves general well-being and quality of life.

Numerous other alternative therapies are claimed by their proponents to improve overall wellness, including acupuncture, Ayurveda, chiropractic, detoxification, homeopathy, massage, naturopathy, osteopathic manipulation, Reiki, Tai Chi, therapeutic touch, traditional Chinese herbal medicine, and yoga. However, there is little meaningful evidence to support these claims.

EBSCO CAM Review Board

FURTHER READING

Dayal, M., et al. "Supplementation with DHEA: Effect on Muscle Size, Strength, Quality of Life, and Lipids." *Journal of Women's Health* 14 (2005): 391-400.

Ellis, J. M., and P. Reddy. "Effects of *Panax ginseng* on Quality of Life." *Annals of Pharmacotherapy* 36 (2002): 375-379.

Graat, J. M., E. G. Schouten, and F. J. Kok. "Effect of Daily Vitamin E and Multivitamin-Mineral Supplementation on Acute Respiratory Tract Infections in Elderly Persons." *Journal of the American Medical Association* 288 (2002): 715-721.

Kjellgren, A., et al. "Wellness Through a Comprehensive Yogic Breathing Program." *BMC Complementary and Alternative Medicine* 7 (2007): 43.

Oken, B. S., et al. "Randomized, Controlled, Six-Month Trial of Yoga in Healthy Seniors: Effects on Cognition and Quality of Life." *Alternative Therapies in Health and Medicine* 12 (2006): 40-47.

Rayman, M., et al. "Impact of Selenium on Mood and Quality of Life." *Biological Psychiatry* 59 (2006): 147-154.

See also: Ginseng; Mental health; Optimal health; Stress; Vitamins and minerals; Wellness, general; Wellness therapies; Yoga.

Well-being: Homeopathic remedies

CATEGORY: Homeopathy

DEFINITION: The use of highly diluted remedies to enhance general well-being.

STUDIED HOMEOPATHIC REMEDY: Human growth hormone

SCIENTIFIC EVALUATIONS OF HOMEOPATHIC REMEDIES

Treatment with human growth hormone (HGH) has been investigated as a potential means for improving energy, body composition (ratio of fat to muscle), and overall quality of life, especially in the elderly. Although HGH has not been proven safe and effective for these goals, a double-blind, placebo-controlled trial suggests that a homeopathic (and therefore safe) version of growth hormone may offer the same potential benefits.

This forty-two-day, double-blind, placebo-controlled, crossover study of sixty-nine people evaluated the effects of two homeopathic preparations made from purified HGH. One remedy had a potency of 6x + 12c (a dilution of one part in 1,012 plus dilution of one part in 1,024). The second remedy had a potency of 6x + 100c + 200c (a dilution of one part in 1,012 plus a dilution of one part in 10,200 plus a dilution of one part in 10,400).

During the twenty-one days of treatment, treated participants showed a significant reduction in body weight and an increase in muscle mass compared with those given placebo. Participants also reported relative improvements in general health, including sleep quality, energy, vision, and skin texture.

However, there is one odd feature of this study: The homeopathic treatment, apparently, produced precisely the same effects as the substance from which it was made. This appears inconsistent with the usual expectations regarding homeopathy: that a diluted and potentized treatment should produce effects opposite to those of the original substance, not the same effects.

TRADITIONAL HOMEOPATHIC TREATMENTS

It is part and parcel of the theory behind classical homeopathy that the use of properly chosen homeopathic remedies can improve overall health. These remedies are chosen based on personal constitution and are generally varied over time as various levels of health are uncovered.

EBSCO CAM Review Board

FURTHER READING

Cartwright, T. "'Getting on with Life': The Experiences of Older People Using Complementary Health Care." *Social Science and Medicine* 64 (2007): 1692-1703.

Teut, M., et al. "Homeopathic Treatment of Elderly Patients." *BMC Geriatrics* 10 (2010): 10.

Witt, C. M., et al. "How Healthy Are Chronically Ill Patients After Eight Years of Homeopathic Treatment?" *BMC Public Health* 8 (2008): 413.

See also: Aging; Elder health; Homeopathy; Mental health; Wellness, general.

Wellness therapies

CATEGORY: Therapies and techniques

RELATED TERMS: Holistic medicine, integrative medicine

DEFINITION: Therapies to increase one's well-being and to minimize the chance of becoming ill.

PRINCIPAL PROPOSED USES: Exercise, lifestyle modification, meditation, nutritional therapies, stress reduction, therapeutic massage

OVERVIEW

Wellness exists on a continuum that ranges from disease and disability to the optimal health that a person can realistically achieve. Wellness therapies are forms of complementary and alternative medicine (CAM). Complementary medicine is a combination of allopathic (conventional) and alternative techniques, whereas alternative medicine is a substitute for allopathic medicine. Wellness therapies differ from other forms of CAM in that they focus on a lifestyle that reduces the risk of illness. Other CAM therapies encompass the diagnosis of an illness determining the underlying cause of that illness and then prescribing a treatment regimen to cure or reduce the impact of a disease.

Wellness therapists assist their clients in periodically assessing their risk of illness. Following this assessment, behavior modifications are determined, which will lower the risk of illness. In essence, wellness therapy is proactive, preventive health care. Both allopathic and CAM practitioners incorporate wellness therapies in their practice.

MECHANISM OF ACTION

Wellness therapies are based on the principle of a healthy physical, mental, emotional, and spiritual lifestyle. A healthy diet, too, is emphasized by wellness therapy. Wellness therapists, for example, often educate their clients about the dangers of refined and preserved foods, which include additives and are often high in sugar, fat, and cholesterol. A wellness regimen may include a vegetarian diet or a reduction in meat consumption, particularly red meat. Dietary plans are developed for persons who are overweight. A regular exercise program is a component of wellness medicine. Stress reduction is another component. Various stress-reduction techniques are employed, including massage, aromatherapy, meditation, and yoga. Allopathic physicians also recommend vaccination for childhood diseases and influenza vaccination for the population as a whole or for persons in high-risk subgroups.

USES AND APPLICATIONS

Exercise. Evidence is accumulating that regular exercise, as little as a brisk walk five days per week for thirty to forty-five minutes, can increase the effectiveness of the body's immune system. This boost can increase the circulation of cells that fight off viral and bacterial infections. Studies show that an increased level of exercise can reduce the number of sick days by 25 to 50 percent.

Many health experts claim that inactivity is as great a health risk as smoking. Even slender men and women who do not exercise are at higher risk of death and disease. Other studies have shown that exercise reduces the risk of diabetes, hypertension (high blood pressure), and breast cancer recurrence and mortality by approximately 50 percent; of stroke by 27 percent; of Alzheimer's disease by about 40 percent; of colon cancer by more than 60 percent; and of depression (as effectively as the antidepressive medication Prozac).

Meditation. Meditation involves entering a state of extreme relaxation and concentration. During meditation, the body is in a restful state and the mind is freed of surface thoughts. Several major religions (such as Buddhism and Daoism) embrace meditation; however, meditation does not necessarily require a religious or spiritual component for practice. Many persons who meditate regularly report that doing so improves their concentration and their ability to deal with the stresses in their lives.

Naturopathic medicine. Naturopathic medicine embraces the concept of whole medicine. The basic concept of naturopathy is that the body has an innate ability to heal and maintain itself. The American

Study on Meditation

The National Center for Complementary and Alternative Medicine reports in a study, published in the journal *Psychiatry Research: Neuroimaging* in 2011, that practicing mindfulness meditation appears to be associated with measurable changes in the brain regions involved in memory, learning, and emotion. Mindfulness meditation focuses attention on breathing to develop increased awareness of the present. Previous research has demonstrated that mindfulness meditation may reduce symptoms of anxiety, depression, and chronic pain, but little is known about its effects on the brain. The focus of this study was to identify brain regions that changed in participants enrolled in an eight-week mindfulness-based stress reduction program.

In this study, researchers took magnetic resonance images of the brains of sixteen participants two weeks before and after they joined the meditation program. (Participants were physician- and self-referred individuals seeking stress reduction.) Researchers also took brain images of a control group of seventeen persons who did not meditate over a similar time period. Participants in the meditation group attended weekly sessions that included mindfulness training exercises and received audio recordings for guided meditation practice at home. They also kept track of how much time they practiced each day. Members of both groups completed a questionnaire, before and after joining the group, which measured five aspects of mindfulness: observing, describing, acting with awareness, nonjudging of inner experience, and nonreactivity to inner experience.

Brain images in the meditation group revealed increases in gray matter concentration in the left hippocampus. The hippocampus is an area of the brain involved in learning, memory, and emotional control, and it is suspected of playing a role in producing some of the positive effects of meditation. Gray matter also increased in four other brain regions (though not in the insula, a region that has shown changes in other meditation studies) in the meditation group. Responses to the questionnaire indicated improvements in three of the five aspects of mindfulness in the meditators, but not in the control group.

The researchers concluded that these findings may represent an underlying brain mechanism associated with mindfulness-based improvements in mental health.

Cancer Society describes naturopathy as "A complete alternative care system that uses a wide range of approaches such as nutrition, herbs, manipulation of the body, exercise, stress reduction, and acupuncture."

Nutritional therapies. A wide range of nutritional therapies are available in all developed nations. Most embrace the concept that a healthy diet is essential to attain and maintain good health. Nutritional therapy is often a component of conventional and allopathic medicine.

Stress reduction. All whole-medicine therapies embrace the concept of stress reduction.

Therapeutic massage. Therapeutic massage involves holding, causing movement, and applying pressure to the body's soft tissue. The manipulations are performed to promote health and wellness by reducing pain, muscle spasm, and stress. Adjunctive therapies, such as aromatherapy or soothing music, often accompany therapeutic massage. Massage therapy has been reported to improve circulation (both blood and lymphatic), reduce muscular pain, reduce joint pain, increase range of motion, relieve stress, relieve tension headaches, enhance postoperative recovery, and promote rehabilitation after an injury.

Traditional Chinese medicine. Traditional Chinese medicine (TCM) is a form of CAM that is commonly practiced in Asia. TCM has advocates in the Western world and is increasing in popularity. TCM is a holistic approach to health that attempts to bring the body, mind, and spirit into harmony. It consists primarily of herbal medicine; however, it also embraces acupuncture, nutritional therapy, and massage.

SCIENTIFIC EVIDENCE

Inasmuch as wellness therapies are based on the principles of a healthy lifestyle, the benefits are clear. Many scientific studies have documented the health hazards of an unhealthy lifestyle. These hazards include smoking tobacco, drinking alcohol to excess, a poor diet, and obesity.

CHOOSING A PRACTITIONER

In the field of allopathic medicine, family practitioners, internists, and obstetrician-gynecologists are the most likely to incorporate wellness therapies into their practices. However, other medical specialists may incorporate wellness therapies pertinent to their specialties. For example, an orthopedic surgeon may recommend an exercise program or a course of physical therapy. CAM practitioners, such as whole-medicine practitioners and naturopaths, often advocate wellness therapies.

The training of practitioners who incorporate wellness therapies ranges from graduate or postgraduate education to no formal training. Persons who want to use wellness therapies should ascertain the credentials of any practitioner, regardless of professional degree. It is appropriate to ask what professional degrees the practitioner holds, where the training occurred, and which professional organizations he or she belongs to.

SAFETY ISSUES

Wellness therapies can become harmful only if done to excess. For example, exercise to the point of exhaustion could result in a heart attack or other medical condition.

Robin L. Wulffson, M.D., FACOG

FURTHER READING

Carlson, Jodi. *Complementary Therapies and Wellness.* New York: Prentice Hall, 2002. Provides practical information about complementary care and wellness.

Ditcheck, Stuart, et al. *Healthy Child, Whole Child: Integrating the Best of Conventional and Alternative Medicine to Keep Your Kids Healthy.* New York: Harper Paperbacks, 2009. A thorough guide for parents who are interested in complementary methods of prevention and healing and who are looking for a reliable text directed at pediatricians unfamiliar with alternative treatments.

Murcott, Tony. *The Whole Story: Alternative Medicine on Trial?* New York: Palgrave Macmillan, 2006. Collects updated evidence on the placebo effect, the randomized-controlled trial, personalized genetic medicine, acupuncture, homeopathy, osteopathy, and more.

See also: Diet-based therapies; Exercise; Massage therapy; Meditation; Mental health; Mind/body medicine; Naturopathy; Optimal health; Relaxation therapies; Traditional Chinese herbal medicine; Transcendental Meditation; Spirituality; Stress; Well-being; Homeopathic remedies; Wellness, general.

Wheat grass juice

CATEGORY: Herbs and supplements
RELATED TERM: *Triticum aestivum*
DEFINITION: Natural plant product used to treat specific health conditions.
PRINCIPAL PROPOSED USES: General health improvement, ulcerative colitis
OTHER PROPOSED USE: Plantar fasciitis

OVERVIEW

Grains such as wheat and barley are ordinarily consumed in their mature state, once their seeds have fully matured. However, use of the deep green, immature forms of these plants has been advocated for health promotion. Wheat grass juice is one of these "green foods." It was popularized in the 1960s by Ann Wigmore, who claimed that use of wheat grass juice had cured her of ulcerative colitis; furthermore, when she gave it to her neighbors, their health improved too. She went on to become a major figure in the natural health movement.

Since the introduction of wheat grass, a succession of "green drinks" have become popular for cleansing the body and improving overall health. Barley magma and blue-green algae both fall within this tradition.

THERAPEUTIC DOSAGES

A typical dosage of wheat grass juice is 100 to 300 milliliters daily.

THERAPEUTIC USES

There is no question that wheat grass juice is a nutritive food containing numerous amino acids, vitamins, and minerals. However, besides known human nutrients, wheat grass also contains a number of other substances that proponents claim provide benefit.

For example, wheat grass, like all leafy plant products, contains chlorophyll, the substance used by plants to create glucose from carbon dioxide and light energy. Chemically purified chlorophyll became a popular health food supplement in the 1960s, when it was promoted as a cure for many diseases. Chlorophyll's central role in the metabolism of plants was somehow supposed to suggest benefit for people. However, animals no more have an obvious use for chlorophyll than plants have use for hemoglobin (the vital substance in red blood cells). It is certainly possible that chlorophyll could, by chemical accident, offer benefit

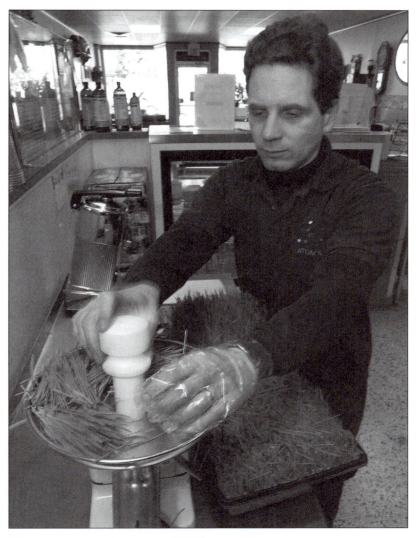

Wheat grass juice being made. (AP Photo)

for animals, but there is no meaningful evidence to indicate that it actually does.

Wheat grass also contains superoxide dismutase (SOD), a substance used by the body as part of its natural antioxidant defense system. SOD is very poorly absorbed by mouth, and it is unlikely that people who consume wheat grass juice receive a meaningful quantity of this substance. Furthermore, the benefit of antioxidants per se has been cast in doubt by the failure of such supplements as vitamin E and beta-carotene to prove effective when tested in enormous double-blind studies.

Proponents of wheat grass also point to a constituent called P4D1 as another source of benefit. However, while P4D1 has shown interesting properties in test-tube studies, there is no real evidence that it offers any benefit.

The only scientifically reliable way to determine whether a medical treatment truly offers medical benefits is to test it in double-blind, placebo-controlled studies. Two such studies have been reported for wheat grass. One found benefit but was seriously flawed; the other failed to find benefit.

The first of these double-blind, placebo-controlled studies enrolled twenty-four people with ulcerative colitis and examined the effects of wheat grass juice taken at a dose of 100 cubic centimeters daily for one month. According to various measures of disease severity, participants given wheat grass juice improved to a greater extent than those given placebo.

This study is interesting, as it tests the initial use of wheat grass popularized by Wigmore. However, the study suffers from two major limitations. One is that it was quite small, limiting the statistical validity of the results. The other is that wheat grass juice is extremely bitter, and therefore it seems unlikely on the face of it that participants and doctors did not know who was getting the wheat grass juice and who was getting the placebo. Indeed, when researchers polled the participants, a majority of those given wheat grass juice were aware of it. Such "unblinding" substantially invalidates a study.

Another double-blind, placebo-controlled study evaluated the potential benefits of a topical wheat grass cream for treating plantar fasciitis, a chronic painful condition of the feet. However, no greater benefit was seen in the treatment group than in the placebo group.

In promotional literature, wheat grass juice is additionally advocated for numerous other conditions, including cancer, arthritis, allergies, fatigue, and diabetes. However, there is no meaningful scientific evidence to support these uses.

SAFETY ISSUES

Wheat grass juice is believed to be safe. However, comprehensive safety studies have not been performed. Maximum safe doses in pregnant or nursing women, young children, and people with severe liver or kidney disease have not been reported.

EBSCO CAM Review Board

FURTHER READING

Ben-Arye, E., et al. "Wheat Grass Juice in the Treatment of Active Distal Ulcerative Colitis." *Scandinavian Journal of Gastroenterology* 37 (2002): 444-449.

Young, M. A., J. L. Cook, and K. E. Webster. "The Effect of Topical Wheat Grass Cream on Chronic Plantar Fasciitis." *Complementary Therapies in Medicine* 14 (2006): 3-9.

See also: Antioxidants.

Whey protein

CATEGORY: Functional foods
DEFINITION: Natural substance promoted as a dietary supplement for specific health benefits.
PRINCIPAL PROPOSED USE: Raising glutathione levels
OTHER PROPOSED USES: Cancer treatment support, cataracts, diabetes, human immunodeficiency virus infection, mental function enhancement, sports performance enhancement, viral hepatitis

OVERVIEW

Whey is one of the two major classes of protein in milk. The other is casein, the "curds" of "curds and whey." Proteins are made of amino acids, and whey contains high levels of the amino acid cysteine. This is the basis for many of its proposed uses. It also contains branched-chain amino acids (BCAAs). However, while there is no question that whey is a highly digestible and rich protein source, there is no meaningful supporting evidence that it provides any specific health benefits.

SOURCES

When milk is converted into cheese, whey is the liquid that is left behind. There is no specific dietary requirement for whey, because the amino acids it contains are present in a wide variety of other foods too.

THERAPEUTIC DOSES

A typical dose of whey protein is 20 to 30 grams per day.

THERAPEUTIC USES

There are no well-documented medicinal uses of whey protein. There is some evidence that whey can raise levels of glutathione. Glutathione is an antioxidant that the body manufactures to defend itself against free radicals. In certain diseases, glutathione levels may fall to below-normal levels. These conditions include cataracts, human immunodeficiency virus (HIV) infection, liver disease, diabetes, and various types of cancer. This reduction of glutathione might in turn contribute to the symptoms or progression of the disease.

To solve this problem, glutathione supplements have been recommended, but glutathione is essentially not absorbed when it is taken by mouth. Whey protein may be a better solution. The body uses cysteine to make glutathione, and whey is rich in cysteine. Meaningful preliminary evidence suggests that whey can raise glutathione levels in people with cancer, hepatitis, or HIV infection. However, while these are promising findings, one essential piece of evidence is lacking: There is no evidence that this rise in glutathione produces any meaningful health benefits.

Whey protein has also been proposed as a bodybuilding aid, based partly on its high content of BCAAs. However, there is no more than minimal evidence that whey protein helps accelerate muscle mass development. Furthermore, there is little evidence that whey protein is more effective for this purpose than any other protein. For example, one small double-blind study found evidence that both casein and whey protein were more effective than placebo at promoting muscle growth after exercise, but whey was no more effective than the far less expensive casein. However, a single small study did find ergogenic benefits with whey compared with casein.

One study looked at whether whey protein could help women with HIV build muscle mass. Study participants were divided into three groups: those who undertook a course of resistance exercise (weight lifting), those who took whey, and those who did both. Resistance exercise alone was just as effective as resistance exercise plus whey, while whey alone was not effective.

Whey contains alpha-lactalbumin, a protein that contains high levels of the amino acid tryptophan. Tryptophan is the body's precursor to serotonin and is thought to affect mental function. In a small double-blind study, the use of alpha-lactalbumin in the evening improved morning alertness, perhaps by enhancing sleep quality. Another small double-blind study found weak evidence that alpha-lactalbumin improved mental function in people sensitive to stress. A third study failed to find that alpha-lactalbumin significantly improved memory in women experiencing premenstrual symptoms.

Weak evidence hints that whey might help prevent cancer or augment the effectiveness of cancer treatment. Infant formula based on predigested (hydrolyzed) whey protein is somewhat less allergenic than standard infant formula; this might reduce symptoms of colic and possibly decrease the risk that the infant will later develop allergies.

SAFETY ISSUES

As a constituent of milk, whey protein is presumed to be a safe substance. People with allergies to milk, however, are likely to be allergic to whey (even to partially hydrolyzed forms of whey).

EBSCO CAM Review Board

FURTHER READING

Agin, D., et al. "Effects of Whey Protein and Resistance Exercise on Body Cell Mass, Muscle Strength, and Quality of Life in Women with Human Immunodeficiency Virus" *AIDS* 15 (2001): 2431-2440.

Borsheim, E., et al. "Effect of an Amino Acid, Protein, and Carbohydrate Mixture on Net Muscle Protein Balance After Resistance Exercise." *International Journal of Sport Nutrition and Exercise Metabolism* 14 (2004): 255-271.

Chromiak, J. A., et al. "Effect of a Ten-Week Strength Training Program and Recovery Drink on Body Composition, Muscular Strength and Endurance, and Anaerobic Power and Capacity." *Nutrition* 20 (2004): 420-427.

Markus, C. R., et al. "Evening Intake of Alpha-Lactalbumin Increases Plasma Tryptophan Availability and Improves Morning Alertness and Brain Measures of Attention." *American Journal of Clinical Nutrition* 81 (2005): 1026-1033.

Marshall, K. "Therapeutic Applications of Whey Protein." *Alternative Medicine Review* 9 (2004): 136-156.

Micke, P., et al. "Effects of Long-Term Supplementation with Whey Proteins on Plasma Glutathione Levels of HIV-Infected Patients." *European Journal of Nutrition* 41 (2002): 12-18.

Szajewska, H., et al. "Extensively and Partially Hydrolysed Preterm Formulas in the Prevention of Allergic Diseases in Preterm Infants." *Acta Paediatrica* 93 (2004): 1159-1165.

See also: Cancer treatment support; Cataracts, Diabetes; Glutathione; Hepatitis, viral; HIV support; Memory and mental function impairment; Sports and fitness support: Enhancing performance.

White willow

CATEGORY: Herbs and supplements
RELATED TERM: *Salix alba*
DEFINITION: Natural plant product used to treat specific health conditions.
PRINCIPAL PROPOSED USES: Back pain, bursitis, dysmenorrhea, migraine headaches, musculoskeletal pain, osteoarthritis, rheumatoid arthritis, tendonitis, tension headaches

OVERVIEW

Willow bark has been used as a treatment for pain and fever in China since 500 B.C.E. In Europe, it was primarily used for altogether different purposes, such as stopping vomiting, removing warts, and suppressing sexual desire. However, in 1828, European chemists made a discovery that would bring together some of these different uses. They extracted the substance salicin from white willow, which was soon purified to salicylic acid. Salicylic acid is an effective treatment for pain and fever, but it is also sufficiently irritating to do a good job of burning off warts. Chemists later modified salicylic acid (this time from the herb meadowsweet) to create acetylsalicylic acid, or aspirin.

THERAPEUTIC DOSAGES

Standardized willow bark extracts should provide 120 to 240 milligrams (mg) of salicin daily.

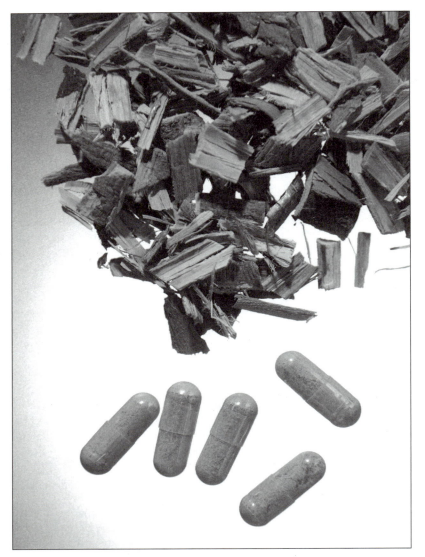

Dried white willow bark and pills. (Olivier Voisin/Photo Researchers, Inc.)

Aspirin and related anti-inflammatory drugs are notorious for irritating or damaging the stomach. However, when taken in typical doses, willow does not appear to produce this side effect to the same extent. This may be partly due to the fact that most of the salicylic acid provided by white willow comes from salicin and other chemicals that are converted to salicylic acid only after absorption into the body. Other evidence suggests that standard doses of willow bark are the equivalent of one baby aspirin daily, rather than a full dose.

This latter finding raises an interesting question: If willow provides only a small amount of salicylic acid, how can it work? The most likely answer seems to be that other constituents besides salicin play a role. Another possibility is that the studies finding benefit were flawed and that it actually does not work.

SCIENTIFIC EVIDENCE

In a four-week, double-blind, placebo-controlled study of 210 individuals with back pain, two doses of willow bark extract were compared against placebo. The higher-dose group received extract supplying 240 mg of salicin daily; in this group, 39 percent were pain-free for at least five days of the last week of the study. In the lower-dose group (120 mg of salicin daily), 21 percent became pain-free. In contrast, only 6 percent of those given placebo became pain-free. Stomach distress did not occur in this study. The only significant side effect seen was an allergic reaction in one participant given willow. Benefits were also seen in a double-blind, placebo-controlled trial of seventy-eight individuals with osteoarthritis of the knee or hip.

However, two subsequent double-blind, placebo-controlled studies performed by a single research group failed to find white willow more effective than placebo. One enrolled 127 people with osteoarthritis

THERAPEUTIC USES

As interest in natural medicine has grown, many people have begun to turn back to white willow as an alternative to aspirin. One double-blind, placebo-controlled trial found it effective for back pain, and another found it helpful for osteoarthritis. White willow is also used for such conditions as bursitis, dysmenorrhea, tension headaches, migraine headaches, rheumatoid arthritis, and tendonitis. However, two recent studies failed to find it effective for rheumatoid arthritis or osteoarthritis.

(OA) of the hip or knee, the other 26 outpatients with active rheumatoid arthritis (RA). In the OA trial, participants received either willow bark extract (240 mg of salicin per day), the standard drug diclofenac (100 mg per day), or placebo. In the RA trial, participants received either willow bark extract at the same dose or placebo. While diclofenac proved significantly more effective than placebo in the OA trial, willow bark did not. It also failed to prove more effective than placebo in the RA study. The most likely interpretation of these conflicting findings is that willow provides at best no more than a modest level of pain relief.

SAFETY ISSUES

Evidence suggests that willow, taken at standard doses, is the equivalent of 50 mg of aspirin, a very small dose. Willow does not impair blood coagulation to the same extent as aspirin, and it also does not appear to significantly irritate the stomach. Nonetheless, it seems reasonable to suppose that if it is used over the long term or in high doses, willow could still cause the side effects associated with aspirin. All the risks of aspirin therapy potentially apply.

For this reason, white willow should not be given to children because of the risk of Reye's syndrome. It should also not be used by people with aspirin allergies, bleeding disorders, or kidney disease. In addition, white willow may interact adversely with blood thinners, other anti-inflammatory drugs, methotrexate, metoclopramide, phenytoin, probenecid, spironolactone, and valproate. Safety in pregnant or nursing women, or in those with severe liver or kidney disease, has not been established.

IMPORTANT INTERACTIONS

Persons should avoid combining white willow with blood-thinning medications such as warfarin (Coumadin), heparin, clopidogrel (Plavix), ticlopidine (Ticlid), and pentoxifylline (Trental); with aspirin, methotrexate, metoclopramide, phenytoin (Dilantin), sulfonamide drugs, spironolactone and other potassium-sparing diuretics; or with valproic acid.

EBSCO CAM Review Board

FURTHER READING

Biegert, C., et al. "Efficacy and Safety of Willow Bark Extract in the Treatment of Osteoarthritis and Rheumatoid Arthritis." *Journal of Rheumatology* 31 (2004): 2121-2130.

Chrubasik, S., et al. "Treatment of Low Back Pain Exacerbations with Willow Bark Extract." *American Journal of Medicine* 109 (2000): 9-14.

Krivoy, N., et al. "Effect of Salicic Cortex Extract on Human Platelet Aggregation." *Planta Medica* 66 (2000): 1-4.

Schmid, B., et al. "Efficacy and Tolerability of a Standardized Willow Bark Extract in Patients with Osteoarthritis." *Zeitschrift für Rheumatologie* 59 (2000): 314-320.

See also: Back pain; Bursitis; Dysmenorrhea; Migraine; Osteoarthritis; Rheumatoid arthritis; Tendonitis.

Whole medicine

CATEGORY: Therapies and techniques
RELATED TERMS: Ayurvedic medicine, complementary and alternative medicine, holistic medicine, integrative medicine, Native American medicine
DEFINITION: A treatment that takes into account the whole person instead of only the specific disease, illness, or condition.
PRINCIPAL PROPOSED USES: Chiropractic, herbal medicine, homeopathy, meditation, naturopathic medicine, nutritional therapy, psychotherapy, stress reduction, therapeutic massage, traditional Chinese medicine, yoga

OVERVIEW

Whole medicine is a treatment that is an alternative to allopathic (conventional) medicine. Whole medicine is a type of complementary and alternative medicine (CAM). Complementary medicine is a combination of allopathic and alternative techniques, and alternative medicine is a substitute for allopathic medicine. Both disciplines evaluate symptoms before making a diagnosis; however, whole medicine searches for the underlying cause or causes of illness. In addition, whole medicine embraces preventive health care to optimize a person's health.

Whole medicine considers the body's systems (circulatory, respiratory, and gastrointestinal) as interdependent components of a person's whole being. One's natural state is considered one of health; illness is deemed to be an imbalance in the body's systems. The whole-medicine approach emphasizes proper nutrition and avoidance of substances that are harmful to one's health. Whole medicine also favors noninvasive techniques and the avoidance of pharmaceuticals.

In general, whole-medicine procedures and treatments are less expensive than those of conventional medicine. Thus, some persons opt for this approach because of financial considerations. Also, many health insurers cover CAM therapies and treatments, especially chiropractic care.

MECHANISM OF ACTION

Whole-medicine practitioners employ the same basic principles of allopathic medicine, which encompass physical health, and they also incorporate mental, emotional, and spiritual well-being. A healthy diet is emphasized by whole-medicine practitioners, and they discourage the use of refined or preserved foods. In addition to having additives, these foods are often high in sugar, fat, and cholesterol. Many practitioners promote a vegetarian diet or, at minimum, a reduction in meat consumption, particularly in the consumption of red meat.

The goal of whole medicine is to bring all aspects of one's life into harmony. This concept includes bringing all the energy flowing within the body into accord. Although noninvasive and pharmaceutical-free treatments are stressed, many whole-medicine practitioners are not averse to the inclusion of allopathic medicine and medications; these practitioners feel that the two disciplines are complementary. For example, most practitioners would agree that an inflamed appendix needs excision, a cancerous tumor needs to be surgically removed, and a diabetic requires insulin. For cases in which allopathic medicine predominates, most whole-medicine practitioners believe that their principles can help the ill person through the situation. They also believe that once the crisis of an acute illness has passed, whole-medicine techniques, which search for underlying causes, can reduce the chance of a negative recurrence.

USES AND APPLICATIONS

Many applications of general medicine exist, and some incorporate whole medicine to varying degrees. Many wellness practitioners incorporate a combination of the following applications in their practice:

Chiropractic. Chiropractic focuses on manipulation of the spinal column under the hypothesis that disorders of the spinal column affect one's health by means of the nervous system. In addition to manipulation of the spine, chiropractic treatment entails manipulation of other joints and soft tissues. Chiropractors often recommend specific exercises to treat a condition and also provide lifestyle counseling.

Herbal medicine. The boundary between pharmaceuticals and herbs is blurred. Many pharmaceuticals are herbal products or are derived from plants. Digitalis, which is used for the treatment of heart conditions, is derived from the foxglove shrub (*Digitalis lanata*). Quinine, which has a number of medicinal uses (such as antimalarial and analgesic), is derived from the bark of the cinchona tree (*Cinchona* species). Herbal products have been used by Asian peoples for medicinal purposes since antiquity. Because herbal products are natural products, they do not fall under the jurisdiction of government regulatory agencies such as the U.S. Federal Drug Administration (FDA). The FDA requires a rigorous testing process before a drug can be made available to the general public. Some herbal products have proven benefits, while others have no proven benefit.

Homeopathy. Homoeopathy involves the use of very small amounts of a substance to stimulate the body's immune system to fight a disease. Homeopathic practitioners use substances such as herbs and metals as a treatment regimen. Some of these substances are toxic if given in higher doses. Homeopathic practitioners embrace the concept of whole medicine in that they treat the whole person rather than focusing on the disease itself. Before prescribing a treatment, they take a detailed history of the patient's likes, dislikes, and habits. Many illnesses are not suitable for homeopathic treatment alone, but in others, homeopathic treatments have been shown to complement traditional medical treatment.

Meditation. Meditation involves entering a state of extreme relaxation and concentration; during meditation, the body is in a restful state, and the mind is freed of surface thoughts. Several major religions (such as Buddhism and Daoism) embrace meditation; however, practicing meditation does not necessarily require a religious or spiritual component. Persons who meditate regularly report that doing so improves their concentration and their ability to deal with the stresses in their lives. People meditate for a variety of reasons, including relaxation, personal insight, and communication with their god.

The Naturopathic Doctor

Naturopathic medicine, practiced by medical doctors, naturopathic specialists, and others with training in naturopathy, have a range of whole-medicine skills and techniques. The U.S. Department of Labor defines the naturopathic doctor as one who does the following:

Diagnoses, treats, and cares for patients, using a system of practice that bases treatment of physiological functions and abnormal conditions on natural laws governing the human body. Utilizes physiological, psychological, and mechanical methods, such as air, water, light, heat, earth, phytotherapy, food and herb therapy, psychotherapy, electrotherapy, physiotherapy, minor and orificial surgery, mechanotherapy, naturopathic corrections and manipulation, and natural methods or modalities, together with natural medicines, natural processed foods, and herbs and natural remedies. Excludes major surgery, the therapeutic use of X-rays and radium, and the use of drugs, except those assimilable substances containing elements or compounds that are components of body tissues and are physiologically compatible to body processes for the maintenance of life.

Naturopathic medicine. Naturopathic medicine embraces the concept of whole medicine. The basic concept of naturopathy is that the body has an innate ability to heal and maintain itself. The American Cancer Society (ACS) describes naturopathy as "A complete alternative care system that uses a wide range of approaches such as nutrition, herbs, manipulation of the body, exercise, stress reduction, and acupuncture." The ACS accepts that portions of naturopathic medicine can sometimes be used with conventional medicine as complementary therapy. Naturopaths include medical doctors with training in naturopathy, naturopathic doctors who have college-level training in naturopathy, and others with lower levels of training.

Nutritional therapies. A wide range of nutritional therapies are available in all developed nations. Most embrace the concept that a healthy diet is essential to attain and maintain good health. Nutritional therapy is often a component of both conventional and allopathic medicine.

Psychotherapy. Psychotherapy embraces the concept of improving one's sense of well-being by talking about problems with a psychotherapist. Psychotherapists include medical doctors with specialized training in psychiatry, clinical psychologists, mental health counselors, and social workers.

Stress reduction. All whole-medicine therapies embrace the concept of stress reduction

Therapeutic massage. Therapeutic massage involves holding, manipulating, and applying pressure to the body's soft tissues. The manipulations have the goal of promoting health and wellness by reducing pain, muscle spasm, and stress. Adjunctive therapies such as aromatherapy or soothing music often accompany therapeutic massage. Types of massage therapy include Swedish massage, which is a gentle, relaxing massage; pressure point therapy, which focuses on a certain portion of the body; and sports massage, which focuses on specific muscle groups. Massage therapy has been reported to improve circulation (both blood and lymphatic), reduce muscular pain, reduce joint pain, increase range of motion, relieve stress, relieve tension headaches, enhance postoperative recovery, and promote rehabilitation after an injury.

Traditional Chinese medicine. Traditional Chinese Medicine (TCM) is a form of CAM that is commonly practiced in Asia. TCM also has advocates in the Western world and is increasing in popularity. TCM is a holistic approach to health that attempts to bring the body, mind, and spirit into harmony. It primarily consists of herbal medicine; however, it also embraces acupuncture, nutritional therapy, and massage.

Yoga. Yoga is a physical and mental discipline that originated in India. It reflects the belief that for one to be in harmony with oneself and the environment, one must integrate the body, the mind, and the spirit. For these three entities to be integrated, emotion, action, and intelligence must be in balance. This balance is accomplished through exercise, breathing, and meditation.

Other practices. Other whole-medicine practices are Ayurvedic medicine and Native American, or indigenous, medicine. Ayurvedic medicine, the traditional medicine of India, emphasizes the reestablishment of balance in the body through a healthy lifestyle and through diet, exercise, and body cleansing. Ayurveda encompasses the body, mind, and spirit. Native American medicine is based on natural remedies derived from the earth. It combines herbs, spirituality, and magic and is overseen by a medicine man or woman.

SCIENTIFIC EVIDENCE

Much of the literature regarding whole medicine lacks a high level of scientific evidence. Valid studies randomly assign persons to a treatment group or to a control group, which is given a placebo (a substance with no pharmacological activity). The largest number of valid studies in whole medicine have been conducted on herbal products. Placebo-controlled studies are easier to conduct on herbal products than on other whole-medicine procedures such as massage and acupuncture. Also, many whole-medicine studies comprise anecdotal reports, in which a participant claims some benefit from the therapy (resulting in a placebo effect).

Aside from limited whole-medicine studies with a high level of evidence, it is well established that good nutrition, stress reduction, and other healthy lifestyle practices embraced by whole medicine are conducive to health. Furthermore, the medical literature contains innumerable well-conducted studies documenting the harmful effects of an unhealthy lifestyle. For example, obesity increases the risk of type 2 diabetes, cardiovascular disease, and many other diseases; smoking tobacco (or marijuana) increases the risk of many types of cancer.

CHOOSING A PRACTITIONER

The training of practitioners of whole-medicine ranges from postgraduate work to no formal training. Persons seeking whole-medicine care should examine the credentials of practitioners, regardless of professional degree. It is appropriate to ask what professional degree or degrees the practitioner holds, where his or her training occurred, and to what professional organizations he or she belongs. An informative resource for locating a whole-medicine practitioner is the American Holistic Medical Association, which maintains a comprehensive list of practitioners in many types of therapies throughout the United States. However, the organization stresses that it is the responsibility of the person seeking care to check a practitioner's credentials before treatment. The American Naturopathic Medical Certification Board (ANMCB) administers certification for whole-medicine practitioners. Practitioners certified by ANMCB must meet certain standards based on their level of certification.

SAFETY ISSUES

Many medical experts are concerned that some persons with serious medical conditions, such as a malignancy, will seek alternative medical care or purchase worthless herbal products rather than seek conventional medical care. In contrast to possible health risks from a whole-medicine regimen, the basic principles of healthy diet and stress reduction, for example, which are embraced by whole medicine, are not only safe but also beneficial to one's health.

Robin L. Wulffson, M.D., FACOG

FURTHER READING

American Holistic Medical Association. http://www.holisticmedicine.org.

Ditcheck, Stuart, et al. *Healthy Child, Whole Child: Integrating the Best of Conventional and Alternative Medicine to Keep Your Kids Healthy.* New York: Harper, 2009. A thorough guide for parents who are interested in complementary methods of prevention and healing and who are looking for a reliable text for pediatricians unfamiliar with alternative treatments.

Lu, Henry C. *Traditional Chinese Medicine: How to Maintain Your Health and Treat Illness.* Laguna Beach, Calif.: Basic Health, 2006. Describes the thirteen syndromes identified in Chinese medicine. Also incorporates more familiar Western medical terminology, resulting in a handbook that straddles both traditions.

Murcott, Tony. *The Whole Story: Alternative Medicine on Trial?* New York: Palgrave Macmillan, 2006. Collects updated evidence on the placebo effect, the randomized-controlled trial, acupuncture, homeopathy, osteopathy, and more.

See also: Alternative versus traditional medicine; Ayurveda; Chinese medicine; Chiropractic; Folk medicine; Herbal medicine; Homeopathy; Integrative medicine; Massage therapy; Meditation; Mind/body medicine; Naturopathy; Optimal health; Traditional Chinese herbal medicine; Traditional healing; Wellness, general; Wellness therapies; Yoga.

Wild cherry

CATEGORY: Herbs and supplements
RELATED TERM: *Prunus serotina*
DEFINITION: Natural plant product used to treat specific health conditions.
PRINCIPAL PROPOSED USE: Cough

OVERVIEW

The bark of the wild cherry tree is a traditional Native American remedy for two seemingly unrelated conditions: respiratory infections and anxiety. European settlers quickly adopted the herb for similar purposes.

THERAPEUTIC DOSAGES

Syrups containing wild cherry should be taken as directed.

THERAPEUTIC USES

Over time, wild cherry has come to be used primarily as a component of cough syrups. It is tempting to connect the two traditional uses of wild cherry by imagining that it functions like codeine to affect both the mind and the cough reflex. However, this is just speculation, as there has been very little scientific evaluation of this herb.

SAFETY ISSUES

Wild cherry is generally regarded as safe when used at recommended dosages. However, since it contains small amounts of cyanide, it should not be taken to excess. It is not recommended for use by young children, pregnant or nursing women, or those with severe liver or kidney disease. Some evidence suggests that wild cherry might interact with various medications by affecting their metabolism in the liver, but the extent of this effect has not been fully determined.

EBSCO CAM Review Board

FURTHER READING

Budzinski, J. W., et al. "An In Vitro Evaluation of Human Cytochrome P450 3A4 Inhibition by Selected Commercial Herbal Extracts and Tinctures." *Phytomedicine: International Journal of Phytotherapy and Phytopharmacology* 7 (2000): 273-282.

See also: Cough.

Wild indigo

CATEGORY: Herbs and supplements
RELATED TERM: *Baptisia tinctoria*
DEFINITION: Natural plant product used to treat specific health conditions.
PRINCIPAL PROPOSED USES: Chronic bronchitis (acute exacerbation, along with antibiotic therapy), colds and flu (in combination with echinacea and white cedar), immune support

OVERVIEW

Like its botanical relative true indigo (*Indigofera tinctoria*), wild indigo has historically been used as a source of a deep blue dye. It was also used medicinally: The natives of North America used it as a topical treatment for nonhealing wounds and infections of the mouth and throat. The root is the part used.

THERAPEUTIC DOSAGES

Combination therapies containing wild indigo, echinacea, and white cedar should be taken according to label instructions.

THERAPEUTIC USES

Currently, wild indigo is primarily used as part of a standardized four-herb combination said to improve immune function. In addition to wild indigo, this combination contains *Echinacea purpurea* root, *E. pallida* root, and white cedar (*Thuja occidentalis*). This combination is hypothesized to have immune-stimulating properties.

In a well-designed double-blind study of 263 people with recent onset of the common cold, use of this combination significantly improved cold symptoms compared with placebo. Recovery occurred approximately three days earlier among people taking the herbal mixture than among those taking the placebo.

Benefits for the common cold were also seen in other double-blind, placebo-controlled studies involving a total of about 250 people.

The same combination therapy has also shown promise for augmenting the effects of antibiotics in people with bacterial infections. For example, in one study, fifty-three people experiencing an acute exacerbation of chronic bronchitis were given either antibiotics plus placebo or the same antibiotics plus this herbal combination. The results showed that participants who received the herbal mixture recovered significantly more quickly than those who were given placebo.

Proponents of this combination therapy claim that it works by "balancing" or "strengthening" the immune system. However, while there is evidence that this herbal mixture affects the immune function, the current state of scientific knowledge is generally inadequate to determine whether any such effects are good, bad, or indifferent.

SAFETY ISSUES

Wild indigo has not undergone comprehensive safety testing. However, in clinical studies, use of the standardized combination therapy has not been associated with any serious harmful effects. Safety in young children, pregnant or nursing women, and people with severe liver or kidney disease has not been established.

EBSCO CAM Review Board

FURTHER READING

Hauke, W., et al. "Esberitox N as Supportive Therapy When Providing Standard Antibiotic Treatment in Subjects with a Severe Bacterial Infection (Acute Exacerbation of Chronic Bronchitis): A Multicentric, Prospective, Double-Blind, Placebo-Controlled Study." *Chemotherapy* 48 (2002): 259-266.

Henneicke-von Zepelin, H., et al. "Efficacy and Safety of a Fixed Combination Phytomedicine in the Treatment of the Common Cold (Acute Viral Respiratory Tract Infection): Results of a Randomised, Double Blind, Placebo Controlled, Multicentre Study." *Current Medical Research and Opinion* 15 (2000): 214-227.

Naser, B., et al. "A Randomized, Double-Blind, Placebo-Controlled, Clinical Dose-Response Trial of an Extract of Baptisia, Echinacea, and Thuja for the Treatment of Patients with Common Cold." *Phytomedicine: International Journal of Phytotherapy and Phytopharmacology* 12 (2005): 715-722.

Wustenberg, P., et al. "Efficacy and Mode of Action of an Immunomodulator Herbal Preparation Containing Echinacea, Wild Indigo, and White Cedar." *Advances in Therapy* 16 (1999): 51-70.

See also: Bronchitis; Colds and flu; Immune support.

Wild yam

CATEGORY: Herbs and supplements
RELATED TERMS: *Dioscorea species*, Mexican yam
DEFINITION: Natural plant product used to treat specific health conditions.
PRINCIPAL PROPOSED USES: None
OTHER PROPOSED USE: Source of female hormones

OVERVIEW

Various species of wild yam grow throughout North and Central America and Asia. Traditionally, this herb has been used as a treatment for indigestion, coughs, morning sickness, gallbladder pain, menstrual cramps, joint pain, and nerve pain. The main use of wild yam in the United States today, however, is based on a fundamental misconception: that it contains women's hormones, such as progesterone and dehydroepiandrosterone (DHEA). In reality, there is no progesterone, DHEA, or any other hormone in wild yam, nor does wild yam contain any substances that have progesterone-like or estrogen-like effects.

To explain this widespread misunderstanding, it is necessary to go back a number of years. When progesterone was first discovered, it was very expensive to produce. The first methods involved direct extraction of progesterone from cow ovaries, a process that required fifty thousand cows to yield 20 milligrams of purified hormone. Other hormones, such as estrogen and DHEA, were also difficult to manufacture. Although doctors wanted to experiment with prescribing these treatments as medicine until a simpler

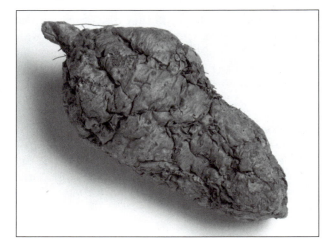

Wild yam. (Geoff Dann/Getty Images)

production method could be developed, it simply was not feasible.

The race to discover a more economical source of hormones was won by a scientist and businessman named Russell Marker. In the 1940s, he perfected a method of synthesizing progesterone from a constituent of wild yam called diosgenin. This process involved several chemical transformations carried out in the laboratory.

Marker focused his attention on two species of yam found in Mexico, *Dioscorea macrostachya* and *D. barabasco*, the latter of which is richer in diosgenin, while the former is much easier to harvest in the wild. He formed a manufacturing company in Mexico that produced progesterone and DHEA from these raw materials.

Corporate competition and difficult labor conditions eventually forced him to close his plant. However, Marker's method of synthesizing progesterone continued to be used, bringing the price down drastically and helping to pave the way for the modern birth control pill. Progesterone continued to be manufactured from wild yam for decades until a cheaper source of raw material was found in cultivated soybeans.

Neither soybeans nor wild yams, however, contain progesterone. They contain only chemicals that chemists can use as a starting point to manufacture progesterone. However, just because chemists can make progesterone out of diosgenin does not mean that the body can do the same. Actually, it is very unlikely, because the steps used by chemists to carry out this conversion do not even remotely resemble natural processes. Thus, any product that claims to contain "natural progesterone from wild yam" is misleading.

Studies involving cells in a test tube have shown that wild yam does not act like estrogen or progesterone. Furthermore, in a double-blind, placebo-controlled study of twenty-three women with symptoms of menopause, use of wild yam did not reduce hot flashes or raise levels of progesterone or estrogen in the body.

Nonetheless, some wild yam products do contain progesterone. Is this a contradiction? Not at all: Manufacturers add synthetic progesterone to these creams. There may be a value to taking progesterone in cream form, but the "wild yam" part of the product is a red herring.

EBSCO CAM Review Board

FURTHER READING

Komesaroff, P. A., et al. "Effects of Wild Yam Extract on Menopausal Symptoms, Lipids, and Sex Hormones in Healthy Menopausal Women." *Climacteric: The Journal of the International Menopause Society* 4 (2001): 144-150.

See also: Women's health.

Witch hazel

CATEGORY: Herbs and supplements
RELATED TERM: *Hamamelis virginiana*
DEFINITION: Natural plant product used to treat specific health conditions.
PRINCIPAL PROPOSED USES: Eczema, hemorrhoids
OTHER PROPOSED USES: Canker sores, cold sores, diarrhea, gum inflammation, minor wounds, varicose veins

OVERVIEW

The bark, leaves, and twigs of the witch hazel shrub were widely used as medicinal treatments by native peoples of North America. Witch hazel was applied topically as a treatment for such conditions as skin wounds, insect bites, hemorrhoids, muscle aches, and back stiffness, and it was taken internally for colds, coughs, and digestive problems. It came into use among European colonists in the 1840s, when a businessperson named Theron Pond marketed an extract of witch hazel as Golden Treasure.

The most common witch hazel product available in the United States is made from the whole twigs of the shrub. Extracts of the bark alone are used in Europe.

THERAPEUTIC DOSAGES

Witch hazel preparations should be used according to label instructions.

THERAPEUTIC USES

Witch hazel is widely marketed for direct application to the skin to relieve pain, stop bleeding, control itching, reduce symptoms of eczema, and treat muscle aches. Pads, ointments, and suppositories containing witch hazel are used for treatment of hemorrhoids. Extracts of the bark and leaf are used in Europe to treat diarrhea, inflammation of the gums, canker

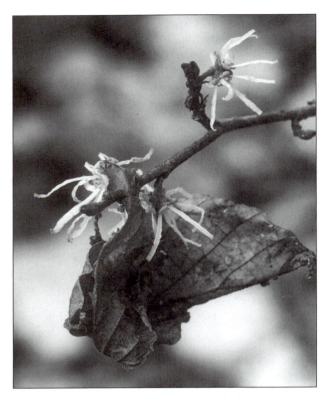

The whole twigs of the shrub are used to make the most common witch hazel product in the United States. (Gail Jankus/Photo Researchers, Inc.)

sores, and varicose veins. However, there is no meaningful evidence that witch hazel is actually effective for any of these conditions.

One small double-blind study is commonly cited as evidence that witch hazel is effective for treatment of eczema. This study compared topical witch hazel ointment to the drug bufexamac and found them equally effective. However, bufexamac itself has not been shown effective for the treatment of eczema, and so this study proves little. A subsequent study failed to find witch hazel more effective than a placebo treatment for eczema.

There are no other meaningful studies of witch hazel. Extremely preliminary evidence hints that it may have anti-inflammatory properties, and even weaker evidence suggests that witch hazel may increase the contractility of veins, potentially making it useful in varicose veins. However, this evidence is far too weak to support using witch hazel for any of these conditions.

SAFETY ISSUES

Witch hazel appears to be a relatively safe substance, but comprehensive safety studies have not been performed. When applied to the skin, it may cause allergic reactions. Witch hazel contains tannins, which can upset the stomach. Safety in pregnant or nursing women, young children, and people with severe liver or kidney disease has not been established.

EBSCO CAM Review Board

FURTHER READING

Hughes-Formella, B. J., et al. "Anti-Inflammatory Effect of Hamamelis Lotion in a UVB Erythema Test." *Dermatology* 196 (1998): 316-322.

Korting, H. C., et al. "Comparative Efficacy of Hamamelis Distallate and Hydrocortisone Cream in Atopic Eczema." *European Journal of Clinical Pharmacology* 48 (1995): 461-465.

See also: Eczema; Hemorrhoids; Canker sores; Diarrhea; Varicose veins.

Wolfberry

CATEGORY: Herbs and supplements

RELATED TERMS: Goji juice, gou qi zi, *Lycium barbarum, L. chinensis, L. fructus,* lycium fruit, Tibetan goji berry

DEFINITION: Natural plant product used to treat specific health conditions.

PRINCIPAL PROPOSED USES: None

OTHER PROPOSED USES: Alzheimer's disease prevention, cancer treatment, diabetes, high cholesterol, life extension, liver protection, enhancement of sexual function in men and in women

OVERVIEW

Wolfberry, the berry of the *Lycium chinensis* plant, has a long history of use in traditional Chinese herbal medicine. Chinese herbal medicine is part of an ancient and complex medical system that analyzes the effects of treatments in terms of their effects on the energy of various organs. Within this system, lycium berry has the effects of nourishing liver and kidneys, moistening the lungs, and supplementing the yin. Typical uses based on these actions include life extension and treatment of dry skin, dizziness, diminished sexual desire, low back pain, and chronic dry cough. The Tibetan goji berry is closely related to Chinese lycium.

THERAPEUTIC DOSAGES

Wolfberry tincture is typically taken in a dose of 3 to 4 tablespoons daily. People taking standardized extracts or other forms of the herb should follow label instructions.

THERAPEUTIC USES

Wolfberry is a nutritious food, containing relatively high levels of numerous vitamins and minerals. However, other proposed uses of wolfberry have no meaningful supporting evidence.

For example, while wolfberry is widely marketed as a life extension aid, there is no scientific evidence that it offers this benefit. In fact, even within the framework of traditional Chinese herbal medicine, the herb's action is far more complex, and it would not be expected to prolong life per se.

Much the same can said regarding the proposed uses of wolfberry to enhance male or female sexual function. Weak evidence from test-tube studies, far too preliminary to rely upon, hints at potential liver-protective, anti-Alzheimer's disease, anticancer, and cholesterol- and blood-sugar-lowering effects.

SAFETY ISSUES

As a widely used food, wolfberry is thought to be relatively safe. However, it has not undergone comprehensive safety testing. Maximum safe doses in pregnant or nursing women, young children, and people with severe liver or kidney disease have not been established.

EBSCO CAM Review Board

FURTHER READING

Luo, Q., et al. "Hypoglycemic and Hypolipidemic Effects and Antioxidant Activity of Fruit Extracts from *Lycium barbarum*." *Life Sciences* 76 (2004): 137-149.

Ram, V. J. Herbal Preparations as a Source of Hepatoprotective Agents." *Drug News and Perspectives* 14 (2003): 353-363.

Yu, M. S., et al. "Neuroprotective Effects of Anti-Aging Oriental Medicine *Lycium barbarum* Against Beta-Amyloid Peptide Neurotoxicity." *Experimental Gerontology* 40 (2005): 716-727.

Zhang, M., et al. "Effect of *Lycium barbarum* Polysac-

charide on Human Hepatoma QGY7703 Cells: Inhibition of Proliferation and Induction of Apoptosis." *Life Sciences* 76 (2005): 2115-2124.

See also: Alzheimer's disease; Cancer treatment support; Diabetes; Cholesterol, high; Liver disease; Sexual dysfunction in men.

Women's health

CATEGORY: Issues and overviews

DEFINITION: The use of nutrients, dietary supplements, herbal extracts, and alternative therapies for preventing and treating health conditions specific to or predominant in women, such as urinary tract infections, menstrual disorders, menopause, and osteoporosis.

OVERVIEW

Although men and women share a majority of health issues, there are many conditions that are specific to women. Women's health issues are those that are unique to the female anatomy and those that are found primarily in women. Men and women may share similar health issues, but these issues can affect women and men in different ways. Although pain relief is the most common reason for its use, complementary and alternative medicine (CAM) is used throughout the spectrum of women's health.

Many women use CAM as a form of medical treatment. According to a 2008 Centers for Disease Control and Prevention (CDC) health study, 42 percent of women surveyed had used some form of CAM. (Men were more likely to adhere to conventional medical practices.) This figure represents an increase in women's CAM use, compared with a similar survey in 2002, which showed that more women were beginning to use CAM. Financial concerns, mistrust of the health care system, toxicity of conventional medicines, and limited access to health care are some of the reasons why women turn to CAM. Women who are thirty to sixty-nine years of age and those with a higher level of education are more likely to use CAM.

An increasing number of studies have examined the efficacy of CAM in women's health. Rigorous scientific-based studies began in earnest in the early 1990s, coinciding with the establishment of the U.S.

Tai Chi and Green Tea Supplements for Osteopenia

The National Center for Complementary and Alternative Medicine reported on the results of a study examining the practice of tai chi and the consumption of green tea polyphenols by postmenopausal women with osteopenia (low bone mineral density). The study, published in 2010 in the journal *BMC Complementary and Alternative Medicine*, also found that practicing tai chi by itself or in combination with green tea polyphenol supplementation may improve quality of life; however, taking green tea supplements by themselves offers no significant improvement in quality of life. Osteopenia may precede osteoporosis, a bone disease characterized by reduced bone strength that can lead to fractures—a significant cause of disability in older people.

Researchers from Texas Tech University randomly assigned 171 women to receive green tea polyphenols (500 milligrams [mg] daily), green tea polyphenols plus tai chi training, placebo pills (500 mg starch daily), or placebo pills plus tai chi training for twenty-four weeks. The tai chi training consisted of three sixty-minute sessions per week. Researchers measured participants' depression (mood) and general health status, as well as liver and kidney function throughout the study. Participants in the tai chi groups reported significant beneficial effects in quality of life in terms of improving their emotional and mental health. The researchers found that green tea supplements did not significantly affect participants' liver enzymes or kidney serum levels and had no effect on quality of life.

The researchers also noted that this is the first placebo-controlled, randomized study to evaluate the safety of long-term use of green tea supplements in postmenopausal women. Based on these findings, the researchers concluded that green tea polyphenols at a dose of 500 mg daily for twenty-four weeks, alone or in combination with tai chi, appears to be safe in postmenopausal women with low bone mineral density.

government's Office of Alternative Medicine, now called the National Center for Complementary and Alternative Medicine (NCCAM). This center serves as the principal government agency for analyzing medical practices that are outside the scope of conventional medicine. NCCAM also scrutinizes and funds evidence-based research on CAM.

Just as NCCAM examines the efficacy of CAM treatments, it also reviews their safety. Many herbal medicines used in combination or used with conventional medications may have adverse side effects. Women who participate in exercise-based treatments may sustain injuries if they are not physically healthy enough or if supervision is improper.

GENITOURINARY INFECTIONS

Genitourinary infections involve the bladder, kidneys, vagina, cervix, and, rarely, uterus. Women experience infections of the bladder and kidneys far more often than do men. The close proximity, in females, of the entrance to the urinary tract (urethra) to the anus makes the risk of urinary infections higher for women than for men. Because urinary tract infections are so common, many women look for inexpensive and convenient treatment options.

Cranberry juice and cranberry-based products have been used by women for decades to treat urinary tract infections (UTIs). There have been no comprehensive, randomized-controlled trials on the use of cranberry juice for UTIs, so there is no scientific evidence to suggest that it is effective. Clinical trials do suggest, however, that cranberry juice may prevent infection in women with recurrent UTIs. A large study sponsored by NCCAM examining the use of cranberry juice for the treatment and prevention of UTIs is currently underway.

Lactobacillus is a probiotic used in the treatment of UTIs, vulvovaginal candidiasis (vaginal yeast infection), and bacterial vaginosis. Probiotics are live microorganisms that are thought to inhibit the growth of unwanted infectious microorganisms. Available clinical data demonstrate that orally and intravaginally administered lactobacillus appears to be effective in treating bacterial vaginosis. The data were inconclusive, however, regarding the effectiveness of lactobacillus probiotics for UTIs and vulvovaginal candidiasis.

MENOPAUSE AND OSTEOPOROSIS

The cessation of ovarian function and, thus, of regular menses is referred to as menopause. Hormonal changes that occur during menopause can cause bothersome effects. Many women experience hot flashes, vaginal dryness, insomnia, and mood disturbances. Because bone density relies in part on estrogen secreted by the ovaries, there is a risk of bone thinning or osteoporosis after menopause. In 2002, the use of hormone replacement therapy drugs containing estrogen dramatically decreased following the announcement of possible health risks. Because of this, many women have turned to alternative medicine to relieve the effects of menopause.

Herbal medicines and nutritional supplements. Black cohosh, evening primrose, soy, gong guai root, ginsing, kava, and DHEA (dehydroepiandrosterone) are products used to treat hot flashes, vaginal dryness, and other symptoms of menopause. The most widely studied and used product is black cohosh. Lacking, however, is scientific evidence supporting the effectiveness of these products in treating menopause.

Soy isoflavones and green tea are widely used in the treatment and prevention of osteoporosis. Soy isoflavones are derived from plant-based soy products and possess estrogen-like activities. Also called phytoestrogens, soy isoflavones are in wide use in many over-the-counter preparations that promote bone health. The *American Journal of Clinical Nutrition* published a large study of isoflavones in March, 2010, and concluded that soy isoflavones did not prevent osteoporosis. Conversely, a large amount of scientific evidence suggests that green tea provides some protection against osteoporosis. Although the antioxidant properties of green tea may be at work, the exact mechanism of action is not known.

Exercise-based therapies. Tai Chi and qigong are traditional Chinese forms of exercise incorporating discrete low-impact movements, breathing, and meditation. In 2010, several large, well-designed studies showed that Tai Chi and presumably qigong were beneficial in preserving bone density in postmenopausal women. In a 2008 randomized clinical trial published in the journal *Menopause*, yoga reduced hot flashes by 30 percent. There have been, however, no double-blind studies. The more aggressive forms of yoga, such as ashtanga, vinyasa, and Iyenger, which incorporate weight-bearing activities, can be effective in preventing bone loss.

PREGNANCY AND INFERTILITY

Many women seek to relieve discomfort during pregnancy and labor without conventional medications and invasive procedures. The prohibitive cost of conventional infertility treatment makes CAM an attractive option.

A Cochrane review of clinical studies using CAM in labor demonstrated that acupuncture and hypnosis were effective methods of pain relief. There was no evidence that massage, acupressure, or aromatherapy used to relieve pain during labor had any benefit. Vitamin C and E supplements have been touted to reduce the risk of high blood pressure during pregnancy. A large study sponsored by the National Institutes of Health, however, did not support this claim.

Yoga and acupuncture practitioners and advocates assert that these two CAM methods can enhance fertility. Promising scientific evidence exists that acupuncture in conjunction with in vitro fertilization can increase rates of pregnancy. Furthermore, numerous studies have demonstrated that yoga improves sex performance anxiety and female sexual desire, which can indirectly enhance fertility. Chasteberry has been used for more than two thousand years by women to treat various gynecological disorders, such as infertility; clinical evidence supporting this claim is lacking, however.

Hyperemesis gravidarum is severe, persistent nausea and vomiting that occurs in early and mid-pregnancy. There are alternative treatments that are used to treat this condition. The most commonly used treatments are acupuncture, acupressure, ginger products, and vitamin B_6. A Cochrane review of twenty-seven randomized controlled trials examined these treatments, but the effectiveness of these modalities could not be determined because the studies were conducted in a way that introduced bias. More well-designed studies are needed.

CANCERS OF THE FEMALE REPRODUCTIVE SYSTEM

The diagnosis of cancer may bring emotional and physical disruptions to a woman's daily life. Many women also have doubts about conventional treatment decisions. It is not uncommon for women to turn to CAM to meet their emotional and physical needs. The use of CAM in women with breast, ovarian, and uterine cancer encompasses prevention, cure, and treatments to minimize the side effects of conventional therapies.

Herbal medicines and nutritional supplements. Antioxidants such as vitamin C, vitamin E, coenzyme Q_{10}, and green tea are thought to prevent cancers of the breast, ovaries, and uterus. Also, soy isoflavones and garlic are thought to prevent these types of cancers. Between the years 2002 and 2009, numerous large clinical trials examined the use of antioxidants, soy products, and garlic in the prevention of cancers in women. These studies provided no sufficient evidence to support the claim that most of these products are protective against cancers.

Studies examining garlic use for ovarian cancer prevention, however, are more promising. Although the National Cancer Institute does not recommend using garlic for cancer prevention, it does recognize that garlic may contain anticancer properties and that more studies are needed to determine this. There are no high-quality studies available that support the use of herbal medicines or nutritional products as a cancer cure.

Physical and mind/body interventions. Meditation, yoga, and hypnosis are often used in conjunction with conventional medicine in the treatment of breast, ovarian, and uterine cancer. Clinical trials have demonstrated that all three modalities are effective in reducing anxiety, pain, and insomnia during cancer treatment, although scientists continue to debate the exact mechanisms of action. Acupuncture may help with nausea during chemotherapy, but more high-quality studies are needed to confirm its efficacy. Art therapy combines the creative process with traditional therapy to allow for the expression of thoughts and feelings. A study of women who had breast cancer showed an improvement of mood disorders when art therapy was applied.

MENSTRUAL DISORDERS

Menstrual cramps and premenstrual syndrome (PMS) may be a monthly source of physical and emotional distress to premenopausal women. About 35 percent of women experience painful menses on a regular basis. Although a majority of women experience some degree of abdominal bloating, anxiety, irritability, and breast tenderness during the premenstrual period, about 2 percent of women have severe disrupting symptoms. Although these symptoms are typically treated with medications and dietary and lifestyle changes, many women find these modalities intolerable or ineffective and so turn to CAM.

Omega-3, rose hip tea, vitamin B_1 (thiamine), magnesium, vitamin B_6, vitamin E, chasteberry, evening primrose, and calcium are used in the treatment of menstrual cramps and PMS. No clinical trials have provided strong evidence supporting the efficacy of most of these products. Calcium supplementation, however, showed promising evidence as a treatment for PMS. A Cochrane database review found promising evidence supporting the use of a Chinese herbal medicine called jingqianping granules for menstrual cramps and PMS; however, more well-designed clinical trials are needed to confirm this. There is clinical evidence as well that chasteberry is effective in treating the symptoms of PMS and breast pain associated with menses; however, more studies are needed. In a 2009 review, acupuncture appeared to be a promising treatment for PMS. In another, similar review study, transcutaneous electrical nerve stimulation and massage therapy were found to be ineffective in treating menstrual cramps.

Endometriosis, a condition in which cells of the uterus grow in other parts of the body, can cause pelvic pain and severe menstrual cramps. Traditional Chinese herbs are used in the treatment of this disorder. The limited reviews that found traditional Chinese herbs helpful were not high-quality randomized-control trials. Therefore, more study is needed to confirm the efficacy of this treatment.

CONCLUSIONS

Despite extensive use of CAM by women, there remains a lack of high-quality scientific evidence to support the effectiveness of most CAM modalities. Rigorous, well-designed clinical trials to determine the effectiveness of CAM therapies for women have become popular only in the twenty-first century. Major studies sponsored by NCCAM are being conducted for a variety of treatment modalities.

Women should not replace traditional medicine for serious medical disorders, such as cancer, with CAM. Women using CAM as a complementary therapy should be aware of the efficacy and safety profile of the treatment before use.

Marie President, M.D.

FURTHER READING

Barnes, P. M., B. Bloom, and R. L. Nahin. "Complementary and Alternative Medicine Use Among Adults and Children: 2007 United States." *National Health Statistics Reports* 12 (December 10, 2008): 1-23. Gives results of the second nationwide health survey in the United States and explains why prayer was excluded from the survey's definitions of CAM modalities.

Carlson, L. E. "Mind-Body Interventions in Oncology." *Current Treatment Options in Oncology* 9, nos. 2/3 (2008): 127-134. Looks at the use of mind/body therapies in the treatment of cancer.

National Center for Complementary and Alternative Medicine. http://www.nccam.nih.gov. The lead U.S.-government agency on CAM. An invaluable resource.

Zoorob, J. R. "CAM and Women's Health: Selected Topics." *Primary Care* 37, no. 2 (2010): 367-387. Looks at CAM use in women from the perspective of primary care medicine.

See also: Bladder infection; Breast enhancement; Breast pain, cyclic; Breast-feeding support; Candida/yeast hypersensitivity syndrome; Cervical dysplasia; Dysmenorrhea; Eating disorders; Endometriosis; Infertility, female; Lupus; Menopause; Morning sickness; Osteoporosis; Polycystic ovary syndrome; Preeclampsia and pregnancy-induced hypertension; Pregnancy support; Premenstrual syndrome (PMS); Premenstrual syndrome (PMS): Homeopathic remedies; Sexual dysfunction in women; Vaginal infection.

Wormwood

Category: Herbs and supplements

Related terms: *Artemisia absinthium*, common wormwood

Definition: Natural plant product used as a dietary supplement for specific health benefits.

Principal proposed use: Crohn's disease

Other proposed uses: Dyspepsia, esophageal reflux, irritable bowel syndrome, parasites

Overview

Artemisia absinthium, or common wormwood, is best known as an ingredient of the alcoholic beverage absinthe. Wormwood is also found in vermouth, but at lower levels. Besides its common function as a flavoring, wormwood also has a long history of medicinal use. A reputed ability to kill intestinal worms gave rise to the herb's name. Other traditional uses include treating liver problems, joint pain, digestive discomfort, loss of appetite, insomnia, epilepsy, and menstrual problems. The leaves and flowers, and the essential oil extracted from them, are the parts used medicinally. Common wormwood is a relative of sweet wormwood (*A. annua*), a source of the malaria drug artemisinin (also called artemesin).

Uses and Applications

Wormwood is sometimes recommended for the treatment of digestive conditions such as intestinal parasites, dyspepsia, esophageal reflux, and irritable bowel syndrome. However, there is no meaningful evidence to indicate that it is effective for any of these conditions. Only double-blind, placebo-controlled studies can show a treatment effective, and only one has been performed using wormwood. This ten-week study conducted in Germany evaluated the potential benefits of wormwood for the treatment of people with Crohn's disease, an inflammatory condition of the intestines. All forty people enrolled in the study had achieved good control of their symptoms through the use of steroids and other medications. One-half were given an herbal blend containing wormwood (500 milligrams [mg] three times daily), while the other one-half were given an identical-appearing placebo. Researchers and study participants did not know who was receiving real treatment and who was not. Beginning at week two, researchers began a gradual tapering down of the steroid dosage used by participants. In subsequent weeks, most of those given placebo showed the expected worsening of symptoms that the reduction of drug dosage would be expected to cause. In contrast, most of those persons receiving wormwood showed a gradual improvement of symptoms. No serious side effects were attributed to wormwood in this study.

These findings are extremely promising. However, many treatments that show promise in a single study fail to hold up in subsequent independent testing. Further research is needed to establish wormwood as a helpful treatment for Crohn's disease. Other proposed uses of wormwood have far weaker supporting evidence. Preliminary indications hint that wormwood essential oil (like many other essential oils) might have antifungal, antibacterial, and antiparasitic actions. Note, however, that this does not mean that wormwood oil is an antibiotic. Antibiotics are substances that can be taken internally to kill microorganisms throughout

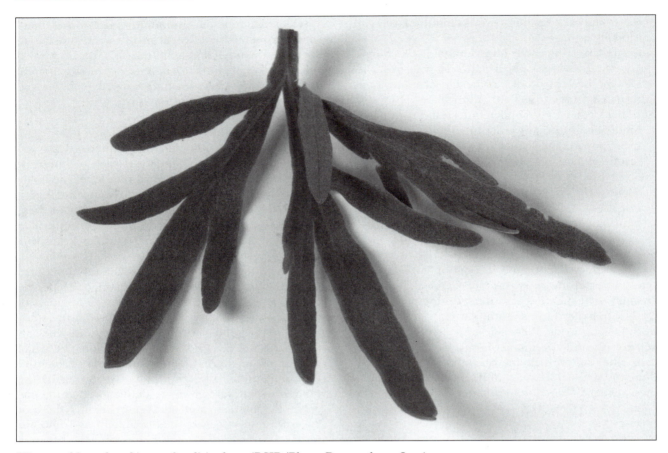

Wormwood has a long history of medicinal use. (BSIP/Photo Researchers, Inc.)

the body. Wormwood oil, rather, has shown potential antiseptic properties, but it also is potentially toxic. Other weak evidence hints that an alcohol extract of wormwood might have liver-protective actions.

DOSAGE

In the foregoing study, wormwood was taken at a dose of 500 mg three times daily. A typical traditional dose of wormwood is three cups daily of a tea made by steeping 2.5 to 5 grams of wormwood in hot water. Wormwood essential oil should not be used. One should not attempt long-term use (more than four weeks) of any form of wormwood except under physician supervision.

SAFETY ISSUES

There are many unsolved questions about the toxicity of wormwood. When absinthe was popular in the late nineteenth and early twentieth centuries, a mental disorder known as absinthism, which involved hallucinations, tremors, vertigo, sleeplessness, and seizures, was associated with it. Wormwood contains thujone, a substance thought to be toxic to nerves when taken at high doses, and thujone has been proposed as a factor contributing to absinthism. However, the symptoms of absinthism are also consistent with mere chronic overuse of alcohol, and absinthe does not appear to contain sufficient thujone to cause harm. Furthermore, animal studies have generally failed to find significant toxicity with wormwood, even at relatively high doses.

Despite the absence of firm evidence, wormwood is still considered a potentially toxic herb, especially if taken over the long term. Wormwood essential oil, which contains thujone at much higher levels than those found in absinthe, should be avoided. Wormwood should not be used by young children, pregnant or nursing women, or people with severe liver or kidney disease.

EBSCO CAM Review Board

FURTHER READING

Kordali, S., et al. "Screening of Chemical Composition and Antifungal and Antioxidant Activities of the Essential Oils from Three Turkish *Artemisia* Species." *Journal of Agricultural and Food Chemistry* 53 (2005): 1408-1416.

Lachenmeier, D. W. "Wormwood (*Artemisia absinthium* L.): A Curious Plant with Both Neurotoxic and Neuroprotective Properties?" *Journal of Ethnopharmacology* 131 (2010): 224-227.

_____ et al. "Thujone: Cause of Absinthism?" *Forensic Science International* 158 (2006): 1-8.

Omer, B., et al. "Steroid-Sparing Effect of Wormwood (*Artemisia absinthium*) in Crohn's Disease." *Phytomedicine* 14 (2007): 87-95

See also: Crohn's disease; Dyspepsia; Functional beverages; Gastroesophageal reflux disease; irritable bowel syndrome (IBS); Parasites, intestinal.

Wounds, minor

CATEGORY: Condition
RELATED TERMS: Cuts, lacerations, scrapes
DEFINITION: Treatment of minor cuts and other injuries to the skin.
PRINCIPAL PROPOSED NATURAL TREATMENT: Careful wound cleaning
OTHER PROPOSED NATURAL TREATMENTS: Aloe vera, amino acid cream, bee propolis, calendula, comfrey, cartilage, essential oils, chamomile, chitosan, garlic, goldenseal, gotu kola, honey, picrorhiza, royal jelly, St. John's wort, vitamin A, vitamin C, vitamin E, zinc

INTRODUCTION

Minor cuts are an ordinary fact of life, and they nearly always heal on their own. There is no evidence that antibacterial gels and creams will help wounds heal faster or prevent infection. By keeping the air away from a wound, these treatments might actually interfere with healing.

The best approach to minor wounds is also the simplest and most natural: Clean the wound well and keep it clean and exposed to the air. If signs of infection develop, such as redness, oozing, or swelling, a physician should be consulted.

PROPOSED NATURAL TREATMENTS

Application of honey (or concentrated sugar preparations) to wounds might help prevent infection and possibly speed healing. Honey is thought to work primarily through its high sugar content, which directly kills microorganisms. However, trace substances contained in it might also be at work. Not all studies show clear benefit, however. One trial found that antibacterial honey (Medihoney) did not significantly improve wound healing in 105 persons with mostly leg ulcers.

Preliminary evidence suggests that the herb gotu kola might have general wound-healing properties and might help to prevent and to treat keloid scars (a particular type of scar that is enlarged and bulging). A small, double-blind, placebo-controlled trial found that the amino acids cysteine, glycine, and threonine applied as a combination cream could help the healing of leg ulcers. A variety of nutrients, including vitamins A, C, and E, and zinc, taken both orally and topically, have also been tried as a treatment for minor wounds, and creams containing A and E are common staples in hospitals. A number of topical herbs also have been tried, including calendula, cartilage, chamomile, chitosan, goldenseal, royal jelly, and St. John's wort, but there is no real evidence that any of these approaches provides any benefits.

Numerous herbs (and their essential oils) have antibacterial properties and for this reason might theoretically be helpful for preventing wound infection. However, this has not been proven. In addition, if a wound is serious enough that infection is a real risk, physician supervision is essential.

The gel of the aloe vera plant has a long folk history in the treatment of skin conditions. There is some evidence from human and animal studies that aloe might be helpful for wound healing, but one study found that aloe gel actually slowed the healing of surgical wounds.

In a well-designed trial, two concentrations of comfrey creams were evaluated for the treatment of fresh abrasions among 278 persons. A 10 percent comfrey formulation was compared to a 1 percent comfrey formulation, which was considered the reference or placebo cream. The topical application of 10 percent comfrey led to significantly faster wound healing than the reference cream after two to three days of application. Although the researchers reported no adverse effects in either group, the use of comfrey has been associated with severe, even life-threatening toxic effects when used orally, and its use over open wounds must be undertaken with extreme caution.

Animal studies suggest that the honeybee product propolis applied topically may be of benefit in healing wounds. Similarly weak evidence hints at benefits with the herb picrorhiza.

EBSCO CAM Review Board

FURTHER READING

Al-Waili, N. S. "Investigating the Antimicrobial Activity of Natural Honey and Its Effects on the Pathogenic Bacterial Infections of Surgical Wounds and Conjunctiva." *Journal of Medicinal Food* 7 (2004): 210-222.

Folstad, Steven G. "Soft Tissue Infections." In *Emergency Medicine: A Comprehensive Study Guide*, edited by Judith E. Tintinalli. 6th ed. New York: McGraw-Hill, 2004.

Pieper, B., and M. H. Caliri. "Nontraditional Wound Care: A Review of the Evidence for the Use of Sugar, Papaya/Papain, and Fatty Acids." *Journal of Wound, Ostomy, and Continence Nursing* 30 (2003): 175-183.

Robson, V., S. Dodd, and S. Thomas. "Standardized Antibacterial Honey (Medihoney) with Standard Therapy in Wound Care." *Journal of Advanced Nursing* 65 (2009): 565-575.

See also: Bruises; Burns, minor; Comfrey; Injuries, minor; Pain management; Soft tissue pain.

X

Xylitol

CATEGORY: Functional foods
DEFINITION: Natural substance promoted as a dietary supplement for specific health benefits.
PRINCIPAL PROPOSED USE: Cavity prevention
OTHER PROPOSED USES: Ear infections, periodontal disease

OVERVIEW

Xylitol, a natural sugar found in plums, strawberries, and raspberries, is used as a sweetener in some "sugarless" gums and candies. Not only does xylitol replace sugars that can lead to tooth decay, it also appears to help prevent cavities by inhibiting the growth of bacteria, such as *Streptococcus mutans*, that cause cavities. Xylitol also inhibits the growth of a related species, *S. pneumoniae*, which is a cause of ear infections. Gums, toothpaste, and candy containing high levels of xylitol are now available in the United States.

USES AND APPLICATIONS

Many studies, including several under the auspices of the World Health Organization, have evaluated xylitol gums, toothpastes, and candies for preventing dental cavities, with good results. In all of these studies, xylitol users developed fewer cavities than those receiving either placebo or no treatment.

Xylitol is thought to prevent cavities by inhibiting the growth of *S. mutans* bacteria. Because a related bacterium, *S. pneumoniae*, can cause ear infections, xylitol has been investigated as a preventive treatment for middle ear infections, with some success. In addition, preliminary evidence suggests that the use of xylitol may offer some protection against periodontal disease (gum disease).

SCIENTIFIC EVIDENCE

Preventing cavities. Double-blind, placebo-controlled studies enrolling almost four thousand people, mostly children, have found that xylitol gum, candy, or toothpaste can help prevent cavities. One study also suggested that the chewy candy "gummy" bears may be an effective alternative method of administering xylitol to children.

A double-blind, placebo-controlled study of 1,677 children compared a standard fluoride toothpaste with a similar toothpaste that also contained 10 percent xylitol. In the three-year study period, children given the xylitol-enriched toothpaste developed significantly fewer cavities than those in the fluoride-only group.

In another trial, a forty-month, double-blind study of 1,277 children, researchers studied gum products containing various concentrations of xylitol or sorbitol, or both. Participants were divided into nine groups: xylitol gum in four different concentrations, two forms of xylitol-sorbitol gum, sorbitol-only gum, sucrose (ordinary sugar) gum, or no gum. The gum with the highest xylitol concentration proved most effective at reducing cavities. However, children in every one of the xylitol-gum and or sorbitol-gum groups showed significant reductions in cavities compared with the sugar gum and no-gum groups. Another series of studies suggests that children acquire cavity-causing bacteria from their mothers; the regular use of xylitol by a mother of a newborn child may provide some protection to the child.

Ear infections. One large, double-blind, placebo-controlled trial of 857 children investigated how well xylitol (in chewing gum, syrup, and lozenges) could prevent ear infections. The gum was most effective, reducing the risk of developing ear infections by a full 40 percent. Xylitol syrup was also effective, but less so. The lozenges were not effective; researchers speculated that children got tired of sucking on the large candies and did not get the proper dose of xylitol. (In addition, the children were able to distinguish between the xylitol and placebo lozenges by taste, making that portion of the study single-blind.)

Similarly positive results had been seen in an earlier double-blind study by the same researchers, evaluating about three hundred children. However, these studies were of short duration and did not test the long-term effect of xylitol in young children and infants, who are most at risk of contracting ear infections.

DOSAGE

In the foregoing studies, dosages for cavity prevention ranged from 4.3 to 10 grams (g) per day. The doses were divided throughout the day, usually after meals. For ear infections, children given xylitol-sweetened gum received 8.4 g of xylitol daily, also in divided doses. Those who took syrup received 10 g daily.

SAFETY ISSUES

Xylitol is believed to be safe, but doses higher than 30 g per day can cause stomach discomfort and possibly diarrhea. In studies, children taking xylitol syrup tended to have more such side effects than those using other forms, possibly because the syrup reached the stomach in a more concentrated dose.

EBSCO CAM Review Board

FURTHER READING

Danhauer, J. L., et al. "National Survey of Pediatricians' Opinions About and Practices for Acute Otitis Media and Xylitol Use." *Journal of the American Academy of Audiology* 21 (2010): 329-346.

Gales, M. A., and T.-M. Nguyen. "Sorbitol Compared with Xylitol in Prevention of Dental Caries." *Annals of Pharmacotherapy* 34 (2000): 98-100.

Hildebrandt, G. H., and B. S. Sparks. "Maintaining *mutans* Streptococci Suppression with Xylitol Chewing Gum." *Journal of the American Dental Association* 131 (2000): 909-916.

Ly, K. A., et al. "Xylitol Gummy Bear Snacks." *BMC Oral Health* 8 (2008): 20.

See also: Cavity prevention; Ear infections; Periodontal disease.

Y

Yarrow

CATEGORY: Herbs and supplements

RELATED TERMS: *Achillea millefolium*, bloodwort, herbe militaire, soldier's wound-wort

DEFINITION: Herbal product used as a dietary supplement for specific health benefits.

PRINCIPAL PROPOSED USES: None

OTHER PROPOSED USES: Colds and flu, stopping bleeding from nosebleeds and minor wounds

OVERVIEW

According to legend, the Greek general Achilles used yarrow to stop the bleeding of his soldiers' wounds during the Trojan War; hence yarrow's scientific name *Achillea* and the common names soldier's wound-wort, bloodwort, and herbe militaire. Yarrow has also been used traditionally as treatment for respiratory infections, menstrual pain, and digestive upsets.

USES AND APPLICATIONS

Like osha, yarrow tea is commonly taken at the first sign of a cold or flu to bring on sweating and, according to tradition, ward off infection. Crushed yarrow leaves and flower tops are also applied directly as first aid to stop nosebleeds and bleeding from minor wounds. However, there are no formal scientific studies determining whether yarrow works for this purpose.

DOSAGE

Yarrow tea is made by steeping 1 to 2 teaspoons of dried herb per cup of water. Combination products should be taken according to label instructions.

SAFETY ISSUES

No clear toxicity has been associated with yarrow. The U.S. Food and Drug Administration (FDA) has expressed concern about a toxic constituent of yarrow known as thujone and permits only thujone-free yarrow extracts for use in beverages. Nonetheless, the common spice sage contains more thujone than

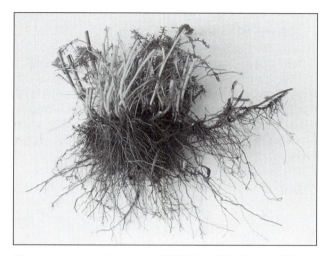

Yarrow roots and stems. (TH Foto-Werbung/Photo Researchers, Inc.)

yarrow, and the FDA lists sage as generally recognized as safe. The safety of yarrow use by young children, pregnant or nursing women, or those with severe liver or kidney disease, however, has not been established.

EBSCO CAM Review Board

FURTHER READING

Benedek, B., et al. "Yarrow (*Achillea millefolium* L. s.l.): Pharmaceutical Quality of Commercial Samples." *Pharmazie* 63 (2008): 23-26.

"Final Report on the Safety Assessment of Yarrow (*Achillea millefolium*) Extract." *International Journal of Toxicology* 20, suppl. 2 (2001): 79-84.

Nemeth, E., and J. Bernath. "Biological Activities of Yarrow Species (*Achillea* spp.)." *Current Pharmaceutical Design* 14 (2008): 3151-3167.

Potrich, F. B., et al. "Antiulcerogenic Activity of Hydroalcoholic Extract of *Achillea millefolium* L.: Involvement of the Antioxidant System." *Journal of Ethnopharmacology* 130 (2010): 85-92.

See also: Colds and flu; Wounds, minor.

Yellow dock

CATEGORY: Herbs and supplements
RELATED TERM: *Rumex crispus*
DEFINITION: Natural plant product used to treat specific health conditions.
PRINCIPAL PROPOSED USES: None
OTHER PROPOSED USES: Constipation, diarrhea, hemorrhoids, minor skin wounds

OVERVIEW

Yellow dock (*Rumex crispus*) is a perennial flowering herb, native to Europe, that grows throughout the United States. Its yellow roots were traditionally thought to have medicinal properties, and its sour-sweet leaves can be used, in moderation, as a salad green.

Historically, the plant has been used to treat a variety of problems, including constipation and diarrhea, as well as dermatitis and venereal diseases. Powdered yellow dock root has also been used as a mouthwash or dentifrice.

THERAPEUTIC DOSAGES

Typical doses of yellow dock root are 2 to 4 grams of the dried root, 2 to 4 milliliters (ml) of the liquid extract, or 1 to 2 ml of the tincture.

THERAPEUTIC USES

Yellow dock root has no established medical uses. However, it contains chemicals called anthroquinones (also found in the more famous herbal laxative senna), which stimulate bowel movements. For this reason, yellow dock is occasionally included in herbal laxative mixtures.

Like many other plants, yellow dock contains a substantial amount of tannins. These have astringent properties that may offer some benefit for treating minor skin wounds and hemorrhoids. Yellow dock is also sometimes recommended for nasal and lung congestion.

SAFETY ISSUES

Comprehensive safety studies of yellow dock have not been performed, and for this reason it should not be used by pregnant or nursing women, young children, or individuals with severe liver or kidney disease. As with any stimulant laxative, yellow dock should not be used if there is an intestinal obstruc-tion. Possible side effects of overuse include cramps, diarrhea, nausea, intestinal dependence on the laxative, and excessive loss of potassium.

In addition, yellow dock (like spinach) contains oxalic acid. Consuming excessive quantities of oxalic acid can cause severe toxic symptoms, including vomiting and abdominal pain, and, in extreme cases, kidney stones or kidney failure. One case of fatal yellow dock poisoning has been documented. The victim, who had diabetes, ingested one kilogram of the raw herb in a salad and died of liver and kidney failure. The liver failure was not explained.

EBSCO CAM Review Board

FURTHER READING

McGuffin, M., ed. *American Herbal Products Association's Botanical Safety Handbook*. Boca Raton, Fla.: CRC Press, 1997.

Reig, R., et al. "Fatal Poisoning by *Rumex crispus* (Curled Dock): Pathological Findings and Application of Scanning Electron Microscopy." *Veterinary and Human Toxicology* 32 (1990): 468-470.

See also: Constipation; Diarrhea; Hemorrhoids.

Yerba santa

CATEGORY: Herbs and supplements
RELATED TERM: *Eriodictyon californicum*
DEFINITION: Natural plant product used to treat specific health conditions.
PRINCIPAL PROPOSED USES: Asthma, bronchitis, common cold, poison ivy, rash

OVERVIEW

Yerba santa is a sticky-leafed evergreen that is native to the American Southwest. It was given its name, which means "holy weed," by Spanish Catholic priests impressed with its medicinal properties. The aromatic leaves were boiled to make a tea to treat coughs, colds, asthma, pleurisy, tuberculosis, and pneumonia, and a poultice of the leaves was applied to painful joints.

Unlike many medicinal herbs, yerba santa actually has a pleasant taste. It has been used as a general food flavoring and in cough syrups to disguise the bad taste of other ingredients.

THERAPEUTIC DOSAGES

Yerba santa tea may be made by adding 1 teaspoon of crushed leaves to a cup of boiling water and steeping for half an hour. However, many of its resinous constituents do not dissolve in water, and for that reason alcoholic tinctures of yerba santa are commonly used.

THERAPEUTIC USES

Yerba santa is often used for the treatment of the common cold, as well as chronic respiratory problems, such as bronchitis and asthma. However, there is no meaningful scientific evidence to indicate that it is effective. About the most that can be said scientifically is that one of its constituents, eriodictyol, might have mild expectorant properties. Also, topical yerba santa has been recommended as a treatment for poison ivy.

SAFETY ISSUES

Yerba santa is on the U.S. Food and Drug Administration's (FDA) Generally Recognized As Safe (GRAS) list for use as a food flavoring. There have been no reports of significant side effects or adverse reactions, except for the inevitable occasional allergic reaction. Nonetheless, safety in young children, pregnant or nursing women, and those with severe liver or kidney disease has not been established.

EBSCO CAM Review Board

FURTHER READING

Tierra, M. *The Way of Herbs*. New York: Pocket Books; 1990.

See also: Asthma; Bronchitis; Colds and flu.

Yoga

CATEGORY: Therapies and techniques
RELATED TERM: Hatha yoga
DEFINITION: A form of exercise based on postures, stretching, breathing, meditation, introspection, and other techniques.
PRINCIPAL PROPOSED USES: Increasing strength, balance, and flexibility; reducing tension and stress
OTHER PROPOSED USES: Asthma, carpal tunnel syndrome, chemical dependency, congestive heart failure, depression, eating disorders, epilepsy, high blood pressure, menopausal symptoms, migraine headaches, obsessive-compulsive disorder, osteoarthritis, schizophrenia, well-being in general

OVERVIEW

Hatha yoga, commonly called yoga in the United States, is an exercise system derived from ancient traditions in India. There are many schools or varieties of yoga, but all of them involve asanas, or postures. Many asanas function as gentle stretching exercises, increasing flexibility. Others encourage the development of strength and balance.

The practice of yoga goes beyond exercise, however. Special breathing techniques are almost always part of the process; in fact, some forms of yoga focus primarily on breathing and, therefore, overlap with traditional breathing practices generally known as *pranayama*. Because yoga originated in traditional Hindu spiritual practice, it can involve meditation, chanting, and philosophical and religious introspection. However, completely secular versions of yoga are widely available.

Yoga is believed by its practitioners to provide benefits above and beyond simple exercise. For example, certain asanas are said to address specific health problems. However, there is only minimal scientific evidence that yoga actually provides any well-defined medical benefits.

USES AND APPLICATIONS

There are numerous specific schools of yoga, including Iyengar yoga, Ashtanga yoga, Kriya yoga, Vini yoga, and Bikram yoga, as well as the "generic" yoga. Yoga is ordinarily learned through inexpensive group lessons, but regular at-home practice is necessary to progress in skill (and to derive potential health benefits). Lessons are commonly available at hospital wellness centers, health clubs, city recreation departments, and private yoga studios. Do-it-yourself yoga DVDs and books are available too, but most serious yoga practitioners caution against learning the technique without an instructor present.

SCIENTIFIC EVIDENCE

Although some evidence exists that yoga may offer medical benefits, this evidence, in general, is not strong. There are several reasons for this (including funding obstacles), but one is fundamental: Even with the best of intentions, it is difficult to properly ascertain the effectiveness of an exercise therapy like yoga.

Finding the Right Type of Yoga and the Right Teacher

The word "yoga" as used in the United States refers to a broad range of different kinds of mental, physical, and spiritual practices. Persons who have a desire to learn should take some time to get acquainted with the different schools and styles to appreciate what various teachers have to offer. Yoga is a most personal kind of exercise, and the benefits accrue slowly and subtly over time.

Many different schools and styles of yoga are taught in the United States. Some teachers have been certified in particular traditions, others offer a synthesis based on their own practice with yoga masters. The various major traditions include the following:

- *Astanga yoga.* This form of yoga, developed by K. Pattabhi Jois, is a demanding form of the practice. This yoga uses a concept of "flow" that has participants moving continuously and jumping from one posture to another, building strength, flexibility, and stamina. Astanga yoga is an intense workout and is not recommended for persons looking for leisurely stretching exercises.

- *Integral yoga.* This form of yoga was developed by Swami Satchidananda. It relies on breathing exercises (*pranayama*) and meditation as much as on postures for the practice.

- *Iyengar yoga.* Iyengar yoga is a style of yoga developed by B. K. S. Iyengar, who systemized his training and certified teachers who have completed an extensive two-to-five-year training program. Iyengar practitioners use props such as blocks and belts to aid them in performing many of the more difficult postures, and great attention is paid to a precise alignment of postures.

- *Kripalu yoga.* This form of yoga places emphasis on "honoring the wisdom of the body" and allowing each student to develop an awareness of mind, body, emotion, and spirit. The practice is delineated into three stages: learning the postures and exploring the body's abilities, holding the postures for an extended time and developing an inner awareness, and moving from one posture to another in a spontaneous movement.

- *Kundalini yoga.* This form of yoga involves postures, meditation, and the coordination of breath.

The practice is said to create a controlled release of kundalini energy, a creative force thought to be at the base of the spine.

- *Viniyoga.* Viniyoga was developed by Krishnamacharya, a teacher whose disciples have created numerous other yoga forms. Viniyoga is a gentle form of flow yoga (continuous movement) that focuses on a student's ability rather than on idealized form.

- *Bikram yoga.* Bikram yoga, founded by Bikram Choudhury, utilizes yoga postures practiced in a heated environment.

- *Sivananda yoga.* This form of yoga involves a set structure that includes relaxation, pranayama (breathing), and classic asana postures.

Many excellent yoga books explain the postures and feature beautiful photographs and illustrations. Teachers, however, can impart an understanding of the poses and the practice of yoga in ways that books cannot. A teacher can also help one develop correct alignment in the various poses so that one gets the greatest benefit and so that internal stretching and healing begin.

While there is still an emphasis on yoga as a physical exercise, many teachers now address the more spiritual aspects of practice too. Other teachers take a holistic or even therapeutic approach with their students, reading their yoga practice as an open book on their personality and behavior.

The kind of relationship one develops with his or her yoga teacher depends on the teacher's philosophy and on what kind of response the student wants. However, certain basic rules should be followed in assessing a yoga teacher's capabilities.

Upon seeing a new student in class, most teachers will acknowledge that the student is new to class and will have a short chat with the student. Teachers also might ask the student if he or she has any injuries so they can recommend alternative poses if they think some routines are too difficult. Good yoga teachers will carefully watch the new student, make adjustments to postures, and push the student beyond perceived limits.

Reviewed by Brian Randall, M.D.

Only one form of study can truly prove that a treatment is effective: the double-blind, placebo-controlled trial. However, it is not possible to fit yoga into a study design of this type. While it might be possible to design a placebo form of yoga, it would be quite difficult to keep participants and researchers "in the dark" regarding who is practicing real yoga and who is practicing fake yoga.

Some compromise with the highest research standards is, therefore, inevitable. However, the compromise used in most studies is less than optimal. In these trials, yoga has been compared to no treatment. The problem with such studies is that a treatment, any treatment, frequently appears to be better than no treatment. It would be better to compare yoga to generic forms of exercise, such as daily walking, but thus far this method has not seen much use. Given these caveats, the following is a summary of what science knows about the possible medical benefits of yoga.

Possible benefits. Yoga, like Tai Chi, has been advocated as a means of increasing strength, balance, and physical function in the elderly. However, there is little scientific proof that yoga offers such benefits or that it is superior to generic exercises such as walking. There is little doubt that yoga, like any form of stretching, will increase flexibility if it is practiced consistently and over a long period of time.

Yoga is also said to relieve tension and stress. In one study of sixty-five women with depression or anxiety (or both), a two-month yoga program specifically designed to address these emotional conditions significantly reduced anxiety (but not depression) compared to enrolled women who were waiting for the program to begin. Another study found that participation in a six-week yoga program was associated with reduced anxiety, depression, and stress in women having radiotherapy for breast cancer. Finally, a trial of 122 healthy pregnant women demonstrated that daily yoga practice incorporating deep relaxation significantly reduced self-perceived stress scores, compared to standard prenatal exercises.

Weak evidence hints that yoga may offer modest benefits for people with chronic obstructive pulmonary disease (COPD) or asthma. For example, in one controlled study, fifty-nine people with mild asthma were randomly assigned to practice yoga and attend a general class or simply to attend the general class. The results showed slight improvements in asthma in the treated group compared to the untreated group.

However, even these modest benefits did not last; assessment two months later showed no difference between the groups. Furthermore, as noted, studies in which the participants in the control group do not receive placebo treatment are inherently unreliable. A small 2009 study of twenty-nine adults with COPD suggests that a twelve-week yoga program may be associated with slight improvement in timed walking distance and self-reported functional ability. A special breathing technique called yogic-style Buteyko breathing may reduce medication use and subjective symptoms, though it does not appear to actually improve lung function.

In another study, forty-two people with carpal tunnel syndrome were randomly assigned to receive either yoga or a wrist splint for eight weeks. The results indicated that the use of yoga was more effective than the wrist splint. However, participants in the control group were simply offered the wrist splint and given the choice of using it or not; it would have been preferable for them to have received a more believable placebo, like other forms of meditative exercise.

In a randomized, controlled trial, eight weeks of daily supervised yoga was modestly more effective than a similar amount of supervised physical exercise in relieving menopausal symptoms (such as hot flashes), decreasing psychological stress, and improving cognitive abilities among 120 perimenopausal women. Only weak evidence has been reported regarding the possible usefulness of yoga for depression, obsessive-compulsive disorder, low back pain, general well-being, migraine headaches, osteoarthritis, and congestive heart failure. A small trial involving fifty-four adolescents with eating disorders found that adding eight weeks of yoga twice weekly to standard therapy was associated with improved eating-disorder-related thoughts and behaviors. Yoga has also been studied for schizophrenia. In one small trial, participants who supplemented their regular treatment with a yoga program lasting four months had improved symptoms, were able to function better, and reported a better quality of life compared to those who engaged in physical therapy.

Yoga also has been promoted as a treatment for epilepsy (seizure disorder), but a review of all published scientific trials concluded that there is no meaningful evidence that it is effective. Some evidence suggests that yoga is not helpful for chemical dependency or high blood pressure.

WHAT TO EXPECT DURING TREATMENT

Yoga classes typically last about one to two hours. Most of that time is spent practicing various asanas; however, other activities such as breathing exercises may take place too. Yoga is generally a gentle, nonaerobic form of exercise. However, some types of yoga, such as Iyengar yoga, are more physically vigorous.

By the end of a yoga class, many people report feeling relaxed and comfortable, and they consider this a meaningful benefit in itself. However, without regular home practice, it is unlikely that performing yoga will provide any long-term benefit. For this reason, instructors generally encourage daily practice, ranging from a few minutes to an hour or more.

SAFETY ISSUES

Yoga is generally as safe as any other stretching-based exercise program. However, there are a few yoga positions, such as the headstand, that can cause injury when they are performed by a person who is not yet sufficiently advanced in yoga or who has certain health problems, such as a detached retina. A properly qualified instructor can help participants avoid injury by taking each person's individual health status into account.

EBSCO CAM Review Board

FURTHER READING

Carei, T. R., et al. "Randomized Controlled Clinical Trial of Yoga in the Treatment of Eating Disorders." *Journal of Adolescent Health* 46 (2010): 346.

Cowie, R. L., et al. "A Randomised Controlled Trial of the Buteyko Technique as an Adjunct to Conventional Management of Asthma." *Respiratory Medicine* 102 (2008): 726-732.

DONEsky-Cuenco, D., et al. "Yoga Therapy Decreases Dyspnea-Related Distress and Improves Functional Performance in People with Chronic Obstructive Pulmonary Disease." *Journal of Alternative and Complementary Medicine* 15 (2009): 225-234.

Duraiswamy, G., et al. "Yoga Therapy as an Add-On Treatment in the Management of Patients with Schizophrenia." *Acta Psychiatrica Scandinavica* 116 (2007): 226-232.

Javnbakht, M., R. Hejazi Kenari, and M. Ghasemi. "Effects of Yoga on Depression and Anxiety of Women." *Complementary Therapies in Clinical Practice* 15 (2009): 102-104.

John, P. J., et al. "Effectiveness of Yoga Therapy in the Treatment of Migraine Without Aura." *Headache* 47 (2007): 654-661.

Kjellgren, A., et al. "Wellness Through a Comprehensive Yogic Breathing Program." *BMC Complementary and Alternative Medicine* 7 (2007): 43.

Oken, B. S., et al. "Randomized, Controlled, Six-Month Trial of Yoga in Healthy Seniors: Effects on Cognition and Quality of Life." *Alternative Therapies in Health and Medicine* 12 (2006): 40-47.

Pullen, P. R., et al. "Effects of Yoga on Inflammation and Exercise Capacity in Patients with Chronic Heart Failure." *Journal of Cardiac Failure* 14 (2008): 407-413.

Satyapriya, M., et al. "Effect of Integrated Yoga on Stress and Heart Rate Variability in Pregnant Women." *International Journal of Gynaecology and Obstetrics* 104 (2009): 218-222.

Sherman, K. J., et al. "Comparing Yoga, Exercise, and a Self-Care Book for Chronic Low Back Pain." *Annals of Internal Medicine* 143 (2005): 849-856.

Vadiraja, H. S., et al. "Effects of a Yoga Program on Cortisol Rhythm and Mood States in Early Breast Cancer Patients Undergoing Adjuvant Radiotherapy." *Integrative Cancer Therapies* 8 (2009): 37-46.

See also: Autogenic training; Exercise; Manipulative and body-based therapies; Meditation; Relaxation response; Stress; Tai Chi; Transcendental Meditation; Walking, mind/body.

Yohimbe

CATEGORY: Herbs and supplements
RELATED TERM: *Pausinystalia yohimbe*
DEFINITION: Natural plant product used to treat specific health conditions.
PRINCIPAL PROPOSED USE: Impotence
OTHER PROPOSED USE: Sexual dysfunction in women

OVERVIEW

The bark of the West African yohimbe tree is a traditional aphrodisiac and the source of yohimbine, a prescription drug for impotence. It appears to be modestly effective, but it also presents numerous safety risks. Yohimbe should not be used except under physician supervision.

THERAPEUTIC DOSAGES

Yohimbe bark is best taken in a form standardized to yohimbine content so people can properly control their dose of the drug. Label claims for yohimbine content have been frequently found to be inaccurate. The usual dose of yohimbine is 15 to 30 milligrams (mg) daily. However, higher doses are not necessarily better, and it appears that some people respond optimally to 10 or even 5 mg daily. Furthermore, although some people appear to respond immediately to a single dose, for others it takes two to three weeks of treatment to provide significant benefits.

THERAPEUTIC USES

Like the drug yohimbine, the bark of the yohimbe tree is widely used to treat impotence. Many herbalists report that the herb is more effective than the purified drug, perhaps because of the presence of other, unidentified active ingredients. However, there have been no studies to evaluate this claim. Furthermore, due to the lack of supervision of herbal products, there are real concerns that herbal yohimbe might contain either too much or too little yohimbine.

Yohimbine (the drug) is only modestly effective at best: better than placebo, but successful only in about 30 to 45 percent of the men who use it. Yohimbine has also been evaluated in combination with the supplement arginine. A double-blind, placebo-controlled trial of forty-five men found that one-time use of this combination therapy an hour or two prior to intercourse improved erectile function, especially in those with only moderate erectile dysfunction scores. Arginine and yohimbine were both taken at a dose of 6 grams.

One small, double-blind study of yohimbine combined with arginine found an increase in measured physical arousal among twenty-three women with female sexual arousal disorder. However, the women themselves did not report any noticeable subjective effects. In addition, only the combination of yohimbine and arginine produced results; neither substance was effective when taken on its own.

An open trial of yohimbine alone to treat sexual dysfunction induced by the antidepressant fluoxetine (Prozac) found improvement in eight out of nine people, two of whom were women. However, in the absence of a placebo group, these results cannot be considered reliable; in addition, there are concerns about the safety of combining yohimbe with antidepressants.

Yohimbe is also sometimes recommended for depression. However, its effectiveness is unknown, and there are much safer herbs for this purpose, such as St. John's wort.

SAFETY ISSUES

The following discussion applies to the drug yohimbine, rather than the herb yohimbe. All risks of the drug apply to the herb, and there are additional risks to consider. For example, the amount of yohimbine in a given sample of the herb may not be accurately reflected on the label. Furthermore, additional constituents contained in the herb besides yohimbine might present unique, and unknown, risks of their own.

Yohimbine in any form should not be used by pregnant or nursing women, or those with kidney, liver, or ulcer disease, or high blood pressure. Intake of more than 40 mg a day of yohimbine can cause a severe drop in blood pressure, abdominal pain, fatigue, hallucinations, and paralysis. (Interestingly, lower dosages can cause an increase in blood pressure.) Since 40 mg is not very far above the typical recommended dose, yohimbine has what is known as a "narrow therapeutic index." This means that there is a relatively small dosing range, below which the herb does not work and above which it is toxic.

Even when taken in normal dosages, side effects of dizziness, anxiety, hyperstimulation, and nausea are common. Finally, yohimbine may interact adversely with numerous medications, including tricyclic antidepressants, buproprion, methamphetamine, phenothiazines, clonidine, and other drugs for lowering blood pressure.

IMPORTANT INTERACTIONS

People who are taking tricyclic antidepressants, bupropion, phenothiazines, clonidine, other drugs for lowering blood pressure, and amphetamines or any other central nervous system stimulants should not use yohimbine.

EBSCO CAM Review Board

FURTHER READING

Haller, C., et al. "Dietary Supplement Adverse Events: Report of a One-Year Poison Center Surveillance Project." *Journal of Medical Toxicology: Official Journal of the American College of Medical Toxicology* 4 (2008): 84-92.

Lebret, T., et al. "Efficacy and Safety of a Novel Combination of L-arginine Glutamate and Yohimbine Hydrochloride: A New Oral Therapy for Erectile Dysfunction." *European Urology* 41 (2002): 608-613.

Meston, C. M., and M. Worcel. "The Effects of Yohimbine Plus L-arginine Glutamate on Sexual Arousal in Postmenopausal Women with Sexual Arousal Disorder." *Archives of Sexual Behavior* 31 (2002): 323-332.

See also: Sexual dysfunction in men; Sexual dysfunction in women.

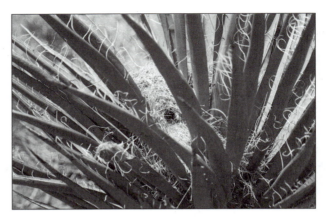

Yucca plant. (Dan Suzio/Photo Researchers, Inc.)

Yucca

CATEGORY: Herbs and supplements
RELATED TERM: *Yucca schidigera* (Mojave yucca) and other species
DEFINITION: Natural plant product used to treat specific health conditions.
PRINCIPAL PROPOSED USES: Osteoarthritis, rheumatoid arthritis

OVERVIEW

Various species of yucca plant were used as food by Native Americans and early California settlers. Yucca contains high levels of soapy compounds known as saponins that also made it a useful natural shampoo and soap.

THERAPEUTIC DOSAGES

The standard dosage is 2 to 4 tablets of concentrated yucca saponins daily.

THERAPEUTIC USES

One double-blind, placebo-controlled trial reported in 1975 concluded that use of yucca reduces arthritis symptoms (both osteoarthritis and rheumatoid arthritis). However, this study was highly preliminary in nature, and there has not been any subsequent confirming evidence.

Animal and test-tube studies suggest that various yucca extracts may have antiviral, antifungal, antiprotozoal, and antibacterial effects, but no human trials have been reported for potential uses based on these actions. Yucca extracts are also widely used to enhance the foaming effect of carbonated beverages.

SAFETY ISSUES

Yucca is generally accepted as safe based on its long history of use as a food. However, it sometimes causes diarrhea if taken to excess. Safety in young children, pregnant or nursing women, or those with severe liver or kidney disease has not been established. Yucca may have slight estrogen-like actions, and for this reason it should not be taken by women who have had breast cancer.

EBSCO CAM Review Board

FURTHER READING

McAllister, T. A., et al. "Studies on the Use of *Yucca schidigera* to Control Giardiosis." *Veterinary Parasitology* 97 (May 22, 2001): 85-99.

Miyakoshi, M., et al. "Antiyeast Steroidal Saponins from *Yucca schidigera* (Mohave Yucca), a New Anti-Food-Deteriorating Agent." *Journal of Natural Products* 63, no. 3 (2000): 332-338.

Wang, Y., et al. "Effect of Steroidal Saponin from *Yucca schidigera* Extract on Ruminal Microbes." *Journal of Applied Microbiology* 88, no. 5 (2000): 887-896.

See also: Osteoarthritis; Rheumatoid arthritis.

Z

Zinc

CATEGORY: Herbs and supplements

RELATED TERMS: Chelated zinc, zinc citrate, zinc gluconate, zinc picolinate, zinc sulfate

DEFINITION: Natural substance of the human body used as a supplement to treat specific health conditions.

PRINCIPAL PROPOSED USES: Colds, general nutritional supplementation, macular degeneration

OTHER PROPOSED USES: Acne, anorexia nervosa, attention deficit disorder, benign prostatic hyperplasia, cold sores, depression, diabetes, diarrhea, eczema, enhancing mental function in seniors, human immunodeficiency virus support, impotence, prostatitis, radiation therapy support, rheumatoid arthritis, sickle cell anemia, tinnitus, ulcers

OVERVIEW

Zinc is an important element that is found in every cell in the body. More than three hundred enzymes in the body need zinc in order to function properly. Although the amount of zinc needed in the daily diet is tiny, it is very important that individuals get it. However, the evidence suggests that many people do not get enough. Mild zinc deficiency seems to be fairly common, and for this reason, taking a zinc supplement at nutritional doses may be a good idea.

However, taking too much zinc is not a good idea—it can cause toxicity. This article discusses the possible uses of zinc at various doses.

REQUIREMENTS AND SOURCES

The official U.S. recommendations (in milligrams, or mg) for daily intake of zinc are as follows:

Infants aged 0 to 6 months (2 mg) and 7 to 12 months (3 mg); children aged 1 to 3 years (3 mg) and 4 to 8 years (5 mg); boys aged 9 to 13 years (8 mg); males aged 14 years and older (11 mg); females aged 9 to 13 years (8 mg) and 14 to 18 years (9 mg); women (8 mg); pregnant girls (13 mg) and pregnant women (11 mg); and nursing girls (14 mg) and nursing women (12 mg).

The average diet in the developed world may provide insufficient zinc, especially in women, adolescents, infants, and the elderly. Thus, it might be a good idea to increase one's intake of zinc.

Various drugs may tend to reduce zinc levels in the body by inhibiting its absorption or increasing its excretion. These include captopril and possibly other angiotensin-converting enzyme (ACE) inhibitors, oral contraceptives, thiazide diuretics, and drugs that reduce stomach acid, including H_2 blockers and proton pump inhibitors. Certain nutrients may also inhibit zinc absorption, including calcium, soy, manganese, copper, and iron. Contrary to previous reports, folate is not likely to have this effect.

Oysters have a very high zinc content; one oyster provides at least the full daily dose of zinc—about 8 to 15 mg. Besides oysters, other types of shellfish, along with poultry and meat (especially organ meats), are high in zinc, providing 1 to 8 mg of zinc per serving. Whole grains, nuts, and seeds provide smaller amounts of zinc, ranging from 0.2 to about 3 mg per serving, and the zinc from them is not as absorbable. Breakfast cereals and nutrition bars are often fortified with substantial amounts of zinc.

Zinc can also be taken as a nutritional supplement in one of many forms. Zinc citrate, zinc acetate, or zinc picolinate may be the best absorbed, although zinc sulfate is less expensive. People who purchase a supplement should be aware of the difference between the milligrams of actual zinc that the product contains (so-called elemental zinc) and the total milligrams of the zinc product, which includes the weight of the sulfate, picolinate, and so forth. All dosages given in this article refer to elemental zinc (unless otherwise stated).

THERAPEUTIC DOSAGES

For most purposes, zinc should simply be taken at the recommended daily requirements of 8 to 15 mg. Some evidence suggests that 30 mg of zinc daily may be helpful for acne. This is a safe dose for most people. However, in most studies of zinc for acne, a much higher dose was used: 90 mg daily or more. Doses this high should be used only under physician supervision. Potentially dangerous doses of zinc have also been recommended for sickle cell anemia, macular degeneration, and rheumatoid arthritis.

For best absorption, zinc supplements should not be taken at the same time as high-fiber foods. However, many high-fiber foods provide zinc in themselves.

Zinc gluconate may be slightly better absorbed than zinc oxide.

When taking zinc for a long time, it is advisable to also take 1 to 3 mg of copper daily because zinc supplements can cause copper deficiency. Zinc may also interfere with magnesium and iron absorption.

Zinc is used topically in lozenge or nasal gel form for the treatment of colds. When using zinc this way, the purpose is not to increase zinc levels in the body but to interfere with the action of viruses in the back of the throat or in the nose. It appears that of the common forms of zinc, only zinc gluconate and zinc acetate have the required antiviral properties. Certain sweeteners and flavorings used in lozenges can block zinc's antiviral action. Dextrose, sucrose, mannitol, and sorbitol appear to be fine, but citric acid and tartaric acid are not. The information on glycine as a flavoring agent is a bit equivocal.

When using zinc nasal gel products, users should not deeply inhale, as this may cause severe pain. Rather, they should simply squeeze the gel into the nose, according to the directions.

THERAPEUTIC USES

Use of zinc nasal spray or zinc lozenges at the beginning of a cold may reduce the duration and severity of symptoms, but study results are somewhat inconsistent. These treatments are thought to work by directly interfering with viruses in the nose and throat, and they involve relatively high doses of zinc used for a short time.

Zinc can also be taken long term at nutritional doses orally to improve overall immunity and reduce risk of infection. However, this approach probably works only if individuals are deficient in zinc to begin with.

A significant body of evidence suggests that oral zinc can reduce symptoms of acne. However, in most studies, potentially toxic doses were used, and in any case, the benefits appear to be rather slight.

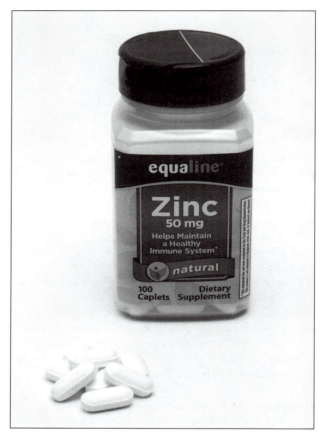

Zinc dietary supplement. (GIPhotoStock/Photo Researchers, Inc.)

Growing evidence suggests that oral zinc, especially in combination with antioxidants, can help slow the progression of macular degeneration. Oral zinc has also shown promise for sickle cell anemia, attention deficit disorder (ADD), and stomach ulcers. Zinc has also been shown to be beneficial for acute diarrhea in children, the most convincing evidence coming from studies done in developing countries. This suggests that zinc is most useful for this condition in the presence of a nutritional deficiency. Topical zinc may be helpful for cold sores.

Zinc has shown some promise for treating dysgeusia (impaired taste sensation). In a study of fifty people with idiopathic dysgeusia (impaired taste sensation of no known cause), use of zinc at a rather high dose of 140 mg daily improved taste ability. Another study enrolled seniors with dysgeusia and gave them either placebo or 30 mg of zinc daily; the results were inconclusive. Dysgeusia can also be caused by radiation therapy in the vicinity of the mouth, but overall, the evidence regarding the use of zinc for this purpose is more negative than positive. Kidney dialysis also impairs taste sensation, but once again zinc supplements failed to prove effective. (The use of any mineral supplement by people undergoing kidney dialysis is potentially dangerous.)

In one study, use of zinc appeared to modestly decrease inflammation of the mucous membranes and skin caused by radiation therapy. Weak, contradictory results have been seen in studies of zinc for anorexia nervosa, depression, rheumatoid arthritis, enhancing sexual function in men on kidney dialysis, tinnitus, and warts.

Some studies have found that persons with human immunodeficiency virus (HIV) infection tend to be deficient in zinc, with levels dropping lower in more severe disease. Higher zinc levels have been linked to better immune function and higher CD4+ cell counts, whereas zinc deficiency has been linked to increased risk of dying from HIV. One preliminary study among people taking azidothymidine (AZT) found that thirty days of zinc supplementation led to decreased rates of opportunistic infection over the following two years. However, other research has linked higher zinc intake to more rapid development of acquired immunodeficiency syndrome (AIDS). Another study failed to find that zinc supplementation reduces diarrhea associated with HIV. People who have HIV should consult their physicians before supplementing with zinc.

Although the evidence that zinc works is not meaningful, the supplement is sometimes recommended for the following conditions: Alzheimer's disease and minor memory loss in seniors, benign prostatic hyperplasia, bladder infection, cataracts, diabetes, Down syndrome, infertility in men, inflammatory bowel disease (ulcerative colitis and Crohn's disease), osteoporosis, periodontal disease, prostatitis, psoriasis, and wound and burn healing. An eight-week, double-blind trial of zinc at 67 mg daily failed to find any benefit for eczema symptoms.

SCIENTIFIC EVIDENCE

Common cold. Lozenges containing zinc gluconate or zinc acetate have shown somewhat inconsistent but generally positive results for reducing the severity and duration of the common cold. For example, in a double-blind trial, one hundred people who were ex-periencing the early symptoms of a cold were given a lozenge that contained either 13.3 mg of zinc from zinc gluconate or a placebo. Participants took the lozenges several times daily until their cold symptoms subsided. The results were impressive. Coughing disappeared within 2.2 days in the treated group versus 4 days in the placebo group. Sore throat disappeared after 1 day versus 3 days in the placebo group, nasal drainage in 4 days (versus 7 days), and headache in 2 days (versus 3 days). Positive results have also been seen in double-blind studies of zinc acetate. While not all studies have been supportive, on balance results appear to favor the effectiveness of zinc lozenges for treating symptoms of the common cold.

It has been suggested that the exact formulation of the zinc lozenge plays a significant role in its effectiveness. According to this view, certain flavoring agents, such as citric acid and tartaric acid, might prevent zinc from inhibiting viruses. In addition, chemical forms of zinc other than zinc gluconate or zinc acetate might be ineffective. Zinc sulfate in particular might not work. Along the same lines, sweeteners, such as sorbitol, sucrose, dextrose, and mannitol, are said to be fine, while glycine has been discussed in an equivocal manner.

Use of zinc in the nose is somewhat more controversial. In addition to showing inconsistent results in studies, use of zinc nasal gel can cause pain and possibly loss of sense of smell.

For example, in a double-blind, placebo-controlled trial of a widely available zinc nasal gel product, 213 people with a newly starting cold used one squirt of zinc gluconate gel or placebo gel in each nostril every four hours while awake. The results were significant: Treated participants stayed sick an average of 2.3 days, while those receiving placebo were sick for an average of 9 days, a 75 percent reduction in the duration of symptoms. Somewhat more modest, but still significant, relative benefits were seen with zinc nasal gel in a double-blind, placebo-controlled study of eighty people with colds. However, another study, this one involving seventy-seven people, failed to find benefit even with near constant saturation of the nasal passages with zinc gluconate nasal spray. Furthermore, a study of ninety-one people using the standard commercially available nasal spray failed to find benefit. Another double-blind, placebo-controlled trial, this one enrolling 185 persons, failed to find benefit with zinc nasal spray. However, this study used a much lower amount of zinc (fifty times lower) per squirt of spray than was used in the studies just described.

Apart from their direct effect on viruses during an infection, zinc supplements (not lozenges) may play a role in reducing the risk of coming down with a cold in the first place. In a review of two randomized trials, which included 394 healthy children, researchers found that the groups who took zinc had fewer colds, school absences, and prescriptions for antibiotics.

Chronic zinc deficiency is known to weaken the immune system. Although low levels of zinc are uncommon in healthy children and adults living in developed countries, deficiencies may be found among the elderly and are widespread among populations in developing countries. A one-year, double-blind study of fifty nursing home residents found that zinc supplements reduced rates of infection compared with placebo. Additionally, in a two-year study of nursing home residents, participants given zinc and selenium developed illnesses less frequently than those given placebo.

Numerous studies in developing countries have also found benefit. For example, a six-month, double-blind, placebo-controlled study of 609 preschool children in India found that zinc supplements reduced the rate of respiratory infections by 45 percent. In addition, more than ten other studies performed in developing countries found that zinc supplements were helpful for preventing respiratory and other infections in children, and that zinc might reduce symptom severity.

Cold sores. Cold sores are infections caused by the herpes virus. One study suggests that topical zinc may be helpful. In this trial, forty-six individuals with cold sores were treated with a zinc oxide cream or placebo every two hours until cold sores were resolved. The results showed that individuals using the cream experienced a reduction in severity of symptoms and a shorter time to full recovery.

Zinc is thought to interfere with the ability of the herpes virus to reproduce itself. As with colds, the formulation of zinc must be properly designed to release active zinc ions. This study used a special zinc oxide and glycine formulation. Some participants in this study experienced burning and inflammation caused by the zinc itself, but this seldom caused a serious problem.

Macular degeneration. Macular degeneration is one of the most common causes of vision loss in the el-

derly. A double-blind, placebo-controlled trial evaluated the effects of zinc with or without antioxidants on the progression of macular degeneration in 3,640 individuals in the early stage of the disease. Participants were randomly assigned to receive one of the following: antioxidants (vitamin C 500 mg, vitamin E 400 international units, and beta-carotene 15 mg), or zinc (80 mg) and copper (2 mg), antioxidants plus zinc, or placebo. Copper was administered along with zinc to prevent zinc-induced copper deficiency. The results suggest that zinc alone, or, even better, with antioxidants, significantly slowed the progression of the disease. Previous studies of zinc for macular degeneration found mixed results, but they were much smaller.

There is also some evidence that individuals who make sure to get their dietary requirements of zinc on a daily basis over many years might reduce their risk of developing macular degeneration later in life. Keep in mind that the dosages of zinc used in most of these studies are rather high and should be used only under a physician's supervision.

Attention deficit disorder. Zinc has shown some promise for treatment of attention deficit disorder (ADD). In a large (approximately four-hundred-participant), double-blind, placebo-controlled study, use of zinc at a dose of 40 mg daily produced statistically significant benefits compared with placebo among children not using any other treatment. This dose of zinc, while higher than nutritional needs, should be safe. However, the benefits seen were quite modest: About 28 percent of the participants given zinc showed improvement compared with 20 percent in the placebo group.

Another, much smaller double-blind, placebo-controlled study evaluated whether zinc at 15 mg per day could enhance the effect of Ritalin. Again, modest benefits were seen. Finally, extremely weak evidence hints that zinc might enhance the effectiveness of evening primrose oil for ADD.

Acne. Studies suggest that people with acne have lower-than-normal levels of zinc in their bodies. This fact alone does not prove that taking zinc supplements will help acne, but several small double-blind studies involving a total of more than three hundred people have found generally positive results.

In one of these studies, fifty-four people were given either placebo or 135 mg of zinc (as zinc sulfate) daily. Zinc produced slight, but measurable, benefits. Similar results have been seen in other studies using 90 to 135 mg of zinc daily. Some evidence suggests that a lower and safer dose, 30 mg daily, may offer some benefits. In some studies, however, no benefits were seen.

Two studies have compared zinc against a standard treatment for acne, the antibiotic tetracycline. One study found that zinc was as effective as tetracycline taken at 250 mg daily, but another found the antibiotic far more effective when taken at 500 mg daily.

Keep in mind that the dosages of zinc used in most of these studies are rather high; case reports indicate that people have made themselves extremely ill by taking zinc in the hope of treating their acne symptoms. Doses of zinc higher than the recommended safe levels should be used only under a physician's supervision.

Sickle cell disease. Children with sickle cell disease often do not grow normally. There is some evidence that people with sickle cell disease are more likely than others to be deficient in zinc. Since zinc deficiency can also cause delayed growth, zinc supplementation at nutritional doses has been suggested for children with sickle cell disease. In a placebo-controlled study, forty-two children (aged four to ten) with sickle cell disease were given either zinc supplements (10 mg of zinc daily) or placebo for a period of one year. Results showed that by the end of the study, the participants given zinc showed enhanced growth compared with those given placebo. Curiously, researchers did not find any solid connection between the severity of zinc deficiency and the extent of response to treatment.

Zinc is thought to have a stabilizing effect on the cell membrane of red blood cells in people with sickle cell disease. For this reason, it has been tried as an aid for preventing sickle cell crisis. In a double-blind, placebo-controlled study of 145 people with sickle cell disease conducted in India, participants received either placebo or about 50 mg of zinc three times daily. During eighteen months of treatment, the zinc-treated subjects had an average of 2.5 crises, compared with 5.3 for the placebo group. However, zinc did not seem to reduce the severity of a crisis, as measured by the number of days spent in the hospital for each crisis.

Sickle cell disease can also cause skin ulcers (nonhealing sores). In a twelve-week, placebo-controlled trial, use of zinc at 88 mg three times per day for twelve weeks enhanced the rate of ulcer healing.

The high dosages of zinc used in the last two studies can cause dangerous toxicity and should be taken (if at all) only under the supervision of a doctor. The nutritional dose described in the first study, however, is safe.

SAFETY ISSUES

Zinc taken orally seldom causes any immediate side effects other than occasional stomach upset, usually when it is taken on an empty stomach. Some forms do have an unpleasant metallic taste. Use of zinc nasal gel, however, has been associated with anosmia (loss of sense of smell). In fact, after receiving more than 130 reports of anosmia, the U.S. Food and Drug Administration (FDA) warned consumers and health care providers in 2009 to discontinue use of certain Zicam Cold Remedy intranasal zinc-containing products, including Zicam Cold Remedy nasal gel, Cold Remedy nasal swabs, and Cold Remedy swabs in children's size. Furthermore, if the gel is inhaled too deeply, severe pain may occur.

Long-term use of oral zinc at dosages of 100 mg or more daily can cause a number of toxic effects, including severe copper deficiency, impaired immunity, heart problems, and anemia. Zinc at a dose of more than 50 mg daily might reduce levels of high-density lipoprotein (HDL, or good) cholesterol. In addition, very weak evidence hints that use of zinc supplements might increase risk of prostate cancer in men.

The U.S. government has issued recommendations regarding tolerable upper intake levels (ULs, in milligrams, or mg) for zinc. The UL can be thought of as the highest daily intake over a prolonged time known to pose no risks to most members of a healthy population. The ULs for zinc are as follows:

Infants aged 0 to 6 months (4 mg) and 7 to 12 months (5 mg); children aged 1 to 3 years (7 mg), 4 to 8 years (12 mg), 9 to 13 years (23 mg), and 14 to 18 years (34 mg); adults (40 mg); pregnant and nursing girls (34 mg); and pregnant and nursing women (40 mg).

Some interactions occur between zinc and certain medications. For example, the use of zinc can interfere with the absorption of the drug penicillamine and also with antibiotics in the tetracycline or fluoroquinolone (Cipro, Floxin) families.

The potassium-sparing diuretic amiloride was found to significantly reduce zinc excretion from the body. This means that if people take zinc supplements at the same time as amiloride, zinc accumulation could occur, which could lead to toxic side effects. However, the potassium-sparing diuretic triamterene does not seem to cause this problem.

IMPORTANT INTERACTIONS

People who are using ACE inhibitors, estrogen-replacement therapy, oral contraceptives, thiazide diuretics, or medications that reduce stomach acid (such as H_2 blockers [Zantac] or proton pump inhibitors [Prilosec]) may need to take extra zinc. In addition, the diuretic amiloride could reduce zinc excretion from the body, leading to zinc accumulation, which could cause toxic side effects. People using amiloride should not take zinc supplements unless advised by a physician.

It may be advisable for people taking manganese, calcium, copper, iron, antacids, soy, or antibiotics in the fluoroquinolone (such as Cipro or Floxin) or tetracycline families to separate their doses of zinc and these substances by at least two hours. Zinc also interferes with penicillamine's absorption, so it may be advisable for people to take zinc and penicillamine at least two hours apart.

Finally, people who are using zinc supplements should also take extra copper and perhaps magnesium because zinc interferes with their absorption. Zinc interferes with iron absorption, too, but people should not take iron supplements unless they know they are deficient.

EBSCO CAM Review Board

FURTHER READING

Bao, B., et al. "Zinc Supplementation Decreases Oxidative Stress, Incidence of Infection, and Generation of Inflammatory Cytokines in Sickle Cell Disease Patients." *Translational Research: The Journal of Laboratory and Clinical Medicine* 152 (2008): 67-80.

Carcamo, C., et al. "Randomized Controlled Trial of Zinc Supplementation for Persistent Diarrhea in Adults with HIV-1 Infection." *Journal of Acquired Immune Deficiency Syndromes* 43, no. 2 (2006): 197-210.

Ebisch, I. M., et al. "Does Folic Acid and Zinc Sulphate Intervention Affect Endocrine Parameters and Sperm Characteristics in Men?" *International Journal of Andrology* 29 (2006): 339-345.

Eby, G. A., and W. W. Halcomb. "Ineffectiveness of Zinc Gluconate Nasal Spray and Zinc Orotate Lozenges in Common-Cold Treatment." *Alternate Therapies in Health and Medicine* 12 (2006): 34-38.

Halyard, M. Y., et al. Does Zinc Sulfate Prevent Therapy-Induced Taste Alterations in Head and Neck Cancer Patients? Results of Phase III Double-Blind, Placebo-Controlled Trial from the North Central Cancer Treatment Group (N01C4)." *International Journal of Radiation Oncology, Biology, Physics* 67 (2007): 1318-1322.

Kurugol, Z., N. Bayram, and T. Atik. "Effect of Zinc Sulfate on Common Cold in Children." *Pediatrics International: Official Journal of the Japan Pediatric Society* 49 (2007): 842-847.

Lazzerini, M., and L. Ronfani. "Oral Zinc for Treating Diarrhoea in Children." *Cochrane Database of Systematic Reviews* 3 (2008): CD005436.

Lin, L. C., et al. "Zinc Supplementation to Improve Mucositis and Dermatitis in Patients After Radiotherapy for Head-and-Neck Cancers." *International Journal of Radiation Oncology, Biology, Physics* 65 (2006): 745-750.

Maylor, E. A., et al. "Effects of Zinc Supplementation on Cognitive Function in Healthy Middle-Aged and Older Adults." *British Journal of Nutrition* 96 (2006): 752-760.

Patro, B., D. Golicki, and H. Szajewska. "Meta-analysis: Zinc Supplementation for Acute Gastroenteritis in Children." *Alimentary Pharmacology and Therapeutics* 28, no. 6 (2008): 713-723.

Prasad, A. S., et al. "Zinc Supplementation Decreases Incidence of Infections in the Elderly: Effect of Zinc on Generation of Cytokines and Oxidative Stress." *American Journal of Clinical Nutrition* 85 (2007): 837-844.

Singh, M., and R. R. Das. "Zinc for the Common Cold." *Cochrane Database of Systematic Reviews* 2 (2011): CD001364.

See also: Acne; Attention deficit disorder; Benign prostatic hyperplasia; Canker sores; Colds and flu; Depression, mild to moderate; Diabetes; Diarrhea; Eczema; HIV support; Macular degeneration; Prostatitis; Radiation therapy support; Rheumatoid arthritis; Sexual dysfunction in men; Sickle cell disease; Supplements, overview; Tinnitus; Ulcers.

APPENDIXES
REFERENCE TOOLS

Glossary

acai: a natural plant product widely marketed for weight-loss and anti-aging purposes.

acerola: a natural plant product promoted as a dietary supplement containing substantial antioxidant properties.

acetaminophen: a common drug used to reduce pain and fever; interactions with chaparral, citrate, co-enzyme Q_{10}, coltsfoot, comfrey, methionine, milk thistle, and vitamin C. *See also* aspirin; ibuprofen; nonsteroidal anti-inflammatory drug.

acetyl-L-carnitine (ALC): *See* carnitine.

acid reflux: *See* gastroesophageal reflux disease (GERD).

acne: a skin condition caused by clogged, inflamed, or infected pores.

acquired immunodeficiency syndrome: *See* AIDS.

active hexose correlated compound: a natural substance advocated primarily as an aid to cancer treatment; also believed to improve survival in people undergoing treatment for liver cancer and other forms of cancer.

acupressure: the noninvasive application of focused touch to specific points of the body.

acupuncture: a treatment in which fine needles are inserted into the skin at designated points.

adenosine monophosphate: a natural substance recommended as a treatment for cold sores, shingles, and photosensitivity.

adrenal extract: a natural substance extract used to strengthen the function of an underperforming or exhausted adrenal gland.

AIDS (acquired immunodeficiency syndrome): a chronic disease caused by the human immunodeficiency virus (HIV), which progressively destroys or damages cells in the immune system, making the body vulnerable to certain cancers and infections.

alcoholism: an addiction to alcoholic beverages.

Alexander technique: an alternative movement therapy that is focused on improving a person's posture and movement.

alfalfa: a natural plant product, high in beta-carotene, various B vitamins, and vitamins C, E, and K, that is promoted for its nutritional support.

allergy: a group of inflammatory reactions that includes allergic conjunctivitis, allergic pharyngitis, allergic rhinitis, allergic sinusitis, hay fever, perennial rhinitis, pollen allergy, and seasonal allergy.

aloe: a natural plant product used to treat burns, diabetes, genital herpes, psoriasis, seborrhea, and other conditions.

alopecia: a medical condition marked by the loss or thinning of hair.

alternative medicine: a complementary or alternative therapy used in place of standard, Western treatments; includes acupuncture, Ayurveda, homeopathy, naturopathy, and traditional Chinese medicine. *See also* integrative medicine.

altitude sickness: an illness caused by the lower pressure and reduced amount of oxygen at high altitudes.

Alzheimer's disease: a medical condition leading to mental and cognitive decline in the elderly.

amenorrhea: a medical condition marked by the absence of menstrual bleeding that is not associated with menopause.

American Academy of Anti-Aging Medicine: a private organization that promotes antiaging medicine and its legitimacy; based in the United States.

amino acids: a group of essential organic compounds that combine to form proteins; amino acids and proteins are the building blocks of life.

aminoglycoside: an intravenous antibiotic that treats certain infections; interactions with calcium, ginkgo, magnesium, N-acteylcysteine, and vitamin B_{12}.

amiodarone: a drug used to restore normal heart rhythm; interactions with chaparral, coltsfoot, comfrey, dong quai, St. John's wort, and vitamin E.

amoxicillin: a relative of the antibiotic penicillin that is modified to have a broader spectrum of effect; interactions with bromelain and vitamin K.

amyotrophic lateral sclerosis (ALS): a nerve disorder that causes progressive muscle weakness; also known as Lou Gehrig's disease.

andrographis: a natural plant product used as a dietary supplement to treat the common cold and to provide immune support.

androstenedione: a hormone believed to enhance sports performance by building muscle and increasing strength.

anemia: a medical condition in which the blood fails to carry enough oxygen to the rest of the body; the most common cause of anemia is not having enough iron in the blood.

angina: a medical condition marked by muscle cramping of the heart.

angiotensin-converting enzyme (ACE) inhibitor: a pharmaceutical that blocks the conversion of a naturally occurring substance, angiotensin, to a more active form; interactions with arginine, dong quai, iron, licorice, potassium, St. John's wort, and zinc.

antacid: a compound that directly neutralizes stomach acid; interactions with calcium citrate, folate, and minerals.

anthroposophic medicine: a holistic, human-centered extension of conventional medical practice that promotes a spiritual understanding of the human being in health and illness.

anti-aging medicine: the practice of complementary and alternative medicine that focuses on the aging process and on the health of the elderly. *See also* American Academy of Anti-Aging Medicine.

antibiotic, general: a substance produced naturally by microorganisms that inhibits the growth of other microorganisms, especially harmful bacteria; interactions with acidophilus, *Bifidobacterium longum*, *Lactobacillus acidophilus*, probiotics, and vitamin K.

antidepressant: a pharmaceutical that primarily affects mood by working on brain chemicals called neurotransmitters, especially serotonin and norepinephrine; other antidepressants work on the neurotransmitter dopamine.

antifungal agent: a medication used to treat fungal infections such as athlete's foot, candidiasis, and ringworm.

anti-inflammatory diet: a type of therapy that uses food with anti-inflammatory properties to treat and prevent chronic degenerative diseases.

anti-inflammatory drug: *See* nonsteroidal anti-inflammatory drug.

antioxidant: an essential natural substance thought to help prevent illness and disease caused by free radicals, molecules that can damage cells. *See also* free radical.

applied kinesiology: the use of techniques such as muscle testing to identify health problems.

arginine: an amino acid found in many foods and used especially as a treatment for cardiovascular diseases, including congestive heart failure.

arjun: an herbal plant product that may have properties that relax blood vessels and may treat angina.

aromatherapy: a form of herbal medicine in which an herb's essential oil is inhaled, applied to the skin, or taken orally.

arrhythmia: a medical condition marked by irregular heart rhythms.

art therapy: the combined use of psychotherapy and creative processes such as painting and drawing to enhance health and well-being.

arthritis: any condition that involves pain in the joints. *See also* gout; osteoarthritis; rheumatoid arthritis.

artichoke: a natural plant product consumed to ease the symptoms of dyspepsia, or indigestion, and to treat elevated levels of "bad" cholesterol.

ashwagandha: a natural plant product used as an adaptogen, a substance said to increase the body's ability to withstand stress of all types.

aspirin: a drug in a group of medications called salicylates; it works by stopping the production of certain natural substances that cause fever, pain, swelling, and blood clots. *See also* acetaminophen; ibuprofen.

astaxanthin: a natural substance used as an antioxidant to treat or prevent a number of health conditions.

asthma: a medical condition involving severe breathing difficulties that are caused by bronchial inflammation and contraction.

Aston-Patterning: a bodywork system involving massage, exercise, movement education, and ergonomics to improve health and well-being.

astragalus: a natural plant product commonly used in Chinese herbal medicine and promoted in the West as an immune stimulant useful for treating colds and flu.

atherosclerosis: a disease in which plaque builds up inside the arteries; plaque is a sticky substance made up of fat, cholesterol, calcium, and other substances found in the blood, whose accumulation leads to various heart diseases.

athlete's foot: a fungal infection of the foot treated primarily with tea tree oil; other proposed treatments include *Ageratina pichinchensis* (snakeroot), essential oils, garlic, ozonized vegetable oil, *Solanum chrysotrichum* (sosa), and various tropical and traditional medicinal plants.

Atkins diet: a diet that emphasizes a drastic reduction in the daily intake of carbohydrates and an increase in protein and fat. *See also* diet-based therapy; Ornish diet; Pritikin diet; South Beach diet.

attention deficit disorder: a psychological condition marked by difficulty sustaining attention or completing tasks and by easy distractibility and impulsive behavior.

autism spectrum disorder: a brain disorder marked by a lack of social interaction skills and unusual and often characteristic behaviors, such as repetitive movements.

autogenic training: a method of self-control therapy that teaches a person to use specific phrases to enter a state of deep relaxation and to achieve healing.

Ayurveda: a holistic medicine system that originated in India in which treatment is highly individualized and incorporates a wide range of methods.

Bach flower remedy: an alternative medical treatment that uses flower extracts.

balneotherapy: an alternative medical treatment using hot and cold baths, saunas, mud packs, and other therapies.

barberry: a plant product traditionally used as a treatment for digestive problems; topical preparations of barberry have been used for the treatment of eczema, psoriasis, and minor wounds.

Bates method: an alternative medical treatment that promotes eye exercises to improve vision.

Beano: the trade name for the enzyme alpha-galactosidase, which is advocated as a treatment for both complex carbohydrate intolerance and ordinary gassiness.

bee pollen: a natural substance produced by bees that is high in protein and carbohydrates and contains trace amounts of minerals and vitamins; it is recommended for a variety of uses, particularly for improving sports performance and relieving allergies.

bee propolis: a natural resinous compound made primarily from tree sap that contains biologically active compounds called flavonoids; it has antiseptic properties, and the flavonoids in propolis may have antimicrobial effects.

bee venom therapy: an alternative therapy that uses bee venom to treat chronic injuries such as bursitis and tendinitis and to treat hay fever, gout, shingles, burns, fibromyalgia, chronic fatigue syndrome, and other health conditions.

belladonna: an herb traditionally used to treat headaches, menstrual symptoms, peptic ulcer disease, allergies, inflammation, and motion sickness.

Bell's palsy: a medical condition marked by a form of facial paralysis.

benign prostatic hyperplasia: an enlarged prostate not caused by cancer.

benzodiazepine: a pharmaceutical used as a muscle relaxant, sedative, and anticonvulsant; interactions with grapefruit juice, hops, kava, passionflower, valerian, melatonin, and pregnenolone.

beta-blocker: any of a class of pharmaceuticals used to treat hypertension and a variety of heart conditions; interactions with chromium, coenzyme Q_{10}, and *Coleus forskohlii*.

beta-carotene: a natural substance promoted as an antioxidant and as a nutritional supplement, specifically vitamin A.

beta-glucan: a soluble fiber found in plants and used to treat high levels of "bad" cholesterol.

betaine hydrochloride: an acidic form of betaine (a natural substance that is found in foods, such as grains) that provides the stomach with extra hydrochloric acid, thought to be beneficial to the stomach.

beta-sitosterol: a natural plant product that contains cholesterol-like compounds called sitosterols and their close relatives, sitosterolins; a mixture used to treat benign prostatic hyperplasia.

bilberry: a natural plant product that contains biologically active substances known as anthocyanosides, which may benefit the retina, strengthen the walls of blood vessels, reduce inflammation, and stabilize tissues containing collagen (such as tendons, ligaments, and cartilage).

bile acid sequestrant drug: any of a class of pharmaceuticals used to lower high levels of cholesterol; interactions with numerous nutrients, including calcium, folate, iron, vitamin A, vitamin B_{12}, and vitamin E.

biochemic tissue salt therapy: an alternative treatment that uses inorganic mineral salts.

bioenergetics: an alternative technique involving the study of energy transfers among all living systems.

biofeedback: an alternative therapy involving simple electronic devices to help a person consciously regulate bodily functions, such as breathing, heart rate, and blood pressure, to improve overall health.

biologically based therapy: a type of alternative therapy that uses natural substances for general well-being and for preventing and treating illness.

biorhythm: a type of alternative medicine based on the belief that natural cycles regulate a person's body, mentation, and emotions.

biotin: a water-soluble B vitamin claimed to provide nutritional support during pregnancy, to help reduce blood sugar levels in people with type 1 or type 2 diabetes, and to possibly reduce the symptoms of diabetic neuropathy.

bipolar disorder: a mental condition marked by alternating periods of psychological mania (highs) and depression (lows).

bitter melon: a natural product widely sold in Asian groceries as a food and used as a folk remedy for diabetes, cancer, and various infections.

bitter orange: a natural plant product primarily used to treat heartburn, nasal congestion, loss of appetite, and unintended weight loss; also is applied to the skin to treat fungal infections such as ringworm and athlete's foot.

black cohosh: an herb used to treat menopausal symptoms.

black tea: a natural plant product used to reduce the risk of heart disease and death from heart disease.

bladder infection: a bacterial infection that causes inflammation of the bladder.

bladderwrack: a type of seaweed used as a common food and as an additive and flavoring in various food products; as a component of kelp tablets or powders, it is used as a nutritional supplement.

blepharitis: a medical condition marked by irritation and inflammation of the eyelids and eyelashes.

blessed thistle: an herb used to treat dyspepsia and poor appetite.

blood sugar: glucose (sugar) found in the blood. *See also* diabetes.

blood thinning medication: any class of pharmaceuticals (anticoagulant or antiplatelet drugs) used to treat heart or blood vessel disease, poor blood flow to the brain, abnormal heart rhythm, and congenital heart defects; also used following heart valve surgery.

bloodroot: an herb used to prevent cavities and periodontal disease and to treat respiratory illnesses and, as a scab-producing paste, warts.

blue cohosh: a toxic, flowering herb used in traditional medicine to induce labor and regulate the menstrual cycle.

blue flag: a natural plant product used to treat digestive problems.

boldo: a natural plant product used to treat liver and bladder disorders, rheumatism, headache, earache, congestion, menstrual pain, and syphilis; also may protect the liver from toxins, stimulate the gallbladder, and reduce inflammation.

boron: a natural substance used to assist in the proper absorption of calcium, magnesium, and phosphorus from foods; it slows the loss of these minerals through urination and may also be helpful for osteoarthritis and osteoporosis.

boswellia: a natural plant product believed to have anti-inflammatory effects; tried for a number of conditions in which inflammation is involved, including painful conditions such as bursitis, osteoarthritis, rheumatoid arthritis, and tendonitis; also tried for asthma and inflammatory bowel disease (ulcerative colitis or Crohn's disease).

botanica: a traditional healer who supplies healing products, sometimes associated with spiritual interventions.

botanical: a plant or plant product used for its flavor, scent, or potential therapeutic properties; includes flowers, leaves, bark, fruits, seeds, stems, and roots.

brahmi: a natural plant product used to improve the mind's functioning and enhance awareness.

branched-chain amino acid: a natural substance of the human body used as a supplement to treat specific health conditions, such as amyotrophic lateral sclerosis (Lou Gehrig's disease) and the loss of appetite in persons with cancer.

bromelain: any of a group of protein-digesting enzymes (also called proteolytic enzymes) found in pineapple juice and in the stem of pineapple plants; used to treat athletic injuries, digestive problems, phlebitis, and sinusitis.

bromocriptine: an herb sometimes used to treat conditions in which there is too much prolactin, a hormone, in the body.

bronchitis: a medical condition marked by inflammation of the major air passageways in the lungs.

bruise: a medical condition in which blood-containing tissue experience damage to blood vessels from injury or surgery.

buchu: a natural plant product used as a part of herbal combinations designed for kidney and bladder problems; said to have a diuretic effect, meaning that it increases the flow of urine.

bugleweed: a natural plant product traditionally used as a sedative, to treat mild heart conditions, and to reduce fever and mucus production in flus and colds; modern use employs it as a treatment for hyperthyroidism and mastodynia, or breast pain.

burdock: a natural plant product used to relieve acne and dry, scaly skin conditions such as eczema and psoriasis.

burning mouth syndrome: a medical condition marked by chronic pain of the tongue and mouth.

bursitis: a medical condition marked by inflammation of the fluid-filled sacs between tissues and bones.

butcher's broom: a natural plant product used as supportive therapy for chronic venous insufficiency and for the treatment of hemorrhoids.

butterbur: a natural plant product used to prevent migraine headaches and to treat allergies, such as hay fever.

caffeine: a natural substance found in the seeds, leaves, and fruit of some plants that affects the body's metabolism and stimulates the central nervous system.

calcium: a natural substance essential for health and used to prevent and treat the symptoms of osteoporosis and to reduce symptoms of premenstrual syndrome.

calcium channel blocker: a pharmaceutical used to treat hypertension, angina, heart arrhythmia, and other heart-related conditions; interactions with calcium, ginkgo, naringen (a citrus bioflavonoid), and vitamin D.

calendula: a natural plant product used to treat canker sores, eczema, hemorrhoids, minor burns, minor wounds, and varicose veins.

CAM on PubMed: a U.S.-government-sponsored research and informational database listing scientific journal citations focused on complementary and alternative medicine; available at http://www.ncbi.nlm.nih.gov/pubmed.

cancer: a large group of different diseases marked by unregulated cell growth in the body that forms malignant (cancerous) tumors.

candida: a yeast infection of moist areas of the body.

candling: an alternative therapy involving the use of a hollow lighted candle to treat specific health conditions of the ear.

candytuft: a natural plant product used, in herbal combinations, to treat dyspepsia.

cannabis (marijuana): a natural plant product with a long history in indigenous medicine; used to relieve pain, nausea and vomiting, anxiety, and loss of appetite; used to treat the symptoms of cancer and the side effects of chemotherapy; its use is prohibited by U.S. federal law, but some states and the District of Columbia permit its use with a physician's prescription for certain medical conditions.

capsaicin: *See* cayenne.

caraway: a natural plant product used to treat dyspepsia and intestinal gas.

carbamazepine: an anticonvulsant drug used primarily to prevent seizures in persons with conditions such as epilepsy; interactions with biotin, calcium, carnitine, dong quai, folate, ginkgo, glutamine, grapefruit juice, hops, ipriflavone, kava, nicotinamide, passionflower, St. John's wort, valerian, vitamin D, and vitamin K.

carbohydrate: a major type of nutrient and the most important source of energy for the body; the digestive system changes carbohydrates into glucose, or blood sugar. *See also* glucose; low-carbohydrate diet.

cardiomyopathy: a medical condition marked by diseased heart-muscle tissue.

carnitine: a natural substance used by the body to turn fat into energy; it is primarily used for heart-related conditions.

carnosine: a natural substance of the human body used as an anti-aging nutrient.

carob: a natural tree product used to treat diarrhea and high cholesterol levels.

carotenoid: the pigments found in fruits and vegetables; the best-known carotenoids include beta-carotene, lutein, lycopene, astaxanthin, and zeaxanthin; used to reduce the risk of cardiovascular disease, age-related vision loss, and some cancers.

cartilage: a natural substance of the body of humans and other animals that is sometimes marketed as a cure for cancer.

cataracts: a medical condition marked by the opaque buildup of damaged proteins in the lens of the eye; causes a decline of vision.

catnip: a natural plant product used for insomnia, for digestive and menstrual problems, as a uterine stimulant in childbirth, and as a symptomatic treatment for colds.

cat's claw: an herb used to treat acquired immunodeficiency syndrome (AIDS), genital and oral herpes, osteoarthritis, rheumatoid arthritis, and shingles.

cayenne: a natural plant product that contains capsaicin, which, when used in a cream, treats painful conditions such as osteoarthritis, peripheral neuropathy, and post-herpetic neuralgia; used orally, capsaicin treats dyspepsia.

cephalosporin: a traditional antibiotic that works similarly to penicillin but has been chemically modified to have a broader spectrum of effect; interaction with vitamin K.

cervical dysplasia: a precancerous stage of cervical cancer.

cetylated fatty acid: a part of a special mixture of fats widely marketed as a treatment for osteoarthritis.

chamomile: a natural plant product used to treat skin inflammation such as eczema and skin inflammation caused by radiation therapy.

chaparral: a natural plant product traditionally used by indigenous peoples of North America to treat joint pain and to eliminate worms; in its tea form, it was applied to painful joints and minor wounds and also used as a mouthwash and hair rinse; later used by European herbalists to treat colds, flu, and intestinal infections.

chasteberry: a natural plant product used to alleviate cyclic breast discomfort, often associated with premenstrual syndrome (PMS) or other PMS symptoms.

chelation therapy: an alternative therapy using ethylenediaminetetraacetic acid (EDTA), a synthetic substance that removes calcium and heavy metals from the body. *See also* EDTA.

Chinese medicine: a complex healing system that seeks to balance the body and free its energy flows. *See also* acupuncture; herbal medicine; qi; traditional Chinese herbal medicine.

Chinese skullcap: a natural plant product used in traditional Chinese herbal medicine to treat conditions such as cancer, liver disease, allergies, skin disorders, and epilepsy.

chiropractic care: an alternative medical technique that involves spinal adjustments and, in some cases, the use of vitamins, herbs, and other alternative treatment methods.

chitosan: a form of fiber chemically processed from crustacean shells and used as an agent to lower cholesterol and reduce weight.

chocolate: a food, rich in antioxidants, made from the cocoa bean and used primarily to prevent cardiovascular disease.

cholesterol: a waxy, fat-like substance that occurs naturally in all parts of the body.

chondroitin: a natural substance of the human body and a major constituent of cartilage, used as a supplement to treat osteoarthritis.

chromium: an essential natural substance of the body that helps regulate the amount of glucose (sugar) in the blood; it is used to as a supplement to improve blood sugar control in people with diabetes.

chronic fatigue syndrome: a chronic disease characterized by debilitating and unexplained low energy, tiredness, and other physical symptoms. *See also* fibromyalgia.

chronic obstructive pulmonary disease (COPD): a chronic lung disease involving coughing and severe shortness of breath.

cinnamon: a natural plant product used to treat type 2 diabetes and high cholesterol.

ciprofloxacin: an antimicrobial pharmaceutical; trade name Cipro.

cirrhosis: a disease of the liver, often caused by alcoholism.

cisplatin: a traditional chemotherapy drug used to treat cancer of the testicles, bladder, lung, stomach, esophagus, and ovaries, as well as other forms of cancer; interactions with acetyl-L-carnitine, antioxidants, black cohosh, ginger, magnesium, melatonin, milk thistle, and potassium.

citrulline: a nonessential amino acid used as a supplement to enhance sports and fitness performance.

Citrus aurantium: a fruit product marketed for weight loss.

citrus bioflavonoid: a natural substance used to treat diseases of the blood vessels and lymph system, including hemorrhoids, chronic venous insufficiency, leg ulcers, easy bruising, nosebleeds, and lymphedema following breast cancer surgery.

cleavers: a natural plant product used primarily for urinary problems and fluid retention, on the basis of its apparent diuretic (urine-stimulating) effects; also used to treat enlarged lymph nodes, tonsillitis, hepatitis, and snake bites.

clinical trial: an observed study of the effect of medications, supplements, vitamins, treatments, and other interventions on the human body.

clomiphene: a pharmaceutical used to enhance female fertility; interactions with N-acetyl cysteine and many herbs used in traditional Chinese herbal medicine.

clonidine: a pharmaceutical often used to reduce blood pressure and to counter symptoms that occur during withdrawal from alcohol and other addictive substances; interactions with coenzyme Q_{10}, *Coleus forskohlii*, and yohimbe.

Codex Alimentarius Commission: a commission of the United Nations that creates international standards for food nutrition, food safety, and fair trade of food and food products.

coenzyme Q10: a natural substance of the human body used as a supplement to treat cardiomyopathy, congestive heart failure, heart attack recovery, hypertension, and nutrient depletion and interference caused by various medications.

cola nut: a natural plant product containing caffeine and used to treat fatigue and to improve mental alertness.

colchicine: a pharmaceutical used to treat attacks of gout and used as a gout preventive; interaction with vitamin B_{12}.

Coleus forskohlii: a natural plant product that includes the substance forskolin, which is used to treat asthma and allergic conditions.

colic: the excessive and frequently inconsolable crying of an infant.

collagen: a strong, flexible protein found in cartilage, tendons, bone, skin, and other connective tissue.

color therapy: an alternative energy therapy based on the use of colored light, the choice of colors in one's personal environment, or Ayurvedic chakra theory. *See also* Ayurveda.

colostrum: a natural substance of a woman's body used as a supplement to treat specific health conditions.

coltsfoot: an herb once approved for the treatment of sore throat; now banned for being potentially toxic to the liver.

comfrey: a natural plant product used to treat back pain and such sports injures as sprains and strains; now banned for oral use but available as a topical cream.

common cold: a common respiratory infection caused by a virus.

complementary and alternative medicine (CAM): a group of nontraditional therapies and techniques based on cultural tradition and not usually part of the canon of Western, science- and evidence-based medicine; includes a broad range of practices and beliefs, such as acupuncture, Ayurveda, folk medicine, chiropractic care, relaxation techniques, massage therapy, herbal remedies, traditional Chinese herbal medicine, homeopathy, integrative medicine, osteopathy, and naturopathy.

complementary medicine: an alternative therapy used along with standard medicine. *See also* alternative medicine; integrative medicine.

compulsive overeating: a pattern of behavior in which a person routinely ingests large quantities of food beyond the feeling of fullness without the ability to stop.

congestive heart failure: a medical condition marked by the weakened pumping ability of the heart.

conjugated linoleic acid: a mixture of different isomers, or chemical forms, of linoleic acid, an essential fatty acid used as a fat-burning dietary supplement.

conjunctivitis: a medical condition marked by inflammation of the conjunctiva, the clear membrane that covers the eyeball.

constipation: a medical condition marked by difficult or infrequent bowel movements.

COPD. *See* chronic obstructive pulmonary disease.

copper: a natural substance of the human body used as a supplement to balance the effects of high zinc intake.

Cordyceps: a dried fungus and larvae combination used to treat various physical illnesses.

Coriolus versicolor: a tree fungus used to treat symptoms of cancer treatment.

corticosteroid: an anti-inflammatory and immune-suppressant medication; interactions with aloe (topical), calcium, chromium, creatine, dehydroepiandrosterone, ipriflavone, licorice, and vitamin D.

corydalis: a natural plant product used to treat soft tissue injuries, menstrual discomfort, and abdominal pain.

cranberry: a natural plant product used to prevent bladder infections.

craniosacral therapy: an alternative therapy involving the placing of hands on a person and working with the skull and spine and its cranial sutures, diaphragms, and fascia to ease the restrictions of nerve passages, to move cerebrospinal fluid through the spinal cord, and to restore misaligned bones.

creatine: a natural substance of the human body that plays an important role in the production of energy in the body; used as a supplement to enhance sports performance.

Crohn's disease: a medical condition marked by a severe bowel disorder; also known as inflammatory bowel disease.

cryotherapy: an alternative therapy involving the use of extreme cold in medical treatment and surgery.

crystal healing: an alternative therapy that employs crystals to effect or facilitate physical, emotional, and psychospiritual healing.

cupping: an alternative skin-surface therapy involving

cupped vessels under vacuum to suction the skin and relieve local congestion.

curandero: a traditional folk healer or shaman originally found in Latin America; curanderos specialize in treating illness through the use of supernatural forces, herbal remedies, and other natural medicines.

cyclosporine: a pharmaceutical that helps to prevent the rejection of a transplanted organ by suppressing the immune system; interactions with berberine (found in goldenseal, Oregon grape, and barberry), *Citrus aurantium,* grapefruit juice, ipriflavone, peppermint oil, St. John's wort, and *Scutellaria baicalensis.*

Cystoseira canariensis: a brown seaweed used to enhance sports performance.

damiana: an herb used to increase male sexual capacity.

dance movement therapy: an alternative body-based technique for enhancing emotional and physical well-being.

dandelion: a natural plant product whose leaves, rich in nutrients, are widely recommended as a food supplement for pregnant women.

deep breathing: an alternative therapy involving slow and deep inhalation through the nose, followed by slow and complete exhalation.

deer velvet: a natural animal product used to treat male sexual dysfunction.

depression: a mental condition marked by mild to moderate emotional distress and apathy.

detoxification: an alternative therapy that involves removing toxins from the body; these toxins include certain chemicals added to food and the mercury in silver dental fillings.

devil's claw: an herb used to treat back pain, gout, loss of appetite, mild stomach upset, muscle pain, osteoarthritis, and rheumatoid arthritis.

DHEA (dehydroepiandrosterone): a naturally occurring substance that is changed in the body to the hormones estrogen and testosterone.

diabetes: a medical condition that causes blood sugar to reach toxic levels and, if left untreated or undertreated, causes damage to tissues and major organs.

diarrhea: a medical condition marked by acute and chronic loose bowel movements.

dietary supplement: a natural product intended to supplement the diet; contains one or more dietary ingredients (including vitamins, minerals, herbs or other botanicals, amino acids, and certain other substances) or their constituents; intended to be taken by mouth in forms such as tablet, capsule, powder, soft gel, gel cap, or liquid.

Dietary Supplement Health and Education Act (DSHEA): a 1994 congressional act that established federal regulations for the manufacture, marketing, and use of dietary supplements in the United States.

diet-based therapy: a complementary and alternative therapy using special diets to improve health, increase longevity, and prevent and treat specific health conditions and diseases. *See also* Atkins diet; Ornish diet; Pritikin diet; South Beach diet.

digoxin: a pharmaceutical used to treat congestive heart failure and other heart conditions; interactions with calcium, *Eleutherococcus senticosus,* ginkgo, hawthorn, horsetail, licorice, magnesium, St. John's wort, and uzara.

diindolylmethane: a natural substance used to prevent various types of cancer, especially breast, cervical, prostate, and uterine cancer.

diverticular disease: a medical condition marked by infected or inflamed pouches in the large intestine.

DMAE (2-dimethylaminoethanol): a natural substance used to treat a number of conditions affecting the brain and central nervous system, including attention deficit disorder.

dong quai: an herb recommended as a treatment for menstrual cramps, premenstrual syndrome, and other problems related to menstruation, and for hot flashes and other menopausal symptoms.

double-blind, placebo-controlled study: a scientific trial in which a fake treatment (a placebo) is used in conjunction with a real treatment and in which participants and researchers, through "blinding," are kept from knowing which participants are receiving real or placebo treatments. *See also* evidence-based medicine; placebo effect; scientific method.

doxorubicin: a chemotherapy drug used to treat many different forms of cancer; interaction with antioxidants.

dysmenorrhea: a medical condition marked by painful menstruation.

dyspepsia: a medical condition marked by digestive problems that have no identifiable physiological cause; also called indigestion.

ear infection: a painful medical condition marked by

infection of the middle ear; most common in infants and young children.

eating disorder: a type of disorder that manifests in three types—anorexia nervosa, bulimia nervosa, and binge eating disorder; anorexia nervosa involves compulsive dieting and exercise to reduce weight, bulimia nervosa is characterized by binge eating followed by purging, and binge eating disorder is marked by binge eating that is not followed by purging.

echinacea: an herbal product used to treat the common cold and influenza.

eczema: a medical condition marked by allergic reactions of the skin.

edema: a medical condition marked by excessive fluid buildup, or swelling, of tissue and caused by congestive heart failure, venous insufficiency, mastectomy, premenstrual syndrome, pregnancy, and other factors.

EDTA (ethylenediaminetetraacetic acid) chelation therapy: an alternative therapy using EDTA, a synthetic substance that removes calcium and heavy metals from the body. *See also* chelation therapy.

elderberry: a natural plant product used as a cold and flu remedy.

elecampane: a natural plant product used to treat asthma, chronic respiratory diseases, and poor digestion.

electromagnetic hypersensitivity: a broad range of symptoms caused by exposure to electrical and magnetic fields in the environment.

Eleutherococcus senticosus: a natural plant product promoted as an adaptogen and used as a dietary supplement to treat stress.

endometriosis: a painful medical condition marked by uterine tissue growth outside the uterus.

energy medicine: an alternative therapy involving the manipulation of energy fields to promote health and well-being.

enzyme potentiated desensitization: an alternative therapy involving the injection of substances to prevent allergies.

ephedra: an herb product used to treat asthma.

epilepsy: a brain disorder that causes recurrent seizures.

essential fatty acids: a class of two essential substances (linoleic and linolenic acid) from foods that help the body in brain development, controlling inflammation, and blood clotting. *See also* linolenic acid.

essential oil: a concentrated liquid that contains aroma compounds from plants.

essential oil monoterpenes: a natural plant product combination that contains cineole from eucalyptus, dlimonene from citrus fruit, and alphapinene from pine; used to treat acute bronchitis, chronic bronchitis, and sinus infections.

estriol: a natural form of estrogen used to treat menopausal symptoms and osteoporosis. *See also* estrogen; phytoestrogen.

estrogen: a hormone that is a natural component of birth control pills and is used for preventing osteoporosis and heart disease in menopausal women. *See also* estriol; phytoestrogen.

ethambutol: a pharmaceutical used with isoniazid in the treatment of tuberculosis; interactions with copper and zinc.

eucalyptus: a natural plant product used as a topical antiseptic and as a lozenge in inhalation therapy for asthma, cough, sore throat, and other respiratory conditions.

evening primrose oil: a natural plant product primarily used to treat conditions involving inflammation, such as rheumatoid arthritis, as well as breast pain associated with menstruation, menopausal symptoms, and premenstrual syndrome (PMS).

evidence-based medicine: the practice of medicine based on the results of double-blind, placebo-controlled trials. *See also* double-blind, placebo-controlled study; placebo effect; scientific method.

exercise-based therapy: an alternative technique involving the use of physical activities to enhance overall health and wellness and to treat specific medical disorders.

eyebright: an herb that contains astringent substances and volatile oils that are probably slightly antibacterial; used to treat conjunctivitis (pink eye) and other eye diseases.

faith healing: an alternative technique involving personal faith to effect physical and psychical healing; the patient is assisted by a practitioner with the charismatic gift or gifts of healing.

false unicorn: an herb believed to balance the female reproductive system, normalizing hormone levels and optimizing ovarian action; recommended for preventing miscarriages and treating infertility, dysmenorrhea, premenstrual syndrome, pelvic inflammatory disease, and morning sickness.

fat, dietary: a type of nutrient that provides energy for the body.

Feldenkrais method: a self-education healing system in alternative medicine that focuses on the relationship between mind and body.

feng shui: an ancient Chinese aesthetic of designing one's environment to enhance one's qi, or energy.

fennel: an herb used to treat infantile colic, dyspepsia, intestinal gas, and menstrual pain.

fenugreek: a natural plant product used to treat constipation, diabetes, and high cholesterol.

feverfew: a natural plant product used primarily for the prevention of migraine headaches.

fiber, dietary: a natural plant product from foods that helps with digestion and helps to prevent constipation.

fibrate drug: any class of pharmaceuticals used to improve levels of cholesterol and related lipids found in the blood; particularly helpful for persons with high levels of triglycerides; interactions with B vitamins and blood thinning supplements.

fibromyalgia: a medical condition of unknown cause that is marked by severe, chronic muscle pain, cognitive impairment, sleep disorders, and fatigue. *See also* chronic fatigue syndrome.

fish oil: a natural, essential substance containing omega-3 fatty acids; promoted as a dietary supplement primarily to prevent heart disease and to treat rheumatoid arthritis.

5-HTP (5-hydroxytryptophan): a natural plant product promoted to treat depression, migraines and other types of headaches.

flavonoid: a type of antioxidant.

flaxseed: a natural plant product used to treat constipation and to prevent heart disease and high cholesterol.

flu (influenza): a common respiratory infection caused by a virus.

fluoride: a chemical compound used to prevent dental cavities.

fluoroquinolone: a type of antibiotic used to treat urinary tract infections and other infectious diseases; interactions with dong quai, fennel, minerals, and St. John's wort.

fluoxetine: a selective serotonin reuptake inhibitor (antidepressant); trade name Prozac.

folate (a B vitamin): an essential natural substance that helps to produce and maintain new cells; used for cancer prevention, depression, heart disease prevention, prevention of birth defects and disorders, and reducing methotrexate side effects.

folic acid: a B vitamin that helps the body make healthy new cells.

folk medicine: a system of alternative and nontraditional beliefs and practices that include home remedies, herbal therapies, and traditional healing.

Food and Drug Administration (FDA): a U.S. government agency that oversees regulations and inspections of the safety and quality of pharmaceuticals and nutritional resources, including food and food products.

free radical: a natural by-product of oxygen metabolism that may contribute to the development of chronic diseases such as cancer and heart disease; the target of antioxidants. *See also* antioxidant.

fructo-oligosaccharide: a natural substance used to improve the user's cholesterol profile.

functional beverage: a juice, water, or soda to which natural additives such as ginseng and ginkgo or other alternative ingredients are introduced to improve health.

functional food: a food marketed as having specific health-promoting benefits.

GABA (gamma-aminobutyric acid): a naturally occurring neurotransmitter that is used within the brain to reduce the activity of certain nerve systems, including those related to anxiety.

gamma oryzanol: a mixture of natural substances derived from rice bran oil; primarily used to treat high cholesterol.

gamma-linolenic acid: one of the two main types of essential fatty acids and promoted as a treatment for diabetic neuropathy. *See also* essential fatty acid.

garlic: an herbal product used to prevent the common cold and heart disease, and used as an insect repellent.

gastritis: a medical condition marked by inflammation of the lining of the stomach.

gastroesophageal reflux disease (GERD): a medical condition that causes stomach acid to enter the esophagus; also known as heartburn, esophageal reflux, and acid reflux.

genistein: a natural chemical present in soy and used for its possible benefits in cancer and heart disease prevention.

gentian: a natural plant product used to increase appetite and to strengthen the digestive system.

GERD. *See* gastroesophageal reflux disease.

germander: a toxic plant product that is especially harmful to the liver; its use is not recommended.

ginger: an herbal product used to treat morning sickness in pregnancy, motion sickness, and postsurgical nausea.

ginkgo: a natural plant product primarily used to treat Alzheimer's disease and to enhance memory and mental function in healthy people, to treat non-Alzheimer's dementia, and to treat intermittent claudication.

ginseng: an herb used to treat the common cold, influenza, and diabetes; to enhance general well-being and mental function; to support the immune system; and to reduce stress.

glaucoma: a medical condition marked by damage to the eye's optic nerve; it leads to impaired vision or blindness.

glucomannan: a dietary fiber used to help reduce high cholesterol and improve constipation, to help regulate blood sugar, and to assist in weight reduction by creating a feeling of fullness.

glucosamine: a natural substance of the human body and a key building block for making cartilage; used as a supplement to treat osteoarthritis.

glucose: the primary source of energy for the cells of the body. *See also* blood sugar; diabetes; low-glycemic-index diet; oral hypoglycemic.

glutamine: an amino acid helpful to the immune system, digestive tract, and muscle cells; used to prevent post-endurance-exercise infections, reduce symptoms of overtraining syndrome, improve nutrition in critical illness, alleviate allergies, and treat digestive problems.

glutathione: a natural substance of the human body that is part of the antioxidant defense system and is used as a supplement to fight free radicals, which are harmful to body tissues.

glycine: an amino acid shown to have some promise as an aid in the treatment of schizophrenia; also may enhance mental function.

goldenrod: a natural plant product used as a supportive treatment for bladder infections, irritation of the urinary tract, and bladder and kidney stones.

goldenseal: a natural plant product used as a topical antibiotic for skin wounds and to treat viral mouth sores and superficial fungal infections, such as athlete's foot.

gotu kola: a natural plant product widely used in Ayurvedic medicine and promoted in the West as a treatment for chronic venous insufficiency, a condition closely related to varicose veins.

gout: a medical condition marked by inflammation and caused by the deposit of uric acid crystals in joints and tissues.

grape seed extract: a natural plant product used for conditions related to the heart and blood vessels, such as atherosclerosis (hardening of the arteries), high blood pressure, high cholesterol, and poor circulation.

grass pollen extract: a natural plant product used to treat prostate enlargement.

greater celandine: a relative of the poppy, a natural plant product that is toxic to the liver and is not recommended for use.

green coffee bean extract: a natural plant product that contains chlorogenic acids, which may reduce blood pressure.

green-lipped mussel: a natural seafood product used to treat conditions caused by inflammation, including arthritis and asthma.

green tea: a natural plant product that contains high levels of substances called catechin polyphenols, known to possess strong antioxidant, anticarcinogenic, antitumorigenic, and even antibiotic properties; used to prevent cancer and heart disease.

guarana: a natural plant product that contains alkaloids in the caffeine family; caffeine is known to reduce pain, treat migraine headaches, and fight fatigue.

guggul: the sticky gum resin from the mukul myrrh tree; used to treat high cholesterol.

guided imagery: an alternative therapy involving the use of imagined scenes and activities to influence body processes.

gymnema: a natural plant product used to help control blood sugar levels in people with diabetes.

H_2 blocker: a pharmaceutical used to decrease the production of stomach acid; interactions with folate, magnesium, minerals, vitamin B_{12}, and vitamin D.

hawthorn: a natural plant product used to treat congestive heart failure.

HDL (high-density lipoprotein) cholesterol: a type of "good" cholesterol. *See also* cholesterol; LDL cholesterol.

he shou wu: an herb widely marketed as a general antiaging herb, said to reduce cholesterol, prevent heart disease, prevent age-related loss of mental function, improve sleep, and extend life span.

headache, cluster: a medical condition marked by severe headaches that strike suddenly after a long time without an episode.

headache, tension: a medical condition marked by aching, dull, and throbbing pain; most commonly felt in the forehead, temples, and base of the skull.

health freedom movement: a collective of organizations, consumers, activists, product manufacturers, and medical practitioners campaigning worldwide for unregulated access to health care.

heart attack: an acute medical condition caused by blocked blood flow to the heart.

heart disease: the diseases of the heart that include angina, atherosclerosis, cardiovascular disease, congestive heart failure, coronary heart disease, hypertension, and peripheral vascular disease.

heartburn. *See* gastroesophageal reflux disease.

Helicobacter pylori: a bacterium that causes, among other illnesses and conditions, stomach ulcers. *See* ulcer.

Hellerwork: an alternative treatment and therapy involving massage, patient education, and patient-practitioner dialogue.

hemorrhoids: a medical condition marked by swollen and inflamed veins in the rectum and caused by constipation, pregnancy, a low-fiber diet, and other factors.

heparin: a blood-thinning drug that is delivered by injection; interactions with chondroitin, garlic, ginkgo, PC-SPES, phosphatidylserine, policosanol, vitamin C, vitamin D, and white willow.

hepatitis, alcoholic: a type of liver disease caused by chronic overconsumption of alcohol.

hepatitis, viral: a viral infection of the liver.

herb: a plant or plant part valued for its medicinal, savory, or aromatic qualities.

herbal medicine: a type of preventive medicine and therapy involving the use of herbs to effect well-being; includes Ayurveda, folk medicine, Native American medicine, indigenous medicine, and traditional Chinese herbal medicine, and, in the West, herbology.

herpes: a medical condition marked by blister-like lesions around the mouth and genitalia and caused by the herpesvirus.

hibiscus: a natural plant product used to lower blood pressure.

histidine: an essential amino acid used as a supplement to treat rheumatoid arthritis.

HIV (human immunodeficiency virus): a virus that progressively destroys or damages cells in the immune system, making the body vulnerable to certain cancers and infections; the virus that causes acquired immunodeficiency syndrome (AIDS). *See also* acquired immunodeficiency syndrome.

hives: a medical condition marked by inflammation of the surface layers of the skin.

holistic medicine: *See* whole medicine.

home health: a method of health promotion that encourage the removal of allergens, pathogens, and other pollutants from the home or other living environment.

home remedy: *See* folk medicine.

homeopathy: an alternative therapy based on the theory that a substance that provokes symptoms in a healthy person can also treat a sick person who has those same symptoms. *See also* provings; symptom picture.

homocysteine: a substance produced when the body breaks down the amino acid methionine.

honey: a natural food promoted as a topical application to treat or prevent infection.

hoodia: a natural plant product used as a supplement for weight loss.

hops: a natural plant product used to treat sleep problems.

horehound: an herb used as a treatment for cough, asthma, and sore throat.

hormone replacement therapy: a medical therapy using female hormones to relieve the symptoms of perimenopause and menopause.

horny goat weed: a natural plant product marketed as a sexual stimulant for both men and women and also as a treatment for menopausal symptoms.

horse chestnut: an herb used as a treatment for venous insufficiency, a condition associated with varicose veins.

horseradish: a natural plant product used to treat acute bronchitis, the common cold, sinusitis, and urinary tract infection.

horsetail: a natural plant product used to prevent or treat osteoporosis and to strengthen brittle nails.

hot flash: a symptom of perimenopause and menopause. *See also* menopause.

human immunodeficiency virus: *See* HIV.

humor and healing: an alternative therapy that uses humor to relieve physical and emotional problems.

huperzine A: a chemical derived from a natural plant and used to treat age-related memory loss, Alzheimer's disease, and other forms of dementia.

hydralazine: a pharmaceutical that dilates the walls of blood vessels; sometimes used to treat hypertension; interactions with coenzyme Q_{10}, *Coleus forskohlii*, and vitamin B_6.

hydrotherapy: an alternative treatment and therapy involving the use of water. *See also* balneotherapy.

hydroxycitric acid: a natural plant product promoted as helpful for weight loss because of its effects on body metabolism.

hydroxymethyl butyrate: a natural substance of the human body used as a supplement to enhance the building of muscles for strength in athletes and bodybuilders.

hypertension: a medical condition marked by abnormal, dangerously high blood pressure.

hyperthyroidism: a medical condition marked by the thyroid gland producing too much thyroid hormone.

hypnotherapy: an alternative technique involving hypnosis to produce a therapeutic benefit.

hypothyroidism: a medical condition marked by the thyroid gland's failure to produce adequate levels of thyroid hormone.

hyssop: a natural plant product used to treat respiratory problems such as the common cold, asthma, acute bronchitis and cough, and to treat digestive problems such as stomach upset and intestinal gas; hyssop tea is recommended as a gargle for sore throat.

IBD: *See* Crohn's disease.

IBS: *See* irritable bowel syndrome.

ibuprofen: a type of nonsteroidal anti-inflammatory drug used to relieve pain, inflammation, and fever. *See also* acetaminophen; aspirin; nonsteroidal anti-inflammatory drug.

imagery exercise: *See* guided imagery.

immune support: any alternative therapy used to increase the effectiveness of the immune system in fighting infection.

indigestion: *See* dyspepsia.

indigo: *See* wild indigo

indole-3-carbinol: a chemical found in vegetables of the broccoli family that is primarily used to prevent cancer.

inflammatory bowel disease: *See* Crohn's disease.

influenza vaccine: a vaccine that decreases the risk of infection with the virus that causes influenza, or the flu; interactions with ginseng.

innate intelligence: the premise that inherent knowledge acquired at birth guides the human body and determines health.

inosine: an essential natural substance of the human body used as a supplementary energy booster for athletes and as a treatment for various heart conditions.

inositol (vitamin B_8): a natural substance of the body that is used primarily as a supplement to treat depression and panic disorder.

insomnia: a medical condition marked by an inability to sleep or to get restful sleep.

insulin: a pharmaceutical injectable used to regulate blood sugar in persons with type 1 diabetes or severe type 2 diabetes; interactions with various herbs and supplements.

integrative medicine: a relationship-centered, complementary care system that combines mainstream medical and alternative therapeutic methods to potentiate the body's innate capacity to heal. *See also* alternative medicine; complementary and alternative medicine; complementary medicine.

intermittent claudication: a medical condition marked by severe muscle pain; caused by blocked arteries in the legs.

interstitial cystitis: a medical condition marked by severe and chronic inflammation of the bladder.

iodine: a natural substance of the human body used as a supplementary treatment for cyclic mastalgia, which is characterized by breast pain and lumpiness that usually cycles in relation to the menstrual period.

ipriflavone: a natural plant product used as a dietary supplement to help slow down and perhaps slightly reverse osteoporosis.

iridology: the alternative medical technique of predicting a person's state of health by examining the iris of his or her eye.

iron: an essential natural substance of the human body used as a supplement to treat iron deficiency and to enhance sports and exercise performance.

irritable bowel syndrome (IBS): a chronic medical condition with no identifiable medical cause; includes diarrhea, constipation, intestinal gas, bloating, and cramping.

isoflavone: a natural plant product primarily used to reduce the risk of cardiovascular disease.

isoniazid: an antibiotic drug used for the treatment of tuberculosis; interactions with vitamin B_3, vitamin B_6, and vitamin D.

isotretinoin: a pharmaceutical related to vitamin A that is used to treat severe acne; interactions with St. John's wort, vitamin A, and vitamin E.

ivy leaf: an herb used to treat asthma, acute bronchitis, chronic bronchitis, colds, flu, and other respiratory problems.

jet lag: a medical condition marked by disruptions to the body's internal clock from air travel across many time zones.

juniper berry: an herb used as a diuretic component of herbal formulas that are designed to treat bladder infections.

Kampo: in Japan, a variation of traditional Chinese herbal medicine.

kava: a member of the pepper family, used to treat anxiety and related conditions.

kelp: a brown algae, or seaweed, used primarily as a nutrient-rich food supplement.

kidney stone: a medical condition marked by crystallized chemicals in the kidneys.

kombucha tea: a natural plant product widely supposed to have miraculous medicinal properties, ranging from curing cancer to restoring gray hair to its original color; other reputed effects include normalizing weight, improving blood pressure, increasing energy, decreasing arthritis pain, restoring normal bowel movements, removing wrinkles, curing acne, strengthening bones, and improving memory.

krill oil: a natural seafood product primarily used to treat dysmenorrhea, high cholesterol, and premenstrual syndrome.

lactose intolerance: a medical condition marked by the absence of the lactose-digesting enzyme known as lactase in the digestive system.

laetrile: an alternative, potentially deadly, cancer cure dismissed as ineffective by the scientific community.

lavender: a natural plant product used to treat anxiety, restlessness, insomnia, depression, headache, upset stomach, and hair loss.

LDL (low-density lipoprotein) cholesterol: a type of "bad" cholesterol. *See also* cholesterol; HDL cholesterol.

lecithin: a natural animal and plant substance used to treat Alzheimer's disease, bipolar disorder, high cholesterol, liver disease, Parkinson's disease, tardive dyskinesia, Tourette syndrome, and ulcerative colitis.

lemon balm: a natural plant product used to treat anxiety, insomnia, nervous stomach, oral and genital herpes, and agitation in persons with dementia.

leukoplakia: a medical disorder of the mucous membranes that manifests in areas such as the mouth, tongue, and female genitals.

levodopa/carbidopa: a drug treatment for Parkinson's disease; interactions with branched-chain amino acids, 5-HTP, iron, kava, policosanol, SAMe, traditional Chinese herbal medicine, and vitamin B_6.

licorice: a natural plant product used to treat asthma, chronic fatigue syndrome, cough, eczema, heartburn, herpes, mouth sores, psoriasis, and ulcers.

life extension: an alternative medicine technique that claims to slow the aging process and increase the human lifespan through medicine, science, technology, and spirituality. *See also* anti-aging medicine.

lignan: a natural chemical substance used for cancer prevention and to treat elevated cholesterol, kidney disease, and menopausal symptoms.

ligustrum: a natural plant product with a long history of use in traditional Chinese herbal medicine; used to enhance and support the immune system.

linden: a natural plant product primarily used to treat common cold.

lipoic acid: an essential natural substance used to treat diabetic neuropathy.

lithium: a pharmaceutical used to treat bipolar disorder; interactions with citrate, herbal diuretics, and inositol.

lobelia: an herb primarily used to treat cigarette addiction.

lomatium: a natural plant product used to treat many types of viral infection, including human immunodeficiency virus (HIV) infection, viral hepatitis, colds and flu, acute bronchitis, sinusitis, and herpes.

loop diuretic: any of a class of pharmaceuticals used to reduce fluid accumulation in the body; interactions with dong quai, licorice, magnesium, potassium, St. John's wort, and vitamin B_1.

low-carbohydrate diet: an alternative treatment claiming that one can attain and maintain a healthy weight through diets that are low in carbohydrates. *See also* carbohydrate.

low-glycemic-index diet: an alternative treatment based on the consumption of certain carbohydrates and low-fat foods that do not create a strong blood sugar and insulin reaction when digested. *See also* carbohydrate; glucose.

lupus: an autoimmune disease in which antibodies develop that aberrantly fight healthy tissue in the body.

lutein: a natural chemical found in green vegetables that is used to help prevent or slow the development of age-related macular degeneration and possibly cataracts.

lycopene: a powerful antioxidant found in tomatoes and pink grapefruit that is used primarily to prevent macular degeneration, cataracts, cardiovascular disease, and cancer.

lysine: an essential amino acid used to help prevent herpes outbreaks such as cold sores and genital herpes.

maca: a natural plant product marketed for improving male sexual function, female sexual function, and both male fertility and female fertility.

macrobiotic diet: a diet that emphasizes whole grains and fresh vegetables, is low in fat and high in protein, and restricts fluid intake.

macular degeneration: a medical condition marked by the gradual deterioration of the macula, an area of the retina.

magnesium: an essential natural substance of the human body, used as a dietary supplement to treat diabetes, hypertension, kidney stones, migraine headaches, and noise-related hearing loss.

magnet therapy: an alternative healing technique using magnets and magnetic fields on or near the body; also known as magnetic healing.

maitake: a medicinal mushroom used to promote robust health.

malic acid: a natural substance of the human body used as a supplement primarily to treat the symptoms of fibromyalgia.

manganese: a natural substance of the human body used as a supplement primarily to treat dysmenorrhea and osteoporosis.

manipulative and body-based practices: a group of alternative manual techniques that release muscle tension and increase circulation to stimulate the body's natural healing abilities.

mannose: a natural substance of the human body used as a supplement to treat urinary tract infections.

marshmallow: a natural plant product used as a dietary supplement to treat asthma, cough, colds, and sore throat; taken as a tea or in capsules, it is recommended for Crohn's disease and ulcers.

massage therapy: an alternative touch-based therapy involving manipulation of the muscles and connective tissues to enhance function and promote relaxation.

maté: a natural plant product traditionally used to enhance alertness and mental function and to treat digestive problems.

medicine man: *See* Native American healer.

meditation: an alternative technique involving an awake, relaxed state of suspending one's stream of thought; characterized by decreased metabolic activity in the body.

medium-chain triglyceride: a natural substance of the human body used as a supplementary fat for persons who have difficulty digesting fat; believed to be helpful for persons with AIDS who need to gain weight but who cannot digest fat easily.

melatonin: a hormone used as a supplement to treat insomnia, jet lag, and other sleep disorders.

menopause: the cessation of a woman's menstrual cycle.

meridian: in traditional Chinese medicine, an invisible pathway that is claimed to circulate energy and maintain balance and harmony throughout the body.

mesoglycan: a natural substance used as a dietary supplement to treat medical conditions such as atherosclerosis, intermittent claudication, and varicose veins.

metabolic syndrome: a medical condition marked by the development of several cardiovascular and other disease risk factors.

metamorphic technique: a gentle-touch alternative healing technique applied to the feet, hands, and head.

methotrexate: a pharmaceutical used in cancer chemotherapy and to treat inflammatory diseases such as rheumatoid arthritis and psoriasis; interactions with citrate, dong quai, folate, ipriflavone, potassium citrate, St. John's wort, and white willow.

methoxyisoflavone: a chemical derivative of ipriflavone, which is a hormonally active substance found in soy and other foods; it is used to enhance sports and fitness performance.

methyl sulfonyl methane: a natural substance used as a dietary supplement to treat osteoarthritis.

methyldopa: a pharmaceutical used to control hypertension; interactions with coenzyme Q_{10} and iron.

migraine: a severe, painful headache with characteristic symptoms that include visual disturbances.

milk thistle: a natural plant product used to treat alcoholic hepatitis, liver cirrhosis, liver poisoning, and viral hepatitis, and to protect the liver in general from the effects of liver-toxic medications.

mind/body medicine: a type of traditional healing that emphasizes the interconnectedness of the mind and the body. *See also* yin and yang.

mistletoe: a natural plant product used as a treatment for cancer; popular in anthroposophic medicine.

mitral valve prolapse: a medical condition caused by the prolapse, or misalignment, of one of the valves of the heart.

molybdenum: an essential trace mineral in food and water used as a supplement to treat female and male sexual dysfunction and insomnia, to prevent tooth decay, and to promote general well-being.

monoamine oxidase (MAO) inhibitor: an antidepressant pharmaceutical; interactions with ephedra, green tea, ginseng, 5-HTP, St. John's wort, SAMe, and scotch broom.

motherwort: a natural plant product used to treat heart conditions.

motion sickness: a feeling of nausea caused by movement, such as in a vehicle or on a boat or ship.

MS: *See* multiple sclerosis.

muira puama: a natural plant product used to treat male sexual dysfunction.

mullein: a natural plant product used to treat asthma, colds, coughs, and sore throats.

multiple sclerosis (MS): a disease that affects the fatty sheath that covers nerve fibers in the brain and spinal cord and leads to the slowing or blocking of nerve signals.

multivitamin: a dietary supplement providing a broad range of nutrients at standard nutritional levels; often combined with minerals.

music therapy: the clinical and evidence-based use of music, including playing instruments and singing, in therapeutic practice.

myrrh: a natural plant product used to treat mouth diseases such as canker sores, gingivitis, halitosis, and sore throats.

N-acetyl cysteine: a natural substance of the human body used as a supplement to treat (in combination with conventional treatment) angina pectoris and chronic bronchitis and to prevent influenza.

narcotic addiction: a medical condition marked by addiction to drugs that include cocaine, heroine, and methamphetamine.

National Center for Complementary and Alternative Medicine (NCCAM): a U.S. government scientific and informational resource on the efficacy and safety of complementary and alternative medical practices and products for consumers, practitioners, and policymakers.

National Health Federation: a nonprofit organization that promotes health education for consumers and seeks to eliminate certain government restrictions on food, water, vitamins, supplements, and alternative medical techniques; based in the United States.

Native American healer: a traditional physical and spiritual healer who transfers knowledge from the "spirit world" to benefit a community. *See also* folk medicine; traditional healing.

natural product: a nonsynthetic substance—such as an herb, a botanical, or a natural substance like an enzyme and a glandular—used to supplement the diet in place of vitamins and minerals.

naturopathy: a complementary and alternative therapy that claims to prevent and treat disease through natural remedies and healing, including nutrition, exercise, and detoxification.

neem: a natural plant product used traditionally, especially in India, to treat a wide variety of health conditions.

nettle: a natural plant product used primarily to treat allergies in its leaf form and benign prostatic hyperplasia in its root form.

nicotinamide adenine dinucleotide (NADH): a natural substance of the human body used as a supplement to treat jet lag.

nitrofurantoin: a pharmaceutical used to prevent bladder infections; interaction with magnesium.

nitroglycerin: a pharmaceutical commonly used to quickly relieve pain associated with angina; interactions with arginine, folate, N-acetyl cysteine, vitamin C, and vitamin E.

nitrous oxide: a gas used as a local anesthetic in dentistry and in certain phases of cardiac bypass surgery; interactions with folate and vitamin B_{12}.

nondairy milk: a type of milk produced from nonanimal sources, such as soy, rice, almond, multigrain, oat, and potato.

noni: a natural plant product promoted for an enormous range of uses, including abrasions, arthritis, diabetes, drug addiction, fever, fractures, malaria, menstrual cramps, stroke, and thrush.

nonsteroidal anti-inflammatory drug (NSAID): any of a class of pharmaceuticals used to treat pain, fever, and inflammation; available both as prescription and over-the-counter medications; interactions with arginine, chondroitin, citrate, cayenne, colostrum, dong quai, feverfew, folate, garlic, ginkgo, licorice, PC-SPES, policosanol, potassium citrate, reishi, St. John's wort, vinpocetine, vitamin C, vitamin E, and white willow. *See also* acetaminophen; aspirin; ibuprofen.

nopal: a type of cactus used primarily to treat the symptoms of hangover from alcohol use.

NSAID: *See* nonsteroidal anti-inflammatory drug.

nutritional therapeutics: an assortment of nutrients and non-nutrients, bioactive food components used as chemopreventive agents, and specific foods or diets used as cancer prevention or treatment strategies.

oak bark: a natural plant product primarily used to treat diarrhea; also used to treat internal hemorrhage, dysentery, cancer, and pneumonia.

oat straw: a natural plant product marketed for enhancing male sexual function; in combination with saw palmetto, it is said to help sexual dysfunction in women and to treat enlargement of the prostate.

obesity: a disease marked by excess body weight—namely, body fat; a serious risk factor for a number of conditions, including diabetes.

obsessive-compulsive disorder (OCD): a mental disorder characterized by recurrent and persistent thoughts or images known as obsessions and resultant repetitive behaviors known as compulsions.

Office of Cancer Complementary and Alternative Medicine (OCCAM): the health consumer hub for U.S. government information on complementary and alternative medicine for persons with cancer and those who treat them.

Office of Dietary Supplements (ODS): a U.S. government office formed to enhance knowledge of dietary supplements to ensure medical understanding and consumer safety.

oligomeric proanthocyanidin (OPC): a natural plant product primarily used to treat chronic venous insufficiency, a condition related to varicose veins.

olive leaf: a natural plant product whose constituents—oleuropein and enolinate—are believed to kill harmful bacteria, viruses, and fungi in the body.

omega-3 fatty acids: a group of polyunsaturated fatty acids that are important for a number of functions in the body; found in foods such as fatty fish and vegetable oils and also available as dietary supplements; used to reduce several cardiovascular disease risk factors and to treat symptoms of rheumatoid arthritis.

oral contraceptive: any of a class of pharmaceuticals used to prevent pregnancy; interactions with androstenedione, dong quai, folate, grapefruit juice, indole-3-carbinol, milk thistle, resveratrol, rosemary, St. John's wort, and soy.

oral hypoglycemic: any of a class of pharmaceuticals used to control blood sugar in persons with type 2 diabetes; interactions with coenzyme Q_{10}, dong quai, ginkgo, herbs and supplements, ipriflavone, magnesium, potassium citrate, St. John's wort, and vitamin B_{12}. *See also* diabetes; glucose.

oregano oil: a natural plant product used to treat yeast hypersensitivity syndrome.

Oregon grape: a natural plant product primarily used as a topical treatment for psoriasis.

Ornish diet: a high-fiber, low-fat, vegetarian diet that promotes weight loss and health by controlling what one eats, not by restricting the intake of calories. *See also* Atkins diet; diet-based therapy; Pritikin diet; South Beach diet.

ornithine alpha-ketoglutarate (OKG): a natural substance of the human body used as a supplement to treat persons recovering from severe physical trauma.

orthomolecular medicine: an alternative medical treatment that calls for eliminating from the body those substances that contribute to malnutrition—such as sugar, salt, and animal fat—and for optimizing the amounts of such substances as vitamins and minerals.

osha: a natural plant product recommended for use at the first sign of a respiratory infection; induces sweating, which could help to avert the common cold; also taken during respiratory infections as a cough suppressant and expectorant.

osteoarthritis: a medical condition marked by damage to joint cartilage.

osteopathic manipulation: an alternative medical treatment involving manipulation of soft tissues and joints outside the spine. *See also* chiropractic care; osteopathy.

osteopathy: a medical field emphasizing soft tissue and joint manipulation outside the spine; osteopathic physicians study and practice the same types of medical and surgical techniques as conventional medical doctors. *See also* osteopathic manipulation.

osteoporosis: a medical condition marked by bone loss that is caused by aging, smoking, lack of exercise, or other factors. *See also* osteoarthritis.

oxerutin: a natural plant substance primarily used to treat venous insufficiency/varicose veins; improves aching, swelling, and fatigue in the legs. *See also* varicose veins; venous insufficiency.

oxygen therapy: an alternative treatment that provides the body with extra oxygen.

PABA (para-aminobenzoic acid): a natural food product used to treat various diseases of the skin and connective tissue, and to treat male infertility.

pancreatitis: a medical condition marked by inflammation of the pancreas.

pantothenic acid and pantethine: a pair of natural food substances used as supplements to treat (in the case of pantothenic acid) rheumatoid arthritis; pantethine is used to treat high triglyceride and high cholesterol levels. *See also* cholesterol; rheumatoid arthritis.

Parkinson's disease: a chronic medical condition caused by the death of nerve cells in certain parts of the brain.

parsley: an herb primarily used to relieve irritation of the urinary tract (such as may occur in a bladder infection) and to aid in passing kidney stones.

passionflower: a natural plant product primarily used as a mildly effective treatment for anxiety and insomnia.

PC-SPES: a formula claimed to include eight natural products (seven herbs and one mushroom) that proponents believed could treat prostate cancer; not recommended for use.

Pelargonium sidoides: a natural plant product in the geranium family primarily used to treat various respiratory problems, including acute bronchitis, the common cold, sinusitis, pharyngitis (sore throat), and tonsillitis.

penicillamine: a pharmaceutical used to treat rheumatoid arthritis and Wilson's disease, an inherited disorder affecting copper metabolism and causing cirrhosis and brain and eye problems; interactions with copper, iron, vitamin B_6, and zinc.

pennyroyal: a natural plant product of the mint family primarily used to treat colds and influenza, coughs, kidney problems, headache, and upset stomach, and used to induce abortion; it is toxic to the liver and should be avoided.

pentoxifylline: a pharmaceutical that makes the blood less "sticky" and is used to increase blood circulation; interactions with chondroitin, garlic, ginkgo, herbs and supplements, PC-SPES, policosanol, reishi, vinpocetine, and white willow.

peppermint: a natural plant product used to treat a variety of health conditions, including dyspepsia and irritable bowel syndrome; peppermint oil is used in aromatherapy.

Perilla frutescens: a natural plant product and member of the mint family used to treat allergic rhinitis (hay fever), primarily, and also depression and rheumatoid arthritis.

periodontal disease: a medical condition marked by gum inflammation that can progress to pockets of infection, bone loss, and loosening of the teeth.

Peyronie's disease: a medical condition in which a thickened, hardened piece of tissue forms on one side of the penis.

Phaseolus vulgaris: a natural plant product made from white kidney beans and sold as a starch blocker; said to interfere with the digestion of carbohydrates and thereby promote weight loss.

phenobarbital: a pharmaceutical used to control seizures; interactions with biotin, dong quai, folate, ginkgo, glutamine, hops, kava, passionflower, St. John's wort, valerian, vitamin D, and vitamin K.

phenothiazine: a pharmaceutical used to treat schizophrenia and other forms of psychosis; interactions with coenzyme Q_{10}, milk thistle, fish oil, ginkgo, vitamin E, vitamin B_6, DHEA, glycine, phenylalanine, kava, St. John's wort and other herbs, and yohimbe.

phenylalanine: a natural substance of the human body used as a supplement primarily to treat depression.

phenytoin: a traditional anticonvulsant agent used primarily to prevent seizures in conditions such as epilepsy; in some cases, combination therapy with two or more anticonvulsant drugs may be used; interactions with biotin, calcium, carnitine, folate, ginkgo, glutamine, hops, ipriflavone, kava, passionflower, valerian, vitamin D, vitamin K, and white willow.

phlebitis: a medical condition marked by serious inflammation of a vein that is often accompanied by blood clots that adhere to the wall of the vein.

phosphatidylserine: a natural substance of the human body primarily used as a supplement to treat age-related memory loss and Alzheimer's disease.

phosphorus: a natural substance of the human body primarily used as a supplement to treat osteoporosis and to provide sports and fitness enhancement.

photosensitivity: a medical condition in which a person sunburns easily or develops certain skin reactions to sunlight.

phyllanthus: a natural plant product proposed to treat chronic hepatitis B.

phytoestrogen: an estrogen-like compound contained in some botanical products, such as soy and red clover; plants rich in phytoestrogens may help relieve some symptoms of menopause. *See also* estriol; estrogen; progesterone.

picrorhiza: a natural plant product traditionally used in Ayurvedic medicine for the treatment of digestive problems, scorpion sting, asthma, liver disease, and febrile infections.

Pilates: a movement therapy that uses physical exercise to strengthen and build control of muscles; integral components include an awareness of breathing and precise control of movements. *See also* yoga.

placebo effect: an observable or measurable improvement in health or relief of symptoms that is attributable to something other than an administered medicine, medical procedure, or treatment. *See also* double-blind, placebo-controlled study; evidence-based medicine; scientific method.

plantain: a natural plant product believed to have an anti-inflammatory effect.

PMS: *See* premenstrual syndrome.

pokeroot: an herb that includes substances that have shown promise for drug development.

policosanol: a natural substance promoted as a dietary supplement to treat high cholesterol.

polycystic ovary syndrome: a chronic endocrine dis-

order in women marked by elevated levels of male hormones, infertility, and other conditions.

polyphenol: a natural plant product used as an antioxidant; common in tea. *See also* antioxidant.

popular health movement: an early nineteenth century health movement in the United States that promoted nontraditional medical treatment, especially the use of herbal remedies, and that opposed traditional medicine.

potassium: a natural substance essential for health and promoted as a dietary supplement primarily to treat hypertension.

potassium-sparing diuretic: any of a class of alternative diuretics used to avoid the potassium loss common with the use of loop and thiazide diuretics; interactions with arginine, magnesium, potassium, white willow, and zinc.

prebiotic: a nondigestible food ingredient that selectively stimulates the growth and activity of microorganisms already present in the body. *See also* probiotic.

preeclampsia and pregnancy-induced hypertension: a medical condition marked by increased blood pressure, protein in the urine, and other symptoms during pregnancy.

pregnenolone: a natural substance of the human body used as a supplement to enhance memory and mental function and to treat aging in general, Alzheimer's disease, depression, fatigue, menopausal symptoms, osteoporosis, Parkinson's disease, rheumatoid arthritis, stress, and excess weight.

premenstrual syndrome (PMS): a medical condition marked by symptoms associated with the onset of menstruation. *See also* menopause.

prickly ash: a natural tree product with a long history of use in Native American medicine; primarily used to treat a variety of conditions such as dry mouth, intermittent claudication, osteoarthritis, Raynaud's syndrome, and toothache.

primidone: a pharmaceutical used to control epileptic seizures; interactions with biotin, dong quai, folate, ginkgo, glutamine, hops, kava, passionflower, St. John's wort, valerian, and vitamins B_3, D, and K.

Pritikin diet: a low-fat diet that emphasizes consumption of foods with a large volume of fiber and water, including vegetables, fruits, beans, and natural, unprocessed grains. *See also* Atkins diet; diet-based therapy; Ornish diet; South Beach diet.

probiotic: a live microorganism that is a "friendly" bacterium; similar to microorganisms normally found in the human digestive tract and that may have beneficial effects; available in foods (such as yogurts) and as a dietary supplement. *See also* prebiotic.

progesterone: a natural substance of the human body used as a dietary supplement synthesized from chemicals found in soy or Mexican yam; used as a replacement for standard progestins, substances similar to progesterone (a female hormone) that are more easily absorbed. *See also* estrogen; phytoestrogen.

progressive muscle relaxation: an alternative technique that promotes physiologic relaxation and reduced stress by systematically tensing and relaxing major muscle groups of the body.

prolotherapy: an alternative treatment involving injections of chemical irritant solutions into the area around a loose ligament.

prostatitis: a medical condition marked by inflammation of the prostate.

protease inhibitor: any of a class of pharmaceuticals used to treat or prevent infection by viruses, including the human immunodeficiency virus (HIV) and the hepatitis C virus; interactions with garlic, glutamine, grapefruit juice, milk thistle, St. John's wort, and vitamin C.

protein: a building block of life, necessary for the body to repair and maintain itself.

proteolytic enzyme: a natural substance of the human body and of plants that is primarily used as a supplement to provide support after surgery and to treat dyspepsia, neck pain and other forms of chronic musculoskeletal pain, osteoarthritis, pancreatic insufficiency, shingles (herpes zoster), and sports injuries.

proton pump inhibitor: a pharmaceutical used to reduce levels of stomach acid; interactions with folate, minerals, St. John's wort, and vitamin B_{12}.

provings: in homeopathy, remedies are chosen according to a detailed list of symptoms sometimes called a symptom picture; these lists are developed through provings, more formally called homeopathic pathogenic trials. *See also* homeopathy; symptom picture.

pseudoscience: a claim that exhibits the superficial appearance of science but lacks its substance. *See also* evidence-based medicine; scientific method.

psoriasis: a skin condition that leads to an intensely itchy rash with clearly defined borders and scales.

pulse diagnosis: an alternative technique used in Asian acupuncture and herbal medicine to assess a person's state of health.

pumpkin seed: a natural food product promoted as a dietary supplement primarily to treat benign prostatic hyperplasia.

pygeum: a natural plant product primarily used to treat benign prostatic hyperplasia but also used to treat impotence, male infertility, and prostatitis.

pyruvate: a natural substance of the human body used as a supplement to enhance weight loss.

qi: in traditional Chinese medicine, the life energy said to animate the body.

qigong: a group of alternative techniques that uses various breathing exercises, mental focus, and gentle physical postures.

quercetin: a natural plant product widely marketed as a treatment for allergic conditions such as asthma, hay fever, eczema, and hives.

radionics: an alternative therapy involving the detection of vital energy patterns from physical matter that are unique to each person, used to diagnose disease and promote healing.

raw foods diet: a vegan diet consisting of uncooked vegetables and fruits, nuts, seeds, and sprouted grains and beans.

Raynaud's phenomenon: a medical condition in which the fingers and toes are extra-sensitive to cold.

recommended daily intake (RDI): the amounts of nutrients people should consume daily, which vary by age and gender; determined by the U.S. Food and Drug Administration.

red clover: an herb promoted to help relieve menopausal hot flashes and other menopausal symptoms.

red raspberry: a natural plant product promoted to prevent complications of pregnancy.

red tea: a natural plant product consumed as a medicinal tea for allergy treatments, cancer prevention, dyspepsia, eczema, infantile colic, insomnia, minor injuries, and warts; also consumed to prevent liver damage.

red yeast rice: a traditional Chinese herbal product used to treat high cholesterol.

reflexology: an alternative therapeutic method of relieving pain and tension by stimulating predefined pressure points on the feet and hands by the use of finger pressure.

Reiki: an alternative type of spiritual healing that involves holding hands in certain positions over parts of the body to transmit qi and improve energy flow trough the body.

reishi: a natural plant product, a tree fungus, with a long history in Asian herbal medicine; primarily used as an adaptogen to improve resistance to stress.

relaxation response: an alternative technique involving a self-induced, peaceful, relaxed mental state.

relaxation therapy: an alternative technique that is claimed to reduce everyday stress.

repetitive transcranial magnetic stimulation (rTMS): an alternative therapy that involves the application of low-frequency magnetic pulses to the brain. *See also* transcutaneous electrical nerve stimulation.

restless legs syndrome: a medical condition in which one feels an intense urge to move one's legs, especially when sitting still or when trying to sleep.

resveratrol: a natural antioxidant found in red wine that is promoted as being able to prevent heart disease and cancer.

retinitis pigmentosa: a progressive eye disease that leads to impaired night vision, decreased peripheral vision, or decreased central and color vision.

reverse transcriptase inhibitor: any of a class of pharmaceuticals used to interfere with actions of the human immunodeficiency virus (HIV); interactions with coenzyme Q_{10} and St. John's wort.

rheumatoid arthritis: a disease in which the immune system attacks tissues in the body, especially cartilage in the joints. *See also* osteoarthritis.

Rhodiola rosea: an herb primarily used as an adaptogen to enhance mental function, reduce fatigue, and improve sports performance.

rhubarb: a natural plant whose root contains a substance with estrogen-like properties; extracts are used to treat menopausal symptoms.

ribose: a natural substance of the human body used to improve exercise tolerance in people with angina; also used to enhance performance in high-intensity anaerobic exercise, such as sprinting.

rifampin: a pharmaceutical used with isoniazid for the treatment of tuberculosis; interaction with vitamin D.

rolfing: an alternative therapy involving vigorous deep-tissue massage that is designed to improve the body's overall skeletal structure and posture through collagen integration.

rosacea: a chronic medical condition of the skin that primarily affects the face.

rose hip: a natural plant product used as an extra source of vitamin C and bioflavonoids.

rosemary: a natural plant product used to treat dyspepsia and, as rosemary oil, to treat joint pain and poor circulation.

royal jelly: an alternative medicine and a nutritional supplement made of a thick, whitish substance that is secreted from a gland of the nurse bee, a young worker bee.

rTMS: *See* repetitive transcranial magnetic stimulation.

SAD: *See* seasonal affective disorder.

saffron: an herbal product promoted as a dietary supplement primarily to treat depression.

sage: a natural plant product primarily used to treat dyspepsia, excessive perspiration (hyperhidrosis), and sore throat.

Salacia oblonga: a natural plant product with a long history of use in Ayurvedic medicine; primarily used to treat diabetes.

salt bush: a natural plant product used to treat type 2 diabetes.

SAMe (S-adenosylmethionine): a natural substance composed of methionine, a sulfur-containing amino acid, and adenosine triphosphate (ATP), the body's main energy molecule; used to treat depression, osteoarthritis, fibromyalgia, and other conditions.

sandalwood: a natural tree product used, in its oil form, as a treatment for bladder infections.

sarsaparilla: a natural plant product promoted as an antifungal and anti-inflammatory, as a cancer preventive, as a treatment for menstrual disorders and sexual dysfunction, and as an enhancer of sports and fitness performance.

sassafras: a natural plant product formerly used to treat influenza and other fever-producing infections, as well as arthritis, urinary tract infections, and digestive disorders; it is toxic to the liver and should not be used.

saw palmetto: a natural plant product whose oil is used to treat benign prostatic hyperplasia.

scar tissue: the fibrous tissue that naturally forms after surgery, disease, or a wound to the skin.

schisandra: a natural plant product with a long history of use in the traditional medicines of Russia and China; believed to prevent cancer, enhance mental function and sports performance, treat hepatitis, and protect the liver.

schizophrenia: a medical condition marked by severe disorder of the brain's structure and chemistry.

sciatica: an often chronic medical condition marked by irritation of the major nerve that extends from the lower spine to the lower buttocks, legs, and feet and often causes severe pain.

scientific method: a formal method to determine truth that involves the elements of laws, hypotheses, experiments, and theories. *See also* double-blind, placebo-controlled study; evidence-based medicine; placebo effect; pseudoscience.

scleroderma: a medical condition that affects the connective tissues of the skin and various organs.

sea buckthorn: a natural plant product used to prevent colds and heart disease, to treat stomach ulcers, and to reduce the side effects of cancer treatment.

seasonal affective disorder (SAD): a form of clinical depression that is most prominent in the late fall and winter months.

seborrheic dermatitis: a medical condition marked by inflammation of the upper layers of the skin.

sedative drugs: a chemical substance, often a pharmaceutical, that induces tiredness.

selective serotonin reuptake inhibitor: *See* SSRI.

selenium: a natural substance essential for health and promoted, especially, to prevent cancer.

self-hypnosis: *See* hypnotherapy.

senna: a natural plant product used to treat constipation.

shaman: a traditional healer. *See also* curandero; folk medicine; Native American healer; traditional healing.

shark cartilage: *See* cartilage.

shiatsu: an alternative technique in which a practitioner applies pressure to specific points on the body to balance the body's flow of energy.

shiitake: a natural product of a mushroom believed to prevent cancer, to provide cancer treatment support and immune support, and to treat genital warts.

shingles: a painful and acute skin infection and continuing irritation of the nerves that develops years after a person has had chickenpox.

sho-saiko-to: an herbal combination with a long history in Chinese medicine; primarily used to treat chronic hepatitis and other liver conditions.

sickle cell disease: an inherited blood disorder characterized by anemia, clogged blood vessels, and organ and tissue damage.

silica hydride: a natural substance combination used as a dietary supplement for disease prevention and general well-being.

silicon: a natural elemental substance used to treat aging skin, brittle hair, and brittle nails.

silver: a natural mineral substance with a long history of use in Ayurvedic medicine; once promoted in the West as an antiseptic; its use should be avoided.

sinusitis: *See* allergy.

Sjögren's syndrome: a medical condition in which the immune system destroys moisture-producing glands.

skullcap: an herb primarily used as a sedative.

slippery elm: a natural plant product with a long history of use in Native American medicine; used to treat cough, dyspepsia, gastroesophageal reflux, gastritis, hemorrhoids, inflammatory bowel disease, and irritable bowel syndrome.

South Beach diet: a diet that distinguishes between "good" and "bad" carbohydrates and fats and that encourages the consumption of whole-grain foods and large amounts of vegetables. *See also* Atkins diet; carbohydrate; cholesterol; HDL cholesterol; LDL cholesterol; Pritikin diet.

soy: a natural food product from the soybean promoted as a dietary supplement primarily to treat high cholesterol.

spinal manipulation: an alternative technique in which a controlled force is applied to a joint of the spine to move that joint beyond its passive range of motion; practiced by chiropractors, osteopaths, and others. *See also* chiropractic care; massage therapy; osteopathic manipulation.

spirituality: a life philosophy that claims the healing power of the transcendent.

spirulina: a natural plant product comprising one or more members of a family of blue-green algae; primarily used as a nutritional support.

spleen extract: a natural substance derived from non-human animals and used as a supplement to strengthen the immune system.

SSRI (selective serotonin reuptake inhibitor): a class of pharmaceuticals used to treat depression and a variety of other conditions; interactions with ephedra, fish oil, 5-HTP, folate, ginkgo, St. John's wort, and SAMe.

St. John's wort: a common herb primarily used to treat mild to moderate depression.

stanols and sterols: a group of natural substances promoted as dietary supplements to reduce high cholesterol. *See also* cholesterol.

statins: a group of pharmaceutical drugs used to improve the body's cholesterol profile; interactions with chaparral, Chinese skullcap, coenzyme Q_{10}, coltsfoot, comfrey, fish oil, grapefruit juice, pomegranate, red yeast rice, St. John's wort, and vitamin B_3. *See also* cholesterol.

stevia: a natural plant product used to sweeten foods and beverages and believed to benefit persons with diabetes and hypertension.

strep throat: a throat infection caused by the bacterium *Streptococcus*.

stroke: a medical condition marked by cell death in the brain; caused by a sudden loss of blood supply. *See also* hypertension.

strontium: a natural substance believed to reduce the incidence of fractures caused by osteoporosis.

sublingual immunotherapy: an alternative treatment of allergies involving the placement of an allergen solution, such as pollen extract, under the tongue.

sulforaphane: a natural chemical found in broccoli sprouts and other cabbage-family vegetables; used to help prevent cancer.

suma: a natural plant product with a long history of use in indigenous medicine; used as an adaptogen to help the body adapt to stress and fight infection.

sunburn: a medical condition marked by burns to the skin; caused by overexposure to the sun.

superoxide dismutase: a natural substance of the human body used to control levels of a chemical called superoxide, which the body manufactures to kill bacteria; excess levels of superoxide can injure healthy cells.

supplement: a dietary additive, such as a vitamin, used to promote health.

sweet clover: a natural plant product whose extract is used to treat symptoms of venous insufficiency, a condition related to varicose veins, and to treat phlebitis and hemorrhoids.

swimmer's ear: an inflammatory medical condition of the external ear canal; commonly caused by a bacterial infection.

symptom picture: in homeopathy, a detailed list of symptoms; these lists are developed through provings. *See also* homeopathy; provings.

Tai Chi: an alternative technique that uses gentle movements to strengthen and balance the body's energy.

tamoxifen: a pharmaceutical that blocks the actions of estrogen and produces some estrogen-like actions; used to prevent and treat breast cancer; interactions with soy isoflavones and tangeretin. *See also* estrogen; phytoestrogen.

tannin: a natural substance that can relieve pain.

tardive dyskinesia: a medical condition marked by mostly uncontrollable bodily movements; caused by side effects of pharmaceuticals used to control schizophrenia and other psychoses.

taurine: a natural substance (an amino acid) of the human body that is used as a supplement primarily to treat congestive heart failure and viral hepatitis.

tea: *See* black tea; green tea; kombucha tea; red tea.

tea tree oil: a natural plant product used externally as an antibacterial or antifungal treatment to treat acne, athlete's foot, nail fungus, and wounds.

temporomandibular joint syndrome (TMJ) syndrome: a chronically painful medical condition marked by inflamed joints of the lower jaw.

tendonitis: a medical condition marked by tendon inflammation.

TENS: *See* transcutaneous electrical nerve stimulation.

tetracycline: an antibiotic used to treat certain infections, such as chlamydia, and to treat acne on a long-term basis; interactions with citrate, dong quai, minerals, and St. John's wort.

therapeutic touch: an alternative technique involving the placement of hands just above a person's body to promote healing.

thiazide diuretic: a commonly used pharmaceutical for treating hypertension; interactions with calcium, coenzyme Q_{10}, licorice, magnesium, potassium, and zinc.

thymus extract: a natural substance from nonhuman animals that is used as a supplement to stimulate or normalize immunity.

thyroid hormone: a supplement used to treat hypothyroidism, a condition caused by deficient secretion of thyroid hormone by the thyroid gland.

Tiger Balm: a topical ointment that contains the aromatic substances camphor, menthol, cajaput, and clove oil, making it a form of aromatherapy; a popular remedy for headaches, muscle pain, and other conditions.

Time to Talk campaign: a U.S. government educational campaign promoting patient and practitioner dialogue about the use of complementary and alternative medicine.

tinnitus: a medical condition marked by chronic ringing or other sounds in the ear.

Tinospora cordifolia: a natural plant product with a long history of use in Ayurvedic medicine; used as a dietary supplement primarily to treat allergic rhinitis, or hay fever.

TMJ: *See* temporomandibular joint syndrome.

tocotrienol: a natural plant substance related to vitamin E; used as an antioxidant. *See also* antioxidant.

tongue diagnosis: an alternative diagnostic technique involving a visual inspection of the tongue.

traditional Chinese herbal medicine: a holistic healing method using herbal combinations tailored to the individual according to complex principles.

traditional healing: an alternative technique marked by holistic indigenous practices to prevent disease and illness and to promote health and healing. *See also* folk medicine.

Trager therapy: an alternative movement therapy in which practitioners apply a series of gentle, rhythmic rocking movements to the joints. *See also* massage therapy; osteopathic manipulation.

tramadol: a non-narcotic and non-anti-inflammatory analgesic medication used to treat moderate pain; interactions with 5-HTP, St. John's wort, and SAMe.

Transcendental Meditation: an alternative technique for relaxing the mind and body through the repetition of a mantra, or a sound without meaning.

transcutaneous electrical nerve stimulation (TENS): an alternative therapy primarily used in the treatment of muscular pain.

Tribulus terrestris: a natural plant product with a long history of traditional medical use in China, India, and Greece; used to enhance sports performance.

tricyclic antidepressant: any of a class of antidepressant medications mostly superseded by selective serotonin reuptake inhibitors (SSRIs); interactions with coenzyme Q_{10}, 5-HTP, St. John's wort, SAMe, and yohimbe.

triglyceride: a component of a group of fat-related substances called lipids; an increase in levels of certain lipids (a condition called hyperlipidemia) contributes to heart disease.

trimethylglycine: a natural substance of the human body used as a supplement to reduce homocysteine levels and improve health among persons with the rare disease cystathionine beta-synthase deficiency.

Tripterygium wilfordii: a natural plant product with a long history of use in traditional Chinese herbal medicine; used primarily to treat rheumatoid arthritis.

turmeric: an herb in the ginger family used as a food spice and as a dietary supplement to treat dyspepsia.

tylophora: a natural plant product primarily used to treat asthma, but also allergies, bronchitis, and the common cold.

tyrosine: a natural substance (an amino acid) of the human body used as a supplement to treat attention deficit disorder, depression, fatigue, and jet lag, and to enhance sports performance and mental function.

ulcer: a "hole" in the tissue of the stomach and duodenum caused by stomach acid.

ulcerative colitis: a medical condition marked by inflammation of the digestive tract.

Unani medicine: the alternative medical practice of balancing defined humors, or components, of the blood to sustain good health.

urinary tract infection: a medical condition marked by infection in the urinary system, which consists of the kidneys, ureters, bladder, and urethra.

uveitis: a medical condition marked by inflammation of the uvea, the middle layer of the tissues surrounding the eyeball.

valerian: an herb primarily used to treat insomnia.

valproic acid: a commonly used traditional anticonvulsant treatment; interactions with biotin, carnitine, dong quai, folate, ginkgo, glutamine, melatonin, St. John's wort, vitamin A, vitamin D, and white willow.

varicose veins: a medical condition that causes damage to veins that are near the surface of the skin. *See also* venous insufficiency.

vega test: an alternative technique that measures the body's electrical resistance at acupuncture points. *See also* acupuncture.

vegan diet: an alternative diet that excludes meat, fish, eggs, honey, and dairy products.

vegetarian diet: an alternative diet that avoids the consumption of meats.

venous insufficiency: a medical condition marked by pooling of fluid in the legs. *See also* varicose veins.

vertigo: a medical condition marked by dizziness accompanied by the sense of movement. *See also* motion sickness.

vervain: an herb with a long history of use in Celtic religious tradition; used to increase the flow of breast milk.

vinpocetine: a natural plant product used to treat Alzheimer's disease and other forms of dementia.

vitamin A: a fat-soluble antioxidant believed to reduce deaths from measles and other infectious illnesses among children in developing countries.

vitamin B complex (vitamins B$_1$, B$_2$, B$_3$, B$_6$, and B$_{12}$): a class of water-soluble organic compounds necessary for human cell metabolism.

vitamin C (ascorbic acid): a natural substance essential for human health and promoted as a dietary supplement; found in some foods; acts in the body as an antioxidant, helping to protect cells from the damage caused by free radicals; also necessary to make collagen, a protein required to help wounds heal; improves the absorption of iron from plant-based foods and helps the immune system work properly to protect the body from disease.

vitamin D: a natural, essential vitamin and hormone; it is a vitamin because the body cannot absorb calcium without it, and it is a hormone because the body manufactures it in response to the skin's exposure to sunlight.

vitamin E: an antioxidant that fights damaging natural substances known as free radicals; works in lipids (fats and oils), which makes it complementary to vitamin C, which fights free radicals dissolved in water.

vitamin K: an organic compound that plays a major role in the body's blood clotting system.

vitiligo: a skin disease that destroys pigment-making cells.

warfarin: an anticoagulant drug used to thin the blood and prevent it from clotting; interactions with alfalfa, bromelain, chamomile, chondroitin, coenzyme Q$_{10}$, cranberry, danshen, devil's claw, dong quai, feverfew, garlic, ginger, ginkgo, ginseng, green tea, ipriflavone, papain, PC-SPES, policosanol, reishi, royal jelly, St. John's wort, soy, vinpocetine, vitamin A, vitamin C, vitamin E, vitamin K, and white willow.

wart: a medical condition marked by benign skin growth; caused by a viral infection.

wheatgrass juice: a natural plant product primarily used to treat ulcerative colitis and to provide general nutrition.

whey protein: a natural substance promoted as a dietary supplement to raise levels of the antioxidant glutathione in the body.

white willow: a natural plant product long used in Chinese medicine to treat back pain, bursitis, dysmenorrhea, migraine headaches, musculoskeletal pain, osteoarthritis, rheumatoid arthritis, tendonitis, and tension headaches.

whole medicine: an alternative medicine that takes into account the whole person instead of only the specific disease, illness, or condition; also called holistic medicine.

wild cherry: an herb used to treat coughs.

wild indigo: a natural plant product used in combination with echinacea and white cedar for immune support and to treat chronic bronchitis, colds, and flu.

wild yam: a natural plant product erroneously thought to contain female hormones, such as progesterone and dehydroepiandrosterone, or DHEA.

witch hazel: a natural plant product traditionally used by indigenous peoples of North America; now used to relieve pain, stop bleeding, control itching, and reduce symptoms of eczema, and to treat muscle aches, hemorrhoids, diarrhea, inflammation of the gums, canker sores, and varicose veins.

wolfberry: a natural plant product with a long history of use in traditional Chinese herbal medicine; used mainly for nutrition, as it contains relatively high levels of numerous vitamins and minerals.

wormwood: a natural plant product used as a dietary supplement to treat digestive conditions such as intestinal parasites, dyspepsia, gastroesophageal reflux, and irritable bowel syndrome.

xylitol: a natural sugar found in plums, strawberries, and raspberries; used as a sweetener in some sugarless gums and candies and believed to prevent cavities by inhibiting the growth of bacteria.

yarrow: an herbal product used, as a tea, to induce sweating and prevent a cold or flu; crushed yarrow leaves and flower tops are also applied directly as first aid to stop nosebleeds and bleeding from minor wounds.

yeast hypersensitivity syndrome: *See* candida.

yellow dock: a natural plant product that contains chemicals called anthroquinones that stimulate bowel movements.

Yerba santa: a natural plant product used to treat asthma, bronchitis, common cold, poison ivy, and rashes.

yerbera: a traditional medicine practitioner with knowledge of the medicinal qualities of plants. *See also* folk medicine; herbal medicine; Native American healer; traditional healing.

yin and yang: the Chinese concept of two opposing yet complementary forces; yin represents the cold, slow, or passive principle, while yang represents the hot, excited, or active principle; according to traditional Chinese medicine, health is achieved by maintaining the body in a balanced state, and disease is caused by an internal imbalance of yin and yang.

yoga: an alternative form of physical and mental exercise based on body postures, stretching, breathing, meditation, introspection, and other techniques. *See also* Pilates.

yohimbe: a natural plant product used to treat impotence.

yucca: a natural plant product used to treat osteoarthritis and rheumatoid arthritis.

zinc: a natural substance of the human body used as a supplement to treat colds and macular degeneration and to provide general nutrition.

Zone diet: a diet consisting of a small amount of low-fat protein, fats, and fiber-rich fruits and vegetables. *See also* Atkins diet; fats, dietary; Pritikin diet; protein; South Beach diet.

Desiree Dreeuws

Homeopathic Remedies for Selected Conditions and Applications

Acetic acid
Surgery support

Aconite
Sports injuries
Surgery support

Aconitum
Common cold

Aconitum napellus
Ear infections
Surgery support

Aesculus
Hemorrhoids

Ambra grisea
Vertigo

Antimonium crudum
Warts

Apis mellifica
Rheumatoid arthritis

Arnica
Bruises
Common cold
Head injury
Sports injuries
Stroke
Surgery support
Venous insufficiency

Arnica montana
Childbirth support
Fibromyalgia
Sports injuries

Arsenicum
Diarrhea

Arsenicum album
Cancer chemotherapy support

Artemisia cina
Common cold

Asafoetida
Irritable bowel syndrome (IBS)

Asclepias vincetoxicum and sulphur
Asthma

Aurum
High blood pressure

Baryta carbonica
High blood pressure

Belladonna
Bladder infections
Breast engorgement
Childbirth support
Common cold
Ear infections
Migraines
Radiation therapy support
Sports injuries
Stroke

Bellis perennis
Sports injuries
Surgery support

Berberis vulgaris
Bladder infections
Rheumatoid arthritis

Bryonia
Breast engorgement
Rheumatoid arthritis
Fibromyalgia

Bryonia cretica
Rheumatoid arthritis

Calcarea carbonica
Osteoarthritis
Premenstrual syndrome (PMS)
Rheumatoid arthritis
Venous insufficiency
Warts

Calcarea fluorica
Osteoarthritis
Rheumatoid arthritis

Calendula
Minor burns
Sports injuries
Surgery support

Cantharis
Bladder infections
Minor burns

Carbo vegetabilis
Surgery support
Tinnitus

Caulophyllum
Childbirth support

Causticum
Rheumatoid arthritis
Warts

Chamomilla
Diarrhea
Premenstrual syndrome (PMS)
Sports injuries

China regia
Surgery support

Chininum sulphuricum
Tinnitus

Cimicifuga
Childbirth support

Cocculus
Vertigo

Collinsonia
Hemorrhoids

Colocynthis
Irritable bowel syndrome (IBS)

Conium
Vertigo

Cuprum
Common cold

Cyclamen
Migraines

Drosera
Common cold

Echinacea
Insect bites and stings

Echinacea angustifolia
Sports injuries

Echinacea purperea
Sports injuries

Equisetum
Bladder infections

Eupatorium perfoliatum
Common cold

Euphorbium
Hay fever

Euphrasia
Common cold

Ferrosi phosphas
Common cold

Ferrum phosphoricum
Ear infections

Galphimia glauca
Hay fever

Gelsemium
Migraines
Stroke

Graphites
Tinnitus

Hamamelis
Hemorrhoids
Sports injuries
Venous insufficiency

Hepar sulphuris calcareum
Sports injuries

Homeopathic cough syrup
Common cold

Homeopathic mouthwash
Cancer chemotherapy support

Human growth hormone
General health and well-being

Hypericum
Sports injuries
Surgery support

Ignatia
Migraines

Isopathic remedies
Hay fever
Insect bites and stings

Kali carbonicum
Osteoarthritis

L52
Flu

Lachesis
Common cold
High blood pressure
Migraines

Ledum
Insect bites and stings
Surgery support

Ledum palustre
Osteoarthritis
Radiation therapy support
Rheumatoid arthritis

Lycopodium
Gastritis
Irritable bowel syndrome (IBS)

Mercurius solubilis
Cancer chemotherapy support
Sports injuries

Millefolium
Sports injuries

Natrum muriaticum
Migraines
Warts

Natrum sulph
Head injury

Nitricum acidum
Hemorrhoids
Warts

Nux vomica
Gastritis

Opium
Surgery support

Oscillococcinum
Flu

Petroleumm
Vertigo

Phosphorus
Common cold
Surgery support

Phytolacca
Common cold

Plantago
Surgery support

Podophyllum
Diarrhea

Pulsatilla
Ear infections
Gastritis
Premenstrual syndrome (PMS)

Raphanus
Surgery support

Raphanus sativus niger
Surgery support

Rhus tox
Fibromyalgia
Osteoarthritis
Sports injuries

Rhus toxicodendron
Osteoarthritis
Rheumatoid arthritis
Sports injuries

Sarcolactic acid
Sports injuries

Sepia
Warts

Silicea
Migraines

Solidago
Common cold

Staphysagria
Bladder infections
Surgery support
Warts

Strychnos nux vomica
Rheumatoid arthritis

Sulphur
Cancer chemotherapy support
Migraines
Radiation therapy support
Warts

Symphytum
Sports injuries

Symphytum officinale
Osteoarthritis

Thuja occidentalis
Warts

Uragoga ipecacuanha
Common cold

Urtica
Insect bites and stings

Bibliography

GENERAL

Albright, Peter. *The Complete Book of Complementary Therapies: The Best Known Alternative Therapies to Relieve Everyday Ailments.* London: Quarto, 1997.

Anderson, John W., Larry Trivieri, and Burton Goldberg, *Alternative Medicine: The Definitive Guide.* 2d ed. Berkeley, Calif.: Celestial Arts, 2002.

Andrews, Synthia, and Bobbi Dempsey. *Acupressure and Reflexology for Dummies.* Hoboken, N.J.: Wiley, 2007.

Audette, Joseph F., and Allison Bailey, eds. *Integrative Pain Medicine: The Science and Practice of Complementary and Alternative Medicine in Pain Management.* Totowa, N.J.: Humana Press, 2008.

Bharadvaj, Daivati. *Natural Treatments for Chronic Fatigue Syndrome.* Westport, Conn.: Praeger, 2007.

Bivins, Roberta E. *Alternative Medicine? A History.* New York: Oxford University Press, 2010.

Cassileth, Barrie R. *The Alternative Medicine Handbook: The Complete Reference Guide to Alternative and Complementary Therapies.* New York: W. W. Norton, 1999.

Colquhoun, David. *Alternative Medicine in UK Universities.* Charlottesville, Va.: Societas, 2008.

"Complementary and Alternative Medicine." In *Current Medical Diagnosis and Treatment 2011,* edited by Stephen J. McPhee and Maxine A. Papadakis. 50th ed. New York: McGraw-Hill Medical, 2011.

Cooper, Edwin L., and Nobuo Yamaguchi, eds. *Complementary and Alternative Approaches to Biomedicine.* New York: Kluwer Academic/Plenum, 2004.

Creagan, Edward T., ed. *Mayo Clinic Book of Alternative Medicine: Making Alternative Therapies Part of Your Healthy Lifestyle.* New York: Time, 2007.

Credit, Larry P., Sharon G. Hartunian, and Margaret Nowak. *Relieving Sciatica: Everything You Need to Know About Using Complementary Medicine.* Garden City Park, N.Y.: Avery, 2000.

_____. *Your Guide to Alternative Medicine: Understanding, Locating, and Selecting Holistic Treatments and Practitioners.* Garden City Park, N.Y.: Square One, 2003.

Crook, William. *Nature's Own Candida Cure.* Summertown, Tenn.: Alive Books, 2002.

Cumming, Allan, Karen Simpson, and David Brown. *Complementary and Alternative Medicine: An Illustrated Color Text.* New York: Churchill Livingstone, 2006.

Davis, Carol M. *Complementary Therapies in Rehabilitation: Evidence for Efficacy in Therapy, Prevention, and Wellness.* 3d ed. Thorofare, N.J.: Slack, 2009.

Deatsman, Colleen. *Inner Power: Six Techniques for Increased Energy and Self-Healing.* Woodbury, Minn.: Llewellyn, 2005.

Ernst, Edzard, et al. *Oxford Handbook of Complementary Medicine.* New York: Oxford University Press, 2008.

Eskinazi, Daniel, ed. *What Will Influence the Future of Alternative Medicine? A World Perspective.* River Edge, N.J.: World Scientific, 2001.

Fontaine, Karen Lee. *Absolute Beginner's Guide to Alternative Medicine.* Indianapolis, Ind.: Sams, 2004.

Forciea, Bruce. *Unlocking the Healing Code: Discover the Seven Keys to Unlimited Healing Power.* Woodbury, Minn.: Llewellyn, 2007.

Goldberg, Burton, and Larry Trivieri, Jr. *Alternative Medicine Guide to Chronic Fatigue, Fibromyalgia, Environmental Illness, and Lyme Disease.* 2d ed. Berkeley, Calif.: Celestial Arts, 2004.

Goldstein, Mark A., Myrna Chandler Goldstein, and Larry Credit. *Your Best Medicine: From Conventional and Complementary Medicine.* Emmaus, Pa.: Rodale, 2009.

Goldstein, Robert S., et al., eds. *Integrating Complementary Medicine into Veterinary Practice.* Hoboken, N.J.: Wiley-Blackwell, 2008.

Gordon, James S. *Manifesto for a New Medicine: Your Guide to Healing Partnerships and the Wise Use of Alternative Therapies.* Reading, Mass.: Perseus Books, 1997.

Gottlieb, Bill. *Alternative Cures: More Than One Thousand of the Most Effective Natural Home Remedies.* New York: Ballantine Books, 2008.

_____ ed. *New Choices in Natural Healing: Over Eighteen Hundred of the Best Self-Help Remedies from the World of Alternative Medicine.* Emmaus, Pa.: Rodale Press, 1997.

Jacobs, Jennifer. *The Encyclopedia of Alternative Medicine: A Complete Family Guide to Complementary Therapies.* Boston: Journey Editions, 1996.

Johnston, Laurance. *Alternative Medicine and Spinal Cord Injury: Beyond the Banks of the Mainstream.* New York: Demos, 2006.

Kail, Konrad, Bobbi Lawrence, and Burton Goldberg. *Allergy Free: An Alternative Medicine Definitive Guide.* Tiburon, Calif.: AlternativeMedicine.com Books, 2000.

Klein, Ruth. *The De-stress Diva's Guide to Life: Seventy-seven Ways to Recharge, Refocus, and Organize Your Life.* Hoboken, N.J.: Wiley, 2008.

Luciani, Joseph J. *The Power of Self-Coaching: The Five Essential Steps to Creating the Life You Want.* Hoboken, N.J.: Wiley, 2004.

_____. *Reconnecting: A Self-Coaching Solution to Revive Your Love Life.* Hoboken, N.J.: Wiley, 2009.

Maniatis, Alice, Jean-François Hardy, and Phillipe van der Linden, eds. *Alternatives to Blood Transfusion in Transfusion Medicine.* 2d ed. Hoboken, N.J.: Wiley-Blackwell, 2010.

Meletis, Chris D. *Liberation from Allergies: Natural Approaches to Freedom and Better Health.* Santa Barbara, Calif.: ABC-CLIO, 2009.

Mitchell, Deborah R., and Paula Maas. *The Natural Health Guide to Headache Relief.* New York: Pocket Books, 1997.

Moser, Isabelle A., and Steve Solomon. *How and When to Be Your Own Doctor.* Boston: IndyPublish.com, 2010.

Murad, Howard. *The Water Secret: The Cellular Breakthrough to Look and Feel Ten Years Younger.* Hoboken, N.J.: Wiley, 2010.

Murray, Michael T., and Joseph E. Pizzorno. *Encyclopedia of Natural Medicine.* Rev. 2d ed. Boston: Little, Brown, 1999.

Natelson, Benjamin H. *Your Symptoms Are Real: What to Do When Your Doctor Says Nothing Is Wrong.* Hoboken, N.J.: John Wiley & Sons, 2007.

Newman, Robert Bruce, and Ruth L. Miller. *Calm Healing: Methods for a New Era of Medicine.* Berkeley, Calif.: North Atlantic Books, 2006.

Odiatu, Uche, and Kary Odiatu. *The Miracle of Health: Simple Solutions, Extraordinary Results.* Hoboken, N.J.: John Wiley & Sons, 2009.

Pagano, John O. A. *Healing Psoriasis: The Natural Alternative.* Hoboken, N.J.: John Wiley & Sons, 2008.

Pelletier, Kenneth R. *The Best Alternative Medicine.* New York: Simon & Schuster, 2007.

Pescatore, Fred. *The Allergy and Asthma Cure: A Complete Eight-Step Nutritional Program.* Hoboken, N.J.: Wiley, 2008.

Peters, David, and Anne Woodham. *Encyclopedia of Natural Healing.* London: DK, 2000.

Rees, Alan, ed. *The Complementary and Alternative Medicine Information Source Book.* Westport, Conn.: Oryx Press, 2001.

Rees, Dewi. *Death and Bereavement: The Psychological, Religious, and Cultural Interfaces.* Philadelphia: Whurr, 2001.

Robson, Terry, ed. *An Introduction to Complementary Medicine.* Crows Nest, N.S.W.: Allen & Unwin, 2003.

Roeder, Giselle. *Healing with Water: Kneipp Hydrotherapy at Home.* Vancouver, B.C.: Alive Books, 2002.

_____. *Sauna: The Hottest Way to Good Health.* Vancouver, B.C.: Alive Books, 2002.

Shealy, C. Norman. *The Complete Family Guide to Alternative Medicine: An Illustrated Encyclopedia of Natural Healing.* Boston: Element, 1996.

Smith, Alan E. *Unbreak Your Health: The Complete Guide to Complementary and Alternative Therapies.* Ann Arbor, Mich.: Loving Healing Press, 2009.

Trivieri, Larry, Jr., and John W. Anderson, eds. *Alternative Medicine: The Definitive Guide.* 2d ed. Berkeley, Calif.: Ten Speed Press, 2002.

Trudeau, Kevin. *More Natural "Cures" Revealed.* Elk Grove Village, Ill.: Alliance, 2010.

_____. *Natural Cures "They" Don't Want You to Know About.* Elk Grove Village, Ill.: Alliance, 2006.

Turner, John L., and Robert F. Spetzler. *Medicine, Miracles, and Manifestations: A Doctor's Journey Through the Worlds of Divine Intervention, Near-Death Experiences, and Universal Energy.* Franklin Lakes, N.J.: Career Press, 2009.

Weil, Andrew. *Natural Health, Natural Medicine: The Complete Guide to Wellness and Self-Care for Optimum Health.* Boston: Houghton Mifflin, 2004.

Whorton, James C. *Nature Cures: The History of Alternative Medicine in America.* New York: Oxford University Press, 2004.

Wider, Barbara, and Kate Boddy. *What Is Complementary and Alternative Medicine?* Charlottesville, Va.: Societas, 2008.

Wood, M. Sandra, and Lillian R. Brazin. *The Guide to Complementary and Alternative Medicine on the Internet.* New York: Haworth Press, 2003.

Yuan, Chun-Su, and Eric J. Bieber, eds. *Textbook of Complementary and Alternative Medicine.* New York: Parthenon, 2002.

Zollman, Catherine, Andrew J. Vickers, and Janet Richardson, eds. *ABC of Complementary Medicine.* 2d ed. Malden, Mass.: Blackwell, 2008.

Aging

Cowden, W. Lee, and Ferre Akbarpour. *Longevity: An Alternative Medicine Definitive Guide.* Tiburon, Calif.: AlternativeMedicine.com Books, 2001.

Kamhi, Ellen, and Eugene R. Zampierson. *Alternative Medicine Definitive Guide to Arthritis: Reverse Underlying Causes of Arthritis with Clinically Proven Alternative Therapies.* 2d ed. Berkeley, Calif.: Celestial Arts, 2006.

Mackenzie, Elizabeth R., and Birgit Rakel, eds. *Complementary and Alternative Medicine for Older Adults: A Guide to Holistic Approaches to Healthy Aging.* New York: Springer, 2006.

Watson, Ronald Ross. *Complementary and Alternative Therapies in the Aging Population.* Boston: Academic Press/Elsevier, 2009.

Wei, Jeanne, and Sue Levkoff. *Aging Well: The Complete Guide to Physical and Emotional Health.* Hoboken, N.J.: Wiley, 2001.

Weil, Andrew. *Healthy Aging: A Lifelong Guide to Your Physical and Spiritual Well-Being.* New York: Anchor Books, 2007.

CANCER

Alschuler, Lise, and Karolyn A. Gazella. *"Alternative Medicine" Magazine's Definitive Guide to Cancer: An Integrated Approach to Prevention, Treatment, and Healing.* Berkeley, Calif.: Celestial Arts, 2007.

American Cancer Society and David Rosenthal. *The American Cancer Society Complete Guide to Complementary and Alternative Cancer Therapies.* Atlanta: American Cancer Society Health Promotions, 2009.

Barraclough, Jennifer, ed, *Enhancing Cancer Care: Complementary Therapy and Support.* New York: Oxford University Press, 2007.

Bognar, David, and David Bonar. *Cancer: Increasing Your Odds for Survival: A Resource Guide for Integrating Mainstream, Alternative, and Complementary Therapies.* Alameda, Calif.: Hunter House, 1998.

Chamberlain, Jonathan. *Cancer Recovery Guide: Fifteen Alternative and Complementary Strategies for Restoring Health.* East Sussex, England: Clairview, 2008.

Diamond, W. John, and W. Lee Cowden. *Alternative Medicine Definitive Guide to Cancer.* Tiburon, Calif.: Future Medicine, 1997.

Hess, David J. *Can Bacteria Cause Cancer? Alternative Medicine Confronts Big Science.* New York: New York University Press, 2000.

Labriola, Dan. *Complementary Cancer Therapies: Combining Traditional and Alternative Approaches for the Best Possible Outcome.* Roseville, Calif.: Prima Health, 2000.

Lerner, Michael. *Choices in Healing: Integrating the Best of Conventional and Complementary Approaches to Cancer.* Cambridge, Mass.: MIT Press, 1996.

Simon, David. *Return to Wholeness: Embracing Body, Mind, and Spirit in the Face of Cancer.* Hoboken, N.J.: Wiley, 1999.

Tovey, Philip, John Chatwin, and Alex Broom. *Traditional, Complementary, and Alternative Medicine and Cancer Care: An International Analysis of Grassroots Integration.* New York: Routledge, 2007.

CHILDREN'S HEALTH

Culbert, Timothy P., ed. *Integrative Pediatrics.* New York: Oxford University Press, 2010.

Ditchek, Stuart, Andrew Weil, and Russell H. Greenfield. *Healthy Child, Whole Child: Integrating the Best of Conventional and Alternative Medicine to Keep Your Kids Healthy.* New York: HarperCollins, 2002.

Kemper, Kathi J. *The Holistic Pediatrician: A Pediatrician's Comprehensive Guide to Safe and Effective Therapies for the Twenty-five Most Common Ailments of Infants, Children, and Adolescents.* Rev. ed. New York: Quill, 2002.

Kurtz, Lisa A. *Understanding Controversial Therapies for Children with Autism, Attention Deficit Disorder, and Other Learning Disabilities: A Guide to Complementary and Alternative Medicine.* Philadelphia: Jessica Kingsley, 2008.

CHRONIC DISEASES AND CONDITIONS

Bailey, Eric J. *African American Alternative Medicine: Using Alternative Medicine to Prevent and Control Chronic Disease.* Westport, Conn.: Bergin and Garvey, 2002.

Bowling, Allen C. *Complementary and Alternative Medicine and Multiple Sclerosis.* New York: Demos Medical, 2006.

Broadhurst, C. Leigh. *Natural Relief from Asthma.* Vancouver, B.C.: Alive Books, 2002.

_____. *Prevent, Treat, and Reverse Diabetes.* Summertown, Tenn.: Alive Books, 2002.

Clark, Carolyn Chambers. *American Holistic Nurses' Association Guide to Common Chronic Conditions: Self-Care Options to Complement Your Doctor's Advice.* Hoboken, N.J.: Wiley, 2003.

Devinsky, Orrin, Stephen Schachter, and Steven Pacia, eds. *Complementary and Alternative Therapies for Epilepsy.* New York: Demos Medical, 2005.

Diamond, Suzanne. *Nature's Best Heart Medicine.* Vancouver, B.C.: Alive Books, 2004.

Guthrie, Diana W. *Alternative and Complementary Diabetes Care: How to Combine Natural and Traditional Therapies. Hoboken, N.J.: Wiley, 2000.

Horwitz, Randy, and Daniel Muller, eds. Integrative Rheumatology. New York: Oxford University Press, 2010.

Kennedy, John M., and Jason Jennings. The Fifteen Minute Heart Cure: The Natural Way to Release Stress and Heal Your Heart in Just Minutes a Day. Hoboken, N.J.: Wiley, 2010.

Lawton, Suzanne C. Asperger Syndrome: Natural Steps Toward a Better Life. Westport, Conn.: Praeger, 2007.

Mirchandani, Moti. Alternative and Complementary Therapies: Recondition Your Body and Feel Better—Reversing and Preventing Heart Disease. Helena, Mont.: Traderoute, 2007.

Stein, Richard A., and Mehmet C. Oz. Complementary and Alternative Cardiovascular Medicine: Clinical Handbook. Totowa, N.J.: Humana Press, 2004.

Vogel, John, and Mitchell Krucoff. Integrative Cardiology: Complementary and Alternative Medicine for the Heart. New York: McGraw-Hill, 2007.

Weintraub, Michael I., and Marc S. Micozzi. Alternative and Complementary Treatment in Neurologic Illness. New York: Churchill Livingstone, 2001.

CRITICISM AND DEBATE

Bausell, Barker. Snake Oil Science: The Truth About Complementary and Alternative Medicine. New York: Oxford University Press, 2009.

Bodeker, Gerard, and Gemma Burford. Traditional Complementary and Alternative Medicine: Policy and Public Health Perspectives. London: Imperial College Press, 2006.

Canter, Peter H. Vitalism and Other Pseudoscience in Alternative Medicine: The Retreat from Science. Charlottesville, Va.: Societas, 2008.

Carroll, Robert Todd. The Skeptic's Dictionary: A Collection of Strange Beliefs, Amusing Deceptions, and Dangerous Delusions. Hoboken, N.J.: Wiley, 2003.

Ernst, Edzard. Healing, Hype, or Harm? A Critical Analysis of Complementary or Alternative Medicine. Charlottesville, Va.: Societas, 2008.

Ernst, Edzard, and Simon Singh. Trick or Treatment: The Undeniable Facts About Alternative Medicine. New York: Norton, 2009.

Fitzpatrick, Michael. Reclaiming Compassion. Charlottesville, Va.: Societas, 2008.

Fontanarosa, Phil B. Alternative Medicine: An Objective Assessment. Chicago: American Medical Association, 2000.

Kelner, Merrijoy, and Beverly Wellman, eds. Complementary and Alternative Medicine: Challenge and Change. New York: Routledge, 2003.

Kirkaldy-Willis, W. H., and A. A. Swartz. Orthodox and Complementary Medicine: An Alliance for a Changing World. Berkeley, Calif.: North Atlantic Books, 2001.

Lejeune, Stephane. Why Is CAM So Popular? Charlottesville, Va.: Societas, 2008.

MacLachlan, Malcolm. Culture and Health: A Critical Perspective Towards Global Health. 2d ed. Hoboken, N.J.: Wiley, 2006.

_____, ed. Cultivating Health: Cultural Perspectives on Promoting Health. Hoboken, N.J.: Wiley, 2000.

Murcott, Toby. The Whole Story: Alternative Medicine on Trial? New York: Macmillan, 2006.

Polevoy, Terry. Chiropractic: Science, Religion, or Political Movement? Charlottesville, Va.: Societas, 2008.

Reisser, Paul C., Dale Mabe, and Robert Velarde. Examining Alternative Medicine: An Inside Look at the Benefits and Risks. Downers Grove, Ill.: Intervasity Press, 2001.

Rose, Leslie B., and Edzard Ernst. CAM and Politics. Charlottesville, Va.: Societas, 2008.

Rosenfeld, Isadore. Dr. Rosenfeld's Guide to Alternative Medicine: What Works, What Doesn't, and What's Right for You. New York: Ballantine Books, 1997.

Smit, Alta, et al. Introduction to Bioregulatory Medicine. New York: Thieme, 2009.

Thornton, Hazel. Patient Choice. Charlottesville, Va.: Societas, 2008.

DIET AND NUTRITION

Cheung, Peter C., ed. Mushrooms as Functional Foods. Hoboken, N.J.: Wiley, 2008.

Dales, Phyllis I., and Bruce Dales. Cranberry: The Cure for Common and Chronic Conditions. Vancouver, B.C.: Alive Books, 2002.

Davis, W. Marvin. Consumer's Guide to Dietary Supplements and Alternative Medicines. New York: Pharmaceutical Products Press, 2006.

Goldberg, Burton, and Editors of Alternative Medicine. Weight Loss: An Alternative Medicine Definitive Guide. Tiburon, Calif.: AlternativeMedicine.com Books, 2000.

Hutchens, Jerry. Total Cleansing: Learn the Secrets for Effective Detox. Summertown, Tenn.: Alive Books, 2008.

Kastner, J"rg. Chinese Nutrition Therapy: Dietetics in Traditional Chinese Medicine. New York: Thieme, 2009.

Miller, Sloane. *Allergic Girl: Adventures in Living Well with Food Allergies.* Hoboken, N.J.: Wiley, 2011.

Skypala, Isabel, and Carina Venter, eds. *Food Hypersensitivity: Diagnosing and Managing Food Allergies and Intolerance.* Hoboken, N.J.: Wiley-Blackwell, 2009.

Stanten, Michele. *Walk off Weight.* Emmaus, Pa.: Rodale, 2009.

Tannis, Allison. *Probiotic Rescue: How You Can Use Probiotics to Fight Cholesterol, Cancer, Superbugs, Digestive Complaints, and More.* Hoboken, N.J.: Wiley, 2008.

Torkos, Sherry. *Winning at Weight Loss: Proven Strategies Based on Diet, Exercise, and Supplements.* Hoboken, N.J.: Wiley, 2004.

2011 PDR for Nonprescription Drugs, Dietary Supplements, and Herbs. Toronto, Ont.: Thomson Health Care, 2010.

DRUG ALTERNATIVES

Balch, James, Mark Stengler, and Robin Young-Balch. *Prescription for Drug Alternatives: All-Natural Options for Better Health Without the Side Effects.* Hoboken, N.J.: Wiley, 2008.

Barceloux, Donald G. *Medical Toxicology of Natural Substances: Foods, Fungi, Medicinal Herbs, Plants, and Venomous Animals.* Hoboken, N.J.: Wiley, 2008.

Brahmachari, Goutam. *Handbook of Pharmaceutical Natural Products.* Hoboken, N.J.: Wiley-VCH, 2010.

Broadhurst, C. Leigh. *Health and Healing with Bee Products.* Vancouver, B.C.: Alive Books, 2000.

David, Thomas. *Miracle Medicines of the Rainforest: A Doctor's Revolutionary Work with Cancer and AIDS Patients.* Rochester, Vt.: Healing Arts Press, 1997.

Gursche, Siegfried. *Coconut Oil: Discover the Key to Vibrant Health.* Summertown, Tenn.: Alive Books, 2002.

_____. *Fantastic Flax: A Powerful Defense Against Cancer, Heart Disease, and Digestive Disorders.* Summertown, Tenn.: Alive Books, 2002.

Lee, Lita, et al. *The Enzyme Cure: An Alternative Medicine Guide.* Tiburon, Calif.: AlternativeMedicine.com Books, 2001.

Mindell, Earl, and Virginia L. Hopkins. *Prescription Alternatives: Hundreds of Safe, Natural, Prescription-Free Remedies to Restore and Maintain Your Health.* 4th ed. New York: McGraw-Hill, 2009.

Rister, Robert. *Healing Without Medication: A Comprehensive Guide to the Complementary Techniques Anyone Can Use to Achieve Real Healing.* Laguna Beach, Calif.: Basic Health, 2003.

2011 PDR for Nonprescription Drugs, Dietary Supplements, and Herbs. Toronto, Ont.: Thomson Health Care, 2010.

Van Straten, Michael. *Home Remedies: A Practical Guide to Common Ailments You Can Safely Treat at Home Using Conventional and Complementary Medicines.* New York: Marlow, 1998.

Zago, Father Romano. *Aloe Isn't Medicine, and Yet . . . It Cures!* Bloomington, Ind.: iUniverse, 2009.

EASTERN MEDICINE

Barnett, Libby, Maggie Babb, and Susan Davidson. *Reiki Energy Medicine: Bringing Healing Touch into Home, Hospital, and Hospice.* Rochester, Vt.: Healing Arts Press, 1996.

Chopra, Deepak, and David Simon. *The Seven Spiritual Laws of Yoga: A Practical Guide to Healing Body, Mind, and Spirit.* Hoboken, N.J.: Wiley 2004.

Elias, Jason, and Katherine Ketcham. *Chinese Medicine for Maximum Immunity: Understanding the Five Elemental Types for Health and Well-Being.* New York: Three Rivers Press, 1999.

Fan, Warner J-W. *Manual of Chinese Herbal Medicine: Principles and Practice for Easy Reference.* Boston: Shambhala, 2003.

Gerber, Richard. *A Practical Guide to Vibrational Medicine: Energy Healing and Spiritual Transformation.* New York: HarperCollins, 2001.

Maciocia, Giovanni. *The Foundations of Chinese Medicine: A Comprehensive Text for Acupuncturists and Herbalists.* 2d ed. New York: Churchill Livingstone/Elsevier, 2005.

_____. *The Psyche in Chinese Medicine: Treatment of Emotional and Mental Disharmonies with Acupuncture and Chinese Herbs.* New York: Churchill Livingstone/Elsevier, 2009.

Manz, Hedwig. *The Art of Cupping.* New York: Thieme, 2008.

Mayor, David F., and Marc S Micozzi, eds. *Energy Medicine East and West: A Natural History of Qi.* New York: Churchill Livingstone/Elsevier, 2011.

Reid, Daniel P. *Shambhala Guide to Traditional Chinese Medicine.* Boston: Shambhala, 1996.

Sharma, Hari M., and Christopher Clark. *Contemporary Ayurveda: Medicine and Research in Maharishi Ayurveda.* Philadelphia: Churchill Livingstone, 1997.

Sheikh, Anees A., and Katharina S. Sheikh. *Healing East and West: Ancient Wisdom and Modern Psychology.* Hoboken, N.J.: Wiley, 1996.

Tsang, Patricia. *Optimal Healing: A Guide to Traditional Chinese Medicine*. San Francisco: Balance for Health, 2008.

Yang, Yifan. *Chinese Herbal Medicines: Comparisons and Characteristics*. New York: Churchill Livingstone/Elsevier, 2009.

Yoga Journal and Timothy B. McCall. *Yoga as Medicine: The Yogic Prescription for Health and Healing*. New York: Bantam Bell, 2007.

Zhou, Jiaju, Guirong Xie, and Xinjian Yan. *Traditional Chinese Medicines: Molecular Structures, Natural Sources, and Applications*. 2d ed. Edited by G. W. A. Milne. Hoboken, N.J.: Wiley 2003.

ETHICS AND LAW

Baum, Michael, and Edzard Ernst. *Ethics and Complementary or Alternative Medicine*. Charlottesville, Va.: Societas, 2008.

Callahan, Daniel. *The Role of Complementary and Alternative Medicine: Accommodating Pluralism*. Hastings Center Studies in Ethics. Washington, D.C.: Georgetown University Press, 2004.

Cohen, Michael H. *Beyond Complementary Medicine: Legal and Ethical Perspectives on Health Care and Human Evolution*. Ann Arbor: University of Michigan Press, 2000.

_____. *Complementary and Alternative Medicine: Legal Boundaries and Regulatory Perspectives*. Baltimore: Johns Hopkins University Press, 1998.

_____. *Legal Issues in Alternative Medicine: A Guide for Clinicians, Hospitals, and Patients*. Victoria, B.C.: Trafford, 2006.

Garrow, John. *CAM in Court*. Charlottesville, Va.: Societas, 2008.

Humber, James M., and Robert F. Almeder, eds. *Alternative Medicine and Ethics*. Totowa, N.J.: Humana Press, 1998.

Jesson, Lucinda E., and Stacey A. Tovino. *Complementary and Alternative Medicine and the Law*. Durham, N.C.: Carolina Academic Press, 2010.

Russo, Ethan B., Fernando Ania, and John Crellin. *Professionalism and Ethics in Complementary and Alternative Medicine*. New York: Haworth Integrative Healing Press, 2001.

Snyder, Lois, ed. *Complementary and Alternative Medicine: Ethics, the Patient, and the Physician*. Totowa, N.J.: Humana Press, 2010.

FITNESS AND EXERCISE

Silver, Julie, and Christopher Morin. *Understanding Fitness: How Exercise Fuels Health and Fights Disease*. Westport, Conn.: Praeger, 2008.

Simon, David. *Vital Energy: The Seven Keys to Invigorate Body, Mind, and Soul*. Hoboken, N.J.: Wiley, 1999.

HERBAL MEDICINE

Al-Achi, Antoine. *An Introduction to Botanical Medicines: History, Science, Uses, and Dangers*. Westport, Conn.: Praeger, 2008.

Dasgupta, Amitava, and Catherine A. Hammett-Stabler, eds. *Herbal Supplements: Efficacy, Toxicity, Interactions with Western Drugs, and Effects on Clinical Laboratory Tests*. Hoboken, N.J.: Wiley, 2011.

Fetrow, Charles W., and Juan R. Avila. *The Complete Guide to Herbal Medicines*. New York: Pocket Books, 2000.

Hobbs, Christopher. *Herbal Remedies for Dummies*. Foster City, Calif.: IDG Books, 1998.

Meletis, Chris D., and Jason E. Barker. *Herbs and Nutrients for the Mind: A Guide to Natural Brain Enhancers*. Westport, Conn.: Praeger, 2004.

Morse, Nancy L. *Evening Primrose Oil: The Healing Power of the Yellow Flower for PMS, Menopause, Skin Problems, and More*. Vancouver, B.C.: Alive Books, 2002.

Mueller, Markus S., and Ernest Mechler. *Medicinal Plants in Tropical Countries: Traditional Use—Experience—Facts*. New York: Thieme, 2005.

Pinn, Graham. *Herbal Medicine: A Practical Guide for Medical Practitioners*. Malden, Mass.: Blackwell, 2003.

2011 PDR for Nonprescription Drugs, Dietary Supplements, and Herbs. Toronto, Ont.: Thomson Health Care, 2010.

White, B. Linda, and Steven Foster. *The Herbal Drugstore*. Emmaus, Pa.: Rodale Press, 2003.

HOLISM

Baum, Michael. *Concepts of Holism in Orthodox and Alternative Medicine*. Charlottesville, Va.: Societas, 2008.

Bendelow, Gillian. *Health, Emotion, and the Body*. Malden, Mass.: Polity Press, 2009.

Collinge, William. *The American Holistic Health Association Complete Guide to Alternative Medicine*. New York: Warner Books, 1997.

Kampner, T. Anthony. *Why Alternative Medicine and Why Now? A Primer on Holistic Medicine*. Victoria, B.C.: Trafford, 2006.

Rustum, Roy. *Science of Whole Person Healing*. Vol. 2. Edited by Meredith Weber. New York: iUniverse, 2004.

HOMEOPATHY

Birch, Kate. *Vaccine-Free Prevention and Treatment of Infectious Contagious Disease with Homeopathy*. 2d ed. Bloomington, Ind.: Trafford, 2007.

Kurz, Chris. *Imagine Homeopathy: A Book of Experiments, Images, and Metaphors*. New York: Thieme, 2005.

Shalts, Edward. *The American Institute of Homeopathy Handbook for Parents: A Guide to Healthy Treatment for Everything from Colds and Allergies to ADHD, Obesity, and Depression*. San Francisco: Jossey-Bass, 2005.

INDIGENOUS AND FOLK MEDICINE

De la Portilla, Elizabeth. *They All Want Magic: Curanderas and Folk Healing*. College Station: Texas A&M University Press, 2009.

Garrett, J. T., and Michael Tlanusta Garrett. *Medicine of the Cherokee: The Way of Right Relationship*. Santa Fe, N.Mex.: Bear, 1996.

Kayne, Stephen B., ed. *Traditional Medicine: A Global Perspective*. London: Pharmaceutical Press, 2010.

INTEGRATIVE MEDICINE

Benjamin, Samuel, and Doris Milton. *Complementary and Alternative Therapies: An Implementation Guide to Integrative Health Care*. Chicago: American Hospital Association, 1999.

Castleman, Michael. *Blended Medicine: How to Integrate the Best Mainstream and Alternative Remedies for Maximum Health and Healing*. Emmaus, Pa.: Rodale Press, 2002.

Elder, Charles, et al. "Integrating Herbs and Supplements in Managed Care: A Pharmacy Perspective." *Permanente Journal* 12, no. 3 (2008): 52-58.

Ernst, Edzard. *Integrated Medicine?* Charlottesville, Va.: Societas, 2008.

Galland, Leo. *Power Healing: Use the New Integrated Medicine to Cure Yourself*. New York: Random House, 1998.

Loo, May, ed. *Integrative Medicine for Children*. St. Louis, Mo.: Saunders/Elsevier, 2009.

Micozzi, Marc S., ed. *Fundamentals of Complementary and Alternative Medicine*. 4th ed. St. Louis, Mo.: Saunders/Elsevier, 2011.

Sierpina, Victor S. *Integrative Health Care: Complementary and Alternative Therapies for the Whole Person*. Philadelphia: F. A. Davis, 2001.

MEN'S HEALTH

Burnett, Arthur L., II, and Norman Morris. *Prostate Cancer Survivors Speak Their Minds: Advice on Options, Treatments, and Aftereffects*. Hoboken, N.J.: Wiley, 2010.

Meletis, Chris D., and Sara G. Wood. *His Change of Life: Male Menopause and Healthy Aging with Testosterone*. Westport, Conn.: Praeger, 2009.

Rona, Zoltan. *Boosting Male Libido Naturally: Natural Alternatives to Viagra*. Vancouver, B.C.: Alive Books, 2002.

MENTAL AND EMOTIONAL HEALTH

Baumel, Syd. *Dealing with Depression Naturally: Alternatives and Complementary Therapies for Restoring Emotional Health*. Los Angeles: Keats, 2000.

Brown, Richard P., Patricia L. Gerbarg, and Philip R. Muskin. *How to Use Herbs, Nutrients, and Yoga in Mental Health Care*. New York: W. W. Norton, 2009.

Engel, Beverly. *Healing Your Emotional Self: A Powerful Program to Help You Raise Your Self-Esteem, Quiet Your Inner Critic, and Overcome Your Shame*. Hoboken, N.J.: Wiley, 2007.

Fosha, Diana, Daniel J. Siegel, and Marion F. Solomon. *The Healing Power of Emotion: Affective Neuroscience, Development, and Clinical Practice*. New York: W. W. Norton, 2009.

Luciani, Joseph J. *Self-Coaching: How to Heal Anxiety and Depression*. Hoboken, N.J.: Wiley, 2002.

_____. *Self-Coaching: The Powerful Program to Beat Anxiety and Depression*. 2d rev. ed. Hoboken, N.J.: Wiley, 2006.

Marohn, Stephanie. *The Natural Medicine Guide to Bipolar Disorder*. Charlottesville, Va.: Hampton Roads, 2003.

_____. *The Natural Medicine Guide to Depression*. Charlottesville, Va.: Hampton Roads, 2003.

Maté, Gabor. *When the Body Says No: Understanding the Stress-Disease Connection*. Hoboken, N.J.: Wiley, 2011.

Schachter, Michael B., and Deborah R. Mitchell. *What Your Doctor May Not Tell You About Depression: The Breakthrough Integrative Approach for Effective Treatment*. New York: Warner Wellness, 2006.

Shannon, Scott. *Handbook of Complementary and Alternative Therapies in Mental Health*. San Diego, Calif.: Academic Press, 2001.

Mind/Body Medicine

Damasio, Antonio R. *The Feeling of What Happens: Body and Emotion in the Making of Consciousness.* San Diego, Calif.: Harcourt, 2000.

Harrington, Anne. *The Cure Within: A History of Mind-Body Medicine.* New York: W. W. Norton, 2008.

Liebler, Nancy, and Sandra Moss. *Healing Depression the Mind-Body Way: Creating Happiness with Meditation, Yoga, and Ayurveda.* Hoboken, N.J.: Wiley, 2009.

Peteet, John R., and Michael N D'Ambra, eds. *The Soul of Medicine: Spiritual Perspectives and Clinical Practice.* Baltimore: Johns Hopkins University Press, 2011.

Samuels, Michael. *Healing with the Mind's Eye: How to Use Guided Imagery and Visions to Heal Body, Mind, and Spirit.* Rev ed. Hoboken, N.J.: Wiley, 2003.

Practice and Research

Cuellar, Norma G. *Conversations in Complementary and Alternative Medicine.* Sudbury, Mass.: Jones and Bartlett, 2006.

Diamond, W. John. *The Clinical Practice of Complementary, Alternative, and Western Medicine.* New York: CRC Press, 2000.

Ernst, Edzard. *Placebo and Other Non-specific Effects: An Important Issue in CAM.* Charlottesville, Va.: Societas, 2008.

Ernst, Edzard, Max H. Pittler, and Barbara Wider, eds. *The Desktop Guide to Complementary and Alternative Medicine: An Evidence-Based Approach.* St. Louis, Mo.: Mosby/Elsevier, 2006.

Fetrow, Charles W., and Juan R. Avila. *Professional's Handbook of Complementary and Alternative Medicines.* 3d ed. Philadelphia: Lippincott Williams & Wilkins, 2004.

Freeman, Lyn. *Mosby's Complementary and Alternative Medicine: A Research-Based Approach.* 3d ed. St. Louis, Mo.: Mosby/Elsevier, 2009.

Hrobjarstsson, Asbjorn. *Research on Complementary and Alternative Medicine: The Importance and Frailty of Impartiality.* Charlottesville, Va.: Societas, 2008.

Jacobs, Bradly P., and Katherine Gundling. *The ACP Evidence-Based Guide to Complementary and Alternative Medicine.* Philadelphia: ACP Press, 2009.

Lee-Treweek, Geraldine, et al. *Complementary and Alternative Medicine: Structures and Safeguards.* New York: Routledge, 2006.

Leskowitz, Eric D., Marc S. Micozzi, and Jon Kabat-Zinn. *Complementary and Alternative Medicine in Rehabilitation.* St. Louis, Mo.: Churchill Livingstone, 2002.

Lewith, G. T., Wayne B. Jonas, and Harald Walach, eds. *Clinical Research in Complementary Therapies: Principles, Problems, and Solutions.* New York: Churchill Livingstone/Elsevier, 2011.

Lyons, Dianne Boulerice. *Planning Your Career in Alternative Medicine: A Guide to Degree and Certificate Programs in Alternative Healthcare.* Garden City Park, N.Y.: Avery, 2000.

Mantle, Fiona, and Denise Tiran. *A-Z of Complementary and Alternative Medicine: A Guide for Health Professionals.* New York: Churchill Livingstone/Elsevier, 2009.

McKone, W. Llewellyn. *Osteopathic Medicine: Philosophy, Principles, and Practice.* Malden, Mass.: Blackwell Science, 2001.

Nurse's Handbook of Alternative and Complementary Therapies. 2d ed. Philadelphia: Lippincott Williams & Wilkins, 2003.

O'Connor, Bonnie Blair. *Healing Traditions: Alternative Medicine and the Health Professions.* Philadelphia: University of Pennsylvania Press, 1995.

Rakel, David, and Nancy Faass. *Complementary Medicine in Clinical Practice.* Sudbury, Mass.: Jones and Bartlett, 2005.

Rees, Dewi. *Healing in Perspective.* Hoboken, N.J.: Wiley, 2005.

Rose, Leslie B. *Evidence in Healthcare: What It Is and How We Get It.* Charlottesville, Va.: Societas, 2008.

Roush, Robert A. *Complementary and Alternative Medicine: Clinic Design.* New York: Haworth Integrative Healing Press, 2003.

Sampson, Wallace, and Lewis Vaughn. *Science Meets Alternative Medicine: What the Evidence Says About Unconventional Treatments.* Amherst, N.Y.: Prometheus Books, 2000.

Seedhouse, David. *Health Promotion: Philosophy, Prejudice, and Practice.* 2d ed. Hoboken, N.J.: Wiley, 2004.

_____. *Total Health Promotion: Mental Health, Rational Fields, and the Quest for Autonomy.* Hoboken, N.J.: Wiley, 2002.

_____. *Values-Based Decision-Making for the Caring Professions.* Hoboken, N.J.: Wiley 2005.

Steiner, Rudolf, and Ita Wegman. *Extending Practical Medicine: Fundamental Principles Based on the Science of the Spirit.* London: Rudolf Steiner Press, 1997.

Stossier, Harald. *Treating Allergies with the F. X. Mayr-Cure: Mobilizing the Body's Self-Healing Powers.* New York: Thieme, 2003.

Strittmatter, Beate. *Identifying and Treating Blockages to Healing: New Approaches to Therapy-Resistant Patients.* New York: Thieme, 2004.

Tovey, Philip, Gary Easthope, and Jon Adams, eds. *Mainstreaming Complementary and Alternative Medicine: Studies in Social Context.* New York: Routledge, 2004.

Vincent, Charles, and Adrian Furnham. *Complementary Medicine: A Research Perspective.* Hoboken, N.J.: Wiley, 1997.

Wainapel, Stanley F., and Avital Fast, eds. *Alternative Medicine and Rehabilitation: A Guide for Practitioners.* New York: Demos Medical, 2003.

SPIRITUALITY AND RELIGION

Anderson, Neil T., and Michael Jacobson. *The Biblical Guide to Alternative Medicine.* Ventura, Calif.: Regal Books, 2003.

Bien, Thomas, and Beverly Bien. *Mindful Recovery: A Spiritual Path to Healing from Addiction.* Hoboken, N.J.: Wiley, 2002.

Cohen, Michael H. *Healing at the Borderland of Medicine and Religion.* Chapel Hill: University of North Carolina Press, 2009.

Dossey, Larry. *Prayer Is Good Medicine: How to Reap the Healing Benefits of Prayer.* San Francisco: HarperSanFrancisco, 1997.

Frohock, Fred M. *Healing Powers: Alternative Medicine, Spiritual Communities, and the State.* Chicago: University of Chicago Press, 1995.

O'Mathuna, Donal, and Walt Larimore. *Alternative Medicine: The Christian Handbook.* Updated ed. Grand Rapids, Mich.: Zondervan, 2006.

Peteet, John R., and Michael N D'Ambra, eds. The *Soul of Medicine: Spiritual Perspectives and Clinical Practice.* Baltimore: Johns Hopkins University Press, 2011.

WOMEN'S HEALTH

Cutler, Winnifred. *Hormones and Your Health: The Smart Woman's Guide to Hormonal and Alternative Therapies for Menopause.* Hoboken, N.J.: Wiley, 2009.

Dale, Theresa. *Revitalize Your Hormones: Dr. Dale's Seven Steps to a Happier, Healthier, and Sexier You.* Hoboken, N.J.: Wiley, 2005.

Goldberg, Burton, and Editors of *Alternative Medicine. Alternative Medicine Guide to Women's Health 2.* Tiburon, Calif.: Future Medicine, 1998.

Hudson, Tori. *Women's Encyclopedia of Natural Medicine: Alternative Therapies and Integrative Medicine for Total Health and Wellness.* New York: McGraw-Hill, 2007.

Marti, James. *Holistic Pregnancy and Childbirth.* Hoboken, N.J.: Wiley, 1999.

Martin, Raquel, and Judi Gerstung. *The Estrogen Alternative: A Guide to Natural Hormonal Balance.* Rochester, Vt.: Healing Arts Press, 2004.

Mitchel, Deborah, and Deborah Gordon. *Breast Health the Natural Way.* Hoboken, N.J.: Wiley, 2002.

Tagliaferri, Mary, Isaac Cohen, and Debu Tripathy. *Breast Cancer: Beyond Convention—The World's Foremost Authorities on Complementary and Alternative Medicine Offer Advice on Healing.* New York: Atria Books, 2003.

Oladayo O. Oyelola, Ph.D.

Resources

NATIONAL AND INTERNATIONAL HEALTH ORGANIZATIONS

Agency for Healthcare Research and Quality (AHRQ)
540 Gaither Road
Rockville, MD 20850
301-427-1104
E-mail: see https://info.ahrq.gov
Web site: http://www.ahrq.gov
   This agency, part of the U.S. Department of Health and Human Services, aims to improve the quality, safety, efficiency, and effectiveness of health care for Americans.

American Botanical Council (ABC)
P.O. Box 144345
Austin, TX 78714-4345
800-373-7105 (512-926-4900 for local calls)
E-mail: abc@herbalgram.org
Web site: http://abc.herbalgram.org
   This independent, nonprofit research and education organization aims to provide accurate and reliable information about herbal medicine to health consumers, health care practitioners, researchers, educators, industry, and the media.

Association for Applied Psychophysiology and Biofeedback (AAPB)
10200 W. 44th Ave., Suite 304
Wheat Ridge, CO 80033
800-477-8892 (303-422-8436 for local calls)
E-mail: aapb@resourcenter.com
Web site: http://www.aapb.org
   This nonprofit organization aims to promote a new understanding of biofeedback and advance the methods used in this practice.

British Medical Acupuncture Society (BMAS)
BMAS House, 3 Winnington Court
Northwich, Cheshire CW8 1AQ, United Kingdom
01606-786782
Fax: 01606-786783
E-mail: admin@medical-acupuncture.org.uk
Web site: http://www.medical-acupuncture.co.uk
   This registered charity encourages the use and scientific understanding of acupuncture within medicine for human benefit.

Center for Food Safety and Applied Nutrition (CFSAN)
5100 Paint Branch Pkwy.
College Park, MD 20740
888-SAFEFOOD (888-723-3366)
E-mail: consumer@fda.gov
Web site: http://www.fda.gov
   This center is one of six product-oriented centers that carry out the mission of the U.S. Food and Drug Administration. It is responsible for the safety of imported and American-produced foods, cosmetics, drugs, biologics, medical devices, and radiological products.

Codex Alimentarius Commission (CAC)
Viale delle Terme di Caracalla
00153 Rome, Italy
+39-06-5705-1
E-mail: codex@fao.org
Web site: http://www.codexalimentarius.net
   This commission was created by the Food and Agriculture Organization of the United Nations and the World Health Organization to develop international food standards, guidelines, and codes of practice.

Institute for Complementary and Natural Medicine (ICNM)
Can-Mezzanine, 32-26 Lomain St.
London, SE1 0EH, United Kingdom
0207-922-7980 (1-561-997-0112 outside)
E-mail: info@icnm.org.uk
Web site: http://www.i-c-m.org.uk
   This registered charity provides the public with information on complementary and natural medicine.

International Society for the Study of Subtle Energies and Energy Medicine (ISSSEEM)
27770 Arapaho Road, Suite 132
Lafayette, CO 80026
303-425-4625
Fax: 866-269-0972
Web site: http://www.issseem.org
   An international nonprofit interdisciplinary organization that is dedicated to exploring and educating the public about energy medicine.

National Center for Complementary and Alternative Medicine (NCCAM)
P.O. Box 7923
Gaithersburg, MD 20898
888-644-6226
TTY: 866-464-3615
E-mail: info@nccam.nih.gov
Web site: http://nccam.nih.gov

This center is the U.S. government's lead agency for scientific research on complementary and alternative medical and health care systems, practices, and products.

Office of Cancer Complementary and Alternative Medicine (OCCAM)
6116 Executive Blvd., Suite 609, MSC 8339
Bethesda, MD 20892
800-4-CANCER (800-332-8615)
TTY: 800-332-8615
E-mail: ncioccam1-r@mail.nih.gov
Web site: http://www.cancer.gov/cam

An office of the National Cancer Institute (NCI) that is responsible for the NCI's research agenda in complementary and alternative medicine as it relates to cancer prevention, diagnosis, treatment, and symptom management.

Office of Dietary Supplements (ODS)
6100 Executive Blvd., Rm. 3B01, MSC 7517
Bethesda, MD 20892-7517
301-435-2920
Fax: 301-480-1845
E-mail: ods@nih.gov
Web site: http://ods.od.nih.gov

An office of the National Institutes of Health that strengthens the knowledge and understanding of dietary supplements by evaluating scientific information, supporting and publicizing research, and educating the public to foster enhanced quality of life and health for the U.S. population.

Therapeutic Goods Administration (TGA)
P.O. Box 100
Woden ACT 2606, Australia
02-6232-8610
TTY: 800-555-677 (then ask for 800-020-653)
Fax: 02-6232-8605
E-mail: info@tga.gov.au
Web site: http://www.tga.gov.au

This organization carries out assessments and monitoring activities to ensure the standards of therapeutic goods, including alternative and complementary medicines and devices, available in Australia.

FOUNDATIONS, SUPPORT GROUPS, AND ADVOCACY GROUPS

Alliance for Natural Health (ANH)
The Atrium, Curtis Road
Dorking, Surrey RH4 1XA, United Kingdom
+44-0-1306-646600
Fax: +44-0-1306-646600
E-mail: see http://www.anh-europe.org/contact
Web site: http://aahf.nonprofitsoapbox.com

This nonprofit, nongovernmental organization merged with the American Association for Health Freedom in 2009 and focuses on promoting natural health care as the primary approach to the management of human health.

Federal Trade Commission (FTC)
600 Pennsylvania Ave., NW
Washington, DC 20580
877-FTC-HELP (877-382-4357 or 202-326-2222 for local calls)
TTY: 866-653-4261

E-mail: see https://www.ftccomplaintassistant.gov
Web site: http://www.ftc.gov

The Federal Trade Commission accepts complaints against misleading advertisements for both alternative and conventional treatments.

National Health Federation (NHF)
P.O. Box 688
Monrovia, CA 91017
626-357-2181
Fax: 626-303-0642
E-mail: contact-us@thenhf.com
Web site: http://www.thenhf.com

This international nonprofit organization for consumer education and health freedom works to protect the individual right to consume healthy food, take dietary supplements, and use alternative therapies without government restrictions.

PROFESSIONAL ORGANIZATIONS

American Academy of Anti-Aging Medicine (A4M)
301 Yamato Road, Suite 2199
Boca Raton, FL 33431
888-997-0112
Fax: 561-997-0112
E-mail: info@a4m.com
Web site: http://www.worldhealth.net
   This nonprofit organization promotes anti-aging medicine and trains and certifies physicians in this specialty. A4M is the first global entity specifically established to unify and coordinate organizations involved in the advancement of progressive preventative medicine.

American Alternative Medical Association (AAMA)
2200 Market St., Suite 803
Galveston, TX 77550-1530
888-764-2237 (409-621-2600 for local calls)
E-mail: office@joinaama.com
Web site: http://www.joinaama.com
   This association is a division of the American Association of Drugless Practitioners Certification and Accreditation Board. It is dedicated to promoting an enhanced professional image among doctors of traditional and nontraditional therapies and methodologies.

American Association of Acupuncture and Oriental Medicine (AAAOM)
P.O. Box 162340
Sacramento, CA 95816
866-455-7999
E-mail: dnewton@aaaomonline.org
Web site: http://www.aaaomonline.org
   This national professional association promotes and advances high ethical, educational, and professional standards in the practice of acupuncture and Oriental medicine in the United States.

American Association of Integrative Medicine (AAIM)
2750 E. Sunshine St.
Springfield, MO 65804
877-718-3053 (417-881-9995 for local calls)
Fax: 417-823-9959
Web site: http://www.aaimedicine.com
   AAIM seeks to promote the development and understanding of integrative medicine and to establish guidelines for professional practices. The group offers educational and certification programs for practitioners.

American Association of Naturopathic Physicians (AANP)
4435 Wisconsin Ave., NW, Suite 403
Washington, DC 20016
866-538-2267 (202-237-8150 for local calls)
Fax: 202-237-8152
E-mail: member.services@naturopathic.org
Web site: http://www.naturopathic.org
   AANP is a national professional society for licensed or licensable naturopathic physicians and students.

American Chiropractic Association (ACA)
1701 Clarendon Blvd.
Arlington, VA 22209
703-276-8800
Fax: 703-243-2593
E-mail: memberinfo@acatoday.org
Web site: http://www.acatoday.org
   ACA is the largest professional association in the world that represents doctors of chiropractic. It provides lobbying, public relations, professional and educational opportunities for practitioners, and funding for research, and offers leadership for the advancement of the profession.

American Herbalists Guild (AHG)
P.O. Box 230741
Boston, MA 02123
857-350-3128
E-mail: ahgoffice@earthlink.net
Web site: http://www.americanherbalistsguild.com
   This nonprofit educational organization represents medicinal herbalists and aims to promote a high level of professionalism and education in the study and practice of herbalism.

American Holistic Medical Association (AHMA)
23366 Commerce Park, Suite 101B
Beachwood, OH 44122
216-292-6644
E-mail: info@holisticmedicine.org
Web site: http://www.holisticmedicine.org
   This organization includes many licensed physicians who practice holistic medicine. The association aims to create fellowship and collaboration among practitioners and to bring about a holistic understanding of health and health care.

American Holistic Nursing Association (AHNA)
323 N. San Francisco St., Suite 201
Flagstaff, AZ 86001
800-278-2462 (928-526-2196 for local calls)
Fax: 928-526-2752
E-mail: info@ahna.org
Web site: http://www.ahna.org

A nonprofit membership association for nurses and other holistic health care professionals. It promotes the education of nurses, other health care professionals, and the public in all aspects of holistic caring and healing.

Energy Medicine Association (EMA)
Bridge House, Neopardy, Crediton
Devon, EX17 5EP, United Kingdom
01363-772992
Fax: 01363-774775
Web site: http://www.energymedicineassociation.com

An international umbrella organization that provides guidelines and a professional body for practitioners who follow the principles of energy medicine.

European Herbal and Traditional Medicine Practitioners Association (EHTPA)
25 Lincoln Close
Tewkesbury, Glos GL20 5TY, United Kingdom
+44-0-1684-291605
E-mail: info@ehpa.eu
Web site: http://ehtpa.eu

The EHTPA is a professional organization comprising multiple professional herbal and traditional medicine associations across Europe.

International Association of Yoga Therapists (IAYT)
P.O. Box 12890
Prescott, AZ 86304
928-541-0004
E-mail: membershipservices@iayt.org
Web site: http://www.iayt.org

IAYT is a professional organization for yoga teachers and therapists worldwide. It supports research and education in the practice of yoga.

International Society for Neurofeedback and Research (ISNR)
1925 Francisco Blvd. East #12
San Rafael, CA 94901

800-488-3867 (415-485-1344 for local calls)
E-mail: office@isnr.org
Web site: http://www.isnr.org

ISNR is a member organization for health professionals, educators, researchers, and students in applied neuroscience.

National Center for Homeopathy (NCH)
101 S. Whiting St., Suite 16
Alexandria, VA 22304
703-548-7790
Fax: 703-548-7792
E-mail: info@nationalcenterforhomeopathy.org
Web site: http://www.homeopathic.org

NCH is an open-membership organization for the promotion of health through homeopathy. It provides general education to the public and specialized education to homeopaths in the United States.

National Herbalists Association of Australia (NHAA)
P.O. Box 45
Concord West, NSW 2138, Australia
02-8765-0071
E-mail: nhaa@nhaa.org.au
Web site: http://www.nhaa.org.au

The oldest natural therapy association in Australia. Its mission is to promote and protect the profession and practice of herbal medicine.

National Institute of Medical Herbalists (NIMH)
Elm House, 54 Mary Arches St.
Exeter EX4 3B, United Kingdom
+44-0-1392-426022
E-mail: info@nimh.org.uk
Web site: http://www.nimh.org.uk

The NIMH is the United Kingdom's leading professional body representing herbal practitioners.

Physicians' Association for Anthroposophic Medicine (PAAM)
1923 Geddes Ave.
Ann Arbor, MI 48104
734-930-9462
E-mail: paam@anthroposophy.org
Web site: http://www.paam.net

This association aims to facilitate communication between physicians and practitioners in anthroposophic medicine.

Yoga Alliance
1701 Clarendon Blvd., Suite 110
Arlington, VA 22209
888-921-YOGA (888-921-9642)
Fax: 571-482-3336
Web site: http://www.yogaalliance.org
A national education and support organization for yoga in the United States that aims to educate the public on the benefits of yoga.

Brandy Weidow, M.S.

Web Sites

ANTI-AGING MEDICINE

A4M (American Academy of Anti-Aging Medicine) Anti-Aging Resource Library

http://www.worldhealth.net/library

This library from the American Academy of Anti-Aging Medicine provides medical news, white papers and official statements, and an alphabetical index of anti-aging related topics in the news.

DIET-BASED THERAPIES

Dietary Supplements Information Bureau

Vitamins and Herbs

http://www.naturalproductsinfo.org

This site includes indexed information on vitamins and herbs, a substance-interaction search engine, an overview of specialty categories (such as fitness supplements and Ayurvedic medicine), and general background information on the use of vitamins and other dietary supplements.

Office of Dietary Supplements

Health Information

http://ods.od.nih.gov/healthinformation

This National Institutes of Health division provides information to consumers on informed decision making, nutrient recommendation reports, safety, and additional resources related to dietary supplements.

Orthomolecular.org

http://orthomolecular.org

This site include an article library, the history of orthomolecular medicine, and detailed information on nutrients.

U.S. Food and Drug Administration (FDA)

Dietary Supplements

http://www.fda.gov/food/dietarysupplements

This information page reviews the FDA's role in dietary supplements and provides general guidance on safe use of supplements.

World Health Organization (WHO)

Monographs on Selected Medicinal Plants, Volumes 1 and 2

http://apps.who.int/medicinedocs

As a result of International Conference of Drug Regulatory Authorities recommendations and requests from WHO's member states for "assistance in providing safe and effective herbal medicines for use in national health-care systems," WHO has published two detailed monographs on selected medicinal plants.

ENERGY MEDICINE

International Center for Reiki Training

What Is Reiki?

http://www.reiki.org/faq/whatisreiki.html

This site provides a brief overview of the philosophy, history, and practice of Reiki.

Yoga Basics

http://www.yogabasics.com

This site reviews the philosophy and basic principles of yoga and provides guidance for poses, meditations, and other aspects of practice. It includes a message board and yoga class finder.

FOLK MEDICINE

Online Archive of American Folk Medicine

http://www.folkmed.ucla.edu

This archive is based on more than fifty years of documentation of beliefs and practices related to folk and alternative medicine. It stems from a collaboration between the University of California, Los Angeles, and folklorists associated with the university.

GENERAL INFORMATION

American Association of Naturopathic Physicians

Your Health

http://www.naturopathic.org

The association's Web site provides an overview of

naturopathic practice, professional education, and licensing. The Your Health page provides a wide range of articles on health topics with a naturopathic perspective.

Holistic Health Now
Resources
http://www.holistichealthnow.org/web/resources.html

This page from the American Holistic Medical Association provides links to more detailed information on various forms of complementary and alternative medicine, a glossary of terms, and a search engine for finding providers.

Holisticonline.com
http://www.holisticonline.com

This site aims to provide comprehensive information on a variety of holistic therapies and on the holistic lifestyle.

Medical News Today
Complementary Medicine/Alternative Medicine News
http://www.medicalnewstoday.com/sections/complementary_medicine

This searchable *Medical News Today* site features updated news reports on complementary and alternative medicine.

National Center for Complementary and Alternative Medicine
http://nccam.nih.gov

This is the site for the National Institutes of Health's division "for scientific research on the diverse medical and health care systems, practices, and products that are not generally considered part of conventional medicine." The site includes an alphabetical directory of health topics, a clinical trials directory, information on grants and training, "herbs at a glance" fact sheets, warnings, an NCCAM events listing, and a monthly newsletter.

National Center for Complementary and Alternative Medicine
Time to Talk Campaign
http://nccam.nih.gov/timetotalk

This site promotes and provides resources for "Time to Talk," a site encouraging patients and providers to communicate about complementary and alternative medicine.

National Center for Complementary and Alternative Medicine
The Use of Complementary and Alternative Medicine in the United States
http://nccam.nih.gov/news/camstats/2007/camsurvey_fs1.htm

This 2008 report by the National Center for Complementary and Alternative Medicine and the National Center for Health Statistics reflects findings specific to complementary and alternative medicine from the National Health Interview Survey.

National Center for Homeopathy
Articles
http://www.homeopathic.org/articles

This searchable articles page provides an overview of homeopathic medicine, its history, related research, and current news items.

Office of Cancer Complementary and Alternative Medicine
http://www.cancer.gov/cam/health_patients.html

This division of the National Cancer Institute provides health information on complementary and alternative medicine of specific interest to cancer patients.

PubMed
Complementary Medicine
http://www.ncbi.nlm.nih.gov/pubmed

The National Center for Complementary and Alternative Medicine and the National Library of Medicine partnered to create a subset within PubMed, in which users can search for journal citations specific to complementary and alternative medicine.

University of Minnesota, Center for Spirituality and Healing
http://www.csh.umn.edu

The center's Web site includes information on whole systems healing and a link to consumer information on alternative therapies, "Taking Charge of Your Health."

WholeHealthMD.com
http://www.wholehealthmd.com

This site provides information on healing centers, healing foods, and international research. It includes an Expert Opinion section (patient questions answered by experts) and a reference library for patients. Information is developed by a team of board-certified physicians and specialists.

MANIPULATIVE AND BODY-BASED PRACTICES

American Association of Acupuncture and Oriental Medicine
http://aaaom.affiniscape.com

This professional organization's site includes a search engine for locating practitioners and links to research and organizations related to acupuncture and Oriental medicine.

American Chiropractic Association
Patient Information
http://www.acatoday.org

This site explains chiropractic medicine and provides information on research and education related to chiropractic medicine, as well as articles and answers to frequently asked questions.

Council of Colleges of Acupuncture and Oriental Medicine
Know Your Acupuncturist
http://www.ccaom.org/downloads/knowyouracu-puncturist.pdf

This PDF fact sheet for the consumer summarizes the levels of education of various practitioners in acupuncture and Oriental medicine.

Feldenkrais Method of Somatic Education
Frequently Asked Questions
http://www.feldenkrais.com/method/frequently_asked_questions

This fact sheet summarizes the basic of the Feldenkrais method, including what to expect from a session and how to find practitioners.

Massage Therapy Research Database
http://www.massagetherapyfoundation.org/researchdb.html

This searchable database contains journal citations on massage therapy research.

National Acupuncture Foundation
http://www.nationalacupuncturefoundation.org

The Web site for this educational and charitable foundation lists books and online documents about acupuncture, information about state regulations, and links to other organizations and resources.

Rolf Institute of Structural Integration
What Is Rolfing Structural Integration?
http://www.rolf.org/about

This page summarizes the concepts behind the rolfing process, how it works, and expected benefits.

What Is Reflexology?
http://www.reflexology-research.com/whatis.htm

This site by expert authors provides an overview of the history and benefits of reflexology, what potential patients can expect from a reflexology session, and research findings.

MIND/BODY MEDICINE

American Society of Clinical Hypnosis (ASCH)
http://www.asch.net

ASCH provides general information for the public on hypnosis, including what it entails, when it may be beneficial, whether common myths have any validity, and how to select a qualified practitioner.

Biofeedback Certification International Alliance
Overview of Biofeedback Areas
http://www.bcia.org

Provides information for the consumer on biofeedback, neurofeedback, and pelvic muscle dysfunction biofeedback.

How to Meditate
http://www.how-to-meditate.org

This site reviews the basics of Buddhist meditation and includes videos for beginners.

Transcendental Meditation Program
http://www.tm.org

This site reviews the basics of Transcendental Meditation, anticipated benefits, and how it differs from other forms of meditation.

SPIRITUALITY

National Cancer Institute (NCI)
Spirituality in Cancer Care
http://www.cancer.gov/cancertopics/pdq/supportivecare

An information page that summarizes the role of spirituality in cancer care, including its connection to quality of life, the elements of a spiritual assessment, and how caregivers can meet patients' spiritual and religious needs.

TRADITIONAL HEALING

National Center for Complementary and Alternative Medicine
Reiki: An Introduction
http://nccam.nih.gov/health/reiki/#moreinfo

This page provides an overview of the practice of Reiki; training, licensing, and certification; and advice for patients considering using Reiki.

National Center for Complementary and Alternative Medicine
Traditional Chinese Medicine
http://nccam.nih.gov/health/whatiscam/chinese-med.htm

This NCCAM site provides an introduction to traditional Chinese medicine, including types of treatment, research findings, safety, and factors for patients to consider.

Traditional Chinese Medicine Basics
Zang Fu Theory
http://www.tcmbasics.com/zangfu.htm

This page summarizes Zang Fu theory, related to body organs and their interrelationships.

Shaman Links
http://www.shamanlinks.net

This resource page reviews topics including the definition of shamanism, what shamans do, specific areas of healing, and an index of resources.

University of Minnesota, Center for Spirituality and Healing
Taking Charge of Your Health: Ayurvedic Medicine
http://www.takingcharge.csh.umn.edu/explore-healing-practices

This overview explains Ayurvedic medicine to interested health consumers.

VISION

I-See.org
Bates Method in a Nutshell
http://www.i-see.org/bates_nutshell

This page reviews the basic steps, first described by William Bates, in using eye exercises and habits to improve vision naturally.

Katherine Hauswirth, R.N., M.S.N.

HISTORICAL RESOURCES

Timeline of Major Developments in Complementary and Alternative Medicine

YEAR	EVENT
2700 B.C.E.	According to Chinese legend, Emperor Shennong (Divine Farmer) composes the *Shennong pen T'sao ching*, or Great Herbal, considered the oldest compilation of Chinese herbal medicine. The oldest surviving copy of the herbal, made about 500 C.E., describes 365 different herbs.
1550 B.C.E.	The Ebers Papyrus, the longest medical treatise to survive from ancient Egypt, describes the use of laxatives and enemas to cleanse the lower bowel of fecal residue, based on the belief that the by-products of normal digestion are toxic. This belief and the associated practice of colon cleansing resurface in Europe and North America in the nineteenth century.
c. 600 B.C.E.	Approximate date of the composition of Psalms 6, 30, 41, 88, and 103, still recited by traditional Jews and many Christians as prayers for healing.
420 B.C.E.	Hippocrates of Cos (c. 460-370 B.C.E.), often considered the founder of Western medicine, recommends bathing in spring water as a treatment for illness. His is one of the earliest known descriptions of hydrotherapy.
c. 200 B.C.E.	Estimated date of composition of the *Charaka Samhita*, the oldest surviving text of Ayurvedic medicine. The book is attributed to a legendary serpent king, or god, who is moved by pity for the sufferings of humankind and assumes human form to reveal the principles of Ayurvedic medicine.
	Rulers of the Han Dynasty in China are buried in ceremonial suits made of small squares of jade joined with gold or silver links in the belief that jade has the power to prevent decomposition of the body. Some scholars think that this belief and the similar use of gemstones in ancient Egyptian tombs mark the origin of the alternative practice of gemstone healing.
c. 150 B.C.E.	Patañjali (fl. second century B.C.E.), a Hindu sage, compiles the Yoga Sutras, a collection of sayings or aphorisms about the practice of yoga. Some scholars believe that portions of the present text of the Yoga Sutras were added as late as 500 C.E.
65 C.E.	Pedanius Dioscorides (fl. c. 40 C.E.), a Greek serving as a physician in the Roman army, compiles a five-volume treatise on plant-based medicines known as *De materia medica*. Considered the world's oldest pharmacopoeia, *De materia medica* remains a standard reference work for physicians in the West until the seventeenth century. A copy made in 512 describes more than five hundred medicinal plants and their uses, including aromatic plants that Dioscorides recommends as an early form of aromatherapy.
c. 70	The writer of the Epistle of James in the New Testament gives biblical sanction to prayers for and ritual anointing of the sick: "Are any among you sick? They should call for the elders of the church and have them pray over them, anointing them with oil in the name of the Lord. And their prayer offered in faith will heal the sick, and the Lord will make them well. And anyone who has committed sins will be forgiven" (James 5:14-15).
1025	Avicenna (Ibn Sin{amacr}; 980-1037), a Persian physician, completes a fourteen-volume medical encyclopedia known as the *Canon of Medicine*. It is used as a textbook in European medical schools as late as 1650. Avicenna is an early proponent of chromotherapy, the belief that color is important in treating disease. The *Canon of Medicine* states that the physician should use the color red to stimulate a patient's blood, the color blue or white to cool or slow the blood, and the color yellow to treat muscle pain and inflammation. Avicenna also describes the use of steam distillation

YEAR	EVENT
1025 (cont.)	to extract essential oils from flowers and aromatic plants; this process facilitates the use of such plants in aromatherapy.
1150	Peter Lombard (c. 1100-1160), one of the most influential theologians of the Middle Ages, defines Extreme Unction as one of the seven sacraments of the Roman Church in his *Four Books of Sentences* (*Libri quattuor sententiarum*), a compilation of theology used as a textbook in European universities until the Reformation. In 1972 the Roman Catholic Church recommended the term "anointing of the sick" to counteract the widespread impression that the sacrament is reserved for the dying. The sacrament is still administered to Catholics who have serious illness.
1484	Peter Schöffer (1425-1503), a German printer and manuscript copyist, produces the first printed book of Western herbalism, the *Herbarius latinus*. The book is reprinted ten times by 1499. Schöffer produces an enlarged German version of the *Herbarius latinus* in 1485.
1683	Willem ten Rhijne (1647-1700), a physician employed by the Dutch East India Company, publishes the first European account of acupuncture, *De acupunctura*, based on his observations of the practice during a two-year stay in Japan.
1774	Franz Anton Mesmer (1734-1815), an Austrian physician, conducts an experiment on a woman in which he has her swallow a preparation containing iron and then attaches magnets to various parts of her body. When the woman is relieved of her symptoms for several hours, Mesmer believes that her relief is caused by a vital force or fluid that he terms *magnétisme animal*, or "animal magnetism." British practitioners of Mesmer's technique refer to his method of treatment as mesmerism.
1796	Samuel Hahnemann (1755-1843), a German physician and the inventor of homeopathy, publishes his first article on the principles of homeopathy in a German medical journal.
1822	Vincenz Priessnitz (1799-1851), a Czech peasant farmer, converts his father's house into a sanatorium for local people who have come to him for healing. Having healed himself of several injuries by pouring cold water on affected limbs, Priessnitz cures some farm animals and his neighbors by the same method. After healing the brother of Emperor Francis II, Priessnitz is given Imperial permission in 1838 to complete the construction of a hydrotherapy spa. Within one year the spa has more than 1,500 visitors.
	Samuel Thomson (1769-1843), a self-taught herbalist practicing in New Hampshire, publishes the first edition of his book *New Guide to Health: Or, Botanic Family Physician*. Thomson then becomes the founder of an alternative medical system known as Thomsonianism, based on the belief that disease results from exposure to cold and that the body's "natural heat" can be maintained by a combination of laxatives and emetics, including lobelia. Thomsonianism evinces an antagonistic attitude toward conventional medicine and is derided in turn by its opponents as the "purge and puke" approach to health.
1833	The Eclectic Medical Institute in Worthington, Ohio, graduates its first class of practitioners. It is the first of one dozen Midwestern medical schools representing eclectic medicine, a movement that combines some elements of Thomsonianism with Native American herbal medicine and more conventional medical practices. The eclectic medicine movement reaches its peak in the 1890s.
1841	James Braid (1795-1860), an eminent Scottish surgeon, attends a demonstration given by a French practitioner of mesmerism named Charles Lafontaine. Convinced that the physical

YEAR	EVENT
1841 (cont.)	changes seen in Lafontaine's mesmerized subjects are genuine, Braid concludes that they result from psychological concentration on the practitioner's words rather than on a magnetic fluid or vital force as described by Mesmer. He describes the technique as "neuro-hypnotism," or simply as "hypnotism," and becomes the first modern practitioner of hypnotism.
1844	The first hydrotherapy facility in the United States is opened by medical doctor Joel Shew (1816-1855) on Barclay Street in New York City.
1848	Three practitioners of homeopathy in Philadelphia open the first school of homeopathy in the United States, the Homeopathic Medical College of Pennsylvania. The school offers the medical doctor (M.D.) degree and the doctor of holistic medicine (H.M.D.) degree. In 1867, the school changes its name to Hahnemann Medical College. Its successor institutions become part of the medical school of Drexel University in 2002.
1866	The Western Health Reform Institute (renamed the Battle Creek Sanitarium in 1903) opens in Battle Creek, Michigan. Based on the vegetarian diet and other health principles advocated by the Seventh-day Adventist Church, the institute is run by John Harvey Kellogg (1852-1943) and his brother, Will Keith Kellogg (1860-1951). Their sanitarium treats persons with hydrotherapy, sunbathing, open-air exercise, colon cleansing conducted with a mixture of water and yogurt instilled by an enema machine, and a high-fiber diet based on grains. The brothers invent what they called corn flakes, a breakfast food for the sanitarium patients, which becomes the first commercially successful, and still common, cold cereal in the United States.
1876	Augustus J. Pleasanton (1801-1894), a general in the Union army during the American Civil War, publishes a pseudoscientific work titled *The Influence of the Blue Ray of the Sunlight and of the Blue Color of the Sky*. Pleasanton, considered the founder of modern chromotherapy, maintains that the color blue can speed the growth of plants and livestock and can heal diseases in humans.
1886	Sebastian Kneipp (1821-1897), a Bavarian priest, publishes a book on hydrotherapy titled *Wasserkur* (*My Water Cure*), describing his method of treating disease through the application of water to the body at different temperatures and levels of pressure. Kneipp, considered one of the founders of naturopathy, recommends combining hydrotherapy with exercise, the use of botanical medicines, spiritual practice, and a plant-based diet with limited amounts of meat.
1892	Andrew Taylor Still (1828-1917), an American physician who becomes disenchanted with mainstream medicine after losing three children to spinal meningitis, founds the American School of Osteopathy in Kirksville, Missouri. The school changes its name several times, opens a second school of osteopathic medicine in Mesa, Arizona, and is finally renamed A. J. Still University in 2007.
1897	Daniel David Palmer (1845-1913), a Canadian-born practitioner of magnetic healing who develops chiropractic as a form of alternative medicine, opens the Palmer College of Chiropractic in Davenport, Iowa. The oldest school of chiropractic in the world, the college eventually opens satellite campuses in San Jose, California, in 1980, and in Port Orange, Florida, in 2002.
1902	Benedict Lust (1872-1945), a German immigrant trained in both osteopathy and homeopathy, opens the American School of Naturopathy in New York City. It is the first school of naturopathic medicine anywhere in the world.
1910	Abraham Flexner (1866-1959) publishes a landmark report on medical education in the United States under the auspices of the Carnegie Foundation. The Flexner Report, which urges the

YEAR	EVENT
1910 (cont.)	standardization of medical education, leads to the closing of most rural medical schools in the United States, all but two African American medical schools, and schools of homeopathy and eclectic medicine.
1918	The Native American Church, which practices a form of peyote religion that uses the hallucinogenic plant *Lophophora williamsii* as part of its communion ritual, is formally incorporated in Oklahoma.
1920	The last nineteenth-century medical school in the United States that teaches homeopathic medicine exclusively closes its doors.
1922	Mikao Usui (1865-1926), a Japanese student of Buddhism and Shinto, has a mystical experience in the course of a twenty-one-day spiritual practice on Mount Kurama, a sacred mountain northwest of Kyoto, Japan. The experience includes a revelation of the principles of Reiki, a form of energy healing. Usui is thought to have intended Reiki as a method for people to attain enlightenment rather than a healing therapy and to have regarded the healing that some of his students experienced as only a "wonderful side effect."
1927	A federal regulatory agency to protect consumers against contaminated or misbranded foods and medicines is established within the U.S. Department of Agriculture and is called the Food, Drug, and Insecticide Organization. In 1930, its name is changed to the Food and Drug Administration (FDA).
1930	Edward Bach (1886-1936), an English homeopath, develops the thirty-eight flower remedies that still carry his name, based on his belief in the healing properties of the specific plants. He makes his remedies by suspending the flowers in spring water and allowing sunlight to pass through them, thus transferring the energy patterns of the flowers to the tinctures.
1931	Margaret "Maud" Grieve (1858-1941) publishes *A Modern Herbal*, a book based on her experiences with growing, drying, and using herbs to meet the demand for plant-based medicines during World War I. A Fellow of the Royal Horticultural Society and the British Science Guild, Grieve founds a medicinal and commercial herb school and farm in Buckinghamshire, England. *A Modern Herbal* is still in print.
1932	Black Elk (1863-1950), a traditional Native American healer of the Lakota Sioux who becomes a Christian catechist (lay teacher), publishes his autobiography *Black Elk Speaks: Being the Life Story of a Holy Man of the Oglala Sioux*. In the book he expresses his belief that there is no contradiction between the traditional religion of his tribe and mainstream Christianity. His descriptions of Sioux rituals spark a revival of interest in Native American rituals and healing practices and are studied intensively by the Swiss psychiatrist Carl Jung (1875-1961).
	Johannes Heinrich Schultz (1884-1970), a German psychiatrist, publishes a book on autogenic training, a form of self-hypnosis intended to promote deep relaxation. Schultz forms the Deutschen Gesellschaft für Ärztliche Hypnose (German Society for Medical Hypnosis) in 1959.
1937	Hawayo Takata (1900-1980), a Japanese American born in Hawaii, is introduced to Reiki in Tokyo after being admitted to a hospital there for gallstones and other gastrointestinal problems. She returns to Hawaii in good health and opens the first Reiki practice in the West. Takata is criticized by some for having turned Reiki into a formal system to increase its appeal to Westerners and for charging large amounts of money for higher-level attunements (initiations).

YEAR	EVENT

1937 (cont.) René-Maurice Gattefossé (1881-1950), a French chemist, publishes the first modern work on aromatherapy, titled *Aromathérapie: Les huiles essentielles, hormones végétales*. Gattefossé had received scientific training in engineering and chemistry, and he had experimented with the use of lavender oil as an anti-infective after burning his hand in a laboratory explosion in 1910. He states explicitly that his goal is to reconcile "forgotten techniques" (*techniques oubliées*) with modern science. Gattefossé is credited with coining the term "aromatherapy."

1938 The U.S. Congress passes the Federal Food, Drug and Cosmetic Act following a tragedy involving the deaths of more than one hundred people from poisoning as the result of an improperly formulated and untested sulfanilamide preparation. The new law empowers the FDA to conduct a review of the safety and effectiveness of all new drugs before marketing, and to regulate cosmetics, medical devices, and drugs.

1939 The last school of eclectic medicine in the United States closes in Cincinnati, Ohio.

1948 Randolph Stone (1890-1981), the Austrian-born founder of polarity therapy, publishes his first book on his eclectic form of energy therapy. The book is called *The New Energy Concept of the Healing Art*.

1950 Jerome I. Rodale (1898-1971), an early advocate of organic farming, begins publication of *Prevention* magazine, a health-related popular periodical focused on preventing illness through plant-based diets, vitamin supplements, natural foods, herbal medicines, and other measures that are promoted by naturopaths in the 1970s and 1980s. In 2010, *Prevention* has a circulation of 2.9 million.

1952 The eminent violonist Yehudi Menuhin (1916-1999) meets an influential teacher of Indian yoga, B. K. S. Iyengar (1918–), at Iyengar's classroom in Pune, India. The two become friends, and Menuhin invites Iyengar to teach classes abroad in London, Paris, and eventually the United States. Iyengar's classes are credited with introducing yoga to the West and with laying the foundation for yoga's subsequent popularity.

Bernard Jensen (1908-2001), a California chiropractor and naturopath, publishes *The Science and Practice of Iridology*, popularizing an alternative method of diagnosis based on the interpretation of streaks, lines, and changes in the color of the iris of the eye. Iridologists claim that various zones in the iris correspond to different parts of the body, and that information gained from examining these zones can be used to predict a person's future health problems and to diagnose present illnesses.

1955 Maharishi Mahesh Yogi (1917-2008) develops a form of mantra-based meditation that he calls Transcendental Meditation (TM). He begins a series of world tours in 1957 to spread information about the technique. TM reaches its peak of popularity in the early 1970s but begins to decline when the Maharishi claimed that practitioners of TM can learn to do "yogic flying," or levitating.

1962 Michael Murphy (1930–), a psychologist interested in comparative religion, and Dick Price (1930-1985), a writer and explorer of altered states of consciousness, cofound the Esalen Institute in Big Sur, California. The institute serves as a laboratory for countercultural and New Age therapies, including gestalt therapy, massage therapy, and art therapy, and as a place for human potential workshops and experimentation with mind-altering drugs.

Year	Event
1966	U.S. Secretary of Defense Robert J. McNamara authorizes the acceptance of doctors of osteopathy (D.O.) into all the medical military services on the same basis as doctors of medicine. In 1996, Ronald Blanck, D.O., becomes the first osteopath to serve as Surgeon General of the Army.
1968	The U.S. Department of Health, Education, and Welfare recommends against expanding Medicare coverage to naturopathic treatments, maintaining that naturopathy is not grounded in medical science.
1969	Stephen Barrett (1933–), an American psychiatrist, founds the Lehigh Valley Committee Against Health Fraud as a nonprofit organization to "combat health-related frauds, myths, fads, fallacies, and misconduct." Barrett develops the Web site Quackwatch in 1996 to serve as a watchdog and critic of most forms of alternative medicine. In 1997, the parent organization changes its name to Quackwatch after the Web site has gained widespread, popular attention.
	The American Medical Association votes to admit doctors of osteopathy to full active membership.
	The Bio-Feedback Research Society is established at a conference held in Santa Monica, California. The society is renamed the Biofeedback Society of America in 1976.
1971	Acupuncture makes headlines in the United States when James Reston (1909-1995), a prize-winning American journalist, is treated with acupuncture for postoperative pain following an emergency appendectomy during a visit to China.
	Ida P. Rolf (1896-1979), originally trained as a biochemist, opens the Rolf Institute of Structural Integration in Boulder, Colorado, to train practitioners in the system of postural improvement and deep tissue manipulation that she developed in the 1940s.
1972	Dolores Krieger (1922–) and Dora Kunz (1904-1999) develop therapeutic touch, a form of energy healing, at Pumpkin Hollow Retreat Center, a Theosophical Society spiritual center in Craryville, New York.
1974	The International Veterinary Acupuncture Society is formed to integrate veterinary acupuncture and Western veterinary science.
	Dolores Krieger offers her first graduate-level course in energy therapy for nursing students, at New York University.
1975	The New England School of Acupuncture, the first school of acupuncture and Oriental medicine to be established in the United States, is opened in Newton, Massachusetts.
	Yoga Journal, a monthly magazine devoted to all schools of classical yoga and their relationships to modern science and nutrition, begins publication. In 2010, the magazine has a paid circulation of 350,000 and a readership estimated at more than one million persons.
1978	The German government establishes Commission E, a body that publishes 380 monographs on the safety and effectiveness of herbal medicines legally approved for use in Germany.
	A group of four naturopaths in the Seattle area found the John Bastyr College of Naturopathic Medicine. Named for a Seattle naturopath and chiropractor who retired in the 1960s, the school becomes a university in 1994. In 2010, it offers degree programs in naturopathy, acupuncture, Oriental medicine, nutrition, herbal sciences, health psychology, midwifery, and exercise science.

YEAR	EVENT
1978 (cont.)	The government of India establishes the Central Council for Research in Ayurveda and Siddha (CCRAS) to conduct studies of that country's traditional medical systems. In 2010, CCRAS comprises thirty-three nationwide research institutes.
	Bernie Siegel, an assistant clinical professor of surgery at Yale-New Haven Hospital in Connecticut, founds Exceptional Cancer Patients, an organization offering spiritual and physical interventions to help persons with cancer strengthen their immune systems and increase their chances of long-term survival. Siegel's first book, *Love, Medicine, and Miracles*, published in 1986, becomes an immediate best seller.
1979	Jon Kabat-Zinn (1944–), a molecular biologist interested in mind/body interventions, introduces the Mindfulness-Based Stress Reduction program at the University of Massachusetts Medical School. By 2010, more than 18,000 people have completed the eight-week program in mindfulness meditation, learning "how to use their innate resources and abilities to respond more effectively to stress, pain, and illness."
	The U.S. Court of Appeals rules in *Malnak v. Yogi* that the teaching of Transcendental Meditation is a form of religious activity within the scope of the establishment clause of the U.S. Constitution and, therefore, is prohibited in public schools on the basis of the First Amendment.
1980	The Biofeedback Certification Institute of America offers the first national examination and the first certification program in biofeedback.
	The American College of Traditional Chinese Medicine opens in San Francisco. It is approved as a degree-granting institution by the state of California in 1986 and becomes the first graduate school in the United States to offer a master's degree in traditional Chinese medicine.
1986	Peter Mandel, a German naturopath, publishes the first volume of his *Practical Compendium of Colorpuncture*, in which he describes an alternative treatment that combines chromotherapy with acupuncture. Mandel's technique involves the application of a small flashlight with a colored tip to the traditional Chinese acupoints on the human body. Mandel maintains that the acupoints have an affinity with various colors, some coordinating with warm colors (red, yellow, orange) and others with cool colors (green, blue, violet). Mandel maintains that pressing on the acupoints with a light source attached to a quartz rod in the appropriate color will correct energy disturbances in the body.
	The National Library of Medicine adds "Alternative and Complementary Medicine" as a subject heading for journal articles.
	The first North American Yogic Flying Contest is held in the Civic Center in Washington, D.C. Twenty-two advanced practitioners of Transcendental Meditation participate in the competition. Reporters describe the participants as simply "hopping" or "bouncing" while seated on foam mattresses in the lotus position. The annual contest is abandoned after 1989.
1988	The Alternative Medicine College of Canada is established in Montreal as the Collège des Médecines Douces du Québec. The college begins with a series of seminars and distance education courses in homeopathy, naturopathy, and acupuncture for French-speaking students. In 2000-2001, the courses are updated and made available in English and French.
	The American Botanical Council is founded in Austin, Texas, to provide health care professionals and the general public with reliable information about the responsible use of medicinal plants.

YEAR	EVENT
1991	The National Institutes of Health establishes the Office of Alternative Medicine.
	The National Cancer Institute establishes a review program called the Best Case Series to evaluate case reports of possible treatments for cancer derived from CAM approaches.
1992	The Agency for Health Care Policy and Research recommends biofeedback as a treatment for urinary incontinence in adults.
1993	Edzard Ernst (1948–) becomes the world's first professor of complementary medicine when he accepts the Laing Chair at the University of Exeter in England. Trained as a medical doctor in Germany, Ernst first practices homeopathy for several years at a homeopathic hospital in Munich. He also receives training in acupuncture, autogenic training, herbal medicine, massage therapy, and spinal manipulation. Ernst acquires a considerable reputation for the rigorous quality of his research and for his willingness to criticize CAM modalities that are ineffective or that have not been sufficiently studied.
	Tapas Fleming, an acupuncturist and practitioner of Chinese medicine in California, invents Tapas acupressure technique (TAT), a form of treatment in which light pressure is applied to four areas on the head (inner corners of both eyes, the back of the head, and a spot half an inch above the space between the eyebrows). Fleming claims that TAT can relieve traumatic stress, clear negative beliefs, and reduce the severity of allergic reactions.
1994	The U.S. Congress passes the Dietary Supplement Health and Education Act, which empowers the FDA to regulate herbal medicines and other botanical preparations as dietary supplements. These products do not require FDA approval before marketing, provided that the manufacturers do not claim that they can be used to treat or cure disease.
	Establishment of the National Center for Jewish Healing follows an upsurge in interest in traditional Jewish resources for spiritual wisdom and comfort in the face of illness. The center is the result of a Jewish healing movement originally led by three rabbis and two lay leaders in the early 1990s. By 2010, more than thirty Jewish healing centers exist in the United States and Canada.
1996	Emily Rosa (1987–) conducts a scientific study of therapeutic touch (TT), a form of energy therapy, carrying out a single-blind experiment for her fourth-grade science fair that shows practitioners of TT do no better than chance in detecting her energy field through a screen. Her study is published in the *Journal of the American Medical Association* in April, 1998, making her the youngest person to have a paper published in a peer-reviewed medical journal.
1997	The James Braid Society is founded in London as a discussion group for hypnotherapists, medical professionals, and others concerned with "the ethical uses of hypnosis."
1998	The Office of Alternative Medicine is renamed the National Center for Complementary and Alternative Medicine and is raised to the status of an NIH center.
	The Office of Cancer Complementary and Alternative Medicine (OCCAM) is founded as part of the division of Cancer Treatment and Diagnosis of the National Cancer Institute (NCI). OCCAM is distinguished from NCCAM by its exclusive focus on cancer therapies. OCCAM's responsibility is defined as conducting research for the NCI in complementary and alternative medicine as it pertains to cancer prevention, diagnosis, treatment, and symptom management.

YEAR	EVENT
1998 (cont.)	An English translation of the German Commission E monographs on herbal medicines is brought into the United States by the American Botanical Council.
	A study published in the *Journal of the American Medical Association* reports that in the United States, 60 percent of the standard medical schools surveyed, 95 percent of osteopathic medical schools, and 84.8 percent of nursing schools are offering courses in some form of CAM along with training in mainstream medicine and surgery.
1999	The Desert Institute School of Classical Homeopathy, the first full-time school of homeopathic medicine to be founded in the United States since 1920, is established in Phoenix, Arizona. The school changes its name to the American Medical College of Homeopathy in 2006. By 2010, twenty-five schools offer instruction in homeopathy in the United States.
2002	Honso USA, the only licensed distributor of Japanese Kampo herbal medicines in the United States, reveals its proprietary herbal formulae to American researchers. Kampo medicines are a variety of traditional Chinese herbal medicines prescribed by Japanese physicians. The herbal formulations began clinical trials for the treatment of hepatitis C at Sloan-Kettering Cancer Center in New York and at the Liver Center of the University of California, San Diego.
2003	Following a six-year study, the Roman Catholic Church publishes a ninety-page monograph titled *A Christian Reflection on the New Age.* The document criticizes crystal healing and similar New Age practices, arguing they have no empirical validity, and criticizes certain beliefs that contradict mainstream Christian teaching.
	A group of practitioners of Ayurveda incorporate the National Ayurvedic Medical Association in New Mexico. By 2010, thirteen schools of Ayurvedic medicine are operating legally in the United States.
	According to the Institute of Medicine, nineteen different institutes and centers within the National Institutes of Health spend $315.5 million on CAM-related research and other activities in this single year.
2005	*Yoga Journal* brings B. K. S. Iyengar to Colorado to teach an extended workshop in yoga. The visit helped make Iyengar's 1966 book, *Light on Yoga,* a basic text for yoga practitioners in the United States. A survey following the workshop estimates that 16.5 million people in the United States practice yoga.
2006	The government of the Netherlands formally ends funding of research into CAM therapies.
2007	The U.S. Food and Drug Administration issues an updated set of guidelines for industry on the FDA's regulation of CAM products, titled "Complementary and Alternative Medicine Products and Their Regulation by the Food and Drug Administration."
	The number of schools of osteopathic medicine in the United States grows to twenty-five, at thirty-one separate locations. The American Osteopathic Association notes that one of every five medical students in the United States is enrolled in a school of osteopathic medicine.
2008	Josephine P. Briggs, M.D., becomes the first woman to be named director of National Center for Complementary and Alternative Medicine. The center's budget for fiscal year 2008-2009 is $122 million.
2009	Lewis Mehl-Madrona, M.D., a member of the Lakota tribe, a graduate of Stanford University School of Medicine, and a practitioner of Native American healing traditions, establishes the

YEAR	EVENT

2009 (cont.) Coyote Institute as a teaching and research center "that looks for ways to encourage people to transform their attitudes towards their own health." The institute is located in South Burlington, Vermont.

Three people die and twenty-one others require medical treatment following a New Age version of a traditional Native American sweat lodge ceremony in Sedona, Arizona. Arvol Looking Horse, the spiritual leader of the Lakota tribe, then publishes an article asking non-Native Americans to stop "copying" or reenacting native ceremonies and charging hefty fees for participation.

New Mexico becomes the first U.S. state to license chiropractors to prescribe medications for certain conditions. Chiropractic remains the largest alternative medical profession in the United States and Canada.

The FDA recalls Pai You Guo, a Chinese herbal formula used as a weight loss supplement, finding that it contains undeclared ingredients known to increase blood pressure and heart rate and, therefore, poses a risk to persons with congestive heart failure and coronary artery disease.

2010 The Office of Dietary Supplements and the National Center for Complementary and Alternative Medicine announce the establishment of five Botanical Research Centers to study the safety, effectiveness, and biological activity of botanical products. The centers, each funded for $1.5 million per year for five years, are opened at the Pennington Biomedical Research Center in Baton Rouge, Louisiana; the University of Illinois, Chicago; the University of Illinois, Urbana-Champaign; the University of Missouri, Columbia; and Wake Forest University Health Sciences in Winston-Salem, North Carolina.

Rebecca J. Frey, Ph.D.

Biographical Dictionary of Complementary and Alternative Medicine Practitioners and Critics

Al-Dinawari (828-896): Kurdish academic and prolific writer who excelled at many fields, including astronomy, botany, metallurgy, and mathematics. Considered the founder of Arabic botany, largely for his book *Kitab al-Nabat* (or *Book of Plants*). Collectively, he described more than 630 plants, many of which reportedly had medicinal properties.

Alexander, Frederick Matthias (1869-1955): Australian actor turned practitioner and teacher of an alternative treatment method that he developed, which came to be known as the Alexander technique. This technique involves teaching persons how to escape self-imposed limitations that were inadvertently acquired during their training for particular skills to enhance their health and reduce pain.

Alexander, Gerda (1908-1994): German-born teacher who developed the alternative method Eutony, which involves awareness and physical exercise to regulate muscle tone and general well-being.

Al-Nabati (fl. twelfth to thirteenth century): Andalusian Arab botanist who introduced the experimental scientific method into the field of the therapeutic properties of healing substances. He developed many empirical techniques in the examination and identification of medicines.

Avicenna (Ibn Sin{amacr}; 980-1037): Persian physician and philosopher who developed chromotherapy (or color therapy), which is an alternative method that uses colors and lights to balance a person's energy, particularly when clinical symptoms are present. He discussed this method in the book *The Canon of Medicine*, in which he claimed that color is a symptom of disease and introduced a color chart for diagnosis purposes.

Bach, Edward (1886-1936): English physician and homeopath practitioner who developed Bach flower remedies. These remedies involve dilutions of various flower components suspended in solution with water or brandy, or both, and are intended to treat various clinical manifestations, especially for emotional and psychological conditions such as depression and anxiety.

Barrett, Stephen Joel (1933–): Retired American psychiatrist, writer, and cofounder of the National Council Against Health Fraud, a nonprofit organization that investigates and reports on health misinformation, fraud, and quackery (fraudulent medical practices). He also is the founder and operator of Quackwatch, which covers health fraud and related issues and focuses on consumer protection, medical ethics, and scientific skepticism. He has argued that alternative medicine practices should be reclassified as genuine, experimental, or questionable, based on the evidence at hand.

Bartenieff, Irmgard (1890-1981): German-born dancer, researcher, writer, teacher, and physiotherapist who developed the Bartenieff fundamentals. Having been a student of Rudolf Laba, she developed this system as an extension of Laban movement analysis. She started an institute to teach her methods in the United States, an institute that remains active.

Bates, Horatio (1860-1931): American eye-care physician who developed the Bates method, which is an alternative therapy for improving eyesight. This technique is based on the assumption that nearly all sight problems are caused by habitual straining of the eyes. Bates asserted that glasses were both harmful and unnecessary for treating or correcting vision problems. He self-published the book *Perfect Sight Without Glasses*, which details his approach and advocates for the use of psychological principles, such as visualization, and movement. He also suggested that exposing the eyes to sunlight alleviated harmful strain.

Bausell, R. Barker (fl. twentieth century): American biostatistician, writer, and skeptic of alternative methods. His book *Snake Oil Science* argues against many popular alternative therapies and methods.

Bowers, Edwin (fl. twentieth century): Medical critic and writer who introduced, to the United States in 1913, along with William Fitzgerald, the precursor to what is now called reflexology. Together they published the book *Zone Therapy*, which was the original name of reflexology until the early 1960s. Reflexology is an alternative or complementary medicine that involves the physical act of applying pressure to the feet and hands, often with the use of lotion or oil, to treat various ailments.

Braid, James (1795-1860): Scottish physician and surgeon who specialized in ocular and muscular conditions. He was a pioneer of hypnotism and hypnotherapy and coined the word "neuro-hypnotism" (nervous sleep), from which both the terms "hypnosis" and "hypnotism" were derived. Braid is often regarded as the first genuine hypnotherapist and has been called the founder of modern hypnotism. He based his practice on mesmerism (or animal magnetism), a similar practice developed by Franz Mesmer and his students and followers. Braid's theory, however, differed from the originators as to how the procedure worked.

Cassileth, Barrie R. (fl. twentieth century): American researcher and educator of complementary and alternative medicine. Cassileth founded the Society for Integrative Oncology and published many studies on alternative cancer therapies.

Charaka (c. 300 B.C.E.): One of the principal contributors to the ancient art and science of Ayurveda (or the "science of life"), a system of medicine and lifestyle developed in ancient India. This alternative traditional medicine system is grounded in metaphysics and involves the intentional balance of three energies, which are often referred to as "wind," "bile," and "phlegm," to sustain a healthy lifestyle. It is a fairly integrative technique that involves exercise, diet, yoga, and meditation. Charaka has been called the founder of anatomy.

Chopra, Deepak (1946–): Indian American physician, writer, and public speaker on Ayurveda, spirituality, and mind/body medicine who began his career as an endocrinologist but later focused his work in alternative medicine. He studied under Maharishi Mahesh Yogi, who developed Transcendental Meditation, for several years before beginning his own career. Chopra has written more than fifty self-help books, translated into more than thirty-five languages, about New Age spirituality and alternative medicine. He is a vocal critic of the over-prescribing of drugs and of prescription drug dependency. He founded the Chopra Center for Wellbeing in California in 1996.

Clarke, John Henry (1853-1931): Prominent English homeopath who acted as a consulting physician to the London Homeopathic Hospital and as the editor of *Homeopathic World*. He was known to self-test various nosodes, or homeopathic remedies comprising pathological samples for treatment of clinical symptoms. He also was said to have promoted urinotherapy, or the use of one's own urine for medical treatment. He also published *A Dictionary of Practical Materia Medica*.

Confucius (551-479 B.C.E.): Chinese scholar acknowledged as a founder of the Scholar qigong tradition, or a system of meditation, breathing, and posture. This method is thought to cultivate intrinsic energy (qi) that can be used to balance health and to aid in healing. In his writings, Confucius alluded to the concepts of qi training as methods of moral training. Many variations of this method are still used as a complementary or alternative approach to treating various ailments.

Corbett, Margaret Darst (d. 1962): American vision educator and practitioner who used the Bates method to treat eyesight issues. After studying under Horatio Bates, the founder of the method, she taught this system at her School of Eye Education in California. She was quoted as saying that "the optic nerve is really part of the brain, and vision is nine-tenths mental and one-tenth physical."

Culpeper, Nicholas (1616-1654). English physician, botanist, herbalist, and astrologer. Culpeper blended traditional medicine with astrology, magic, and folklore. Despite the controversy surrounding some of his methods, his books *The English Physician* and *Complete Herbal* were popular.

Dawkins, Richard (1941–): British ethologist, evolutionary biologist, professor, and popular science writer of such books as *The Selfish Gene* and *The Extended Phenotype*. He has been a vocal critic of alternative medicine and has defined it as a "set of practices which cannot be tested, refuse to be tested, or consistently fail tests." Dawkins wrote the foreword to John Diamond's book *Snake Oil and Other Preoccupations*, which focuses on debunking alternative medicine.

De Bondt, Jacob (1599-1631): Dutch surgeon who went to Asia as an envoy of the Dutch East India Company. During his travels, he observed the practice of acupuncture and then became one of the first to write about its use. He had two published books, *De medicina indorum libri IV* and *Historiae naturalis et medicae Indiae Orientalis libri VI*, which discussed alternative medicine techniques.

Diamond, John (1953-2001): British broadcaster and journalist who was a critic of alternative medicine. His posthumously published book *Snake Oil and Other Preoccupations* focused on debunking alternative medicine.

Dioscorides, Pedanius (c. 40-90): Greek physician, pharmacologist, botanist, and influential writer. In the first century, he wrote a five-volume encyclopedia *De materia medica* (*Regarding Medical Materials*) about herbal medicine and related practices. The work was a cornerstone of various complementary and alternative medical fields over the centuries.

Eden, Donna (fl. twentieth century): Writer, teacher, lecturer, and pioneer in the alternative field of energy therapy (also known as magnetic therapy or energy healing). Eden wrote *Energy Medicine*, which has further defined this field and often serves as a guide for practitioners. Energy medicine is based on the idea that an imbalance in the body's energy field causes ailments and that rebalancing the body restores health.

Eijkman, Christiaan (1858-1930): Dutch physician and professor of physiology who demonstrated in chickens that beriberi (a nervous system disorder) is caused by a poor diet (specifically, thiamine deficiency). His work ultimately led to the discovery of vitamins. One year later, Frederick Hopkins postulated that some foods contain what he called accessory factors (vitamins) that are necessary for the functions of the human body. Eijkman and Hopkins were awarded the Nobel Prize for Physiology or Medicine in 1929 for their discovery of several vitamins.

Ekken, Kaibara (also known as Kaibara Ekiken or Atsunobu; 1630-1714): Japanese neo-Confucian botanist and philosopher who advanced the beginning of empirical science in Japan. He wrote *Yojokun* (*Precepts for Health Care*), which discussed medicine and nutrition and the association of the two. He also wrote a number of self-help manuals on topics such as Confucian virtues, study, and writing, and on precepts for daily life. Ekken was said to have inspired George Ohsawa, who formalized macrobiotics.

Engel, George Libman (1913-1999): American psychiatrist who is best known for proposing the biopsychosocial model. This model is based on the idea that biological, psychological, and social factors all affect health, illness, and healing.

Ernst, Edzard (1948–): First professor of complementary medicine in the United Kingdom and editor of two medical journals, *Alternative and Complementary Therapies* and *Perfusion*. He has researched complementary medicine approaches with a focus on their safety and efficacy. He has suggested that approximately 5 percent of alternative medicine is supported by meaningful evidence, whereas the rest is either insufficiently characterized or not supported by the existing evidence.

Feldenkrais, Moshe Pinchas (1904-1984): Israeli physicist and writer who developed the Feldenkrais method, which is designed to improve human functioning and to decrease pain or limitations in movement by increasing self-awareness through movement. He published a number of articles and books on this and related topics.

Felke, Pastor (1856-1926): German minister and therapist who contributed to the field of natural healing, or homeopathy. He interwove various medical and alternative methods to advance healing. In particular, he combined elements of air, light, water, and earth with homeopathy for treatment.

Finsen, Niels Ryberg (1860-1904): Danish physician who is considered to be the founder of modern phototherapy (light therapy), which involves the use of natural or derived radiation for the treatment of various physical and psychological ailments (such as acne and seasonal affective disorder). He developed the first artificial light source for this purpose and used his invention to treat lupus. In 1903, he received the Nobel Prize in Physiology or Medicine.

Fitzgerald, William H. (1872-1942): Ear, nose, and throat specialist often considered the "rediscoverer" of reflexology because he introduced the precursor of what is now known as reflexology to the United States in 1913. Fitzgerald claimed that applying pressure had an anesthetic effect on other areas of the body. With Edwin Bowers, he published the book *Zone Therapy* (the name by which reflexology was known until the early 1960s) in 1917.

Gattefosse, Rene-Maurice (1881-1950): French chemist who is considered the founder of aromatherapy. In 1937, he included the first known usage of the term "aromatherapy" in his book *Aromathérapie: Les Huiles Essentielles, Hormones Végétales*. Sources suggest he first discovered aromatherapy when he was working in a laboratory after he burned his hand and doused it with a nearby liquid: lavender oil. His hand healed more quickly than expected, which led him to investigate other similar aromatic oils.

Gautama, Siddhartha (also known as Gautama Buddha; c. 563-483 B.C.E.): Historical spiritual teacher from India who founded Buddhism. He is said to have achieved enlightenment while meditating under a tree, after which he founded the monastic way of life. Hundreds of specific Buddhist meditative methods have been derived from his ancient teachings.

Gerard, John (1545-1611): English herbalist and surgeon. He translated or cowrote *The Herball: Or, General History of Plants* (1597), although his level of contribution to this work is debated.

Gerson, Max (1881-1959): German physician and orthomolecularist who developed Gerson therapy, which involves using an alternative dietary system with the intent of curing various chronic diseases and cancer. Gerson described his approach in the book *A Cancer Therapy: Results of 50 Cases.* However, the American Medical Association and the National Cancer Institute consider this method to be ineffective and unsupported.

Gram, Sylvester (1794-1851): American Presbyterian minister and early advocate of dietary reform, with a particular emphasis on vegetarianism and the temperance movement.

Hackett, George S. (fl. twentieth century): American physician who is often called the founder of prolotherapy, which involves injecting an otherwise nonpharmacological solution into the body to strengthen weakened connective tissues and to alleviate musculoskeletal pain. He developed the technique in the 1940s.

Hahnemann, Samuel (1755-1843): German physician who first proposed homeopathy, or the use of highly diluted preparations. He developed a practical healing system based on an *ipse dixit* axiom, which he called the law of similars (or the natural law of like cured by like).

Hemwall, Gustav (1908-1998): American pioneer and practitioner of prolotherapy, which involves injecting an otherwise nonpharmacological solution into the body to strengthen weakened connective tissues and to alleviate musculoskeletal pain. He began his studies and treatments in the 1950s and continued until the mid-1990s.

Hippocrates (c. 460-370 B.C.E.): Ancient Greek physician who is often called the founder of Western medicine. One of his writings, *Airs, Waters, and Places,* includes the earliest recorded use of the term "macrobiotics." In this text, he used the word to describe people who were healthy and long-lived. He also advocated the use of a few simple herbal drugs, along with fresh air, rest, and proper diet. In addition, Hippocrates spoke of cupping as a therapeutic procedure.

Hopkins, Frederick Gowland (1861-1947): English biochemist who postulated that some foods contain what he called accessory factors (or vitamins) that are necessary for the functions of the human body. Hopkins and Christiaan Eijkman, another researcher in the field, were awarded the Nobel Prize for Physiology or Medicine in 1929 for their discovery of several vitamins. Hopkins also discovered the amino acid tryptophan in 1901.

Hufeland, Cristoph Wilhelm (1762-1836): German physician, researcher, professor, and notable writer who introduced the term "macrobiotic" in his book *Makrobiotik: The Art of Prolonging Life* (1797) in the context of food and health. He was friends with Samuel Hahnemann, who founded homeopathy.

Hyashi, Chujiro (1880-1940): Japanese physician, teacher, and disciple of Mikao Usui. Hyashi was a practitioner of Reiki (or palm healing) and played an important role in simplifying and demystifying Reiki techniques and teachings, which facilitated their worldwide transmission from Japan.

Ibn al-Baitar (1188-1248): Andalusian scientist, physician, botanist, and pharmacist who described more than 1,400 different plants, foods, and drugs, more than three hundred of which were his own discoveries.

Ishizuka, Sagen (1850-1909): Japanese physician who pioneered the concept of food education (called *shokuiku*) and the macrobiotic diet. He theorized that a natural diet, in which foods are eaten in season and have a correct balance of potassium and sodium, and acid and alkaline, leads to good health. He performed many clinical trials and published two large volumes of his work.

Jacobson, Edmund (1888-1983): American physician and psychologist who introduced the progressive muscle relaxation method to treat diverse psychophysiological disorders (such as hypertension). He also developed biofeedback, or the instrument-aided process of being aware of physiological functions. He invented hardware to measure electromyograph (EMG) voltages over time and showed that cognitive activity affects EMG levels. He wrote *Progressive Relaxation* (1929) and *You Must Relax* (1934).

Jarvis, William T. (fl. twentieth century): Professor of public health and preventive medicine who was critical of various alternative practices. He was also a member of the National Council Against Health Fraud and a contributor to Quackwatch, an organization that focuses on exposing health-related fraud and fallacy.

Jensen, Bernard (1908-2001): A leading American iridologist, chiropractor, nutritionist, and entrepreneur, and the writer of numerous books and articles on health and healing.

Kellogg, John Harvey (1852-1943): American physician who managed a sanitarium that used holistic methods, largely based on his Seventh-day Adventist religious upbringing. He focused on treating persons with a combination of nutrition, exercise, and enemas. He advocated vegetarianism and is best known for inventing the still-popular cereal Kellogg's Corn Flakes with his brother.

Klenner, Frederick Robert (1907-1984): An American physician and medical researcher. He is most notable for his work in the 1940s that explored using large doses of vitamin C to treat a wide range of illnesses, most notably polio.

Krieger, Dolores (1922–): American holistic nurse and educator who developed, with Dora Kunz, the practice of therapeutic touch, otherwise known as noncontact therapeutic touch, the healing touch, or distance healing. This method is an energy therapy claimed to promote healing and to reduce pain and anxiety levels; in this technique, practitioners place their hands on, or near, a patient to detect and manipulate the patient's energy field.

Kunz, Dora (1904-1999): American writer and healer who promoted theosophy and was a president of the Theosophical Society in America. With Dolores Krieger, she developed the practice of therapeutic touch, otherwise known as noncontact therapeutic touch, the healing touch, or distance healing. This method is an energy therapy claimed to promote healing and to reduce pain and anxiety levels; in this technique, practitioners place their hands on, or near, a patient to detect and manipulate the patient's energy field.

Laban, Rudolf (also known as Josh Mason and Rudolph von Laban; 1879-1958): Hungarian theorist and dancer who developed the fundamentals that led to the introduction of Laban movement analysis. This body movement system overlaps with kinesiology and other therapies to reduce body pain, to rehabilitate, and to enhance general well-being.

Laozi (c. 400 B.C.E.): Chinese philosopher and central figure in Daoism who described using both meditative training and physical exercises to increase longevity and to access higher realms of existence.

Lee, Yao Wu (fl. twentieth century): Chinese American doctor of Oriental medicine who reportedly opened the first acupuncture clinic in the United States (in Washington, D.C., in 1972). He also is noted for establishing the first legal clinic in a medical school setting.

Leonard, Jim (1955-2008): American writer, educator, and pioneer of what he termed "vivation," which involves meditation and breathing (or "breathworks") for the treatment of psychological issues such as anxiety and other negative emotions.

Lind, James (1716-1794): Scottish surgeon who discovered that citrus foods helped to prevent scurvy in what is said to be the first clinical trial on record. In 1753, Lind published his *Treatise on the Scurvy*, which recommended consuming lemons and limes to avoid the ailment. His was a key finding in using food products to avoid disease.

Ling, Per Henrik (1776-1839): Swedish medical-gymnastic practitioner who is said to have befriended a Chinese man who taught him about Asian fighting, exercising, and health philosophies. Ling reportedly healed himself of rheumatism and joint issues by applying exercises of pressure, pulling, and squeezing and stretches he had learned from the man. The version of massage that was popularized in the United States in the mid-nineteenth century was based on Ling's techniques. Also, Swedish massage is based on his system.

Lundberg, George D. (fl. twentieth century): An American physician, pathologist, and pioneer of Internet medicine. He is also the former editor of the Web site Medscape and of the *Journal of the American Medical Association*. He is a vocal critic of complementary and alternative medicines that are not supported by sufficient and convincing scientific evidence.

Lust, Benedict (1872-1945): German cofounder of naturopathic medicine, which focuses on using natural remedies and body's natural ability to heal and maintain itself. He is often considered the founder of naturopathy in the United States.

Lux, Johan Joseph Wilhelm (1773-1849): German veterinary surgeon who invented, in the 1830s, isopathy, a therapy derived from homeopathy. Isopathy differs from homeopathy in that its remedies, which are sometimes referred to as homeopathic vaccines, are made of disease-causing agents (pathogens) or from products of disease, such as pus.

Manabu, Nishibata (fl. twentieth century): Japanese pupil of George Ohsawa (the founder of the macrobiotic diet) who brought the macrobiotic theory to the United States in the 1960s. Manabu, and Michio Kushi, expanded the theory to bring it to its present version.

Mann, Felix (1931–): German-born acupuncturist and writer noted for his publications in and contributions to that field. He also was the founder and president of the Medical Acupuncture Society, the first president of the British Medical Acupuncture Society, and writer of the first English-language acupuncture textbook, *Acupuncture: The Ancient Chinese Art of Healing* (1962). He won the German Pain Prize in 1995.

Mehlmauer, Leonard (fl. twentieth century): Naturopathic physician and researcher who practiced various types of iridology, which is based on the idea that markings in the irises and whites of the eyes are connected to overall human health. He coined the term "eyology" to simplify the description of the practice and combined terminologies of the alternative eye sciences.

Mencius (c. 372-289 B.C.E.): Chinese scholar and famous Confucian acknowledged as a possible founder of the Scholar Qigong tradition, which is rooted in physical and mental exercises and controlled breathing. In his writings, he alluded to the concepts of qi training as methods of moral training.

Meschalkin, E. N. (fl. twentieth century): Russian researcher who cofounded intravenous laser blood irradiation and introduced it into clinical practice in 1981. Originally, this method was used in the treatment of cardiovascular abnormalities; it has since been used for other ailments.

Mesmer, Franz Anton (also known as Friedrich Anton Mesmer; 1734-1815): German physician and astrologist who developed the theory of what he called *magnetisme animal* ("animal magnetism") and other forces, which were commonly grouped under the term "mesmerism." This practice was based on the idea that a magnetic force or "fluid" exists within the universe that influences the health of the human body. Mesmer experimented with magnets to influence this field and cause healing, and subsequently concluded that the same effect could be created by the hands.

Metchnikoff, Ilya Ilyich (also known as Elie Metchnikoff; 1845-1916): Ukrainian biologist, zoologist, protozoologist, and Nobel laureate. He developed the theory that the aging process results from the activity of proteolytic microbes that produce toxins in the bowels, which eventually led to the usage of probiotics.

Meyeus, Philippus (also known as Philip Meyen von Coburg; fl. seventeenth century): German physician who first explicitly described iridological principles in his book *Chiromatica medica* (1665). This technique is based on characterizing the iris of the eye with the intent to determine information about a person's health.

Mizuno, Namboku (fl. eighteenth century): Japanese physiognomic (one who assesses outer appearance to predict inner characteristics), teacher, and writer who taught that diet, lifestyle, and environment govern a person's health and fortune. His teachings inspired George Ohsawa to formalize the field of macrobiotics.

Ohsawa, George (also known as Nyoichi Sakurazawa; 1893-1966): Japanese philosopher, teacher, and writer who founded the macrobiotic diet. His intention was to create a diet and philosophy to help people live full lives. He introduced macrobiotics to Europe from Japan.

Oschman, James (fl. twentieth century): Researcher and authority on Reiki, or hands-on healing, which aims to rebalance the body's energy field to restore health. He wrote the book *Energy Medicine*, which surveys the existing research evidence in the field.

Palmer, Bartlett Joshua (1881-1961): Canadian-born pioneer of chiropractic who trained with his father, Daniel Palmer, the founder of the field.

Palmer, Daniel David (1845-1913): Canadian-born magnetic healer who founded the chiropractic field in the 1890s. He moved to the United States and eventually founded a chiropractic school based on his work. Palmer hypothesized that vertebral joint misalignments affected the body's functions and its ability to heal itself.

Park, Robert L. (1931–): American professor, writer, and skeptic of alternative medicines or science that have not been evidenced by appropriate studies. In his book *Voodoo Science: The Road from Foolishness to Fraud*, he argues against alternative techniques, including homeopathy, and other scientific findings.

Pascoe, Friedrich (1867-1930): German chemist who produced many homeopathic medicines. He often collaborated with Pastor Felke, an authority in natural medicine, to produce remedies.

Patanjali (c. 150 B.C.E.): Ancient sage and writer who is widely regarded as the founder of formal Yoga philosophy. Patanjali's yoga is known as Raja yoga, which is a system for control of the mind. His writings also became the basis for a system referred to as Ashtanga yoga (meaning "eight-limbed" yoga).

Rolf, Ida Pauline (1896-1979): American biochemist and the creator of structural integration, or rolfing, which is considered an alternative technique that involves a "holistic system of soft tissue manipulation and movement education that organizes the whole body in gravity."

Sampson, Wallace (fl. twentieth century): American professor and editor of the *Scientific Review of Alternative Medicine*. Sampson studied and taught about unscientific medical systems and aberrant medical claims. He has been on the board of directors of the National Council Against Health Fraud and is affiliated with many organizations that protect consumers from bogus healthcare claims and products.

Scheel, John (fl. eighteenth to nineteenth century): European naturopathist who coined the term "naturopathy" in 1895 and later "sold" the term to Benedict Lust, now considered the founder of American naturopathy.

Sergievskiy, V. S. (fl. twentieth century): Russian researcher who codeveloped intravenous laser blood irradiation and introduced it into clinical practice in 1981. The method was originally applied in the treatment of cardiovascular abnormalities and has since been used for treating other ailments.

Shermer, Michael (1954): American science writer, founder of the Skeptics Society, and editor of the magazine *Skeptic*. He is a vocal critic of many alternative medical treatments and wrote the book *Why People Believe Weird Things*.

Slavicek, John (fl. twentieth century): Czech native who claimed to have created an eye cure that improves eyesight in three days, borrowing from ancient yogic eye exercises, visualizations, and the Bates method. Slavicek's self-published manual, *Yoga for the Eyes*, however, was rejected by an ophthalmologist who evaluated it and was disavowed by the World Health Organization.

Steiner, Rudolf (1861-1925): Austrian philosopher and architect who codeveloped anthroposophical medicine, which involves using exercises in self-determination, dignity, and autonomy to strengthen a person's being and individuality, to improve health and healing.

Stopfel, Eunice Ingham (1889-1974): Nurse and physiotherapist who further modified reflexology in the 1930s and 1940s. In her book *Stories the Feet Can Tell* (1938), she claimed that the feet and hands were especially sensitive, and she mapped the entire body into reflexes on the feet.

Sutherland, William (1873-1954): Physician who originated cranial osteopathy in about 1900. He used the term "reciprocal tension membrane system" to describe the three Cartesian axes held in reciprocal tension, which create the cyclic movement of inhalation and exhalation of the cranium.

Takada, Hawayo (1900-1980): Reiki practitioner and teacher and originally a student of Chujiro Hayashi. Takada established several Reiki clinics in the United States.

Ten Rhyne, Wilhelm (also known as Wilhelm ten Rhijne; 1649-1700): Dutch physician, botanist, and writer who first introduced acupuncture to Europe in his book *De acupunctura* (1683) after he studied acupuncture for two years in Japan. It has been suggested that he first coined the term "acupunctura." He also wrote about moxibustion, which is the burning of herbs for clinical purposes.

Thomson, Samuel (1769-1843): America herbalist and founder of the Thomsonian system of medicine. It has been suggested that he, more than any other researcher in the United States, was likely the foremost contributor to the science of herbs, although he was not formally trained in medicine.

Tiller, William A. (fl. twentieth century): Professor, proponent of crystal therapy, and a pioneer of psychoenergetics. Tiller claims to have discovered a new class of natural phenomena generated through what he called subtle energies, which he claims are manifested in the practices of healers and other paranormal practitioners. He defines the term "psychoenergetics" as the study of these energies in relation to the application of human consciousness, and has described his ideas in his book *Science and Human Transformation*.

Trager, Milton (1908-1997): American physician and educator who developed the Trager approach, a mind/body system for educating a person about movement to promote better health. This system involves using rhythmic movement to promote general well-being and to decrease body pain. It also involves personal exploration of natural, free movement (called Mentastics) to promote optimal body performance. Trager was said to encounter the principles of this system somewhat serendipitously during exercising, around the age of eighteen years.

Usui, Mikao (1865-1926): Japanese Buddhist who developed, in 1922, Reiki, the spiritual practice that involves using palm healing to treat physical and mental ailments. Through the use of this technique, practitioners claim they can transfer healing energy to patients through the palms. Many of Usui's disciples furthered the field and continue to practice this system.

Valnet, Jean (1920-1995): French physician, surgeon, and a pioneer of using aromatherapy and herbs for medicinal purposes. He is said to have used oil-based antiseptics in the treatment of wounded soldiers during World War II.

Vogel, Marcel (1917-1991): American research scientist, inventor, and proponent of crystal therapy for medicinal purposes. He designed the Vogel crystal, which he claims focuses "universal life force" by concentrating it to a higher level to enhance health.

Wegman, Ita (1876-1943): Indonesian-born Dutch medical doctor who codeveloped anthroposophical medicine, which involves using exercises in self-determination, dignity, and autonomy to strengthen one's being and individuality and to improve health and healing. She also developed rhythmical massage and other therapeutic strategies.

Weil, Andrew T. (1942–): American physician, writer, and practitioner of integrative medicine in the United States. He is known for popularizing and coining the term "integrative medicine." He is the founder and program director of the Arizona Center for Integrative Medicine and also founded a company that promotes using integrative medicine to promote general health.

Yogi, Maharishi Mahesh (also known as Mahesh Prasad Varma; 1914-2008): Indian philosopher and teacher who developed the Transcendental Meditation technique, which combines mantra meditation and spiritual techniques. Yogi has been called the guru of this technique, which has more recently been termed a "spiritual movement." He also was a mentor to Deepak Chopra, a popular Indian American physician, writer, and public speaker.

Brandy Weidow, M.S.

INDEXES

Category Index

Drug interactions

Functional foods

Homeopathy

Issues and overviews

Category Index

Personages Index

Note: Page numbers in **bold** indicate the main discussion.

Subject Index

Note: Page numbers in **bold** indicate the main discussion.

rice-source policosanol, 1056
rickets, 1381
rifampin, **1151**
Riley, Joe Shelby, 1122
risperidone, 593
Ritalin, 106, 608
ritonavir, 554, 1092, 1093
rofecoxib, 405, 556
Rolf, Ida, 1152
rolfing, 95, 849, **1152–1153**
Romano, John, 469
Rooibos tea (red tea), **1119–1120**
rosacea, 606, **1153–1154**
rose hips, 775, 1144, **1154–1155**
rosemary, **1155–1157**; estrogen, 483–484; narcotic addiction, 926, 1156; oral contraceptives, 974, 1156
rosmarinic acid, 1028, 1156
rotator-cuff injury, 117
roundworm, 1011–1012
royal jelly, 1075, **1157–1158,** 1403
rTMS. *See* repetitive transcranial magnetic stimulation
rubbing alcohol, 1273
rumalaya, 117
Russian ginseng. *See also Eleutherococcus senticosus*
Ruta graveolens, 1271
rutin, 1000

Saccharomyces boulardii, 556
safety testing, 1127
saffron, 402, **1159–1160**
safrole, 1169
sage, **1160–1161**; herpes, 649; periodontal disease, 1029; sunburn, 1264
Saiboku-to, 91, 1305
Saiko-keishi-to, 1306
Saint-Pierre, Gaston, 889
Sakurazawa, Yukikazu (George Ohsawa), **967–968**
Salacia oblonga, **1161–1162**
salai guggal, 1144
salicin, 988, 1255
salicylic acid, 705, 1417, 1418.

See also aspirin (acetylsalicylic acid)
salmon, 87
salt bush, **1162–1163**
salt intake, 425, 698, 699
SAMe, **1163–1166**; alcoholic hepatitis, 642; alcoholic liver damage, 30, 31; cirrhosis, 322; depression, 399–400, 1163, 1165; glutathione, 591; levodopa/carbidopa, 793; liver disease, 807; osteoarthritis, 987, 1163–1164; Parkinson's disease, 1014, 1164, 1165; SSRIs, 1235–1236; tramadol, 1313; tricyclic antidepressants, 1316; trimethylglycine, 1320
Sampson, Wallace, **1166**
sandalwood, **1166–1167**
sand rat *(Psammomys obesus),* 1162
sanpaku, 967
Santhuff, Patricia J., 498, 499
saponins, 953, 1168
saquinavir, 665, 1093
sargassi, 962
sarsaparilla, **1167–1169**
sassafras, 645, **1169**
Satchidananda, Swami, 1440
satiety: glycemic index, 815; obesity, 958
saturated fat consumption, 425–426, 914
saw palmetto, **1169–1171**; benign prostatic hyperplasia, 139, 141, 878; prostate disorders, 938, 1092, 1104, 1169, 1170
scar tissue, **1171–1172**
Scheer, James F., 708
schisandra, **1172–1173**
schistosomiasis, 919–920
schizophrenia, **1173–1176**; fish oil, 508; glycine, 592, 593, 594; magnet therapy, 841
Schultz, Johannes H., 110
sciatica, **1176–1177**
Science and Human Transformation: Subtle Energies, Intentionality, and Consciousness (Tiller), 1295

Science-Based Medicine (Web site), 1166
scientific method, **1177–1178**
scientific-sounding language, 1099
scleroderma, 1003, **1178–1179**
scoliosis, 296
scotch broom, 908
scurvy, 1374
Scutellaria baicalensis (Chinese skullcap), **290–291,** 389, 1211
Scutellaria lateriflora (European skullcap), **1210–1211**
sea buckthorn, 238, 239, **1180–1181**
sea cucumber, 1030
seal oil, 1101
Sears, Barry, 635
seasonal affective disorder, **1181–1182**; melatonin, 865–866; St. John's wort, 1182, 1243
seaweed, 962
seborrheic dermatitis, 40, **1182–1183**
secretin, 109
sedative drugs: ashwagandha, 87; lemon balm, 790–791; passionflower, 1018; proteolytic enzymes, 1097; sandalwood, 1167; skullcap, 1211; valerian, 1343. *See also* insomnia; sleep
seizures: biotin, 162; epilepsy, **474–478**; ginkgo, 576; hyssop, 710
selective serotonin reuptake inhibitors. *See* SSRIs
selenium, **1184–1187**; cancer risk reduction, 227–228; diabetic blood sugar control, 411; HIV/AIDS support, 664; hypothyroidism, 708; male fertility, 880; prostate cancer, 877–878; psoriasis, 1101; recommended intake levels, 1395
self-care, **1187–1188**
self-correction, 1099
Selfish Gene, The (Dawkins), 395
senior health. *See* aging; elder health